D1608934

Pediatric, Adolescent, & Young Adult Gynecology

Pediatric, Adolescent, & Young Adult Gynecology

EDITED BY

Albert Altchek MD, FACS, FACOG, FNYAM

Clinical Professor with Tenure of Obstetrics, Gynecology and Reproductive Science
Chief, Pediatric and Adolescent Gynecology
Attending Obstetrician and Gynecologist
Mount Sinai School of Medicine and Hospital and
Lenox Hill Hospital
New York, NY, USA

Liane Deligdisch MD, FCAP

Professor of Pathology
Professor of Obstetrics, Gynecology and Reproductive Science
Member of the French National Academy of Medicine
Mount Sinai Medical Center
New York, NY, USA

FOREWORD BY

Alan deCherney MD

Head, Program in Reproductive and Adult Endocrinology
National Institute of Child Health and Human Development
National Institutes of Health

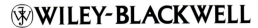
WILEY-BLACKWELL
A John Wiley & Sons, Ltd., Publication

BMJ|Books

This edition first published 2009, © 2009 by Blackwell Publishing Ltd

BMJ Books is an imprint of BMJ Publishing Group Limited, used under licence by
Blackwell Publishing which was acquired by John Wiley & Sons in February 2007. Blackwell's publishing program
has been merged with Wiley's global Scientific, Technical and Medical business to form Wiley-Blackwell.

Registered office: John Wiley & Sons Ltd, The Atrium, Southern Gate, Chichester, West Sussex, PO19 8SQ, UK

Editorial offices: 9600 Garsington Road, Oxford, OX4 2DQ, UK
The Atrium, Southern Gate, Chichester, West Sussex, PO19 8SQ, UK
111 River Street, Hoboken, NJ 07030-5774, USA

For details of our global editorial offices, for customer services and for information about how to apply for
permission to reuse the copyright material in this book please see our website at www.wiley.com/wiley-blackwell

Library of Congress Cataloging-in-Publication Data
Pediatric, adolescent, and young adult gynecology / edited by Albert Altchek, Liane Deligdisch.
     p. ; cm.
   Includes bibliographical references.
   ISBN 978-1-4051-5347-8
   1. Pediatric gynecology.   2. Adolescent gynecology.   I. Altchek, Albert, 1925–   II. Deligdisch, Liane.
   [DNLM: 1. Genital Diseases, Female.   2. Adolescent.   3. Child. WS 360 P3702 2008]
   RJ478.P335 2008
   618.92′098–dc22

                                                                                                2008039503

ISBN: 978-1-4051-5347-8

A catalog record for this book is available from the British Library.

Set in 9/12 pt Minion by Aptara® Inc., New Delhi, India
Printed and bound in Malaysia by Vivar Printing Sdn Bhd

1   2009

Contents

Contributors

Paula J. Adams Hillard MD
Professor of Obstetrics and Gynecology
Stanford University School of Medicine
Stanford, CA, USA

Jeremy T. Aidlen MD
Assistant Professor of Surgery and Pediatrics
The Warren Alpert School of Medicine of Brown University
Hasbro Children's Hospital
Providence, RI, USA

Ivanya L. Alpert
Clinical Assistant Professor, Department of Pediatrics
Mount Sinai School of Medicine
New York, NY, USA

Albert Altchek MD, FACS, FACOG, FNYAM
Clinical Professor with Tenure of Obstetrics, Gynecology and Reproductive Science
Chief, Pediatric and Adolescent Gynecology
Attending Obstetrician and Gynecologist
Mount Sinai School of Medicine and Hospital and
Lenox Hill Hospital
New York, NY, USA

Jennifer Aranda MD
Clinical Instructor, Department of Dermatology
University of Texas Southwestern Medical Center
Dallas, TX, USA

Marc S. Arkovitz
Columbia University
New York, NY, USA

Charles J. Ascher-Walsh MD, MS
Director of Gynecology
Mount Sinai School of Medicine
New York, NY, USA

Janice L. Bacon MD
Professor and Chair, Edward J. Dennis III MD Endowed Chair
of Obstetrics and Gynecology
University of South Carolina School of Medicine
Columbia, SC, USA

David A. Baker MD
Professor of Obstetrics, Gynecology and Reproductive
Medicine, and Director, Division of Infectious Diseases
Stony Brook University Medical Center
New York, NY, USA

Frank M. Biro MD
Professor of Pediatrics, University of Cincinnati College of
Medicine, and Director, Division of Adolescent Medicine
Cincinnati Children's Hospital Medical Center
Cincinnati, OH, USA

Leslie R. Boyd MD
Fellow, Division of Gynecologic Oncology
Department of Obstetrics and Gynecology
New York University School of Medicine
New York, NY, USA

William Bradley III MD
Senior Clinical Fellow, Division of Gynecologic Oncology
Mount Sinai School of Medicine
New York, NY, USA

Michael Brodman MD
Professor and Chairman of Obstetrics, Gynecology and
Reproductive Science
Mount Sinai School of Medicine
New York, NY, USA

K. Robin Carder MD
Clinical Assistant Professor, Department of Dermatology
University of Texas Southwestern Medical Center
Dallas, TX, USA

Alan B. Copperman MD
Director, Division of Reproductive Endocrinology,
Vice-Chairman, Department of Obstetrics, Gynecology and
Reproductive Science, Mount Sinai Medical Center
Co-Director, Reproductive Medicine Associates of New York
New York, NY, USA

George Creatsas MD, FACS, FRCOG
Professor of Obstetrics and Gynecology, 2nd Department of
Obstetrics and Gynecology, University of Athens
Aretaieion Hospital, Athens, Greece

John P. Curtin MD, MBA
Professor and Chair, Department of Obstetrics and Gynecology
New York University School of Medicine
New York, NY, USA

Robert A. Cusick MD
Assistant Professor of Pediatric Surgery, Children's Hospital
of Omaha, University of Nebraska Medical Center
Omaha, NE, USA

Liane Deligdisch MD, FCAP
Professor of Pathology, Professor of Obstetrics, Gynecology and
Reproductive Science, Member of the French National Academy
of Medicine
Mount Sinai Medical Center
New York, NY, USA

Efthimios Deligeoroglou MD, PhD
Associate Professor of Obstetrics and Gynecology, 2nd
Department of Obstetrics and Gynecology, University of Athens
Aretaieion Hospital, Athens, Greece

Angela Diaz MD, MPH
Jean C. and James W. Crystal Professor of Adolescent Health
Director, Mount Sinai Adolescent Health Center
New York, NY, USA

Stephen E. Dolgin MD
Chief, Pediatric Surgery, Schneider Children's Hospital, North
Shore-Long Island Jewish Hospital, and Professor of Clinical
Surgery and Pediatrics, Albert Einstein College of Medicine,
Bronx
New York, NY, USA

Hinde El Fatemi MD
Pathologist, Hassan II Teaching Hospital, Fez, Morocco

Monica S. Epelman MD
Assistant Professor of Radiology, University of Pennsylvania
Philadelphia, PA, USA

Wassim Essamet MD
Department of Pathology, Centre Jean Perrin
Clermont-Ferrand, France

Emanuel A. Friedman MD, ScD
Professor Emeritus of Obstetrics, Gynecology and Reproductive
Biology
Harvard Medical School
Boston, MA, USA

Rhea G. Friedman JD (retired)
New York State Family Court Judge
New York, NY, USA

Alvin F. Goldfarb MD (deceased)
Professor of Obstetrics and Gynecology
Jefferson Medical College of Thomas Jefferson University
Philadelphia, PA, USA

Christopher P. Houk MD
Director, Pediatric Endocrine Unit
Mercer University School of Medicine
Savannah, GA, USA

Yasmin Jayasinghe MBBS, FRANZCOG
Consultant Gynaecologist
Department of Gynaecology
Royal Children's Hospital
Melbourne, Australia
Research Collaborator
Department of Pediatric and Adolescent Medicine
Mayo Clinic, Rochester, MN, USA

Nathan Kase MD
Professor, Department of Obstetrics, Gynecology and
Reproductive Science, and
Professor, Department of Medicine, and Dean Emeritus
Mount Sinai School of Medicine
New York, NY, USA

Raymond H. Kaufman MD
Professor, Department of Obstetrics and Gynecology
Weil Medical College, Cornell University, New York
Professor Emeritus, Department of Obstetrics and Gynecology
The Methodist Hospital and Baylor College of Medicine, and
Houston, TX, USA

Nancy D. Kellogg MD
Professor of Pediatrics
University of Texas Health Science Center at San Antonio
San Antonio, TX, USA

Genna W. Klein MD
Fellow, Division of Pediatric Endocrinology and Diabetes
Mount Sinai School of Medicine
New York, NY, USA

Peter A. Lee MD
Professor of Pediatrics, Department of Pediatrics
Indiana University School of Medicine
Indianapolis, IN, USA

Kenneth A. Levey MD, MPH
Clinical Assistant Professor of Obstetrics and Gynecology
New York University Medical Center
Department of Obstetrics and Gynecology
New York, NY, USA

Karen Lin-Su MD
Assistant Professor of Pediatrics, Pediatric
Endocrinology/Adrenal Steroid Disorders Program
Mount Sinai School of Medicine
New York, NY, USA

Elizabeth Lorde-Rollins MD, MSc
Assistant Professor of Pediatrics
Assistant Professor of Obstetrics and Gynecology
Mount Sinai Adolescent Health Center
New York, NY, USA

Ali Mahdavi MD, FACOG
Fellow and Clinical Instructor, Division of Gynecologic
Oncology, Department of Obstetrics and Gynecology
University of California Irvine Medical Center
Irvine, CA, USA

Diane F. Merritt MD
Director of Pediatric and Adolescent Gynecology, Professor of
Obstetrics and Gynecology, Washington University School of
Medicine, Washington, and
Barnes-Jewish Hospital, Saint Louis Children's Hospital,
Missouri Baptist Medical Center,
St Louis, MO, USA

Claude Migeon MD
Professor of Pediatrics, Pediatric Endocrinology
Johns Hopkins Children's Center
Baltimore, MA, USA

Rachel J. Miller MD
Pediatric and Adolescent Gynecology
Children's Hospitals and Clinics of Minnesota
Minneapolis, MN, USA

Mara Minguez MD
Assistant Clinical Professor, Department of Pediatrics and
Heilbrunn Department of Population and Family Health
Columbia University
New York, NY, USA

Florence Mishellany MD
Pathologist, Anticancer Center, Service Anatomie Pathologique,
Centre Jean Perrin, Clermont-Ferrand, France

Khush Mittal MD
Director of Surgical and Gynecologic Pathology, New York
University Medical Center and Bellevue Hospital
New York, NY, USA

Bradley J. Monk MD, FACOG, FACS
Associate Professor, Department of Obstetrics and Gynecology,
Division of Gynecologic Oncology
University of California Irvine Medical Center
Irvine, CA, USA

Maria I. New MD
Professor of Pediatrics, Mount Sinai School of Medicine
New York, NY, USA

Camran Nezhat MD FACOG FACS
Fellowship Director, Center for Special Minimally Invasive
Surgery
Stanford University Medical Center
Palo Alto, CA, USA

Ceana Nezhat MD
Fellowship Director, Atlanta Center for Special Minimally
Invasive Surgery, Associate Professor of Obstetrics and
Gynecology (Adj. Clinical), Atlanta, GA, and
Stanford University School of Medicine
Palo Alto, CA, USA

Farr R. Nezhat MD, FACOG
Director, Minimally Invasive Surgery and Gynecologic
Robotics Chief, St Luke's-Roosevelt Hospital Center
University Hospital of Columbia University
New York, NY, USA

Saroj Nimkarn MD
Assistant Professor of Pediatrics, Adrenal Steroids Disorders
Program
Mount Sinai School of Medicine
New York, NY, USA

Anne Nucci-Sack MD
Assistant Professor in Pediatrics, Medical Director
Mount Sinai Adolescent Health Center
New York, NY, USA

Kara Pappas MD
Pediatric Endocrinology, Johns Hopkins University
Baltimore, MA, USA

Frédérique Penault-Llorca MD, PhD
Head, Department of Pathology, Centre Jean Perrin
Clermont-Ferrand, France

Jamal Rahaman MB, BS, DGO FACS, FACOG
Fellowship Director, Division of Gynecologic Oncology
Mount Sinai School of Medicine
New York, NY, USA

Robert Rapaport MD
Professor of Pediatrics, Emma Elizabeth Sullivan Professor of
Pediatric Endocrinology and Diabetes, and Director, Division of
Pediatric Endocrinology and Diabetes
Mount Sinai School of Medicine
New York, NY, USA

Aaron R. Rausen MD
Professor of Pediatrics, Founding Director Stephen D.
Hassenfeld Children's Center for Cancer and
Blood Disorders, New York University Medical Center, and
Adolescent Health Center
Ralph Lauren Center for Cancer Care and Prevention
New York, NY, USA

Irmi Rey-Stocker MD, Phd, Fellow ISSVD
Senior Lecturer
University of Lausanne
Switzerland

Erika Rivera-Serrano MD
Department of Pathology, Centre Jean Perrin
Clermont-Ferrand, France

Mary Rojas PhD
Assistant Professor of Pediatrics and Health Policy
Director of Research
Mount Sinai Adolescent Health Center
New York, NY, USA

Sabah Servaes MD
Assistant Professor
The Children's Hospital of Philadelphia
Philadelphia, PA, USA

Alireza A. Shamshirsaz MD
Third Year Resident, Department of Obstetrics and Gynecology
University of Iowa Hospital and Clinics
Iowa City, IA, USA

Patricia Simmons MD
Professor of Pediatrics, Mayo Medical School, Pediatric and
Adolescent Gynecology, Mayo Clinic
Rochester, MN, USA

Don Sloan MD
Clinical Associate Professor, Department of Obstetrics and
Gynecology
New York Medical College
New York, NY, USA

Rhoda Sperling MD
Vice Chair, Obstetrics, Gynecology and
Reproductive Science
Mount Sinai School of Medicine
New York, NY, USA

Michelle Tham MD
Chief Resident, Mount Sinai Medical Center
New York, NY, USA

Albert George Thomas Jr MD, MS,
FACOG
Associate Professor of Obstetrics and Gynecology, Senior
Consultant Family Planning Services, Mount Sinai School of
Medicine, and
Chief of Obstetrics and Gynecology
North General Hospital, Bronx VA Medical Center
New York, NY, USA

Gazi Yildirim MD
Assistant Professor, Department of Obstetrics
and Gynecology
Yeditepe University Medical Faculty,
Istanbul, Turkey

Robert K. Zurawin MD
Associate Professor, Baylor College of Medicine
Houston, TX, USA

Preface

In August 1972 I was the Guest Editor of the Symposium on Pediatric and Adolescent Gynecology for the *Pediatric Clinics of North America* (WB Saunders, Philadelphia). There was a great demand for that issue of the journal. Since then I have dreamed about a book, more comprehensive and personal.

The subject of pediatric and adolescent gynecology is not taught because it is multidisciplinary. Gynecology house staff rarely see young patients. Correspondingly, pediatric house staff are not adequately taught about gynecologic problems. It should be emphasized that the young patient is completely different from the usual mature adult gynecologic patient in all aspects. Thus there is a need for postgraduate education in the field of pediatric and adolescent gynecology.

I have always enjoyed teaching and have lectured extensively in the US and abroad. I have conducted pediatric and adolescent gynecology clinics at three hospitals, including a weekly clinic at Lenox Hill Hospital for 20 years. I was a founding member of the North American Society for Pediatric and Adolescent Gynecology.

In the early 1970s I started the annual postgraduate course on Pediatric and Adolescent Gynecology at Mount Sinai Hospital in New York City. It was the first continuous course in the US on the subject. In recent years I have added young adult gynecology. This course is given yearly to an ever-increasing audience and it is intended that this book will be a companion for the course.

My continuing private consultations observing the same patients over a number of years have given me the unique advantage of being able to discover certain conditions such as prepubertal distal vaginal longitudinal folds (which mimics molestation and rhabdomyosarcoma); prepubertal unilateral labium majus tumor (which mimics a malignancy); subacute atopic dermatitis of the vulva (which mimics molestation and is frequent, chronic,

has disturbing symptoms and is overlooked because it has not been described previously). I have also been able to devise psychologic support for congenital absence of the vagina and uterus.

Unique aspects of this book

The book is unique:
- in describing new findings, some not yet published elsewhere, based on personal observations over many years
- in its personal style as it guides the reader on the approach, evaluation and basic management of problems of the young patient, especially when the patient is apprehensive
- in emphasizing the psychologic aspects which are associated with almost every gynecologic problem, especially congenital anomalies
- in giving prompt, concise help which will benefit practical office or clinic care
- in the quality of the chapters by the contributing authors, who are great teachers
- in concentrating on common problems which can be readily managed and alerting the reader to possible dangerous situations where expert help is appropriate
- in having a detailed chapter on the McIndoe procedure, the most common surgery for congenital absence of the vagina in the US. It describes the many unappreciated problems which may destroy an otherwise good result, including detailed pre- and postoperative care. It is based on a large series performed and followed by myself
- in emphasizing the concept of education for life, self-esteem, avoiding unwanted pregnancy and school dropout, maintenance of good health, continuous routine care and standard vaccinations
- in being edited by a clinician and pathologist.

This is the first book on the subject to include the concept of the young adult. The timing of the change from adolescent to young adult varies with the individual. Furthermore, there is no standard definition regarding when the young person is considered to be a young adult. Ideally the physician should encourage continuing routine medical care as a lifelong habit. The problems of the young adult begin in adolescence, such as contraception, avoiding sexually transmitted disease, education, responsibility, long-range plans, etc. Another aspect is continuity of care. Adolescents tend to drift away from medical care as they become young adults. They tend to neglect their health and appropriate routine vaccinations as they develop an independent lifestyle.

Most colleges in the US require health evaluation and routine vaccinations prior to entry. There is usually a college medical office. The confidentiality of college medical records should be maintained. In the US there may be a problem for the young adult in paying for health insurance because of expenses, living independently, traveling for occupation and/or study, relatively good health, and a feeling of invincibility. In some countries with routine universal healthcare there may be less of a problem.

The readership

The book is a practical guide for the busy clinician who sees young patients, including the obstetrician-gynecologist, pediatrician, adolescent medicine physician, and primary care (family) physician. In addition, the book will be useful for nurse practitioners who are progressively rendering an increasing amount of patient care and who greatly appreciate education. The book should be in emergency rooms, clinics and libraries in every hospital as well as in private offices.

Disturbing reports of social tragedies

The physician should be aware of important social problems. A 2008 *New York Times* editorial ("More Kids Dying", July 18) indicated that between the ages of 15 and 24, deaths from drug overdoses have more than doubled between 1999 and 2005. The most common drugs were oxycodone and vicodin.

Another editorial on July 19 2008 was entitled "Help for Victimized Children." Among children who run away from home because of neglect or abuse, "tens of thousands will spend time working for sexual predators." The average age is between 11 and 14.

The coeditor

Professor Liane Deligdisch, the coeditor of the book, is a gynecologic pathologist who originally practiced obstetrics and gynecology and therefore has a clinical perspective. She was recently elected to the prestigious French National Academy of Medicine. She has made important contributions to clinical care by translational studies in the pathology of trophoblastic tumors, HPV infection in adolescents, the two types of endometrial cancers each requiring different management, the effects of hormones on the endometrium, the diagnosis of early ovarian cancer and the precursor stages of ovarian cancer.

Acknowledgments

We are indebted to the contributing authors for their excellent chapters in this multidisciplinary subject. We also wish to acknowledge the excellent help of Joseph Samet, medical photographer and illustrator, and Angelica M. Mares MD, research and editorial assistant.

Albert Altchek MD

Foreword

This comprehensive text addresses an often unrecognized and underappreciated population that comes under the aegis of the gynecologist. With increasing specialization and subspecialization, this group seems to be left out of any traditional curriculum. Therefore, Altchek and Deligdisch have done a great job and provided a much needed service. They have discussed the issues in a chronologic fashion, starting out with the evaluation of the newborn, including ambiguous genitalia and congenital adrenal hyperplasia. Also included are bridging diseases: androgen insensitivity and ovarian dysgenesis.

The gynecologic approach to the child, adolescent, and young adult is covered, with subareas being vulvovaginitis, vaginal bleeding in the child, and ovarian cysts in infants and children.

The difficult area of genital trauma, sexual abuse, and adolescent sexuality is also discussed in great detail in a sensitive and insightful fashion.

The endocrine aspects of this age group are thoroughly addressed, looking at puberty and its problems, including primary and secondary amenorrhea and precocious puberty.

Then, as this population approaches adulthood, pelvic pain, endometriosis, chronic pelvic pain, and the disorders of menstrual bleeding are covered. The book therefore presents a comprehensive approach to this patient group. This is the only text that one would need to care for this group of patients. This would be a valuable book for residents, fellows, and practitioners.

My hope would be that, in the future, this group of patients receives greater recognition since these problems are more readily diagnosed and significant treatment can be utilized with advancing surgical techniques and genetic recognition of these entities, coupled with new medications. These therapeutic entities will be geared to signaling and epigenetic errors; this is a virgin field for research and translational work and the application of these new understandings to this group is on the horizon. I learned in medical school that children are not little adults and this has certainly become more apparent as science marches on and unfolds many of its mysteries.

A unique element to this book is that it represents years of experience on the part of the authors. This is intangible information and raises the awareness that, no matter how great the technology gets, there is nothing better than experience. This vignette is a gem.

This is an important text; it addresses, in a unified and chronologic fashion, an important group of patients who deserve intensive care and understanding.

Alan DeCherney MD

Dedication to John Dewhurst and Hugh Barber

In December 2006 two world-famous gynecologists passed away. They were personal friends, teachers, and pioneers in their special interests. They were humble, dedicated clinicians, surgeons, researchers, and role models for integrity. They loved taking care of people and were revered by all whose lives they touched.

John Dewhurst (1920–2006)

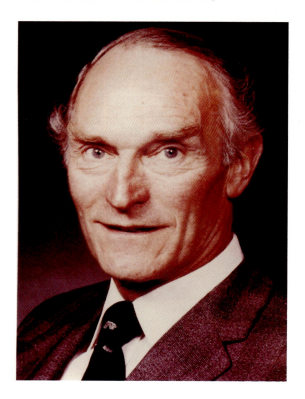

Christopher John Dewhurst was a friend, teacher, and world pioneer in pediatric and adolescent gynecology. He served in World War II in the Royal Naval Volunteer Reserve (Surg. Lieut. 1943–1946) following which he entered obstetrics and gynecology. Sir John ("Jack") Dewhurst FRCS, FRCOG, Hon FACOG (and five other honorary degrees) was President of the Royal College of Obstetricians and Gynaecologists (1975–1978) (when he was knighted), and Professor of Obstetrics and Gynaecology, University of London at Queen Charlotte's Hospital for Women (1967–1985) where Albert Altchek had the honor of working with him. He made it into an international center for postgraduate training. His classic 1963 book *The Gynaecological Disorders of Infants and Children* was followed by many landmark books including *Royal Confinements* (1980), a history of midwifery.

He founded and edited the original journal *Pediatric and Adolescent Gynecology* (1983). This developed into the present *Journal of Pediatric and Adolescent Gynecology* when it became the official journal of the North American Society for Pediatric and Adolescent Gynecology in 1988.

Dewhurst retired in 1986 to enjoy cricket, gardening, and music at his home in Harefield, Middlesex, but continued to be active in medicine and wrote several books.

Hugh Barber (1918–2006)

Hugh R.K. Barber was Director of Obstetrics and Gynecology at Lenox Hill Hospital for an unprecedented 34 years from 1963 to 1997 at the insistence of the entire attending staff. He was a leading authority on ovarian cancer and was invited to lecture all over the world. He was one of the first to point out the vague gastrointestinal symptoms of early ovarian cancer. He was the founding editor of the journal *The Female Patient*. He edited 20 books, published 400 medical papers, and received numerous medical awards. He was Professor and Chair at New York Medical College and Professor at Cornell Medical College and New York University Medical School. He was also Honorary

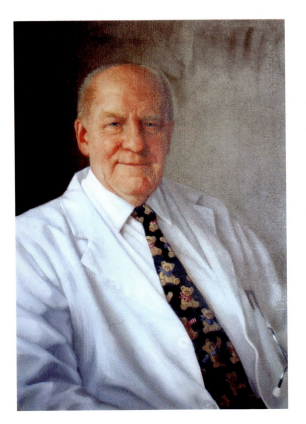

Professor of Obstetrics-Gynecology and Gynecologic Oncology at Beijing Medical School, Beijing, China from 1985. He was one of the first in the US to open a domestic violence center. The annual Hugh R.K. Barber MD lectureship was established by the Society of Gynecologic Oncologists.

Not only was he always a brilliant student but he was also captain of the victorious Columbia University College football team. This background gave him the physical stamina for his intense lifestyle of surgeries, travel, teaching, research, and writing. He dedicated himself to his profession, being the first in the hospital in the morning and the last to leave at night. The patients sensed his compassion and all said "he gave me hope." He served as a medical officer in the US Navy (Lt. JG) from 1946 to 1948, mainly at sea, following which he continued his extensive clinical and research training.

After retiring he was appointed Emeritus Director and continued his activities. An endowed Academic Chair was established in his honor under the direction of his successor Dr Michael Y. Divon.

On June 6 2007, the first *Dr Hugh R.K. Barber Annual Memorial Lecture* organized by Dr Irving Butterman was given by Dr Richard C. Boronow.

CHAPTER 1

Introduction

Albert Altchek

Mount Sinai School of Medicine and Hospital, New York, NY, USA

Why there is a need for this book

Pediatric, adolescent, and young adult gynecology is not taught because of our traditional compartmentalized system of medical school education. Our gynecologic residents never see children and would be ill equipped to evaluate a pediatric gynecologic problem. Our pediatric house staff rarely learn about gynecologic problems or how to evaluate those problems in their young patients. There are only a handful of fellowships in the USA in pediatric and adolescent gynecology. Nevertheless, it is important for the clinical physician to have a basic, practical understanding of diagnosis and management of common problems and to know when to suspect a possibly dangerous situation.

In the future, medical school curricula will develop a multidisciplinary approach and will include this subject. The specialty examinations for obstetrics/gynecology and pediatrics in the USA now have questions on the subject. This enables the student to immediately understand the relevance of a preclinical science such as gynecologic pathology. In our school it is now taught with clinical case presentation, physical examination, ultrasound diagnosis, and management.

The child is completely different from the adult in every aspect including approach, evaluation, and management. Their illnesses are different, such as tumors, problems of growth and development, future fertility, and delayed and precocious puberty. As an example, whereas the first procedure for abnormal bleeding in the menopause is usually endometrial sampling or dilation and curettage of the uterus, in the adolescent this procedure is the last choice. The reason is that menopausal bleeding may be due to endometrial cancer which is extremely rare in the adolescent. In addition, in the latter it may result in emotional and possibly local physical damage.

Adolescent ovarian malignancies are usually of the germ cell variety. These have a different biology from the usual adult ovarian surface serous papillary cancer. The latter immediately spreads to the opposite ovary and is usually detected in an advanced stage. Chemotherapy often appears successful but after a negative second look there is often a recurrence. The germ cell malignant tumor of the child rarely spreads to the opposite ovary. Without treatment, it is rapidly fatal. However, with removal of the involved ovary and adjacent tube, resection of metastatic lesions and with current chemotherapy (different from that for the adult), most cases can be cured and fertility preserved.

In former years the rare vaginal rhabdomyosarcoma was usually fatal within two years unless it was discovered early and a pelvic exenteration performed. At present, with early diagnosis, local resection and chemotherapy, most cases are cured.

Unfortunately, humans develop sexual and reproductive ability in adolescence before achieving an adult sense of responsibility, completing basic education, and achieving financial independence. Despite education, sexual activity occurs and with it come problems of sexually transmitted infection and emotional stress. The USA has a high rate of unwanted pregnancy because of a lack of contraception information and access. Pregnancy complications may present unexpectedly such as ectopic pregnancy, miscarriage, and hydatidiform mole.

The adolescent may be exposed to substance abuse (smoking, alcohol, drugs), being overweight, eating disturbances (anorexia nervosa, bulimia) and automobile

Pediatric, Adolescent, & Young Adult Gynecology. Edited by A. Altchek and L. Deligdisch. © 2009 Blackwell Publishing, ISBN: 978-1-4051-5347-8.

accidents (when allowed to drive). She often fears that she is not developing normally, and struggles to be independent. Although not common, adolescent suicide is of concern. The US Centers for Disease Control and Prevention reported for 2003–2004 that the suicide rate for ages 10–24 increased by 8%, the largest rise in 15 years, to 4599 or 7.32 per 200,000. The increase was especially high in female adolescents. There are differences of opinion over whether this was a statistical fluctuation or the start of a trend, whether the reduction in prescriptions for antidepressants was a factor, and whether it was related to increased use of alcohol or drugs. A similar suicide increase also occurred in The Netherlands [1].

In the standard adult gynecology practice, many patients can be seen in a relatively short time because of the ease of history taking, examination, evaluation and explanation to the patient. Dealing with the young patient takes more time in obtaining a history from the patient (if old enough) and/or parents, and requires a quiet, unhurried individualized, nonintimidating approach and a sense of privacy for the apprehensive adolescent. The physician should be aware of legal aspects and cultural and family traditions. Nevertheless, there comes a time when complete privacy of the adolescent should be maintained, even from the parents. This is necessary because otherwise the adolescent may not report dangerous activities. The adolescent has to develop a personal sense of individual responsibility for her well-being. There should be separate clinic times for young patients and ideally the staff should have empathy for and like young patients.

When the adolescent is covered by the parent's health insurance, this may raise concern about the secrecy of health records and tests.

Despite the difficulties of caring for the young patient, the provider will derive great personal satisfaction helping youngsters have a happy, healthy, motivated, productive life with high self-esteem. This will stimulate their seeking higher education, assuming leadership roles if desired, and avoiding unwanted pregnancy.

Thus the roles of medical care include education, prevention of illness, treatment, and promoting good physical and emotional health.

Why this book is different

This book is a current, concise, clinical, practical, reader-friendly overview and guide for common problems. It is directed to the practicing obstetrician, gynecologist, pediatrician, adolescent medicine physician, and concerned primary care physician. It emphasizes diagnosis and management. Clinical chapters are structured to give an immediate overview for an urgent problem and further details for when more time is available. Throughout the book there are Quick Take boxes that list critical points. Thus, when the apprehensive mother and patient burst into your consultation room screaming "She is hemorrhaging! Do something!" you will not panic.

Recommendations are given regarding referral for complex, rare, urgent or possible serious problems.

For many years I have conducted an annual postgraduate course with an ever-increasing audience on "pediatric and adolescent gynecology." Recently I have added the "young adult." Many gynecologic problems which begin in the adolescent continue into young adulthood. These include menstrual disturbances, dysmenorrhea, pelvic pain, polycystic ovarian syndrome, anovulation, obesity, eating disturbances, and early diabetes. With sexuality, there are problems of unwanted pregnancy, disruption of education, sexually transmitted disease (STD), papilloma virus (HPV), and immunodeficiency virus (HIV, AIDS). There are also the emotional stresses of puberty such as depression and the temptation of substance abuse (smoking, alcohol, drugs) and gambling. In the USA, there is significant mortality and morbidity from automobile accidents. Furthermore, there is no uniform agreement on the boundary between puberty and young adult. There are many criteria including chronologic age, menstrual age, bone age, sexual development, emotional maturity, etc. Different populations and individuals in each population may vary in maturation. Different cultures have different definitions of adulthood. Young adulthood as a topic itself has been overlooked and in addition the young adult tends to avoid routine care.

This book is intensely personal, based on many years of solo private practice in the same office in New York City (Manhattan), with continuous voluntary academic affiliation at Mount Sinai Hospital and with additional affiliation to help the initiation of the new Albert Einstein College of Medicine in the Bronx, New York City. In addition, I conducted three pediatric gynecology clinics at three hospitals. The one at Lenox Hill Hospital was held weekly for a continuous 20 years. My large private consultation practice continues where the same patients are seen continuously over many years.

Thus this book is the first to describe new observations, including the following.

• The prepubertal unilateral, rapidly growing enlargement of the labium majus without a border simulating a malignancy: "prepubertal unilateral fibrous hyperplasia of the labium majus, report of eight cases and review of the literature" (Chapter 25) [2].

• The prepubertal distal longitudinal vaginal folds which may be confused with rhabdomyosarcoma and sexual molestation (Chapter 26) [3].

• The first description of subacute atopic dermatitis of the vulva which may be confused with sexual molestation. Dermatologists erroneously think it rarely involves the vulva. Atopic dermatitis is increasing in the USA and industrial areas (Chapter 7) [4].

• The first reported case of xanthogranuloma of the vagina which, despite benign histology, requires close follow-up (Chapter 8) [5].

• The first report of using human cultured bilayered newborn foreskin to line the vaginal dissection in Rokitansky syndrome (congenital absence of the vagina and uterus in a young adult). It had been thought that laboratory-cultured skin would lose its antigenicity and not be rejected by another human. Immediate early rejection did not occur but late slow rejection occurred two weeks later. Nevertheless, there was a good long-term result due to the extraordinary multiple growth stimulation factors which speeded the inward ascent of histologic vaginal cells from the 2 cm patch of the vaginal dimple (remnant of the embryologic urogenital sinus) (Chapter 24) [6].

• Successful *in vitro* culture of human skin and vaginal mucosa from the vaginal dimple and vagina in a three-dimensional, relatively thick layer of bovine collagen. This should withstand the pressure of the soft vaginal surgical mold and later use of a firm stent for the Rokitansky syndrome (and other reconstructive surgery) and be transplanted to the original donor without rejection. It would be easier to handle and less susceptible to trauma than the usual delicate epidermal skin culture for use in burn victims which cannot tolerate pressure and which often heals with scarring (Chapter 24) [7].

Because of wide experience of about 100 cases of Rokitansky syndrome, treated mainly by the modified McIndoe technique, there is a chapter describing in detail the psychologic, surgical, and follow-up care. A small error at any stage can cause a poor result (Chapter 24).

Evolving practice concepts

Concepts and practice are constantly changing and evolving. Laparoscopy has a role for benign ovarian cystectomy and is also beginning to be utilized in malignancy (Chapters 20, 26, 37). Pelvic and renal ultrasound may expand to include perineal and transrectal approaches. Magnetic resonance imaging (MRI) is being used especially for anomalies. Serum tumor markers are increasingly utilized. There is a fetal protective approach to congenital adrenal hyperplasia (CAH). The more common, atypical, late-onset CAH is being appreciated as a factor in infertility, polycystic ovarian syndrome, acne, hirsutism and scalp balding of the adult (Chapter 4).

Herpes simplex type 2 is increasing in incidence. Most cases are asymptomatic but nevertheless may shed virus and be infective to their consort. Management of pregnant women now includes herpes simplex type 2 antibody status. If negative and the partner is positive, he may be shedding virus and should consider taking medication to prevent spread. If the patient is positive, should she take suppressive therapy at the end of pregnancy to avoid a vulval ulcer in labor and a cesarean section (Chapter 38)?

The American College of Obstetricians and Gynecologists (ACOG) recommends that the first visit to the obstetrician-gynecologist should be between the ages of 13 and 15 years with the mother present. The visit is the start of a physician–patient relationship with a discussion of preventive healthcare, education and guidance, and any specific individual concerns of the patient. At the initial visit usually there is no physical or pelvic examination unless indicated. A simple approach might be a concise introduction followed by referral to group educational talks by nurse practitioners and/or appropriate books or educational videos. If feasible, try to schedule repeat visits perhaps at six-monthly intervals without interrupting school, and when other patients of a similar age group are being seen. The patient and her parents should be aware that regarding confidentiality, the law requires that the risk of bodily harm and physical or sexual abuse of minors is reported. Educational topics might include puberty development, menstruation, menstrual diary, dysmenorrhea, prevention of pregnancy, condoms, emergency contraception, prevention of STD, and avoiding substance abuse, eating problems, and mental health problems (anxiety, depression). A preinterview questionnaire as well as visual teaching aids are helpful. A visual general body evaluation, including visual breast evaluation and axillary and pelvic hair with perineum visualization, might be done at the initial or later visit to evaluate development, depending on patient anxiety and medical indication. If the patient is sexually active, she should be screened for STD including new urine STD screening if needed to avoid the need for a vaginal speculum.

The ACOG recommends that the first Pap cervix cytology and HPV cervix test be delayed until three years after the first coitus (or by age 21) because the first HPV infection may cause an over-reported cytology which may provoke surgical procedures which might disturb future pregnancy and because by three years most HPV tests become negative (see Chapters 38, 40, 45). However, other tests may be performed when there is sexual activity, including gonorrhea, chlamydia, etc. [8].

A problem in the USA is the multiple insurance companies which administer health maintenance organizations and managed care. There may be unavoidable physician changes as the parents alter their insurance companies with employment changes. This may mean a new physician introduction with associated stresses. Despite good intentions, adolescents are often lost to medical care.

Another problem is that a significant proportion of the population does not have health insurance.

Vaccination for human papilloma virus

In addition to preserving good health, vaccinations is a method of encouraging continuity of routine care [9]. It gives the opportunity for guidance in avoiding risk-taking behavior and substance abuse, especially for adolescents with poor self-esteem, depression, stress, and inadequate social support [10].

The high-risk type of papilloma virus, hrHPV (of which there are many), is a sexually transmitted disease. Although most sexually active young people acquire HPV, usually without symptoms, most spontaneously cure themselves within three years. In about 10% it may persist and may cause cervix dysplasia and later cervix cancer. In the USA there is an approved vaccine which will prevent most types of high-risk virus and is recommended for girls prior to sexual activity. It has not as yet been approved for boys. It is highly recommended by the medical profession to reduce the chance of cervix cancer by about

75% [11, 12]. The vaccine requires three separate injections and is expensive. Vaccination is approved for ages 9–26 regardless of previous sexual activity (Chapter 40).

The trade name of the quadrivalent HPV type 6, 11, 16, 18 recombinant vaccine is Gardasil®. The US Food and Drug Administration approved it for females aged 9–26 years in 2006. The Advisory Committee on Immunization Practices recommended vaccination at ages 11 or 12. The ideal situation is vaccination before sexual activity. The original recommendation of the manufacturer (Merck & Co., Inc.) was that vaccination would not do any good once there is a positive hrHPV cervical cytology test. The vaccine is given in three doses at 0, two and six months by injection.

The current viewpoint is that vaccination is helpful despite previous sexual activity, cervix dysplasia, and positive hrHPV. The reason is that most cases of hrHPV infection are with one or, rarely, two genotypes of hrHPV. The standard hrHPV test does not specify which genotype is present and will give a positive result for any of about 15 hrHPV genotypes. Although less effective in preventing later possible cervix cancer, it is now thought appropriate to give the vaccination despite a positive hrHPV test.

About 15 hrHPV genotypes are associated with cervical cancer. About 70% of cervical cancer is associated with hrHPV genotypes 16 and 18. About 90% of genital warts (which are usually not malignant) are associated with HPV genotypes 6 and 11.

In 2008 a vaccine was approved to prevent vaginal and vulvar cancer. Despite vaccination, standard cytology screening should be continued, starting three years after first coitus in the adolescent or no later than age 21. Routine cytology and HPV screening should be performed at age 30 [13]. If hrHPV is positive at this stage, the patient must be carefully followed because cervical cancer may result from persistent hrHPV. Cytology is not always reliable so even a report of atypical squamous cells of unknown significance (ASCUS) merits consideration of colposcopy and biopsy. Some advise colposcopy and biopsy even with negative cytology. In addition, consider simultaneous endocervical curettage, especially for atypical glandular cells on cytology which could indicate primary endocervical glandular neoplasia which is increasing in young women. It tends to be discovered late because it is not palpable, often has false-negative cytology, is not visible to direct view on ultrasound, and has a relatively poor prognosis.

Another concern is sexuality in later years. About half of marriages end in divorce in the USA. Widows and single women over 30 may have new sexual exposure and with it sexually transmitted infection. Although the FDA approval for HPV vaccination is up to age 26, this is simply because the over-26 year age group has not been sufficiently studied. Logically this group should consider vaccination.

For children, the physician should emphasize that vaccination is considered a standard recommendation used to prevent cervical cancer. It does not promote promiscuity.

HPV vaccination is not FDA recommended for pregnant women.

Most vaccinations are given to those with insurance coverage. Unfortunately, in the USA a significant proportion do not have medical insurance. However, with extensive use of cervical cytology (Papanicolaou) testing, cervical cancer rates and deaths have been greatly reduced in the USA.

In underdeveloped countries with poverty and poor-quality medical care, there is a lack of screening for cervical cytology and a much higher rate of cervical cancer and deaths than in the affluent countries. These countries would benefit even more than the affluent countries if HPV vaccination became available to them.

The Centers for Disease Control (CDC) in the USA now emphasize vaccination for both HPV and meningococcus for adolescents by age 18 [12, 13].

The adolescent or young adult patient should also consider vaccination or update for the following: hepatitis B and A, diphtheria, tetanus, pertussis, measles, mumps, rubella, varicella, meningococcus, pneumococcal, yearly influenza, (haemophilus influenzae type b), meningitis, and inactivated polio.

Education for life

As part of normal customary schooling, the young patient should be instructed in "education for life," emphasizing good general physical and emotional health including exercise, diet, and avoiding obesity and substance abuse. In addition, she should understand the importance of good education, self-esteem, empowerment and having aspirations for adult life, including the later choice of a mate. Learning human biology is important. Because sexual development occurs before adulthood, the young patient requires early guidance.

A recently recognized concern is universal increasing obesity in developed countries which often starts in adolescence. It results from a combination of a genetic tendency to "truncal obesity" (waist-to-hip ratio), intolerance to the refined carbohydrates of affluent societies, and lack of exercise. This may affect up to 30% of all humans. Obesity predisposes to diabetes and cardiovascular disease. The lack of exercise compounds the problem [14].

A school course on contraception is often met with opposition. If it is presented as part of an overall program on "education for life," it is more acceptable. Parents and school administrators sometimes erroneously believe that it may encourage promiscuity. The USA has a high rate of adolescent unwanted pregnancy. Other developed countries have similar rates of adolescent sexuality but without unwanted pregnancy because of the use of contraception. Correspondingly we have high rates of abortion. Unwanted pregnancy is an important reason for school drop-outs as well as emotional stress. Teaching abstinence alone usually is ineffective.

The educator should not be judgmental and yet not condone sexuality. The young girl should be advised that she controls her own body and is empowered to do whatever she wishes, and that is not to have sex if she doesn't wish to. She can always say "I'm not ready for it yet." If she is sexually active she needs contraceptive advice.

Even though one hears that "everyone is doing it," early sexual activity has hazards. First, there is the possibility of unwanted pregnancy. Even with oral contraceptives, there is a difference between the small theoretical risks of pregnancy compared to the actual risk in use, which is much higher because of forgetfulness. An unwanted pregnancy is usually a high-risk pregnancy associated with prematurity, disruption of education, substance abuse, and persistence of poverty.

Second, there is the possibility of sexually transmitted disease (STD) also called sexually transmitted infection (STI). STD may leave a legacy of infertility, ectopic pregnancy, pelvic pain, and AIDS. Condoms will tend to reduce the risk and therefore should be used in addition to more effective contraception. In addition, the number of consorts should be kept to a minimum. Routine testing for STD should be performed even in the absence of symptoms. Females acquire the HIV (AIDS) virus more readily than males because of a large susceptibility area of vaginal mucosa which frequently has microabrasions.

Even if the boyfriend is in apparently good health, he may be a carrier of STD.

The theoretical ideal would be to have the consort tested for all STD (STI) (Chapters 38, 39, 40). Early AIDS is asymptomatic. About one-third of the population in the USA have herpes simplex type 2 infection. Most are asymptomatic but can still shed virus and be infective. Syphilis and hepatitis are also of concern. Unfortunately although in many parts of the USA in previous years a blood test for syphilis was required for a marriage license, at present many communities do not require any testing (Chapter 44).

From a practical point of view the potential partner should be asked about previous number of partners, any past history or symptoms of STD (STI), drug addiction, sharing of intravenous needles, and hemophilia with many blood transfusions before complete blood testing was available.

From a legal viewpoint there have been law suits against adults for failing to report a history of herpes simplex type 2 to the partner who later developed it.

Personal observations

Dermatologic lesions of the vulva may be readily misinterpreted as molestation, especially with lichen sclerosus, atopic dermatitis, and distal longitudinal vaginal folds (Chapters 7, 34, 35).

Recurrent urinary tract infection may be due to a urogenital sinus, congenital adrenal hyperplasia (CAH), labial fusion, agglutination of the labia minora or microperforate hymen with the opening near or under the urethra. It may also occur from increased anal bacteria colonization in the vestibule and periurethral area in atopic dermatitis. Any vulvitis may cause vulvar dysuria with infrequent voiding and "holding it in." Voiding in warm water may be helpful.

Recurrent prepubertal vaginitis may be due to atopic dermatitis with perianal fissures allowing anal bacteria to reach the anestrogenic vagina. It may also result from rubbing the vulva because of pruritus. Recurrent atopic dermatitis may occur from secondary bacterial infection. Other causes include recurrent foreign bodies, congenital vaginal anomalies, and wearing of tights.

Recurrent and severe labia minora agglutination is often due to atopic dermatitis. Topical estrogen cream once daily at night usually will cause spontaneous separation of the labia minora within two weeks. If the child requires diapers then the cream is removed when the child is cleaned. Therefore the cream should be applied three times daily. If the cream is used for several months it may be absorbed and cause breast stimulation, pain and tenderness, darkening of the vulva skin and vulva hair growth. If the labia minora have been agglutinated for about six months or longer, fibrous tissue may grow in and surgery may be required. It is best done by someone with experience because the urethra is just under the closed labia minora, especially if the labia appear to be completely closed. It may cause urinary tract infections, distortion of the voided urine stream, and postvoid dribbling. On examination there seems to be no exit for urine. With careful inspection, the most anterior section will be found to have a 1–2 mm opening with a watery appearance.

Agglutination which is less than half with an anterior opening not distorting the urinary stream usually does not require surgery.

In former years some physicians would rip apart the labia with both thumbs. This causes pain, bleeding, and a very disturbed patient and mother. In addition, the new jagged edges promptly reattach.

Some physicians recommend avoiding any treatment in anticipation of pubertal estrogen opening the labia. In this case, the latter remain closed for years and do not open at puberty because of agglutination being replaced by fibrous tissue.

For mild cases of labia minora agglutination, try good hygiene and topical petroleum jelly (Vaseline®).

House physicians never see children with agglutination of the labia minora because they are not hospitalized. The differential diagnosis includes CAH. Sometimes with atopic dermatitis, the foreskin traps smegma under the clitoris, causing severe local pain, or sometimes it causes swelling of the clitoris prepuce foreskin, simulating a large clitoris. With labial agglutination, this may simulate congenital adrenal hyperplasia.

Premature thelarche (prepubertal isolated nonprogressive breast development) is more common than true precocious puberty. Breast enlargement is seen in both. Although many experts recommend investigation with sometimes frightening x-ray of the left wrist for bone age, and extensive (and expensive) serum hormone tests, the latter may be difficult to interpret because of lack of biologic activity of elevated gonadotropin which is not infrequent in the young child. I have found that most cases can be managed by examination, vaginal swab maturation index (or using centrifuged voided urine if not feasible), and periodic observation. Pelvic ultrasound may be performed to rule out an estrogen-secreting ovarian neoplasm (Chapters 43, 49, 52). Severe hypothyroidism may precipitate an increase of prolactin which may stimulate the breasts. The vaginal mucosa is more sensitive to estrogen than the breast. In the usual case of premature thelarche, the vaginal mucosa is anestrogenic, prepubertal, and thin and the cytology shows predominantly parabasal cells which are small, oval and contain a large nucleus.

With true central nervous system precocious puberty there is increase in serum gonadotropin and estradiol, and the vaginal mucosa is thick and has superficial, large, flat polygonal epithelial cells with a small dark nucleus. The vaginal mucosa changes before the breasts enlarge. The educated observer can confirm this immediately by a wet microscopic swab without staining. With an atrophic smear there is no estrogen from true central nervous system activation or rare ovarian neoplasm. With premature thelarche both breasts may enlarge simultaneously or one may enlarge followed by the other in a few months. The breast enlargement ceases spontaneously and does not get larger than stage 3. It is thought that premature thelarche may result from a previous transient elevation of active gonadotropin. Therefore there are rare in-between cases (Chapters 18, 27).

Old autopsy reports of rhabdomyosarcoma show that recurrences always present at the original site. This suggests that the site should be tested after therapy. I performed a local vaginal resection of a lesion high on the anterior wall in an 11-month-old girl. A simultaneous deep bladder biopsy showed the tumor in the vesico-vaginal septum. After appropriate chemotherapy, it was thought that the tumor was cured. However, repeated vaginoscopy showed recurrences at the site which had repeated excisions. For the next year there were repeated courses of chemotherapy. The local recurrences persisted and after one year radiation and anterior exenteration had to be undertaken. She has remained tumor free after 20 years (Chapters 8, 37, 49).

Almost every gynecologic problem in the young patient has a psychologic component (Chapter 13).

If surgery can be accomplished without excessive delay following torsion of the ovary or adnexa, despite an ominous dark blue color and swelling, detorsion plus careful observation for the next 5–10 minutes will often show that circulation is restored or improved and the structures can be preserved. A predisposing dermoid cyst should be resected to prevent recurrence of torsion. There are differences of opinion regarding pexy of one or both ovaries (Chapters 26, 32, 33, 36).

Cervical histology of the adolescent shows the dramatic, initial HPV infection. The marked reaction explains the often alarming cytology which may lead to overly aggressive surgery (Chapter 45). Initial viral infection sites tend to have violent reactions as the host mounts a vigorous immune response. This is analogous to a primary genital type 2 herpes simplex virus infection. Later biopsies are subdued. The current concept is to defer cytology to about 2–3 years after the first coitus by which time, in the vast majority, the cytology returns to normal and the DNA test for HPV becomes negative by an unknown normal body defense mechanism. Nevertheless, tests for other STD should be performed with the first coitus and repeated periodically, as well as education regarding contraception, pregnancy complications, and AIDS (Chapters 38, 39, 40).

Sometimes, often after a broken partnership, if the asymptomatic patient requests tests for all STD, consider doing cervical cultures or DNA tests for gonorrhea and chlamydia, serum tests for syphilis, HIV (AIDS), herpes simplex type 2 specific antibody, hepatitis screen, lymphogranuloma venereum or any other STD suggested by cultural or geographic factors. In addition, consider inspection of the throat and skin and palpation for inguinal adenopathy (Chapters 39, 40).

The use of ultrasound (sonogram) may reveal unsuspected fetal ovarian cysts which often persist into the early months of infancy. Most of these are benign follicular cysts which are reminiscent of the approximately 10% incidence of postmenopausal asymptomatic, benign, small simple ovarian cysts which may come and go and are discovered by coincidental transvaginal ultrasound. It is not unusual for follicular cysts to develop in the prepubertal child. These are usually asymptomatic and tend to disappear within six weeks to a few months (Chapters 9, 36, 50).

Often coincidental pelvic ultrasound may reveal a "complex ovarian cyst" in an adolescent or young adult. These are usually benign asymptomatic hemorrhagic corpus luteum cysts which usually recede in six weeks. Some are associated with early pregnancy. In the postmenopausal woman, a "complex ovarian cyst" should arouse concern (Chapter 36, 41).

Although polycystic ovarian syndrome (POS) is associated with oligomenorrhea and amenorrhea in the young adult, I have noticed that in the adolescent it may manifest by irregular, heavy vaginal bleeding. This is understandable because anovulatory dysfunctional uterine bleeding (ADUB) may manifest by irregular heavy bleeding or, less often, by a characteristic three months of amenorrhea followed by one month of continuous irregular bleeding. About 5% or more cases of ADUB, especially those with heavy irregular bleeding, may never ovulate and may later be diagnosed as POS. About 5–25% of POS may be due to atypical late-onset CAH (Chapters 23, 32). Apart from immediate care, POS has implications for later general health and therefore for preventive care.

Most vaginal bleeding in the child is due to local causes rather than precocious puberty. Even children with signs suggestive of puberty may have bleeding from a local cause (Chapter 8, 10, 11).

Chronic pelvic pain is not rare. Sometimes the etiology is uncertain and often it is attributed to a coincidental benign simple small unilocular ovarian cyst. Not infrequently, there is a gastrointestinal etiology suggested by bilateral continuous or intermittent crampy pain, tympanic abdomen on percussion and palpable right colon and sometimes sigmoid colon. It may be associated with lactose intolerance, food allergies, regional ileitis (spastic colon), irritable bowel syndrome, intestinal parasites, and celiac sprue. Sensitive skin stroking may suggest neurologic or fascial origin. Do not rush to perform a laparoscopy for recurrent pelvic pain if the patient has had several previous laparotomies or laparoscopies. There may be adhesions, nongynecologic cause of pain, and an increased chance of surgical complications.

Fellowship development

Co-ordinated advanced training is almost nonexistent in the USA outside a handful of fellowships, each of which is different. There is a need to develop a consensus standard fellowship program which would include two aspects: nonsurgical education, and surgical aspects for those with surgical privileges.

The main limiting factor for advanced training is the relatively few reconstructive procedures for congenital anomalies in one hospital done annually.

Personal concept of collaborative fellowship

Pediatric and adolescent gynecology, although a small subspecialty, is being recognized by all large hospitals and clinics as an important service. Each institution has different strengths for teaching programs. Surgical procedures are infrequent, especially for congenital anomalies. Thus it would take a relatively long time for a fellow to achieve sufficient experience at one hospital. Institutions are reluctant to close certain services in order to give complete care in one institution. The logical approach is to establish a collaborative fellowship in which the fellow will rotate through different institutions and in addition scrub in or observe surgery for unusual cases as they present themselves. In addition to training, such collaboration could facilitate research planning, data collection, and collaborative hospital educational conferences. At a certain stage, the fellow might even be a consultant for emergency rooms.

Since most hospitals are territorial in philosophy in an attempt to give full service, the ideal would be a collaborative rotating fellowship with one base co-ordinating hospital. This is especially true for New York City with its five medical schools and numerous competing "children's hospitals."

Central Europe has had a long traditional interest in advanced training (Chapter 52). There is a standard test and certification which could be used as the basis for a curriculum, test, and certification in the US.

Concerns associated with particular age groups

Fetus

Occasionally, by coincidence, a large simple follicular cyst of the ovary is discovered by routine ultrasound in pregnancy. The usual management is periodic observation by repeat ultrasound for the remainder of the pregnancy and after birth. Most cysts are asymptomatic and spontaneously disappear in a few months after birth. Infrequently surgery is performed in the newborn or infancy if there is evidence of malignancy or torsion (Chapter 9).

Newborn to about two weeks

• Atypical-appearing genitalia (ambiguous external genitalia) (Chapter 3)

- Congenital adrenal hyperplasia, salt-losing form may cause sudden death at one week (Chapter 4)
- Androgen insensitivity (Chapter 5). Family history of amenorrhea, infertility; bilateral inguinal hernia sometimes containing a testis; feminine vulva; short vagina; no cervix or uterus; karyotype 46,XY
- Ovarian dysplasia (gonadal dysgenesis, XO syndrome, Turner syndrome): karyotype 45,X mosaic; anomalies (cardiac, coarctation of aorta, renal, extremities), edema of the dorsum of the hands and feet; broad chest; excessive pigmented nevi (Chapter 5)
- Microperforate hymen (small orifice just below urethra) (Chapter 25)
- Imperforate hymen: sometimes bulging from excess endocervical mucus due to over-reaction to maternal estrogen (Chapter 25)
- Midvaginal complete transverse septum may result in a huge upper vaginal distension with cardiorespiratory distress (Chapter 25)
- Cyst of introitus (paraurethral cyst) present at birth concealing urethra and vagina, attached to distal anterior vagina and distal posterior urethral meatus (Chapter 25)
- No opening to vagina despite mucosal dimple – possible Rokitansky syndrome of absent vagina and uterus; test patency with adult urethral catheter (Chapter 24)
- Polyps of the hymen, usually small at 6 o'clock, may shrivel and disappear in a few days when maternal estrogen effect is lost. Some may persist and require removal for cosmetic reasons or bleeding from trauma (Chapter 25)
- Unusual vulva rashes due to secondary syphilis acquired in late pregnancy following early pregnancy negative serology (Chapter 7, 40)
- Associated anomalies – rectum, low back, spina bifida, renal anomalies, ectopic ureter (Chapter 25)
- Physiologic leukorrhea and bleeding due to maternal estrogen stimulation and later withdrawal bleeding
- Trichomonad vaginitis and urethritis acquired from maternal vagina after vaginal delivery can cause a heavy white discharge and sterile pyuria (Chapter 7)
- Labial edema due to breech presentation
- Rare vaginal rhabdomyosarcoma presenting as a polyp and/or bleeding with the base above the hymen. The surface may have normal vaginal mucosa with the neoplasm being submucosal; therefore the entire polyp must be removed rather than a surface mucosal biopsy (average age for rhabdomyosarcoma is about 11 months) (Chapters 8, 37, 49).

- Bilateral slight breast enlargement, 1 cm cystic-feeling breast tissue, sometimes with galactorrhea ("witch's milk"). Do not massage breasts which may provoke infection. If surgery performed for abscess, do not excise breast bud (Chapter 27).

Infant (about 2 weeks to 2 years)
- Diaper rash (Chapters 7, 36, 37)
- Atopic dermatitis (Chapters 7, 36, 37)
- Seborrheic dermatitis (Chapters 7, 36, 37)
- Agglutination of labia minora, often associated with atopic dermatitis (Chapter 7)
- Vulvar and perianal condyloma: may be acquired from vaginal birth exposure to maternal vaginal papilloma virus and/or by caretaker cleansing, especially if there is sensitive skin. It may be sexually transmitted (Chapters 7, 38, 39, 40, 45)
- Premature thelarche, unilateral or bilateral (Chapters 18, 27; also see above p. 6)
- Many newborn concerns

Young child (about 3–6 years)
- Trauma (climbing, running, falling) (Chapter 10)
- Foreign body causing persistent, foul bloody discharge, usually due to wads of toilet tissue deep in the vagina (Chapter 7)
- Agglutination of labia minora (Chapter 7)
- Vulvovaginitis (Chapter 7)
- Atopic and seborrheic dermatitis (Chapter 7)
- Prolapsed urethra (Chapters 1, 8)
- Ovarian follicular cysts (usually asymptomatic), coincidental discovery (Chapters 9, 50)
- Premature adrenarche (pubic hair, may be familial) (Chapter 18, 27)
- True central nervous system precocious puberty, with ovulation, high follicle-stimulating hormone (FSH) and estradiol (Chapter 18)
- Rare rhabdomyosarcoma of vagina (Chapter 8, 37, 49)
- Rare hormone-producing ovarian cystic tumors (granulosa cell) causing precocious puberty without ovulation, elevated estrogen, and no increase in FSH (Chapters 18, 47)

Prepubertal (about 7–10 years)
- Vulvovaginitis (Chapter 7)
- Vaginal bleeding (foreign body, rare rhabdomyosarcoma) (Chapter 8)

- Trauma (Chapters 8, 10, 11)
- Ovarian follicular cysts: usually asymptomatic, discovered by coincidental ultrasound, done for nonspecific lower abdominal cramps. A simple, small unilateral cyst may be coincidental. Usually repeat ultrasound after about two months shows resolution (Chapters 9, 36, 50)
- Complex ovarian cysts (dermoid, hemorrhagic) may undergo torsion with adjacent tube (Chapters 9, 36, 50)
- Sexual molestation (Chapters 10, 11)
- Rare hormone-producing ovarian neoplasm (Chapters 41, 47)
- Ectopic ureter exiting into vagina causing constant watery purulent leakage (Chapters 7, 25)
- Beginning "education for life" courses, including puberty development and preparation for menses (see above)
- Rare unilateral rapid enlargement of labium majus (Chapter 25)

Puberty (about 10–17 years)
- Anxiety, emotional stresses
- "Am I developing normally?" (Chapters 13, 15, 27)
- Menstrual problems: irregularity, menorrhagia, dysmenorrhea, primary and secondary amenorrhea (Chapters 15–22, 24, 25)
- "Education for life", including contraception, avoiding STD (sexually transmitted infection – STI), continuing education, self-esteem, finding a partner, career development, obesity, substance abuse, development of a sense of responsibility, vaccination update (Chapters 15, 28, 29; also see above)
- Onset of manifestation of POS (Chapter 31) sometimes with excessive bleeding in adolescence and secondary oligoamenorrhea in young adulthood
- Acute pelvic pain: torsion of ovarian cysts (associated with long ligaments and heavy cysts) with tube (Chapters 32, 33, 47), rupture of malignant cyst, ectopic pregnancy, pelvic inflammatory disease, acute appendicitis
- Pelvic and abdominal masses (Chapters 32, 33, 47)
- Chronic pelvic pain (Chapters 20, 21)
- Ovarian simple cysts, hemorrhagic cysts (hemorrhagic cysts may have the ultrasound appearance of "complex cyst" – repeat ultrasound in 6–8 weeks; "complex cyst" in menopause is of concern) (Chapter 36)
- Continuity of care, need for general health vaccinations which promotes continuity (see above)

- Consideration of HPV vaccinations (series of three injections) (Chapter 40; also see above)
- Ovarian neoplasms: dermoid cysts (mature benign teratoma), malignant germ cell tumors (rapid growth, large, pain) (Chapter 47)
- Understanding adolescent labor (Chapter 30)
- Confusing congenital anomaly symptoms: amenorrhea in a normal-appearing adolescent (Rokitansky syndrome; Chapter 24); severe dysmenorrhea not relieved by oral contraceptives ("no eponym" syndrome of uterus didelphys; Chapter 25)

Young adult (about 18–25 years)
- Continuation of adolescent concerns including: menstrual disturbances, sexuality, STD, avoiding unwanted pregnancy (Chapters 12, 15–23, 24, 25, 29, 30, 35, 40, 42, 47) as well as obesity and substance abuse
- Abortion (Chapters 29, 43, 44)
- Pregnancy complications: miscarriage, ectopic pregnancy, hydatidiform mole (Chapters 33, 48)
- Ovarian cysts and neoplasm including dermoid (mature teratoma); rare germ cell malignancies; adnexal torsion (Chapters 32, 35, 47, 48, 50)
- Asymptomatic "complex ovarian cysts" usually managed by repeat ultrasound in 6–8 weeks in proliferate phase (Chapter 36)
- Chronic and acute pelvic pain (Chapters 20, 21, 32, 33)
- Pelvic and abdominal masses (Chapters 32, 33, 47, 52)
- Understanding adolescent labor (Chapter 30)
- "Education for life" courses (see above)
- Finding a partner
- Advanced education
- Career development
- Developing a sense of responsibility
- Does she need vaccinations? (see above)
- Primary care doctor or gynecologist for continuing care and vaccination update (see above)

References

1. Gibbon RD, Brown CH, Hur K et al. Early evidence of the effects of regulators' suicidality warnings on SSRI prescriptions and suicide in children and adolescents. *Am J Psychiatry* 2007;**164**:9.
2. Altchek A, Deligdisch L, Norton K et al. Prepubertal unilateral fibrous hyperplasia of the labium majus: report of eight cases

and review of the literature. *Obstet Gynecol* 2007;**110**(1):103–108.

3. Altchek A, Wasserman B, Deligdisch L. Update on prepubertal distal longitudinal vaginal mucosal folds. *J Pediatr Adolesc Gynecol* 2007;**20**(2): 127–128.

4. Altchek A. The subacute stage of vulva atopic dermatitis. *J Pediatr Adolesc Gynecol* 2007;**20**(2):131.

5. Altchek A, Brovender B, Green I et al. The first case report of xanthogranuloma of the prepubertal vagina. *J Pediatr Adolesc Gynecol* 2006;**19**(2):158–159.

6. Altchek A, Brem H. Case report: the first reported successful use of human skin equivalent (APLIGRAF®) to line new vagina in Rokitansky syndrome. *J Pediatr Adolesc Gynecol* 2005;**18**:215–218.

7. Doillon CJ, Altchek A, Silver FH. Method of growing vaginal mucosal cells on a collagen sponge matrix. Results of preliminary studies. *J Reprod Med* 1990;**35**(3):203–207.

8. ACOG Committee Opinion # 335. The initial reproductive health visit. *Obstet Gynecol* 2006;**107**:1215–1219.

9. Rupp R, Rosenthal S, Middleman A. Vaccination: an opportunity to enhance early adolescent preventative services. *J Adolesc Health* 2006;**39**:461–464.

10. Mazzaferro KE, Murray PJ, Ness RB et al. Depression, stress, and social support as predictors of high-risk sexual behaviors and STIs in young women. *J Adolesc Health* 2006;**39**:601–603.

11. Society for Adolescent Health. Position statement – human papillomavirus (HPV) vaccine. *J Adolesc Health* 2006; **39**(4):620.

12. Recommended immunization schedules for persons aged 0–18 years – United States, 2007. *MMWR Quick Guide* 2007; **55**:nos 51, 52.

13. ACOG Committee Opinion # 344. Human papilloma vaccine. *Obstet Gynecol* 2006;**108**(3,1):699–705.

14. Wood L. Obesity, waist–hip ratio and hunter-gatherers. *BJOG* 2006;**113**:1110–1116.

Further reading

Altchek A, Brem H. The first reported successful use of human skin equivalent (APLIGRAF®) to line a new vagina in Rokitansky syndrome. *J Pediatr Adoles Gynecol* 2005;**18**:215–218.

Altchek A, Deligdisch L, Norton K et al. Prepubertal unilateral soft-fibrous tumor of labium majus without palpable border in girls. *Obstet Gynecol* 2006;**107**(4):205.

Balen AH. *Paediatric and Adolescent Gynecology: A Multidisciplinary Approach.* Cambridge, UK: Cambridge University Press, 2004.

Emans SJH, Laufer MR, Goldstein DP. *Pediatric and Adolescent Gynecology*, 5th edn. New York: Lippincott, Williams and Wilkins, 2005.

Sanfilippo JS, Muram D, Dewhurst J, Lee PA. *Pediatric and Adolescent Gynecology*, 2nd edn. New York: WB Saunders, 2001.

CHAPTER 2

Evaluation of the Newborn

Albert Altchek

Mount Sinai School of Medicine and Hospital, New York, NY, USA

There are two types of evaluation. The more common is a routine part of the general evaluation, which may be nothing more than adequate visualization. The other is a specific consultation by an expert because of unusual findings or because of a suspicious family or personal history.

The family history, past history, and prenatal observations should be reviewed. These may give a clue to androgen insensitivity (female relatives who did not menstruate or become pregnant), congenital adrenal hyperplasia (family history, hirsutism, short women), sexual ambiguity, and progestin or androgen hormone therapy in pregnancy or endogenous progestin from functional ovarian cyst or an androgen-secreting ovarian neoplasm or fetal ovarian cyst. Was a routine late pregnancy test done for syphilis or HIV? Was the mother's serum herpes type 2-specific antibody negative early in pregnancy and could the consort be positive despite lack of symptoms? Pertinent items should be impartially noted on the chart without making any judgment.

The examination should be scheduled with the nursery in advance to avoid feeding time or just after feeding when the child might vomit. The mother's consent is assumed if it is understood as a routine procedure. If a special consultation is suggested by the initial pediatric evaluation, the mother should give at least verbal consent and be told the name of the consultant. The consultant should introduce himself or herself in advance, especially if photography may be done which might require written consent.

The examination area should not be visible from the outside corridor. There must be good light; some consultants use a headlight and 2.5 optical loop. An aide

should be present for legal protection, for assistance, and to hold the child still if necessary. A restraining board should be available. Other items to consider are sterile gloves, cotton-tipped applicator stick, provision for cytology (for suspicion of vaginal malignancy), surgical lubricating jelly, and an adult urethral soft bladder catheter to probe the vagina.

The abdomen is gently palpated for abdominal and pelvic masses and inspected for distension. The low back is inspected. The inguinal area is inspected and palpated for hernia and masses (testes or ovaries). The urethra is inspected for prolapse of the urethra, bladder polyp or ureterocele. The labia majora are inspected and palpated. Bilateral labial enlargement may result from pressure edema of fetal breech presentation. The vestibule (just outside the hymen) is inspected as well as the opening of the hymen. Rarely an ectopic urethra exits just below the urethral meatus.

The urethra and vagina may be hidden by a 0.5–3 cm milk-white paraurethral cyst with "capillary" bright red tiny vessels in its covering membrane (see Chapter 26). At first glance, there may not seem to be a urethra or vagina. The clue is that the edge of the posterior hymen may be visible. With a dry cotton-tipped applicator, gently pull the cyst posteriorly which will reveal the urethral meatus. Gentle anterior traction will reveal the posterior opening of the hymen. Gentle probing reveals a 3–4 cm vagina. These cysts are not rare but their incidence is under-reported because they are missed at initial examination or because they often spontaneously rupture within a week or two, leaking a thick milky-white liquid, and within 1–2 minutes the cyst completely collapses and disappears.

If there does not appear to be an opening into the vagina, use the cotton-tipped applicator stick technique to retract the anterior hymen (just underneath the

Pediatric, Adolescent, & Young Adult Gynecology. Edited by A. Altchek and L. Deligdisch. © 2009 Blackwell Publishing, ISBN: 978-1-4051-5347-8.

urethra) posteriorly, which may reveal another opening – the microperforate hymen. Releasing the anterior hymen causes the microperforate hymen to disappear under the urethra.

If there is a possibility of patent anus (apparently only a dimple), the usual procedure is a small-finger digital examination. This may cause a small tear and slight bleeding. Another approach is passage of an adult urethral catheter. Examine the low back for anomalies. Purulent skin rashes should be cultured and a Gram stain slide made.

Lack of a patent hymen may be due to an imperforate hymen. If so, and if there has been excessive fetal endocervical mucus production, the hymen may bulge (see Chapter 26). Even with a patent hymen, it is worth passing an adult urethral catheter into the vagina to measure the depth and get an idea of the width. With the Rokitansky syndrome (see Chapter 25), there is no vaginal opening or, less often, a short (up to 2 cm) vagina ("vaginal dimple") which is "blind" (no cervix or uterus present).

The usual newborn vagina is about 4 cm in length. Under 3 cm requires investigation. With androgen insensitivity (see Chapter 5), the vulva is also normal female but usually there is a short, "blind" vagina. With experience, a small narrow endoscope can be inserted into the vagina which may be gently distended with saline to inspect the upper vagina. Another approach is to use a miniature bivalve vaginal speculum and an optical loop with attached headlight. Veterinary otoscopes have a long narrow speculum of 4 cm length (see Chapter 6).

Polyps of the newborn hymen are not rare. Most are on the posterior lip and vary from small mucoid 3 mm projections to longer narrow forms extending 2 cm. Some are 1–3 cm cysts. These are usually benign. Some small polyps spontaneously regress in a few days with reduction of exogenous maternal estrogen (see Chapter 26). Polyps of the hymen are usually benign. Some may be large, persist and may bleed with trauma. Polyps whose origin is in the vagina (especially anterior) above the hymen and present through the hymen opening are considered possibly malignant, especially if growing rapidly and bleeding (rare rhabdomyosarcoma), and should be removed rather than

simply performing a microsurgical surface biopsy (see Chapter 8).

The posterior anal (natal) cleft is inspected as well as the low back for a hairy patch, pilonidal cyst, skin defect or spina bifida (with paralysis of the lower extremities in severe cases).

Immediate consultation is recommended for possible urgent or serious conditions such as congenital adrenal hyperplasia (see Chapter 4) (large clitoris, single perianal opening), ambiguous external genitalia (atypical-appearing genitalia), vaginal rhabdomyosarcoma (see Chapters 8, 37, 49), spina bifida, lower extremity paralysis, and gross anatomic distortion (imperforate anus, double vulva, absent lower abdominal wall, etc.). If there is cause for concern, the pediatrician should be notified before the mother, who might react with extreme anxiety or significant emotional disturbance. For uncertain findings, some pediatricians may feel that the mother should not be informed until confirmatory tests are performed. This is a judgment call. Nevertheless, a brief objective note should be placed on the chart to alert all caregivers.

Pelvic ultrasound is considered for Rokitansky syndrome and for possible complete transverse midvaginal septum, especially with distension of the upper vagina from excess endocervical mucus secretion which may simulate an ovarian cyst on ultrasound and, if severe, may present as abdominal swelling causing cardiorespiratory distress (see Chapters 25, 26, 41).

Many significant gynecologic anomalies are associated with renal anomalies. With Rokitansky syndrome about 25% or more have an absent or pelvic kidney. With the "no eponym" syndrome of double uterus, cervix, and vagina with one distal vagina obstruction, there is almost always a 100% ipsilateral absent kidney. In some families there is a predisposition to an absent kidney or uterus didelphys, as separate entities.

In general, if there is any question it is wise to call a consultant, even if only for the emotional benefit for the pediatrician, obstetrician and parents, as well as good practice. It also reassures the (often anxious) parents that the newborn is under proper care and enhances the reputation of the pediatrician.

CHAPTER 3

Early Diagnosis and Management of Atypical-Appearing Genitalia

Genna W. Klein & Robert Rapaport
Mount Sinai School of Medicine and Hospital, New York, NY, USA

Introduction

The birth of an infant with atypical-appearing (formerly known as "ambiguous") genitalia is accompanied by an enormous amount of parental anxiety, concern, and questioning. The importance of a carefully coordinated, thoughtful, sensitive, deliberate and confident approach on the part of the healthcare team cannot be overemphasized. The swift mobilization of pertinent subspecialists, support personnel, and laboratory and radiological diagnostics is crucial for diagnosis, treatment, and management of the infant, including, when appropriate, correct sex assignment as early as possible.

A recent meeting of expert participants representing the Lawson Wilkins Pediatric Endocrine Society and the European Society for Paediatric Endocrinology was convened with the purpose of deriving a consensus statement. The document was based on a broad, comprehensive, and critical review of the literature and of cumulative experiences of the participants regarding the diagnosis and life-long management of patients with "intersex" disorders. Advances in the understanding of sex determination, sex differentiation, and psychosexual development, new surgical techniques and availability of longer-term outcome data were addressed with careful attention to ethical concerns and patient advocacy.

A new term, "disorders of sex development (DSD)," was proposed for the complex group of congenital disorders that often result in the phenotypic appearance of atypical genitalia. Formerly referred to as hermaphroditism, pseudohermaphroditism, intersex and sex reversal, DSD confers an unbiased, inclusive description, demonstrating that atypical sex differentiation can occur anywhere along the developmental pathway, including chromosomal, gonadal or anatomic sex. Previous terms were imprecise, often used incorrectly, with associated pejorative subtexts that often implied incorrectly that such individuals cannot lead normal, healthy, and satisfying lives. The incidence of DSD is 1 in 2000–3000 live births but there are some disorders, such as complete androgen insensitivity syndrome, that may be diagnosed later in life. This chapter will focus on the diagnosis and management of DSD with atypical-appearing genitalia presenting in the newborn period. We propose a new term, "atypical-appearing genitalia" to replace "ambiguous genitalia" as a more appropriate and possibly more comprehensive term.

With the easy availability of modern prenatal sonographic and genetic technology, many parents and their families opt for prenatal notification of gender. The distress associated with a baby born with genitalia that are unexpected and discrepant from the prenatally assigned gender is amplified by the parental concern regarding notification of family and friends, circumstances regarding religious rituals and other social issues. Furthermore, with delivery rooms permitting the presence of multiple family members with their readily available photographic equipment, information regarding initial sex assignment that is communicated with joyous alacrity may prove imprecise.

Pediatric, Adolescent, & Young Adult Gynecology. Edited by
A. Altchek and L. Deligdisch. © 2009 Blackwell Publishing,
ISBN: 978-1-4051-5347-8.

Box 3.1 Physical findings that could suggest DSD in the newborn period

- Overt atypical appearance of the genitalia in an apparently phenotypic male:
  - Bilaterally undescended testes in full-term male
  - Micropenis
  - Hypospadias
    - (Severe) perineal hypospadias
    - Hypospadias with undescended testis

- In an apparently phenotypic female:
  - Clitoromegaly
  - Posterior labial fusion
  - Rugated labia
  - Inguinal/labial mass

- Abnormal number or position of perineal openings
- Abnormal position or fusion of labioscrotal folds
- Hyperpigmentation of genital area
- Discrepancy with prenatally assigned sex
- Family history of DSD (common is androgen insensitivity syndrome)

Approach to the patient and family

The obstetrician or midwife is usually the first individual to observe the external genitalia and announce the sex of the newborn. As first impressions are carried with families indelibly, it cannot be overemphasized that the situation with the birth of a baby with atypical genitalia be handled cautiously. If a physical finding such as those noted in Box 3.1 casts any doubt on the sex of the baby, assignment should be deferred, with careful explanation and demonstration on the baby as to where the atypical finding is located. In cases in which early pediatric consultation is requested in the delivery room prior to sex assignment, any doubt should result in deferral of assignment. If the pediatrician's examination yields doubt subsequent to gender having already been assigned, it is important to not rescind the assignment but to explain why questions have arisen and counsel the family regarding the temporary suspension of further notification to friends and relatives. Confidence should be instilled at the outset that either a male or female sex assignment will be made and that a baby with DSD can grow up to be a fully functional member of society.

Although many questions exist in the immediate postnatal period, the specialist team will work closely with the family to aid in all decision-making processes as information becomes available. The infant whose sex is not yet assigned should be referred to as "your baby" as opposed to "he," "she" or "it." If appropriate, the family should be reassured that the baby is otherwise healthy with an otherwise apparently normal physical exam. Every attempt should be made to allow for normal bonding to occur between the parents and baby.

Early development

The notion that discordance between genetic sex and phenotypic sex occurs and is compatible with a healthy, normal lifestyle is often difficult to fully comprehend. To explain to a family that DSD can occur secondary to incomplete development at any stage requires an understanding of the nomenclature and integration of genetic and hormonal aspects of normal sexual development. Table 3.1 lists relevant terminology; many influences and interactions are still unknown. Genes and transcription factors, many of which have been identified, are expressed at variable times along the pathway.

The union of gametes determines gonadal differentiation which, in turn, determines the development of internal and external genitalia. It should be emphasized that male and female embryos contain primordial bipotential structures that could produce either male or female genitalia and that, under the influence of genetic and hormonal factors, will undergo differentiation. At about four weeks postconception, primordial germ cells migrate from the yolk sac to the urogenital ridge, which also contains undifferentiated cells that will become follicular or Sertoli cells and theca or Leydig cells. The adrenal glands and gonads develop simultaneously, with the steroidogenic cells for both originating from identical embryologic tissue. The expression of genes and transcription factors common to the adrenal gland and gonad explains how mutations can affect their development. There are genes common to the gonad and kidney that are implicated in the development of certain syndromes affecting the two. Figure 3.1 illustrates the pathway of sexual differentiation from chromosomal sex to phenotypic sex, including some genes whose roles are well described.

Alterations in chromosomes, genes, transcription factors, hormones, and receptors can all be implicated in DSD. Some of the factors that play a role in psychosexual

Table 3.1 Nomenclature in sexual development

Anatomic development	Influenced by genes, hormones, and transcription factors
Chromosomal sex	Determined at the time of conception and governs gonadal differentiation
Gonadal sex	Presence of an ovary or testis from the undifferentiated gonad
Phenotypic sex	The appearance of the internal and external genitalia, having been determined by the differentiated gonad
Psychosexual development	**Influenced by androgen exposure, sex chromosome genes, brain structure, societal and family dynamics**
Gender identity	A person's self-representation as either male or female*
Gender role	Psychologic characteristics and behaviors that are generally classified as either male or female*
Sexual orientation	Direction(s) of erotic interest
Gender dissatisfaction	Displeasure with assigned sex or sex of rearing

*With the caveat that some do not identify with one or other.

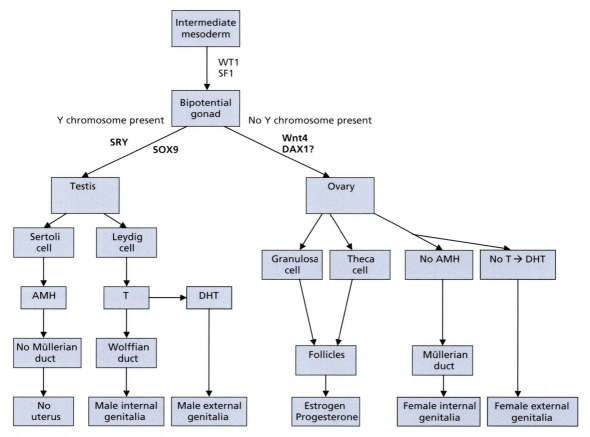

Figure 3.1 Outline of sexual differentiation. SRY, sex-determining region on Y chromosome; AMH, anti-Müllerian hormone; T, testosterone; DHT, dihydrotestosterone; WT1, Wilms' tumor suppressor gene; SF1, steroidogenic factor 1; SOX9, SRY-like HMG-box; Wnt4, Wnt = a group of secreted signaling molecules that regulate cell-to-cell interactions during embryogenesis; DAX1, DSS-AHC critical region on the X chromosome. Adapted from Ogilvy-Stuart AL, Brain CE. *Arch Dis Child* 2004;**89**(5):401–407.

Box 3.2 Members of the team responsible for caring for newborn with DSD

- Pediatric endocrinologist
- Pediatrician/neonatologist
- Geneticist
- Pediatric radiologist
- Pediatric urologist and/or surgeon
- Psychologist/psychiatrist
- Social worker
- Nurses
- Medical ethicists
- Gynecologist

development are indicated in Table 3.1. Information regarding the relative contributions of these factors is based on studies of childhood play, limited availability of longer-term follow-up of children born with DSD, and animal studies. Fetal androgen exposure may affect psychosexual development but this is modified by degree, timing, and type of exposure, as well as social and family environment. Genes specific to sex chromosomes may directly influence brain structure and psychosexual development independent of hormonal influence. Imaging studies do reveal differences in certain brain structures between the sexes; however, it remains unknown how genes, hormones, and even experiences mold these structures. At this time brain structure imaging is not used to help assign sex.

Evaluation, investigation, diagnosis, and management

The care of the newborn with atypical genitalia is best undertaken at a tertiary institution with multiple pediatric subspecialists (Box 3.2) who are experienced in the diagnosis, treatment, and ongoing management of disorders of sex development. A team approach is crucial, as the parents and family should be given current and correct information that is consistent among the consultants. Parents should be given a broad, comprehensive, and understandable summary of the biology of sexual development and how DSD could occur. They should be informed regarding the tests that will be performed on the baby and the meaning of the results as they are available.

Finally, they should be notified regarding what treatments will be required, the time frame for helping them decide on sex of rearing as soon as possible, how best to communicate information to family members and the availability, timing, and advisability of surgical procedures. These points must be delivered with honesty, sensitivity, and ongoing psychosocial support. Team members should make it a priority to designate as much time with the family as needed. The parents' thoughts, cultural and religious beliefs, background, understanding of the situation, anxieties, and decisions must be entertained, respected in strict confidence, and sought repeatedly.

The team, often led by a pediatric endocrinologist, should include a geneticist, pediatric radiologist, pediatric urologist, neonatologist, pediatrician, psychologist/psychiatrist, gynecologist, and social worker (see Box 3.2). Although the family should meet with all team members as much as desired, one team member should be assigned to conduct the majority of communication with the family. It is important for the team to educate and advise other healthcare workers directly involved in the newborn's care regarding initial management so that their approach can be equally sensitive and consistent with the overall plans for the baby and family. Routine nursing and clerical practices in the nursery, such as utilization of pink or blue bassinet identification and immunization cards, assignment of "baby boy or baby girl" as the child's first name for hospital records, and the completion of state forms (e.g. birth certificate, newborn screen), should be handled sensitively and consistently to avoid confusion and distress for the family.

Evaluation

Due to the complexities involved in the pathogenesis of the multiple possible diagnoses, it is best to refrain from speculating to the family at the outset, although a brief and simplistic differential diagnosis may help to reinforce to parents the biologic plausibility of the occurrence. Although much progress has been made in understanding the genetics of sexual development, with over 30 genes identified that are involved in DSD, molecular diagnosis remains unknown in the majority of babies. It is often challenging to explain to the family that sex of rearing can be decided upon even in the absence of a definitive molecular diagnosis.

Multiple algorithms exist to aid in formulating a diagnosis. In practice, however, diversity in presentation,

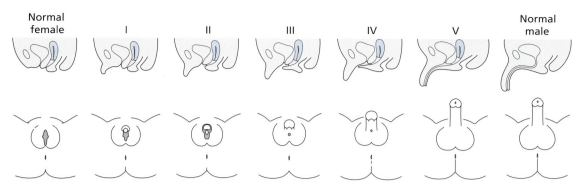

Figure 3.2 Differential virilization of the external genitalia using the staging system of Prader, from normal female (left) to normal male (right). Sagittal (upper panel) and perineal (lower panel) views shown.

findings, and turn-around time for diagnostic results render it difficult to use any one strategy. For instance, initial unconfirmed chromosomal analysis may be available from prenatal chorionic villus sampling (CVS) or amniocentesis or from postnatal X- and Y-specific probe testing prior to the 17-hydroxyprogesterone (17-OHP) result; sometimes the abdominal/pelvic ultrasound is the first to be reported, even prior to consultation.

The first step is always to obtain a careful history and perform a complete physical examination. The history should include thoughtful questions regarding maternal use of exogenous hormones or maternal virilization (both of which could virilize an XX baby), consanguinity (which increases the likelihood of an autosomal recessive condition), family history of genital atypia and early neonatal deaths (which could represent the unrecognized salt-wasting crisis of congenital adrenal hyperplasia (CAH), especially in male infants). The physical examination should be thorough, with observation of associated dysmorphic features and examination of all body systems, as some babies with DSD may, as part of a recognized syndrome, have observable facies, orthopedic abnormalities or cardiac defects. Midline defects associated with pituitary abnormalities can confer a small penis due to hypogonadal hypogonadism, and should serve as an alert to coincidental pituitary deficiencies such as cortisol and thyroid deficiencies. Examination of the genitals for features outlined in Box 3.1 should be done with careful measurements of the anatomy based on normal values. The degree of masculinization of the external genitalia has been described by Prader (Fig. 3.2).

A detailed description of the anatomy should include presence of gonads, degree of hyperpigmentation, degree of rugosity of labioscrotal folds, length, width and symmetry of erectile tissue, presence of chordee (would imply length is actually greater than measurable), presence and degree of hypospadias, degree of labioscrotal fusion and rotation. A well-developed phallus with extensive labioscrotal rugosity indicates that significant testosterone (and dihydrotestosterone (DHT)) were present *in utero*. Asymmetry of the virilization implies that the testosterone is being preferentially secreted from a gonad on the more virilized side, with the contralateral side either containing a malformed testis or, in the case of true ovotesticular DSD, an ovary. Examination for gonads should be done carefully with the fingertips of one hand milking downward from the inguinal area toward the fingertips at the other hand at the labioscrotal fold. This maneuver can often be facilitated by the use of a water-soluble lubricant to eliminate friction. Hyperpigmentation occurs due to excess adrenocorticotropic hormone (ACTH) in CAH and can best be visualized in the region of the genitals, areolae and, in some cases, the earlobes. Documentation of the position of the urethral meatus is aided by observation of urinary stream if possible. Routine catheterization is not recommended, especially if a genitogram will be performed.

Investigations

Results of the history and physical examination offer clues to guide laboratory and imaging studies. Box 3.3 outlines the tests to be done first, results of which should be available within 48 hours, allowing enough information for a

---

Box 3.3 Initial diagnostic studies in the assessment of DSD

- Karyotype
  - X- and Y-specific probes
  - Confirmatory classic karyotype
- 17-hydroxyprogesterone (17-OHP)
- Abdominal/pelvic ultrasound
- Testosterone
- Gonadotropins
- Anti-Müllerian hormone
- Serum electrolytes
- Urinalysis

Box 3.4 Secondary diagnostic studies in the assessment of DSD

- Genitogram
- Genetic testing for mutation analysis
- hCG test
- ACTH test with measurement of steroid intermediates
- Magnetic resonance imaging (MRI)
- Abdominal/pelvic laparoscopy
- Gonadal/skin biopsy

---

working diagnosis and to allow a decision regarding sex of rearing to be made in many cases.

Genetic analysis should include both X- and Y-specific probe testing as well as a confirmatory classic karyotype even in cases where prenatal karyotype results are available. Probe testing results are available within 48 hours; however, probe testing is not definitive and since it only comments on the presence of X and Y material, it cannot rule out mosaicism. The karyotype should examine a larger than usual number of cells to exclude mosaicism, a process which may take up to a week. Mosaicism not apparent in blood cells may, on occasion, be identified in subsequent skin or gonadal biopsies. Hormone studies should be performed in a laboratory with validated assays and with gestational/chronologic age normal values. Some tests need to be repeated and assessed serially.

The quality of the ultrasound of the abdomen and pelvis is technician dependent. An experienced pediatric radiologist may be able to clearly delineate the presence of a uterus, vagina, rectum, urethra, urogenital sinus, and gonads if present in the inguinal canal or labioscrotal structure. Gonadal structures on ultrasound can have sonographic appearances that are more consistent with testes or ovaries, although definitive determination and/or the presence of an ovotestis is not straightforward. Intraabdominal gonads are often not visualized in the neonate and their absence does not mean that they do not exist. Magnetic resonance imaging (MRI), laparoscopy or hormonal stimulation evaluation (such as hCG testing) may be required. Baseline assessment of the kidneys should be done by ultrasound and urinalysis since DSD due to WT1 mutation results in syndromes with accompanying renal

abnormalities. Serum electrolytes are usually not helpful in the first few days since the electrolyte abnormalities seen in the salt-wasting crisis of CAH usually do not occur until later.

Other tests included in certain algorithms that are often performed secondarily are listed in Box 3.4. The genitogram is often undertaken as part of the initial evaluation as it will better delineate internal structures. The information is useful both in the immediate postnatal period, to help with assignment of sex of rearing based on anatomy, and to guide possible surgical management. While some clinical laboratories offer some of the genetic tests, many others are performed at this time only in research laboratories. The hCG test (for which various protocols exist) is performed in some cases at variable times in the diagnosis and management pathway in order to determine the presence of functional Leydig cells capable of testosterone production; in other cases it is used to diagnose a defect in testosterone or DHT biosynthesis. An ACTH test is performed in some cases to assess the adrenal steroid profile when the diagnosis is not obvious from baseline steroid hormone levels, especially if a milder defect in steroidogenesis exists.

Diagnosis

The integration of the results of the initial physical examination, hormone levels, and genetic and radiologic testing is often sufficient to determine sex of rearing within several days (in most cases) to a week of birth. A true molecular diagnosis is not made in a large proportion of patients who present with atypical genitalia and DSD despite improved current genetic understanding of these disorders. Gonadal inspection and biopsy may be required later on for more definitive diagnosis. As DSD is a relatively new

Table 3.2 Proposed revised nomenclature

Previous	Proposed
Intersex	DSD
Male pseudohermaphrodite, undervirilization of an XY male, and undermasculinization of an XY male	46,XY DSD
Female pseudohermaphrodite, overvirilization of an XX female, and masculinization of an XX female	46,XX DSD
True hermaphrodite	Ovotesticular DSD
XX male or XX sex reversal	46,XX testicular DSD
XY sex reversal	46,XY complete gonadal dysgenesis

Reproduced with permission from Lee et al. *Pediatrics* 2006;**118**(2).

term for the group of disorders, the manner in which its associated nomenclature may be used to classify both general and specific disorders is illustrated in Tables 3.2 and 3.3 which were taken from the consensus statement. Still, many practitioners find it helpful to consider the diagnosis in terms of the presumed "appearance" (histology)

of the baby's gonads based upon available information. The gonadal type and function is one factor which contributes to determination of sex of rearing with regard to fertility and development. A simplified differential based on gonadal "appearance" is shown in Table 3.4.

Management

Determination of sex of rearing

Multiple factors contribute to the team's recommendation regarding sex of rearing. This decision is made with the family, and it is important from the outset to explain to the family that they will be given the facts and interpretations necessary to help them arrive at the best possible decision. Most physicians and experts in the field agree that unambiguous sex assignment and resultant sex of rearing be assigned as early as possible. There is a vocal minority, however, composed of some adult patients with DSD and other advocates, who believe that sex assignment and especially nonreversible reconstructive surgery should be delayed until the patient is able to contribute to the decision. Recommendations for sex of rearing should

Table 3.3 An example of a DSD classification

Sex Chromosome DSD	46,XY DSD	46,XX DSD
45,X (Turner syndrome and variants)	Disorders of gonadal (testicular) development: (1) complete gonadal dysgenesis (Swyer syndrome); (2) partial gonadal dysgenesis; (3) gonadal regression; and (4) ovotesticular DSD	Disorders of gonadal (ovarian) development: (1) ovotesticular DSD; (2) testicular DSD (e.g., SRY+, duplicate SOX9); and (3) gonadal dysgenesis
47,XXY (Klinefelter syndrome and variants)	Disorders in androgen synthesis or action: (1) androgen biosynthesis defect (e.g., 17-hydroxysteroid dehydrogenase deficiency, 5αRD2 deficiency, StAR mutations); (2) defect in androgen action (e.g., CAIS, PAIS); (3) luteinizing hormone receptor defects (e.g., Leydig cell hypoplasia, aplasia); and (4) disorders of anti-Müllerian hormone and anti-Müllerian hormone receptor (persistent Müllerian duct syndrome)	Androgen excess: (1) fetal (e.g., 21-hydroxylase deficiency, 11-hydroxylase deficiency); (2) fetoplacental (aromatase deficiency, POR [P450 oxidoreductase]); and (3) maternal (luteoma, exogenous, etc.)
45,X/46,XY (MGD, ovotesticular DSD)		Other (e.g., cloacal exstrophy, vaginal atresia, MURCS [Müllerian, renal, cervicothoracic somite abnormalities], other syndromes)
46,XX/46,XY (chimeric, ovotesticular DSD)		

Although consideration of karyotype is useful for classfication, unnecessary reference to karyotype should be avoided; ideally, a system based on descriptive terms (e.g., androgen insensitivity syndrome) should be used wherever possible. StAR indicates steroidogenic acute regulatory protein.
Reproduced with permission from Lee et al. *Pediatrics* 2006;**118**(2).

Table 3.4 Principal causes of ambiguous genitalia according to gonadal histology

- Ovary
  - CAH
  - Placental aromatase deficiency
  - Maternal source of virilization
- Testis
  - Leydig cell hypoplasia
  - Testosterone biosynthesis defect
  - 5-α-reductase deficiency
  - Androgen insensitivity
- Ovary and testis
  - Ovotesticular DSD
- Dysgenetic gonads
  - Gonadal dysgenesis
  - Denys-Drash and Frasier syndromes
  - Smith-Lemli-Opitz syndrome
  - Camptomelic dwarfism

Adapted from American Academy of Pediatrics, Committee on Genetics. Evaluation of the newborn with developmental anomalies of the external genitalia. *Pediatrics* 2000;**106**:138–142.

be accompanied by reassurances that the patient and family will not be abandoned by the team, that the patient and family will require ongoing follow-up with the medical and mental health members of the team, and that they will be given ongoing guidance as to necessary medications, future tests and monitoring, as well as recommendations for optimal time for surgical reconstruction, if needed.

One concern for families is that sex of rearing will be assigned but that contrasexual secondary sex characteristics will develop as the child grows or enters puberty. It is helpful to reinforce that careful endocrine follow-up and adherence to hormone therapy when indicated will ensure that the chosen sex of rearing is manifested phenotypically.

Multiple factors are considered when recommending gender assignment in a baby with DSD, including diagnosis (if known), appearance of internal and external genitalia, gonadal function and requirement for lifelong replacement therapy, potential for fertility, sexual function, surgical options, malignant potential of the gonad with resultant gonadectomy requirement, family views and cultural practice, and prenatal imprinting. Advances in reproductive technology have allowed for individuals

previously regarded as infertile to reproduce, either with their own sperm/ova or with donor assistance, and potential advances in stem cell research may introduce even more alternatives in the future.

Consideration of underlying diagnosis in assigning gender takes into account many of the factors mentioned, along with available longer-term follow-up information for some patients with diagnoses who are now adults. There is variable contribution by each factor depending on the diagnosis. Although evidence-based long-term data are few, the Consensus Statement on Management of Intersex Disorders discusses general rearing guidelines for several diagnoses. Most babies with 46,XX CAH (even those who are significantly virilized) who are assigned to the female gender in infancy go on to identify as females. These patients all have the capacity for fertility as females, while many other diagnoses result in either reduced or absent fertility. Studies examining the role of intrauterine androgen exposure in girls with CAH indicate a male play pattern in some children. Thus, the potential role of androgen imprinting must be discussed with the family of a 46,XX child with CAH or other babies with intrauterine androgen exposure who may be raised as female. Patients with 46,XY complete androgen insensitivity syndrome (CAIS) assigned female also identify as females, yet since the effect of genes on behavior remains unknown, extra caution and counseling should accompany the recommendation of assignment that is different from chromosomal sex.

More than half of 5α-reductase (5αRD2)-deficient patients who are assigned female at birth but reassigned male during pubertal virilization go on to live as males. When diagnosed in infancy, families with babies with 5αRD2 and perhaps 17β-hydroxysteroid dehydrogenase deficiencies should be advised that most demonstrate male gender identity and that there is potential for fertility as a male (documented in the former condition). Evidence demonstrates gender dissatisfaction in approximately 25% of patients with partial androgen insensitivity syndrome (PAIS), androgen biosynthetic defects and incomplete gonadal dysgenesis, regardless of whether reared as male or female. Available information supports assigning babies with micropenis to male gender (despite equivalent satisfaction reported whether assigned male or female) due to the fact that surgery would not be required and there is potential for fertility. In ovotesticular DSD, in which there is ovarian and testicular tissue, the decision should be based upon fertility potential according to the histology of the gonads and anatomy, provided that there is consistency with chosen sex. In mixed gonadal dysgenesis (MGD), one must consider phallic size, gonadal location, androgen exposure and testicular function. In cloacal exstrophy, more than half of individuals assigned to female in infancy live as females.

Although it might appear straightforward that the presence of a gonad with normal function, placement, and histology should dictate gender assignment, there are illustrative cases that refute this. For example, a most rare diagnosis, aphallia (also known as penile agenesis), with 46,XY karyotype and normal scrotum and testes, poses the challenges of complex surgical reconstruction to either gender in order to allow for optimal sexual function and psychologic adaptation. Other cases that demonstrate challenges in assignment are those patients with DSD that result in dysgenetic testes, female-appearing internal genitalia including uterus and vagina, yet sufficient testosterone *in utero* for a normal phallus with hypospadias to have formed. Testosterone levels, even if significant at birth, tend to fall. In such cases, the external anatomy, relative ease of reconstruction, and androgen imprinting favor a male gender assignment, while the internal structures favor female assignment, especially if cultural

views allow for the patient to utilize an egg donor to have children in the future.

Surgical management

The pediatric surgeon or urologist is a crucial member of the team that meets with the family at the outset. Complexity of surgery is a contributing factor in determining sex of rearing. The surgeon must outline for the parents the timing, course, complexity, and sequence of procedures that may be required from infancy through adulthood. Cosmesis and optimization of function and sensation are the goals of urogenital surgical intervention. Surgical experience and expertise in the care of children with DSD are essential. Beyond issues surrounding reconstructive surgery, the surgeon is also involved in issues surrounding the possible need for explorative laparotomy, gonadal biopsy or gonadectomy in cases where there is significant malignant potential, and surgical removal of nongonadal internal structures. Table 3.5 lists DSDs with the associated risk of malignant transformation. As with all other information, full disclosure regarding the necessity and proper timing is warranted as soon as possible. In general, there is insufficient evidence-based data to resolve issues regarding optimal timing of reconstructive surgery, efficacy of techniques, and outcomes including

Table 3.5 Risk of germ cell malignancy according to diagnosis

Risk group	Disorder	Malignancy risk, %	Recommended action	Patients, *n*	Studies, *n*
High	GD[a] (+Y)[b] intraabdominal	15–35	Gonadectomy[c]	12	>350
	PAIS nonscrotal	50	Gonadectomy[c]	2	24
	Frasier	60	Gonadectomy[c]	1	15
	Denys-Drash (+Y)	40	Gonadectomy[c]	1	5
Intermediate	Turner (+Y)	12	Gonadectomy[c]	11	43
	17-β-hydroxysteroid	28	Watchful waiting	2	7
	GD (+Y)[b] scrotal	Unknown	Biopsy[d] and irradiation?	0	0
	PAIS scrotal gonad	Unknown	Biopsy[d] and irradiation?	0	0
Low	CAIS	2	Biopsy[d] and ???	2	55
	Ovotesticular DSD	3	Testicular tissue removal?	3	426
	Turner (−Y)	1	None	11	557
No (?)	5αRD2	0	Unresolved	1	3
	Leydig cell hypoplasia	0	Unresolved	1	2

[a]Gonadal dysgenesis (including not further specified, 46,XY, 46,X/46,XY, mixed, partial, and complete).
[b]GBY region positive, including the TSPY (testis-specific protein Y encoded) gene.
[c]At time of diagnosis.
[d]At puberty, allowing investigation of at least 30 seminiferous tubules, preferentially diagnosis on the basis of OCT3/4 immunohistochemistry.
Reproduced with permission from Lee et al. *Pediatrics* 2006;**118**(2).

sexual function and quality of life. Some studies suggest benefit of early surgery. Outcome data are blurred by inconsistencies in diagnosis and the evaluation of multiple surgical techniques together. Advances in surgical techniques will further change management and treatment choices in the future.

Medical management and hormone replacement

Babies with CAH require special consideration, with medical treatment focusing on prevention of the salt-wasting crisis that accompanies the classic form of 21-hydroxylase deficiency. Since the 17-OHP measurement may not be available right away, any baby with atypical-appearing genitalia in which CAH is a possible diagnosis is best managed conservatively. The salt-wasting crisis does not usually occur until 4–15 days postnatally due to the presence of maternal aldosterone (and cortisol) and fluid and sodium excess. Pre-emptive transfer to the neonatal intensive care unit should be undertaken but can usually be postponed until initial parent–infant bonding begins in the routine care nursery. The 17-OHP level is usually markedly elevated. The description of specific treatment of CAH is beyond the scope of this chapter but it includes administration of hydrocortisone, sodium chloride, and fludrocortisone. Serial measurements of electrolytes, plasma renin activity and 17-OHP levels, along with clinical evaluation and careful monitoring of growth, will help guide changes in doses. A treated baby will demonstrate a reduction in hyperpigmentation and virilization. The infant will require lifelong corticosteroid replacement, close monitoring of growth and hormone levels by a pediatric endocrinologist, and instructions regarding the need for stress dose steroids in cases of moderate to severe illness and stress.

Sex steroid replacement therapy in those patients with hypogonadism due to dysgenetic gonads, sex steroid biosynthesis defects and androgen resistance is initiated at variable times and will allow for normal progression through puberty, including development of secondary sexual characteristics, pubertal growth spurt, and accrual of bone mineral density. Testosterone can be given intramuscularly in depot form or transdermally, with doses that depend on the underlying disorder. Females will require estrogen supplementation for breast development and menses, with the later addition of a progestin if a uterus is present. Future studies will help elucidate the role of dehydroepiandrosterone (DHEA) replacement in individuals with this hormone deficiency.

Initiation of early surveillance, monitoring, and appropriate subspecialist referral for potential comorbidities and malignancies is the responsibility of the healthcare team. Certain DSDs are associated with cardiac conditions, renal abnormalities, nongonadal tumors, mental retardation, and developmental disorders. The consensus statement includes a table of genes known to be involved in DSD and associated features.

Psychosocial management

The role of the mental health specialists on the multidisciplinary team cannot be overemphasized, in both the acute period surrounding birth and diagnosis and long-term continued management with the family and patient. Professionals with experience in working with these children and families can offer their services in a manner that allows for open dialog, having the ability to ask appropriate questions if the family and patient are reticent, and offer an empathetic ear when there is much to say. At the time of diagnosis, close psychosocial support is paramount, offering coping strategies and helping the parents to bond with their baby and establish the foundation for the love and support that the infant will require as she or he grows into a confident and grounded individual. The mental health team can also help identify any unrecognized family issues or misconceptions about the diagnosis and management. Psychosocial support should be an ongoing process during the infant's lifetime.

Certain groups involved with DSD patients hold the position that patients should be given maximum autonomy with no gender assignment and especially no reconstructive surgery until an age is reached at which the patient can decide. The alternative point of view is that the psychosexual development and normal adaptation of these children will be compromised due to ambiguity in early development. While one side believes that it is unethical for parents to make such decisions, the majority are in accord with parental determination of management as is the case with most other health-related aspects of a minor. A separate issue is if, when and how to inform the patient of the condition. Consensus is that age-appropriate information be given by skilled professionals, and that the patient be given the opportunity at any time to have office visits and counseling sessions separate from the parents.

It is important to ask direct questions that will gather information about play preference, gender identity, social interactions, relationships, gender satisfaction, objects of affection, sexual attraction, sexual function, and sexual pleasure at the appropriate developmental stages. General questions about mood, coping practices, resilience, and depression that may accompany any chronic condition should also be incorporated into the health maintenance program. Often it is the child or adolescent who will guide the initiation as well as the depth of the information flow.

Conclusion

There is consistent agreement that the affected newborn with DSD and family are to be approached, counseled, treated, and supported with sensitivity, expertise and professionalism. Individualized care that addresses the medical, psychologic, and social needs, while at the same time maintains awareness of patient advocacy, is the goal of the specialized treatment team. Much has been elucidated regarding the etiology of DSD but there is still a paucity of information concerning longer-term, evidence-based patient follow-up and outcome data. Future studies and developments will help narrow the knowledge gap and will contribute to continued improvements in optimizing the care of the infant with DSD.

Further reading

American Academy of Pediatrics, Committee on Genetics. Evaluation of the newborn with developmental anomalies of the external genitalia. *Pediatrics* 2000;**106**:138–142.

Blizzard RM. Intersex issues: a series of continuing conundrums. *Pediatrics* 2002;**110**(3):616–621.

Frader J, Alderson P, Asch A et al. Health care professionals and intersex conditions. *Arch Pediatr Adolesc Med* 2004;**158**(5):426–428.

Lee PA, Houk CP, Ahmed SF, Hughes IA, International Consensus Conference on Intersex organized by the Lawson Wilkins Pediatric Endocrine Society and the European Society for Paediatric Endocrinology. Consensus statement on management of intersex disorders. *Pediatrics* 2006;**118**(2):e488–500.

Levine LS, White PC. Disorders of the adrenal gland. In: Behrman RE, Kliegman R, Jenson HB (eds) *Nelson Textbook of Pediatrics*, 17th edn. Philadelphia, PA: Saunders, 2004.

Ogilvy-Stuart AL, Brain CE. Early assessment of ambiguous genitalia. *Arch Dis Child* 2004;**89**(5):401–407.

Rapaport R. Disorders of the gonads. In: Behrman RE, Kliegman R, Jenson HB (eds) *Nelson Textbook of Pediatrics*, 18th edn. Philadelphia, PA: Saunders, 2007.

Rapaport R, Grant R, Hyman SJ, Stene M. Laboratory methods in pediatric endocrinology. In: Sperling M (ed) *Pediatric Endocrinology*, 3rd edn. Philadelphia, PA: Saunders, 2008.

Stein MT, Sandberg DE, Mazur T, Eugster E, Daaboul J. A newborn infant with a disorder of sexual differentiation. *J Dev Behav Pediatr* 2004;**25**(5 suppl):S74–78.

CHAPTER 4

Diagnosis and Management of Congenital Adrenal Hyperplasia

Karen Lin-Su, Saroj Nimkarn, & Maria I. New
Mount Sinai School of Medicine and Hospital, New York, NY, USA

Introduction

Congenital adrenal hyperplasia (CAH) is a family of inherited errors of steroidogenesis, each disorder characterized by a specific enzyme deficiency that impairs normal steroid synthesis by the adrenal cortex. The most common of these enzyme deficiencies is 21-hydroxylase, which accounts for over 90% of CAH cases. Less frequent causes of CAH include deficiencies of 11β-hydroxylase, 3β-hydroxysteroid dehydrogenase, 17α-hydroxylase/17,20-lyase, and the steroidogenic acute regulatory protein (lipoid hyperplasia). This chapter will focus on 21-hydroxylase deficiency (21-OHD).

CAH due to 21-OHD can be classified as either classic or nonclassic (NC). The classic form is characterized by more severe symptoms of hyperandrogenism, including *in utero* masculinization of the female genitalia and the potential for life-threatening adrenal crises. Classic CAH is further categorized into salt-wasting (SW) or simple-virilizing (SV) forms. The SW form is characterized by insufficient aldosterone, which places patients at risk for salt-wasting crises, whereas the SV form retains the ability to conserve salt. The milder NC-CAH causes postnatal symptoms of hyperandrogenism that are not apparent at birth [1].

Screening studies indicate that the worldwide incidence of classic 21-OHD is 1:14,000 live births [2], of which approximately 75% are salt wasters. The frequency of NC-CAH is considerably higher at 1:1000, with an even higher frequency among selected ethnic groups, most notably Ashkenazi Jews [3,4].

Diagnosis

Pathophysiology of 21-hydroxylase deficiency

The production of cortisol occurs in the zona fasciculata of the adrenal cortex through five enzymatic steps as shown in Figure 4.1. Deficiency of the 21-hydroxylase enzyme causes blockage of cortisol production in the adrenal glands. Insufficient cortisol then signals the hypothalamus and pituitary to increase respective production of corticotropin-releasing hormone and adrenocorticotropic hormone (ACTH). High ACTH levels induce the adrenal glands to become hyperplastic and to produce excess sex hormone precursors that do not require 21-hydroxylation for synthesis (such as Δ^4-androstenedione). Once secreted, these hormones are further metabolized to testosterone and dihydrotestosterone (active androgens) and, to a lesser extent, estrogens. Therefore, excessive androgens are found in varied degrees in all three forms of 21-OHD and are attributable to the severity of the enzyme defect.

Differential diagnosis

In a typical case when all the symptoms related to *in utero* androgen excess occur along with a salt-wasting crisis and there is a family history suggestive of a recessive mode of inheritance, the diagnosis can be established on clinical grounds and further confirmed by hormonal or genetic

Pediatric, Adolescent, & Young Adult Gynecology. Edited by
A. Altchek and L. Deligdisch. © 2009 Blackwell Publishing,
ISBN: 978-1-4051-5347-8.

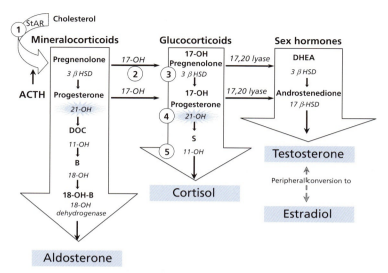

Figure 4.1 Adrenal steroidogenesis. Five enzymatic steps necessary for cortisol production are shown in numbers. 1 = 20,22 desmolase, 2 = 17-hydroxylase (17-OH), 3 = 3β-hydroxysteroid dehydrogenase (3β-HSD), 4 = 21-hydroxylase (21-OHD), 5 = 11β-hydroxylase (11-OH). In the first step of adrenal steroidogenesis, cholesterol enters mitochondria via a carrier protein called StAR. ACTH stimulates cholesterol cleavage, the rate-limiting step of adrenal steroidogenesis.

testing. However, when the full clinical presentation is not apparent, clinicians must consider other possibilities that can cause each of these manifestations. Table 4.1 shows possible etiologies of each presentation.

Hormonal diagnosis

Biochemical diagnosis of 21-OHD can be confirmed by hormonal evaluation. In a randomly timed blood sample, a very high concentration of 17-hydroxyprogesterone

Table 4.1 Differential diagnosis of each clinical presentation of 21-OHD CAH

Clinical presentation	Source of hormone excess or deficit	Possible causes
Ambiguous genitalia in 46,XX fetus	Maternal exposure to androgens during pregnancy	Medications
		Unknown sources
	Fetal adrenal enzyme defects	11β-hydroxylase deficiency CAH
		3β-hydroxysteroid dehydrogenase deficiency
		P450 oxidoreductase
Salt-wasting crisis	Aldosterone production defect	CMO type 1 and 2
		Adrenal hypoplasia congenita
		Adrenal hemorrhage
		Addison disease
	Unresponsiveness of end-organ to aldosterone	Pseudohypoaldosteronism
		Mineralocorticoid antagonist such as spironolactone
Postnatal virilization	Androgens originate from adrenal	Virilizing adrenocortical tumors
		ACTH-producing tumor; pituitary and ectopic sources
		hCG-producing tumors
	Androgens originate from gonad	Central precocious puberty
		Gonodotropin-producing tumor (choriocarcinoma, chorioepithelioma, dysgerminoma, hepatoblastoma, hepatoma and teratoma)
		Virilizing ovarian tumors (adrenal rest tumor, hilar cell tumor, Leydig cell/Sertoli cell tumor and hCG-producing germ cell tumor)
		Testicular tumor (Leydig cell tumor)
		Ovarian hyperthecosis
		Polycystic ovarian syndrome
	Androgens from other sources	Environmental
		Drug induced

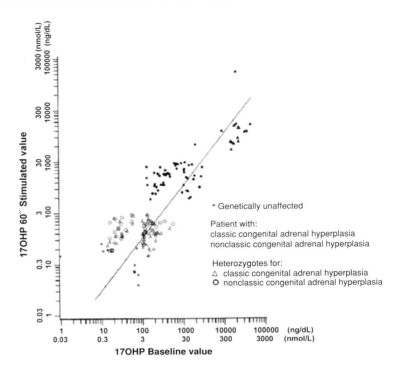

Figure 4.2 Nomogram relating baseline to ACTH-stimulated serum concentrations of 17-hydroxyprogesterone (17-OHP). The scales are logarithmic. A regression line for all data points is shown.

(17-OHP), the precursor of the defective enzyme, is diagnostic of classic 21-OHD. Such testing is the basis of the newborn screening program developed to identify classically affected patients who are at risk for life-threatening salt-wasting crises before the disease becomes clinically apparent. The concentration of 17-OHP is measured on a filter paper blood spot sample obtained by heel-stick, which is also used for newborn screening of other disorders. The universal newborn screening program for 21-OHD has been implemented in 47 out of 51 states in the US and also in many countries worldwide. The majority of screening programs use a single screening test without retesting of samples with questionable 17-OHP concentrations. To improve efficacy of screening, a small number of screening programs re-evaluate samples with borderline first-tier test results with a second-tier test. For example, because of the high false-positive rate of immunoassay methods, some programs measure the concentration of different hormones (17-OHP, Δ^4-androstenedione, and cortisol) by liquid chromatography-tandem mass spectrometry as a second-tier test of samples with positive first-tier test results [5].

False-positive results are, however, common in premature infants [6] or even in term newborns if the samples are taken in the first 24 hours [7]. Appropriate references based on weight and gestational age are therefore in place in many screening programs. False-negative results may be observed in neonates receiving dexamethasone for management of unrelated problems. The newborn screening program is not designed to detect nonclassic patients, although some may have borderline to high 17-OHP values.

The gold standard for establishing hormonal diagnosis is the corticotropin stimulation test (250 μg cosyntropin intravenously), measuring levels of 17-OHP and Δ^4 androstenedione at baseline and 60 min. These values can then be plotted in the published nomogram to ascertain disease severity (Fig. 4.2) [8]. The corticotropin stimulation test is crucial in establishing hormonal diagnosis of the nonclassic form of the disease since early-morning values of 17-OHP may not be sufficiently elevated to allow accurate diagnosis. Measurement of other adrenal steroids confirms 21-OHD and excludes other forms of CAH (Table 4.2).

Table 4.2 Adrenal enzyme deficiencies leading to congenital adrenal hyperplasia

Deficiency	Precursor(s)*	Product(s)	Androgen	Mineralocorticoid	Approximate %
STAR (steroidogenic acute regulatory) protein	Mediates cholesterol transport across mitochondrial membrane		Deficiency[1]	Deficiency[2]	Rare
3β-HSD (3β-hydroxysteroid dehydrogenase)	Δ^5Steroids (pregnenolone, 17-OH pregnenolone, DHEA)	Δ^4Steroids (progesterone, 17-OHP, Δ^4-androstenedione)	Deficiency[1]	Deficiency[2]	Rare
17α-hydroxylase	Pregnenolone Progesterone	17-OH pregnenolone 17-OH progesterone (17-OHP)	Deficiency[1]	Excess[3]	Rare
21-hydroxylase	Progesterone 17-OH progesterone	Deoxycorticosterone (DOC) 11-deoxycortisol	Excess[4]	Deficiency[2]	90–95%
11β-hydroxylase	Deoxycorticosterone	Corticosterone	Excess[4]	Excess[3]	5%
P450 oxidoreductase**	Important for electron transfer from NADPH to both 17- and 21-hydroxylase enzymes. Urinary steroid excretion indicates a combined deficiency of both		Excess in females, deficiency in males[1,4]		Rare

Notes: 1. Males are undervirilized at birth, 2. Associated with salt wasting, 3. Associated with hypertension, 4. Females are virilized at birth or later. **Phenotypes may include Antley-Bixler syndrome. *Marked elevation of the precursors leads to diagnosis of adrenal enzyme defects.

Molecular genetics

CYP21A2, the gene encoding 21-hydroxylase enzyme (MIM number 201910), is mapped to the short arm of chromosome 6 (6p21.3). The inactive pseudogene for *CYP21A2*, denoted *CYP21A1P*, is 98% homologous to the active *CYP21A2* gene. The pseudogene is located 30 kilobases (kb) away from the active gene and contains deleterious mutations that render it nonfunctional. The majority of mutations found in *CYP21A2* derive from the pseudogene during either meiotic recombination or gene conversion. *De novo* mutations in the active gene can also occur but account for a small percentage of the transmission. To date, more than 100 mutations have been described, including point mutations, small deletions, small insertions, and complex rearrangements of the gene [9]. Approximately 95–98% of the mutations causing 21-OHD have been identified through molecular genetic studies of gene rearrangement and point mutations arrays [10]. Hormonally and clinically defined forms of 21-OHD CAH are associated with distinct genotypes characterized by varying enzyme activity demonstrated through *in vitro* expression studies. The classic phenotype is predicted when a patient carries two severe mutations. The nonclassic phenotype is caused by a mild/mild or severe/mild genotype, as is expected in an autosomal recessive disorder. Table 4.3 demonstrates the common mutations in *CYP21A2* and their related phenotypes. It is not always possible, however, to accurately predict the phenotype on the basis of the genotype – such predictions have been shown to be 90–95% accurate with some nonconcordance [11].

Clinical features

Clinical presentation

In the classic forms of 21-OHD (SW and SV), virilization begins *in utero*; thus, females are born with genital ambiguity (termed 46XX, disorder of sex development) [12]. Males with classic 21-OHD do not present with sexual ambiguity, but may demonstrate hyperpigmentation of the genitalia due to ACTH excess.

Individuals with the nonclassic (NC) form of 21-OHD have only mild to moderate enzyme deficiency and present postnatally with signs of hyperandrogenism; most notably, females with NC 21-OHD do not have virilized genitalia at birth. Patients with NC 21-OHD may present as children with precocious development of axillary hair or odor, pubic hair, acne or tall stature with an advanced bone age that may eventually result in adult short stature.

Table 4.3 Common mutations in *CYP21A2* gene and their related phenotypes

Exon/intron	Mutation type	Mutation	Phenotype	Severity of enzyme defect (% enzyme activity)	References
Nonclassic mutations					
Exon 1	Missense mutation	P30L	NC	Mild (30–60%)	Tusie-Luna [31]
Exon 7	Missense mutation	V281L	NC	Mild (20–50%)	Speiser [32]
Exon 8	Missense mutation	R339H	NC	Mild (20–50%)	Helmberg [33]
Exon 10	Missense mutation	P453S	NC	Mild (20–50%)	Helmberg [33]
Classic mutations					
Deletion	30 kb deletion	–	SW	Severe (0%)	White [34]
Intron 2	Aberrant splicing of intron 2	656 A/C-G	SW, SV	Severe (ND)	Higashi [35]
Exon 3	Eight-base deletion	G110 Δ8nt	SW	Severe (0%)	White [36]
Exon 4	Missense mutation	I172N	SV	Severe (1%)	Tusie-Luna [37], Amor [38]
Exon 6	Cluster mutations	I236N, V237E, M239K	SW	Severe (0%)	Tusie-Luna [37], Amor [38]
Exon 8	Nonsense mutation	Q318X	SW	Severe (0%)	Globerman [39]
Exon 8	Missense mutation	R356W	SW, SV	Severe (0%)	Chiou [40]
Exon 10	Missense mutation	R483P*	SW	Severe (1–2%)	Wedell [41]

Women may also present with oligomenorrhea, amenorrhea, polycystic ovaries, infertility, hirsutism, or male-pattern baldness. Table 4.4 summarizes the clinical features of classic versus nonclassic forms of 21-OHD CAH.

Classic CAH

Diagnosis at birth of a female with classic CAH usually is made immediately due to the genital ambiguity arising from prenatal exposure to excess androgens. Because adrenocortical function begins around the seventh week of gestation, a female fetus with classic CAH is exposed to adrenal androgens at the critical time of sexual differentiation (approximately 9–15 weeks gestational age). This exposure to androgens causes varying degrees of genital virilization, including clitoromegaly, a urogenital sinus, a

Table 4.4 Clinical features in individuals with classic and nonclassic 21-hydroxylase deficiency CAH

	21-Hydroxylase deficiency congenital adrenal hyperplasia	
Feature	Classic	Nonclassic
Prenatal virilization	Present in females	Absent
Postnatal virilization	Males and females	Variable
Salt wasting	~75% of all individuals	Absent
Cortisol deficiency	~100%	Rare

scrotalization of the labia majora, labial fusion or, in rare cases, a penile urethra. Degrees of genital virilization are classified into five Prader stages [13] (Fig. 4.3).
- Stage I: clitoromegaly without labial fusion
- Stage II: clitoromegaly and posterior labial fusion
- Stage III: greater degree of clitoromegaly, single perineal urogenital orifice, and almost complete labial fusion
- Stage IV: increasingly phallic clitoris, urethra-like urogenital sinus at base of clitoris, and complete labial fusion
- Stage V: penile clitoris, urethral meatus at tip of phallus, and scrotum-like labia (appear like males without palpable gonads)

The female genital abnormalities are present only in the androgen-responsive external genitalia. Because females with CAH have normal ovaries and do not produce anti-Müllerian hormone (AMH), the internal genitalia (uterus and fallopian tubes) develop normally from the Müllerian ducts. Therefore, females with 21-hydroxylase deficiency have the potential for fertility.

If glucocorticoid replacement therapy does not begin postnatally, the clitoris may continue to enlarge because of excess adrenal androgens, and pseudoprecocious puberty can occur. Signs of hyperandrogenism in children affected with CAH include early onset of acne, facial, axillary hair and odor, pubic hair, and rapid linear growth. This early growth spurt is accompanied by premature epiphyseal maturation and closure, resulting in a final height that is typically below that expected from parental heights. CAH

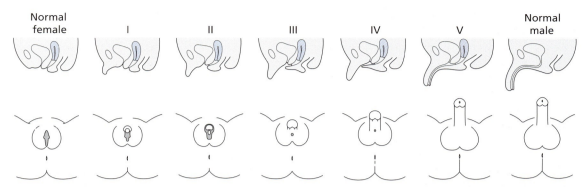

Figure 4.3 Different degrees of virilization according to the scale development by Prader. Reproduced with permission of Springer Science and Business Media.

patients are often tall as children but are short as adults. In adolescents and adults, signs of hyperandrogenism may include temporal balding, severe acne or infertility, and in women, irregular or absent menses and hirsutism. Males with classic CAH, particularly if poorly treated, have been found to have reduced sperm counts [14,15], small testes due to suppression of gonadotropins, and sometimes intratesticular adrenal rests. All of these complications may result in diminished fertility.

When classic CAH is diagnosed and adequately treated in infancy, the onset of puberty in both girls and boys usually occurs at the expected chronologic age. However, studies suggest that excess adrenal androgens (aromatized to estrogens) may inhibit the pubertal pattern of gonadotropin secretion by the hypothalamic–pituitary axis. Although the expected age of menarche may sometimes be delayed in females with classic CAH, many who are adequately treated have regular menses after menarche. Some females, especially those in poor hormonal control, may have oligomenorrhea or secondary amenorrhea with or without hirsutism. Primary amenorrhea or delayed menarche can occur if a woman with classic CAH is untreated, inadequately treated or excessively treated with glucocorticoids. Fertility problems in females with classic CAH may arise for various reasons, including anovulation, secondary polycystic ovarian syndrome, irregular menses, nonsuppressible serum progesterone levels or an inadequate introitus. Adequate glucocorticoid therapy is probably an important variable with respect to fertility outcome.

Approximately 75% of classic CAH patients are considered to have the SW form due to inadequate secretion of the mineralocorticoid aldosterone. Aldosterone secretion is insufficient for the reabsorption of sodium by the distal renal tubule and can result in a salt-wasting crisis, characterized by hyponatremia, hyperkalemia, inappropriate natriuresis, and low serum and urinary aldosterone with concomitantly high plasma renin activity (PRA). In addition, hormonal precursors of 21-hydroxylase may act as mineralocorticoid antagonists and provoke salt wasting [16]. Untreated infants with salt wasting have poor feeding, weight loss, and dehydration, which can progress to azotemia, vascular collapse, shock, and death. Salt-wasting crises in the newborn period may occur as early as 1–7 weeks of life. The other 25% of classic CAH patients, who make adequate aldosterone, are considered to have SV-CAH. It is important to recognize that the extent of virilization in an affected female may be the same in SV- and SW-CAH. Thus, even a mildly virilized newborn with 21-hydroxylase deficiency should be observed carefully for signs of a potentially life-threatening crisis within the first few weeks of life.

Nonclassic CAH

NC-CAH may present at any age after birth with a variety of hyperandrogenic symptoms, excluding ambiguous genitalia. This form of CAH results from a mild deficiency of the 21-hydroxylase enzyme and is diagnosed by serum elevations of 17-OHP that plot on the nomogram between the range for unaffected individuals and for classic patients (see Fig. 4.2). Similar to classic CAH, NC-CAH may cause premature development of pubic hair, advanced bone age, and accelerated linear growth velocity in both males and females. Severe cystic acne has also been attributed to NC-CAH.

Women may present with symptoms of androgen excess, including hirsutism, temporal baldness, and infertility. Menarche in females may be normal or delayed, and secondary amenorrhea is a frequent occurrence. Further virilization may include hirsutism, male habitus, deepening of the voice or male-pattern alopecia (temporal recession). Polycystic ovarian syndrome may also be seen as a secondary complication in these patients. It is thought to be due to excessive levels of adrenal androgens that disrupt gonadotropin release and have direct effects on the ovary, ultimately leading to the formation of androgen-producing cysts.

In males, early beard growth, acne, and growth spurt may prompt the diagnosis of NC-CAH. A clinical indication of an adrenal, as opposed to testicular, source of androgens is the small size of the testes compared to the phallus that results from suppression of the hypothalamic–pituitary–gonadal axis. In untreated males, the testes may remain small due to suppression of gonadotropins. They may also develop intratesticular adrenal rests, which can cause infertility, although some untreated men have been fertile [14]. Symptoms in adult males with NC-CAH may be limited to short stature or oligozoospermia and diminished fertility.

Management of congenital adrenal hyperplasia

Pregnancy

Prenatal diagnosis and treatment of an affected fetus

Since Jeffcoate et al. identified an affected fetus by elevated concentrations of 17-ketosteroids and pregnanetriol in amniotic fluid, prenatal diagnosis has continued to be an important endeavor that has improved in sensitivity and technique over the years [17]. Past investigators were able to conduct prenatal diagnosis by measuring hormone levels in the amniotic fluid during pregnancy, specifically elevated 17-OHP levels, though Δ^4-androstenedione could also be employed as an adjunctive diagnostic assay. Amniotic fluid testosterone levels may not necessarily be outside the normal range in affected males. Measuring hormone levels in amniotic fluid, however, only detects severe

cases, and it has essentially been replaced by molecular diagnosis.

HLA genotyping of amniotic fluid cells was also historically used as a means of diagnosis, but it has now been superseded by direct molecular analysis of the 21-hydroxylase locus, *CYP21A2*. With the advent of chorionic villus sampling (CVS), evaluation of the fetus at risk is now possible in the first trimester at 10–12 weeks gestation. Amniocentesis may also provide fetal DNA for prenatal diagnosis, but cannot be done until the fetus is 16–18 weeks gestation. Because of improved accuracy and earlier diagnosis, molecular analysis of fetal DNA is now the method of choice for prenatal diagnosis.

Treatment with dexamethasone, which crosses the placenta to the fetus, can be employed in pregnancies at risk for 21-hydroxylase deficiency. When properly administered, dexamethasone is effective in preventing ambiguous genitalia in the affected female. The current recommendation is to treat the mother with a pregnancy at risk for 21-hydroxylase deficiency with dexamethasone in a dose of 20 μg/kg (maximum daily dose of 1.5 mg) divided into two or three doses daily. Since differentiation of the external genitalia and urogenital sinus begins around the gestational age of 9 weeks, institution of dexamethasone therapy is recommended as soon as pregnancy is confirmed and no later than 9 weeks after the last menstrual period in order to effectively suppress adrenal androgen production and allow normal separation of the vaginal and urethral orifices, in addition to preventing clitoromegaly. The need to initiate at such an early date means that treatment is blind to the status of the fetus. If the fetus is determined to be male by karyotype or FISH or an unaffected female upon DNA analysis, treatment is discontinued. Otherwise, treatment is continued to term.

Between 1978 and 2002, our group conducted prenatal diagnosis and treatment in 595 pregnancies at risk for 21-OHD, of which 108 babies were affected with classic 21-OHD. Of these, there were 51 females treated prenatally with dexamethasone. Dexamethasone treatment initiated at or before 9 weeks of gestation was shown to be effective in reducing virilization, thus avoiding postnatal genitoplasty [18]. No significant or enduring side effects were noted in either the mothers (other than greater weight gain and a higher incidence of striae and edema than untreated mothers) or the fetuses. Another report, in contrast, noted some significant maternal side effects, including excessive weight gain, cushingoid facial features,

Medication	Glucocorticoid	Mineralocorticoid	Growth-suppressing
Cortisone acetate	0.8	0.8	0.8
Hydrocortisone	1	1	1
Prednisone	4	0.8	5
Prednisolone	4	0.8	16
Methylprednisolone	5	none	8
9-α-Fludrocortisone	16	160	unknown
Dexamethasone	40	none	80

Table 4.5 Relative potencies of glucocorticoid preparations

severe striae resulting in permanent scarring, and hyperglycemic response to oral glucose administration [19]. All the mothers in our report who took prenatal dexametasone stated they would take it again in the event of a future pregnancy. In our study and in others, no cases have been reported of cleft palate, placental degeneration or fetal death, though these complications have been observed in a rodent model [20].

A long-term follow-up study of 44 children treated prenatally in Scandinavia demonstrated normal *in utero* and postnatal growth compared to matched controls [21]. In our study, prenatally treated newborns did not differ in weight, length or head circumference from untreated, unaffected newborns [18,22]. A survey of 174 children prenatally exposed to dexamethasone (ages one month to 12 years) compared to 313 unexposed children found no differences in cognitive or motor development between the two groups [23]. Therefore, we believe that proper prenatal treatment of fetuses at risk for CAH can be considered effective and safe. Long-term studies on the psychologic development of patients treated prenatally are currently under way.

Management of CAH during pregnancy

As described above, females with 21-OHD have normal internal female structures and reproductive capability. Despite genital reconstruction of the external genitalia, many females with classic CAH may have difficulty with a vaginal delivery and will require cesarean section. Due to the physical stress of labor and delivery, particularly if anesthesia is administered, all females with known 21-OHD should receive stress-dose hydrocortisone during labor and delivery.

Preferably, the carrier status of the partner should be ascertained prior to pregnancy. If the patient's partner is a carrier of a severe mutation, placing the fetus at risk

for classic 21-OHD, the patient should receive prenatal dexametasone as described above until CVS or amniocentesis is performed. If the partner is found to be genetically unaffected, then the glucocorticoid of choice is hydrocortisone, which does not cross the placenta. Inactivation of prednisone by the placenta is unpredictable. Thus, prednisone is not an optimal glucocorticoid for use during pregnancy. Our group monitors adrenal hormones, including 17-OHP and androgens, throughout the pregnancy. However, 17-OHP is a necessary hormone for the maintenance of pregnancy, and the target levels to maintain during pregnancy should not be as rigid as in the nonpregnant state. For the most part, the pre-pregnancy dose of hydrocortisone (or the equivalent dose) is adequate to continue throughout pregnancy.

Hormone replacement

The goal of therapy in CAH is to replace the deficient hormones. In 21-OHD, replacing cortisol both corrects the deficiency in cortisol secretion and suppresses ACTH overproduction. Proper treatment with glucocorticoid reduces stimulation of the androgen pathway, thus preventing further virilization and allowing normal growth and development. Some synthetic steroids, such as dexametasone and prednisolone, are substantially more growth suppressing even at the same glucocorticoid equivalency and if possible should be avoided in growing children. Available pharmacologic forms of glucocorticoids and their relative potencies are shown in Table 4.5. Because hydrocortisone does not suspend evenly, liquid preparations of hydrocortisone are not reliable and should not be used. The usual requirement of hydrocortisone (or its equivalent) for the treatment of classic CAH is about 10–15 mg/m^2/day divided into two or three doses per day. Dosage requirements for patients with NC-CAH may be less. Titration of the dose should be aimed at maintaining androgen levels at age- and sex-appropriate levels and 17-OHP levels of <1000 ng/dL. Concurrently, overtreatment should be avoided because it can lead to growth suppression and iatrogenic Cushing syndrome. Depending on the degree of stress, stress-dose coverage may require doses of up to 50–100 mg/m²/day.

Patients with salt-wasting 21-OHD have elevated PRA in response to the sodium-deficient state, and they require treatment with the salt-retaining steroid 9α-fludrocortisone acetate. In addition to 9α-fludrocortisone acetate, infants with salt-wasting CAH require supplemental sodium of about 8–10 meq/kg/day because the sodium content in formula and breast milk is extremely low. The total daily dose of sodium chloride can be dissolved in water, then divided into four doses and added to small amounts of formula or breast milk for administration. Thereafter, dietary salt is usually sufficient for the 9α-fludrocortisone acetate to be effective.

Although aldosterone levels are not deficient in patients with the SV and NC forms of 21-OHD, the aldosterone to renin ratio (ARR) has been found to be lower than normal, though not to the degree seen in the salt-wasting form [24]. It has not been customary to supplement conventional glucocorticoid replacement therapy with the administration of salt-retaining steroids in the SV and NC forms of 21-OHD, though there has been some suggestion that adding fludrocortisone to patients with elevated PRA may improve hormonal control of the disease [25]. Oversuppression of the PRA should be avoided, however, to prevent complications from hypertension and excessive mineralocorticoid activity.

New treatment strategies

Glucocorticoid replacement has been an effective treatment for CAH for the past 50 years and remains its primary therapy; however, the management of these patients presents a challenge because inadequate treatment as well as oversuppression can both cause complications.

Adult short stature is frequently encountered in patients with CAH despite adequate glucocorticoid treatment. Data from our group and others have shown that patients with CAH are about 10 cm shorter than their parentally based target height [26,27]. Our group was recently able to demonstrate that the combination of growth hormone and luteinizing hormone-releasing hormone (LHRH) analog improved final adult height by

8 cm when compared to CAH subjects treated only with glucocorticoid and mineralocorticoid therapy [28].

Some data show that children may be treated with lower doses of hydrocortisone if an androgen receptor antagonist (flutamide) and an aromatase inhibitor (testolactone) are utilized [29]; however, the safety profile of the use of these medications in children has not been well studied. Antiandrogen treatment may also be useful as adjunctive therapy in adult women who continue to have hyperandrogenic signs despite good adrenal suppression.

Bilateral adrenalectomy is a radical but effective measure in some cases. A few patients who were extremely difficult to control with medical therapy alone showed improvement in their symptoms after bilateral adrenalectomy [30]. Because this approach renders the patient completely adrenal insufficient, however, it should be reserved for extreme cases and is not a good treatment option for patients who have a history of poor compliance with medication.

Gene therapy, currently in development, is a promising future treatment strategy.

Conclusion

The pathophysiology of the various types of CAH (the most common being 21-OHD) can be traced to discrete, inherited defects in the genes encoding enzymes for adrenal steroidogenesis. Treatment of CAH is targeted to replace the insufficient adrenal hormones. With proper hormone replacement therapy, normal and healthy development may often be expected. Prenatal diagnosis of 21-OHD is now possible and highly accurate with the advent of molecular diagnosis. Prenatal treatment has been shown to be both effective and safe. Long-term follow-up of both mothers and offspring who received prenatal dexamethasone is currently under way. Glucocorticoid and, if necessary, mineralocorticoid replacement has been the mainstay of treatment for CAH, but new treatment strategies continue to be developed and studied to improve care.

References

1. New MI. Nonclassical 21-hydroxylase deficiency. *J Clin Endocrinol Metab* 2006;**91**(11):4205–4214.
2. Pang SY, Wallace MA, Hofman L et al. Worldwide experience in newborn screening for classical congenital adrenal

hyperplasia due to 21-hydroxylase deficiency. *Pediatrics* 1988;**81**(6):866–874.

3. Speiser PW, Dupont B, Rubinstein P, Piazza A, Kastelan A, New IM. High frequency of nonclassical steroid 21-hydroxylase deficiency. *Am J Hum G*enet 1985;**37**:650–667.

4. Sherman SL, Aston CE, Morton NE, Speiser P, New MI. A segregation and linkage study of classical and nonclassical 21-hydroxylase deficiency. *Am J Hum Genet* 1988;**42**:830–838.

5. Minutti CZ, Lacey JM, Magera MJ et al. Steroid profiling by tandem mass spectrometry improves the positive predictive value of newborn screening for congenital adrenal hyperplasia. *J Clin Endocrinol Metab* 2004;**89**(8):3687–3693.

6. al Saedi S, Dean H, Dent W, Stockl E, Cronin C. Screening for congenital adrenal hyperplasia: the Delfia Screening Test overestimates serum 17-hydroxyprogesterone in preterm infants. *Pediatrics* 1996;**97**(1):100–102.

7. Allen DB, Hoffman GL, Fitzpatrick P, Laessig R, Maby S, Slyper A. Improved precision of newborn screening for congenital adrenal hyperplasia using weight-adjusted criteria for 17-hydroxyprogesterone levels. *J Pediatr* 1997;**130**(1):128–133.

8. New MI, Lorenzen F, Lerner AJ et al. Genotyping steroid 21-hydroxylase deficiency: hormonal reference data. *J Clin Endocrinol Metab* 1983;**57**(2):320–326.

9. Stenson PD, Ball EV, Mort M et al. Human Gene Mutation Database (HGMD): 2003 update. *Hum Mutat* 2003;**21**(6):577–581.

10. Wilson RC, Wei JQ, Cheng KC, Mercado AB, New MI. Rapid deoxyribonucleic acid analysis by allele-specific polymerase chain reaction for detection of mutations in the steroid 21-hydroxylase gene. *J Clin Endocrinol Metab* 1995;**80**(5):1635–1640.

11. Wilson RC, Mercado AB, Cheng KC, New MI. Steroid 21-hydroxylase deficiency: genotype may not predict phenotype. *J Clin Endocrinol Metab* 1995;**80**(8):2322–2329.

12. Hughes IA, Houk C, Ahmed SF, Lee PA. Consensus statement on management of intersex disorders. *Arch Dis Child* 2006;**91**(7):554–563.

13. Prader A, Gurtner HP. [The syndrome of male pseudo-hermaphrodism in congenital adrenocortical hyperplasia without overproduction of androgens (adrenal male pseudo-hermaphrodism).]. *Helv Paediatr Acta* 1955;**10**(4):397–412.

14. Cabrera M, Vogiatzi M, New M. Long term outcome in adult males with classic congenital adrenal hyperplasia. *J Clin Endocrinol Metab* 2001;**86**(7):3070–3080.

15. Bonaccorsi A, Adler I, Figueiredo J. Male infertility due to congenital adrenal hyperplasia: testicular biopsy findings, hormonal evaluation, and therapeutic results in three patients. *Fertil Steril* 1987;**47**(4):664–670.

16. Kuhnle U, Land M, Ulick S. Evidence for the secretion of an antimineralocorticoid in congenital adrenal hyperplasia. *J Clin Endocrinol Metab* 1986;**62**(5):934–940.

17. Jeffcoate T, Fleigner J, Russell S, Davis J, Wade A. Diagnosis of the adrenogenital syndrome before birth. *Lancet* 1965;**2**:553.

18. New M, Carlson A, Obeid J et al. Update: prenatal diagnosis for congenital adrenal hyperplasia in 595 pregnancies. *Endocrinologist* 2003;**13**(3):233–239.

19. Pang S, Clark AT, Freeman LO et al. Maternal side-effects of prenatal dexamethasone therapy for fetal congenital adrenal hyperplasia. *J Clin Endocrinol Metab* 1992;**76**:249–253.

20. Goldman A, Sharpior B, Katsumata M. Human foetal palatal corticoid receptors and teratogens for cleft palate. *Nature* 1978;**272**(5652):464–466.

21. Lajic S, Wedell A, Bui T, Ritzen E, Holst M. Long-term somatic follow-up of prenatally treated children with congenital adrenal hyperplasia. *J Clin Endocrinol Metab* 1998;**83**(11):3872–3880.

22. Carlson AD, Obeid JS, Kanellopoulou N, Wilson RC, New MI. Prenatal treatment and diagnosis of congenital adrenal hyperplasia owing to steroid 21-hydroxylase deficiency. In: New MI (ed) *Diagnosis and Treatment of the Unborn Child.* Reddick, FL: Idelson-Gnocchi Ltd, 1999:75–84.

23. Meyer-Bahlburg H, Dolezal C, Baker S, Carlson A, Obeid J, New M. Cognitive and motor development of children with and without congenital adrenal hyperplasia after early-prenatal dexamethasone. *J Clin Endocrinol Metab* 2004;**89**(2):610–614.

24. Nimkarn S, Lin-Su K, Berglind N, Wilson RC, New MI. Aldosterone-to-renin ratio as a marker for disease severity in 21-hydroxylase deficiency congenital adrenal hyperplasia. *J Clin Endocrinol Metab* 2007;**92**(1):137–142.

25. Rosler A, Levine LS, Schneider B, Novogroder M, New MI. The interrelationship of sodium balance, plasma renin activity and ACTH in congenital adrenal hyperplasia. *J Clin Endocrinol Metab* 1977;**45**(3):500–512.

26. Rivkees S, Crawford J. Dexamethasone treatment of virilizing congenital adrenal hyperplasia: the ability to achieve normal growth. *Pediatrics* 2000;**106**(4):767–773.

27. Di Martino-Nardi J, Stoner E, O'Connell A, New MI. The effect of treatment on final height in classical congenital adrenal hyperplasia (CAH). *Acta Endocrinol* 1986;**279**(suppl):305–314.

28. Lin-Su K, Vogiatzi MG, Marshall I et al. Treatment with growth hormone and luteinizing hormone releasing hormone analog improves final adult height in children with congenital adrenal hyperplasia. *J Clin Endocrinol Metab* 2005;**90**(6):3318–3325.

29. Merke D, Keil M, Jones J, Fields J, Hill S, Cutler G. Flutamide, testolactone, and reduced hydrocortisone dose maintain normal growth velocity and bone maturation despite elevated

androgen levels in children with congenital adrenal hyperplasia. *J Clin Endocrinol Metab* 2000;**85**(3):1114–1120.

30. Gmyrek G, New M, Sosa R, Poppas D. Bilateral laparoscopic adrenalectomy as a treatment for classic congenital adrenal hyperplasia attributable to 21-hydroxylase deficiency. *Pediatrics* 2002;**109**(2):E28.

31. Tusie-Luna MT, Speiser PW, Dumic M, New MI, White PC. A mutation (Pro-30 to Leu) in CYP21 represents a potential nonclassic steroid 21-hydroxylase deficiency allele. *Mol Endocrinol* 1991;**5**(5):685–692.

32. Speiser PW, New MI, White PC. Molecular genetic analysis of nonclassic steroid 21-hydroxylase deficiency associated with HLA-B14,DR1. *N Engl J Med* 1988;**319**(1):19–23.

33. Helmberg A, Tusie-Luna M, Tabarelli M, Kofler R, White P. R339H and P453S: CYP21 mutations associated with nonclassic steroid 21-hydroxylase deficiency that are not apparent gene conversions. *Mol Endocrinol* 1992;**6**(8):1318–1322.

34. White PC, New MI, Dupont B. HLA-linked congenital adrenal hyperplasia results from a defective gene encoding a cytochrome P-450 specific for steroid 21-hydroxylation. *Proc Natl Acad Sci (USA)* 1984;**81**(23):7505–7509.

35. Higashi Y, Tanae A, Inoue H, Hiromasa T, Fujii-Kuriyama Y. Aberrant splicing and missense mutations cause steroid 21-hydroxylase [P-450(C21)] deficiency in humans: possible gene conversion products. *Proc Natl Acad Sci (USA)* 1988;**85**(20):7486–7490.

36. White PC, Tusie-Luna MT, New MI, Speiser PW. Mutations in steroid 21-hydroxylase (CYP21). *Hum Mutat* 1994;**3**(4):373–378.

37. Tusie-Luna M, Traktman P, White PC. Determination of functional effects of mutations in the steroid 21-hydroxylase gene (CYP21) using recombinant vaccinia virus. *J Biol Chem* 1990;**265**(34):20916–20922.

38. Amor M, Parker KL, Globerman H, New MI, White PC. Mutation in the CYP21B gene (Ile-172-Asn) causes steroid 21-hydroxylase deficiency. *Proc Natl Acad Sci (USA)* 1988;**85**:1600–1607.

39. Globerman H, Amor M, Parker KL, New MI, White PC. Nonsense mutation causing steroid 21-hydroxylase deficiency. *J Clin Invest* 1988;**82**(1):139–144.

40. Chiou SH, Hu MC, Chung BC. A missense mutation at Ile172-Asn or Arg356-Trp causes steroid 21-hydroxylase deficiency. *J Biol Chem* 1990;**265**(6):3549–3552.

41. Wedell A, Luthman H. Steroid 21-hydroxylase (P450c21): a new allele and spread of mutations through the pseudogene. *Hum Genetics* 1993;**91**:236–240.

CHAPTER 5

Androgen Insensitivity and Gonadal Dysgenesis

Claude Migeon & Kara Pappas

Johns Hopkins University, Baltimore, MA, USA

Introduction

Sex determination and differentiation during fetal life is a very complex phenomenon involving the action of multiple gene products.

The first step is determination of the genetic sex. This is the result of the fertilization of a 23,X egg by either a 23,X or 23,Y sperm. The second step is the formation of organs common to both sexes: gonads, internal sex ducts both male (Wolffian) and female (Müllerian), and female-appearing external genitalia. This requires a series of transcription factors such as LIM-1, SF-1, WT-1, DAX-1, SOX-9, and many others.

The next step is gonadal differentiation. If the sex-determining region of the Y chromosome (SRY) is present, the gonads will differentiate into testes. In its absence, the gonads will differentiate into ovaries. The fourth step is hormone production by the testes. This includes biosynthesis of testosterone from cholesterol by the Leydig cells and the secretion of Müllerian inhibiting factor (MIF). The testosterone will enhance growth of the male ducts and MIF will suppress the female ducts. In the absence of testosterone and MIF, female ducts will develop and male ducts will disappear.

In the final step, testosterone reaches the target cells of the external genitalia. The 5α-reductase enzyme of these cells metabolizes testosterone into dihydrotestosterone (DHT) which will bind tightly to a specific pro-

tein, the androgen receptor (AR). The locus of the AR gene is Xq11-12. The complex DHT/AR will promote the masculinization of the external genitalia (Fig. 5.1). In its absence, the genitalia will remain feminine.

Abnormalities of sex differentiation can occur at any of the steps mentioned above. Any loss of a sex chromosome will result in Turner syndrome. Any complete abnormality in XY subjects will result in a female phenotype; a partial abnormality will usually result in ambiguous genitalia.

In this chapter, we will consider:
- loss of a sex chromosome (Turner syndrome, 45,X0)
- absence of gonad formation or abnormal SRY gene (complete gonadal dysgenesis with 46,XY or 46,XX karyotype)
- mutation of the AR gene (androgen insensitivity syndrome).

Turner syndrome: 45,X0

Turner syndrome (TS) is a disorder in which females lack all or part of one X chromosome. TS occurs in approximately 1 in 2500 female live births [1]. Turner syndrome is characterized by short stature and gonadal dysgenesis (hypergonadotropic hypogonadism), with a wide array of associated congenital anomalies occurring in varying degrees.

History

In 1938, Henry H Turner observed seven female subjects with what he called "a syndrome of infantilism, congenital webbed neck, and cubitus valgus" [2]. In 1942, Albright et al observed similar patients but added primary

Pediatric, Adolescent, & Young Adult Gynecology. Edited by A. Altchek and L. Deligdisch. © 2009 Blackwell Publishing, ISBN: 978-1-4051-5347-8.

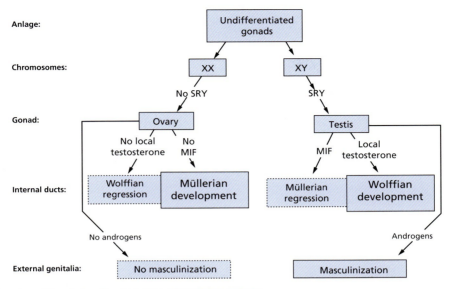

Figure 5.1 Normal sex differentiation. Flowchart of sex differentiation pathway.

ovarian insufficiency with elevated gonadotropins to the description [3]. In 1959, Ford et al reported that Turner patients were lacking one X chromosome, with a karyotype 45,X0 [4]. Then, Turner syndrome was defined as: karyotype of 45,X0, external genitalia completely female, internal ducts completely female, streak gonads with elevated gonadotropin levels, and variable somatic abnormalities, with short stature.

Since then, several variant karyotypes have been shown to result in TS, including mosaicism 45,X0 and structural abnormalities of one X chromosome [5].

Genetics

In subjects with 45,X0 TS, the single X chromosome is maternal in origin in about two-thirds to three-fourths of cases and paternal in the rest [1]. Mosaicism of 45,X0 with other cell lines is common in cases of TS, such as 45,X0/46,XX or 45,X0/46,XXX (Table 5.1). In addition, about 6–9% patients have mosaicism with a 46,XY line.

The duplication of the long arm of X along with the loss of the short arm (isochromosome Xq) will result in many Turner characteristics (Table 5.2). Ring chromosomes or partially deleted X chromosomes are also commonly found [6]. It should be noted that TS makes up to 3% of all conceptuses and 10–15% of all spontaneous abortions [1,7]. Over 90% of all TS conceptuses are spontaneously aborted, suggesting that all TS patients who survive gestation may have some degree of undetected 46,XX mosaicism.

Clinical presentation

Stature

Short stature is the most recognizable feature of TS. Almost 100% of 45,X0 subjects and those with mosaic

Table 5.1 Frequency of karyotypes in Turner syndrome and corresponding origins of the X chromosome. Also shown is the incidence per 100,000 female live births. Reproduced with permission from Reference [4]

Karyotype	Frequency in 902 cases (%)	Normal maternal X (%)	Incidence per 100 000 female live births
45,X0	50	78	11.8
46,Xi(Xq)	10	37.5	3.3
46,Xd(Xq)	9	–	0.9
46,Xd(Xp)	2	–	0.5
45,X0/46,XX	15	–	3.3
45,X0/46,Xi(Xq)	8	64	1.7
45,X0/46,Xr(X)	2	75	0.4

	46,X0	45,X0/46,XX n = 79	46,X,i(Xq) (n = 11) and 45,X0/46X,I(Xq) (n = 24)	46,X,r(X) n = 36
Short stature	98	75	100/100	100
Primary amenorrhea	93	60–75	90/75	79
Low nuchal hairline	70	49	80/40	63
Shield chest	55	63	55/–	55
Pigmented nevi	60	49	80/60	58
Cubitus valgus	60	54	80/90	64
Webbed neck	40	26	0/0	20
Short metacarpal	40	40	60/70	45
High arched palate	40	29	70/80	59
Renal abnormalities	40	16	–	30
Lymphedema	35	26	0	0
Hypertension	25	7	–	0
Cardiovascular anomalies	25	6	0	8

Table 5.2 Clinical features of Turner syndrome associated with various karyotypes. Data summarized from Summit 1979, Lippe 1990, Simpson 1992, Davidenkova *et al* 1978, Berkovitz *et al* 1983

karyotypes exhibit short stature (see Table 5.2). Untreated, TS girls will have a height averaging 144–148 cm, compared to the normal female average height of 165 cm.

TS patients are at the low end of the normal range for height at birth, but their growth velocity is fairly normal early in life. Growth deficiency is often recognized at age two or three years, but may be mild enough to go unnoticed until later, such as when the growth spurt fails to occur in puberty.

There is no evidence that a lack of growth hormone (GH) is involved but with GH treatment, TS patients may gain 6–10 cm in height [8]. Whether or not exogenous growth hormone creates a state of GH levels above normal in order to permit extra growth is unclear.

Cardiac

Cardiac abnormalities occur in almost 25% of patients, 6% in those with mosaicism and is extremely rare in cases with chromosome structural abnormalities. Anomalies include bicuspid coarctation of the aorta, aortic valve, aortic stenosis or regurgitation, and dilation of the aorta [6]. Recent studies suggest that dilation of the aorta occurs frequently in Turner patients. It is unclear whether cardiac malformations are due to haploinsufficiency of X-linked genes or are a secondary effect of disrupted embryonic development. In addition, girls with TS have a threefold higher risk of having hypertension than the regular population [1].

Skeletal

A wide range of skeletal abnormalities are found in TS, including micrognathia, short neck, high arched palate, cubitus valgus, short metacarpals, genu valgum, and Madelung deformity. Kim et al reported the prevalence of scoliosis to be 11.6% in TS subjects, compared to 2.4% in normal girls. The onset of scoliosis was 3–13 years [9].

It has been reported that TS patients also have an increased risk for both osteoporosis and fractures. However, Landin-Wilhemson et al indicated that both are uncommon before age 45 years [10]. Estrogen deficiency may play a role, as it is related to low bone mineral density. It has also been suggested that the body composition of TS girls (lower lean body mass and higher BMI) or the low physical activity of TS patients contributes to this risk.

Renal

A large study done by Lippe et al found renal malformations in 33% of TS patients. Abnormalities included horseshoe kidneys, double collecting system, missing kidney, pelvic kidney, crossed ectopia, ureteropelvic junction obstruction, and ureterovesicular junction obstruction [11]. Other reported abnormalities include kidney stones, multicystic kidneys, abnormal renal vascular supply, and malrotation of the kidneys. Vascular abnormalities may contribute to hypertension [8].

Gonadal dysgenesis

Over 90% of TS subjects have some degree of gonadal dysgenesis. In normal female development, the peak number of germ cells in the ovary is 6 million, reached at 16–20 weeks of gestation. Germ cell attrition by apoptosis is a normal phenomenon in female fetuses and later in childhood and adulthood. At birth only 2 million remain. In girls with Turner syndrome, the rate of apoptosis in the fetal ovary is much higher than normal [12]. At birth, few or no germ cells remain in TS girls.

Most TS patients present with streak gonads and a hypoplastic uterus. At puberty, they remain sexually immature until estrogen replacement is instituted. About 2–5% of patients begin puberty spontaneously but they experience only a few menstrual cycles prior to entering a very premature menopause.

There is some debate about the timing of estrogen supplementation – it is advantageous to delay the onset of puberty to possibly increase final adult height. However, it is suggested that delaying puberty may aggravate already existing social problems of some patients due to physical and psychologic differences [6]. It can also be deleterious to bone development.

There have been a few reports of spontaneous pregnancy in TS patients, although it is extremely rare. Otherwise, pregnancy is possible with oocyte donation. However, there is a high risk of miscarriage as well as chromosomal anomalies in the offspring. In addition, a high incidence of hypertensive disorders during pregnancy leads to a high rate of premature births as well as intrauterine growth restriction [13]. In most of these pregnancies, delivery is by cesarean section.

Lymphatic

Irregularities in the development of the lymphatic system cause several TS features, including neck webbing, low hairline, and congenital lymphedema of hands and feet. Congenital lymphedema manifests *in utero* but usually resolves spontaneously within a few years. Accumulation of fluid in the neck causes a noticeable increase in nuchal thickness around 10–14 weeks of development, which can be detected on fetal ultrasound [8].

Thyroid

A high prevalence of autoimmune hypothyroidism is associated with TS [14]. It has been reported that 25% of TS patients have hypothyroidism [15]. A large study done by Mederios et al found that 16% of TS girls were hypothyroid, 24% were positive for thyroid antibodies, and 34% had thyromegaly [16].

Thyroid problems present usually after 10 years of age. Elsheikh et al report that 83% of TS patients with isochromosome (Xq) have positive thyroid autoantibodies, compared to 0–35% incidence in TS patients with other karyotypes [15].

Dermatology

There is an increased incidence of benign melanocytic nevi affecting many patients. The nevi are typically found on the face, back, and extremities, and increase with age. Although increased numbers of nevi are linked to higher incidence of melanoma, TS patients seem to have a low incidence of melanoma. The origin of the large number of nevi is unknown, with no link thus far to X-linked genes, human growth hormone use or female sex hormone supplementation.

TS patients also may be at higher risk for keloid development so cosmetic surgery for webbed neck is usually discouraged [17].

Hearing loss

Frequent otitis media, conductive hearing loss, and sensorineural hearing loss are common features of TS. In a large study done by Barrenäs et al, auricular anomalies and hearing loss were more frequent and more severe in 45,X0 karyotypes; 10% of the women studied had middle ear surgery due to recurring otitis media, and 12% of the patients used hearing aids. Abnormalities of the growth of the cranial base may predispose TS patients to the chronic otitis media [18].

Neurologic

TS patients generally have normal intelligence with normal performance in school. Verbal skills are normal but visual-spatial abilities are impaired [19]. Mental retardation may occur in subjects with a marker (66%) or ring (30%) X chromosome [8]. This is observed when the abnormal X is missing its X-inactivation center, resulting in disomy of some of the X genes [20]. Other difficulties reported include gross and fine motor dysfunction and atypical handedness pattern. Estrogen deficiency may play a role in motor deficits [21]. There is a higher prevalence of attention-deficit hyperactivity disorder (ADHD) in Turner subjects, probably secondary to atypical brain development due to X chromosome deficiency [1]. Although TS girls are not at higher risk for mental health problems, social awkwardness may be increased by the attention deficits, immaturity, anxiety, and lower self-esteem [8].

Etiology of X haploinsufficiency

Turner syndrome is caused by haploinsufficiency of X-linked genes. Those genes in the pseudo-autosomal regions (PARs) of the X chromosome that have homologous counterparts on the Y chromosome, and escape inactivation in normal females, are absent. Zinn et al studied 29 patients with varying deletions of Xp. They found that deletions of Xp11.2-22.1 were linked to short stature and ovarian failure, and possibly high arched palate and autoimmune thyroid disease as well [23].

A gene located in the PAR on Xp, SHOX, is involved in short stature and other physical anomalies (Madelung deformity, short metacarpals, short neck, scoliosis, and mesomelia). During embryonic development, SHOX is expressed in the developing limbs and the first and second pharyngeal arches. The lack of two doses of SHOX in TS may also account for micrognathia, high arched palate, and recurrent otitis media in Turner patients.

Management

Patients with Turner syndrome must be monitored by cardiology, nephrology, endocrinology, and other specialties as needed. Endocrine management includes growth hormone therapy until final adult height is reached. The dose of growth hormone is usually 0.3 mg/kg/week, 1/6 of the weekly dose being given SQ, on six days of each week.

Growth hormone therapy has also the advantage of permitting earlier estrogen replacement therapy rather than waiting for possible additional height. The sex hormone supplementation at puberty is administered in a progressive fashion. We usually prescribe Premarin, 0.3 mg two days a week, then every other day, and later daily. After 1.5–2 years, consideration is given to a contraceptive pill. We prefer the PCP with the lowest amount of estrogen, on the assumption that it will decrease the risk of breast cancer or endometrial pathology [24].

45,X0/46,XY mosaicism

A Y chromosome loss through nondisjunction can account for this mosaicism. This appears to occur more frequently if the Y chromosome presents a deletion or insertion. The frequency of 45,X0/46,XY mosaicism is about 6–9% of Turner cases. About 90% of these subjects have a normal male phenotype with normal male genitalia. However, 25% of them have abnormal gonads [25].

About 10% of subjects with this mosaicism present ambiguous external genitalia and are raised in either the male or female gender, depending on the extent of the genital ambiguity.

Recently, it has been observed that a Y chromosome or a derivative Y is present in 6% of Turner patients. Another 3% have marker chromosomes that may be derived from the Y. Several recent studies have shown that the prevalence of Y material in TS patients may be higher than previously thought. Studies have found that a total of 14 out of 98 subjects (14%) had some Y material [26–28].

The risk of gonadoblastoma and malignant tumor is known to be quite high in 46,XY subjects with abdominal testes. It is also the case in 45,X0 subjects who carry a 46,XY line. Medleg et al propose that in the developing embryo, expression of Y genes initiates the development of cells in the gonad that do not undergo the usual rapid atresia of germ cells in TS. These may go on to develop and divide into a gonadal tumor [26].

These observations underline the importance of checking carefully for 45,X0/46,XY mosaicism in subjects diagnosed with TS as gonadectomy should be advised in these patients.

46,XY gonadal dysgenesis

46,XY gonadal dysgenesis is a disorder that presents as a completely normal female phenotype to an ambiguous male phenotype.

Complete gonadal dysgenesis (CGD), also known as Swyer syndrome, is characterized by the presence of streak gonads, well-developed Müllerian structures with no Wolffian structures, and a completely female phenotype. Partial gonadal dysgenesis (PGD) includes a wide range of phenotypes, characterized by dysgenetic gonads, mixed Müllerian and Wolffian derivatives, and ambiguous genitalia [29].

Clinical manifestations

The complete form includes bilateral streak gonads, normal female external genitalia, and presence of normal Müllerian structures, including a vagina, uterus, and fallopian tubes. Usually there are no somatic abnormalities. Many patients are diagnosed at puberty while being evaluated for delayed puberty and primary amenorrhea. The patients typically have no breast development and somewhat sparse pubic hair.

As amniocentesis is now frequent, a situation may arise where the karyotype is 46,XY but the fetal external genitalia remain female. The differential diagnosis will include complete gonadal dysgenesis, complete androgen insensitivity syndrome (AIS) as well as complete deficiency of testosterone secretion due to one of the steroid biosynthetic enzymes.

The streak gonads resemble ovarian stoma with no follicles. However, there is a variety of ovarian-like structures seen and in rare cases a few primordial follicles are present. This range of gonadal phenotype suggests that either the primary gonadal anlage does not develop or that ovaries had formed with premature loss of germ cells and follicles. In addition, several patients have been reported in whom seminiferous tubules were found in the gonad, suggesting some testicular development had occurred *in utero*.

Concentrations of serum LH and FSH are elevated early in life sometimes starting at 6–7 years of age. In adolescents and adults, there is no estrogen secretion.

Gonadal tumor formation

Gonadoblastoma are tumors that arise often (and almost exclusively) in dysgenetic gonads that contain a Y chromosome. The tumor is composed of germ cells and sex cord cells [30]. The frequency of gonadoblastoma is approximately 30% in XY females, and they are also found in patients with 45,X0/46,XY Turner syndrome. The tumor can develop into a malignant germ cell tumor. Page proposed that there is a gonadoblastoma locus on the Y chromosome (GBY) that has a normal function in the testis but may act as an oncogene in a dysgenetic gonad [31]. The risk of developing gonadoblastoma increases with age in patients with gonadal dysgenesis [32]. It is extremely rare before pubertal age.

Etiology of CGD

Mutations of SRY are detected in only 15–25% of CGD patients [33]. In the other subjects, mutations of genes for transcription factors involved in the formation of undifferentiated gonads and in the testis-determining pathway also result in CGD. A number of genes have been implicated, including WT1, SOX9, SF1, DAX-1, and loci on chromosomes 2q, 9p, and 10q [29]. In addition, Canto et al reported three cases of gonadal dysgenesis produced by a mutation in the desert hedgehog gene (DHH) [34].

Most cases of gonadal dysgenesis are sporadic, although there are a few familial cases. Both autosomal recessive and autosomal dominant patterns of inheritance have been observed. Le Caignec et al reported a family displaying an autosomal dominant pattern of inheritance, but displaying marked variation in phenotype, from complete to partial gonadal dysgenesis [35].

Mitchell and Harley reported that the *de novo* mutations of SRY reduce DNA-binding ability more than the familial mutations [33].They suggest that a threshold of SRY's ability to bind DNA is necessary for testis development. Familial mutations may reduce the binding activity to close to this threshold, with various other factors determining if and to what extent testes develop, explaining the variation in family phenotype.

Other families have been reported with normal fathers transmitting the mutation to offspring, resulting in some normal males and some XY females. Cases of paternal SRY mosaicism have been reported in other families [29]. An X-linked form of gonadal dysgenesis has also been reported [36].

The great variability in genetic etiology of CGD is most probably related to the fact that mutations of a series of genes can result in the same phenotype.

Other forms of 46,XY gonadal dysgenesis

Partial gonadal dysgenesis

Mutations of the same genes responsible for complete gonadal dysgenesis can result in the partial form. Partial gonadal dysgenesis results in a mixture of male and female internal ducts with ambiguous external genitalia. The degree of ambiguity varies widely, from mostly female to mostly male. Gonads are generally found in the abdomen, and sometimes a bifid scrotum is present.

Two specific gonadal patterns of PGD have been observed. Mixed gonadal dysgenesis consists of a streak gonad on one side, a dysgenetic testis on the other. The streak gonad may have some ovarian-like stroma and is usually associated with a Müllerian duct. The dysgenetic testis may contain some germ cells which disappear at puberty and is associated with Wolffian ducts. Bilateral dysgenetic testes show marked but variable disruption of testicular histology, sometimes including some ovarian stroma. Generally, there are poorly developed seminiferous tubules.

Twenty-five percent of PGD subjects show signs of TS. These patients do not have SRY gene mutations, suggesting a hidden 45,X0/46,XY mosaicism [5].

Ovotesticular disorder of sex development (true hermaphroditism)

True hermaphroditism is characterized by the presence of both well-developed testicular tissue and well-developed ovarian tissue. Approximately one-half of subjects have an ovary on one side and a testis on the other. The other half have an ovotestis on one side accompanied by an ovary, testis or ovotestis on the other side. The ovotestes may contain varying amounts of ovarian and testicular tissue. Most patients are born with ambiguous genitalia and a mixture of Müllerian and Wolffian structures.

This condition is known to occur in subjects with various karyotypes: 65% with 46,XX; 15% with 46,XY; 5% 46,XY/47,XXY; and 10% related to 46,XX/46,XY chimera.

The cause of ovotesticular disorder of sexual development may be related to partial gonadal dysgenesis.

Embryonic testicular regression syndrome

This condition is characterized by a 46,XY karyotype, normal male external genitalia, and male ducts but absence of gonads. Loss of testicular function after 20 weeks of gestation is a probable cause of this disorder. Testis loss occurs after the initiation of testis determination and male sex differentiation. The cause for the disappearance of the testis is not clear. This condition is sometimes called "vanishing testes."

Association with multiple congenital anomalies

Several syndromes have been reported in which gonadal dysgenesis is associated with multiple somatic congenital anomalies. Wilms tumor is associated with aniridia, gonadal dysgenesis, mental retardation, and a 46,XY karyotype in 2% of patients. Denys-Drash syndrome is defined by 46,XY karyotype, Wilms tumor, renal failure, and gonadal dysgenesis. Some 46,XY patients with camptomelic dwarfism also present gonadal dysgenesis, in addition to craniofacial and limb abnormalities. Deletions of 9p have resulted in gonadal dysgenesis as well as other varying anomalies. Another example is the CHARGE syndrome [5].

46,XX (ovarian) gonadal dysgenesis

These subjects present a completely female phenotype at birth and into childhood. However, at puberty, these patients are characterized by absence of secondary sexual characteristic and primary amenorrhea. Streak gonads are present, resulting in hypergonadotropic hypogonadism. This is a heterogeneous disorder that can be associated with neurosensory hearing loss (Perrault syndrome).

There are familial forms of 46,XX gonadal dysgenesis, usually inherited as an autosomal recessive trait [37,38]. In some families, brothers of affected patients show germ cell aplasia. As with 46,XY complete gonadal dysgenesis, 46,XX gonadal dysgenesis can result from an abnormality in the genesis of the undifferentiated gonads or a problem with one of the multiple factors required for the formation of the ovaries.

With hormone replacement, these women can menstruate and become pregnant with oocyte donation, as can occur in 46,XY CGD.

Androgen insensitivity

Androgen insensitivity syndrome (AIS) is a condition in which subjects with a 46,XY karyotype present a normal-appearing female phenotype and successfully adopt a female gender. The frequency of the syndrome is difficult to determine but is estimated to be between 1 in 15,000 and 1 in 60,000 live births [39]. Typically AIS subjects are considered as presenting the complete form (CAIS) but some exhibit partial masculinization (PAIS), and these two forms will be discussed separately.

History

The story of Hermaphroditus, the child of Hermes, the messenger god, and Aphrodite, the goddess of love, was told in Greco-Roman times. It is of interest that the art of the time represented Hermaphroditus with a beautiful feminine face and breasts along with normal male external genitalia. The Talmud contains reports of the Do-kayi family in which most of the women had no menstrual flow, no reproduction, and no body hair.

In the late 1940s, Wilkins coined the term "hairless woman with testes" to describe a patient who did not

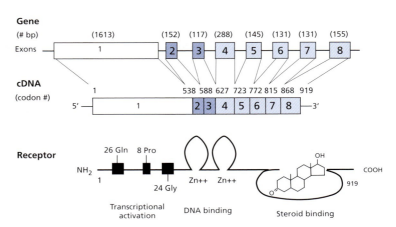

Figure 5.2 The androgen receptor gene. **Top:** the number of nucleotide base pairs in each exon. **Middle:** the AR complementary DNA, with the number of codons in the open reading frame. *Open areas* indicate cDNA coding functional domains for transcriptional activation. *Dark blue areas* indicate DNA-binding regions. *Light blue areas* indicate steroid-binding regions. **Bottom:** the AR protein, which includes 919 amino acids in total. The N-terminal contains a polymeric repeat, the center has cysteine zinc finger motifs, and the C-terminal contains the androgen-binding site. Reproduced with permission from reference [1].

masculinize upon androgen administration, recognizing her insensitivity to male hormones. Thereafter, Morris reviewed several cases of the literature and introduced the term "testicular feminization" [40]. In the mid-1970s, Money and our group proposed the term "androgen insensitivity syndrome" (AIS) as more acceptable to patients and quite specific of its etiopathology.

Jacobs et al showed that AIS subjects had a 46,XY karyotype [41] and later the trait was reported to be X-linked in rodents [42] and humans [43]. French et al reported that CAIS individuals had plasma concentrations of androgen similar to a normal adult male [44].

In 1975, Keenan et al showed the presence of androgen receptors with high binding affinity in cultured human sex skin fibroblast and reported their absence in AIS subjects [45]. In 1988, Lubahn et al and Chang et al reported the cloning and sequence of the androgen receptor gene [46,47].

Androgen secretion

In males, testosterone is primarily synthesized from cholesterol by the Leydig cells of the testes. In both sexes, the adrenal cortex produces androstenedione and about 10–15% of it is metabolized peripherally into testosterone. This is the major source of testosterone in women.

Most of the circulating testosterone is bound to the testosterone estradiol-binding globulin (TEBG). Less than 5% of the total blood testosterone is unbound and therefore available to the target cells. In the cytosol of many target cells, testosterone is metabolized to dihydrotestosterone (DHT).

Androgen receptor: its structure and role

To express their effects, androgens must bind to a specific protein, the androgen receptor (AR). The locus of the AR gene is Xq11-12 [5]. The gene is composed of eight exons and a single promoter with two initiation sites, a GC box, a purine-rich region and a 3′,5′-cyclic adenosine monophosphate response element (CRE) (Fig. 5.2). The transcribed protein contains 910–919 amino acids.

Exon 1, or the transactivation domain, is the largest and shows the most physiologic variation. It transcribes several repeats (26 glutamines, eight prolines, 24 glycines). This part of the AR protein is essential to transactivation. Deletion of amino acids 142–239 decreases its activity; deletion of amino acids 199–239 increases its activity.

Exons 2 and 3 represent the DNA-binding domain which includes two zinc fingers. These are sites of binding of the AR protein to the steroid-responsive elements (SRE) of the genes which are responsive to androgen. The distal part of exon 3 plays a role in the AR protein dimerization required for the activation of SRE.

The junction of exons 3 and 4 is called the hinge region. It is necessary for translocation of the AR/androgen complex through the pores of the nuclear membrane.

Exons 4–8 are the steroid-binding domain. In the absence of the steroid ligand, the AR protein represses gene activation but with the presence of an androgen, it induces transactivation. Dihydrotestosterone has a greater binding activity than testosterone and will therefore have priority for binding to the AR protein.

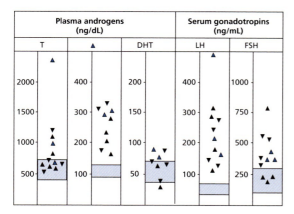

Figure 5.3 Plasma concentration of androgen and serum gonadotropin in CAIS subjects. T, testosterone; Δ, androstenedione; DHT, dihydrotestosterone. Shaded areas represent average concentration +/− one standard deviation for normal adult males. Reproduced with permission from reference [2].

Steroid-responsive elements (SRE)

These are the site of binding of the AR/androgen complex to the promoter of the androgen-responsive genes. The SRE include the consensus sequence TGTTCT. It has two half-sites for the binding of two AR/androgen complexes. In addition, there are also several coactivators and corepressors which modulate the transcription of the androgen-responsive genes.

Complete androgen insensitivity syndrome (CAIS)

Clinical appearance

CAIS subjects appear entirely female at birth. However, a number of these patients will come to medical attention because of bilateral inguinal herniae which, at surgery, are found to contain immature testes. At that point, a 46,XY karyotype will confirm the diagnosis.

In other patients, puberty results in normal breast development but absence of pubic or axillary hair and no menses. Blood study will show elevated gonadotropins, particularly LH, normal to elevated estrogen levels and at the same time testosterone levels in the adult male range (Fig. 5.3). Here again a 46,XY karyotype will make the diagnosis of CAIS.

As already noted, the patients are entirely feminine throughout childhood and adulthood (Fig. 5.4). However, as adults, they tend to be somewhat taller than normal

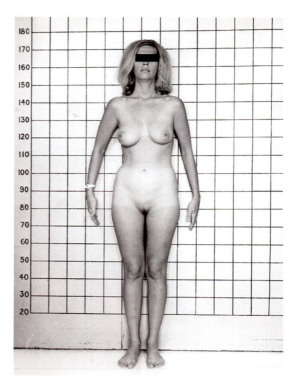

Figure 5.4 Woman with complete androgen insensitivity syndrome. Reproduced with permission from reference [3].

women (Fig. 5.5). This may be related to a somewhat slow pubertal development.

At puberty, CAIS women do not experience acne and about 50% have complete absence of sexual hair, the rest having no axillary hair but a small amount of hair limited to the labia. However, the development of breasts is quite normal.

Gonads and sex ducts

The external genitalia in CAIS is undistinguishable from a normal female at birth and during childhood. In adults, however, the labia may appear somewhat infantile. All CAIS women have a normal introitus but about 40% present a short vaginal cavity of 4–5 cm depth. In all cases the vagina ends blindly because of lack of cervix and uterus.

Before puberty, gonads are described as premature testes. In adults, the testes are small in size and histologically they show poorly developed tubules and few

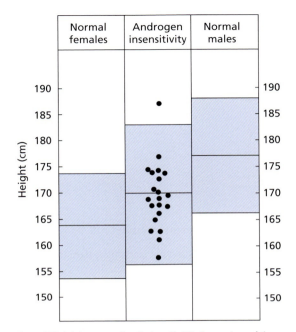

Figure 5.5 Adult stature of patients with AIS. Comparison of the adult height of patients with androgen insensitivity to normal males and females. Shaded areas indicate the average height +/− two standard deviations of each group. Reproduced with permission from reference [59].

germ cells with maturation arrest. Because of the absence of scrotum formation, the testes are intra-abdominal or tend to descend in the labial folds, appearing as inguinal herniae.

The development of the internal genital ducts is generally limited, whether Müllerian or Wolffian ducts. The Wolffian ducts are limited to epididymis and short vas deferens ending blindly. Seminal vesicles and prostate are totally absent. Close to the gonads, a cystic or spermatocele formation can be observed. As to the Müllerian ducts, they are expected to be fully suppressed by the secretion of MIF by the Sertoli cells. However, in half of the cases, there are some fallopian tube remnants located in the back of the bladder.

Hormonal secretion

Androgens

As shown in Figure 5.3, postpubertal patients have plasma testosterone and androstenedione concentrations which are equal or higher than those of normal young adult males. The ratio of testosterone to dihydrotestosterone tends to be somewhat lower than normal, suggesting a slightly decreased 5α-reductase activity.

Gonadotropins

Simultaneously, there is a significant increase of serum LH and FSH levels. LH levels in CAIS women are 4–5 times the normal male average.

Estrogens

The secretion of estradiol in CAIS is approximately twice that of normal men. It has been shown that most of the estrogens are actually secreted by the gonads rather than being derived from aromatization of testosterone peripherally; these estrogens are responsible for breast development in CAIS women.

Testosterone estradiol- and thyroxine-binding globulins (TEBG and TBG)

It is well established that increased estrogen levels result in higher levels of TEBG and TBG. This is the situation in CAIS subjects. It has been suggested that increased TEBG could be a diagnostic tool for AIS.

Müllerian inhibiting factor (MIF)

The presence of some Müllerian duct remnants in about half of CAIS subjects suggests that MIF secretion and/or action is not completely normal in fetal life. At birth and in the first year of life, MIF levels are usually at the levels of normal male infants.

Pathophysiology of AIS

In 1948, Wilkins demonstrated that a CAIS patient was insensitive to the administration of pharmacologic amounts of androgens [2].

In the early 1970s, Lyon and Hawkes recognized the X-linkage of the disorder in mice (tfm) [4] while Gehrig et al detected a mutation in the dihydrotestosterone receptor in tfm mice [48].

As discussed at the beginning of this chapter, androgen effects are expressed in a specific step-wise mechanism:

1 secretion of androgen

2 transcription of the AR gene of the X chromosome to produce the AR protein

3 binding of the AR protein and androgen

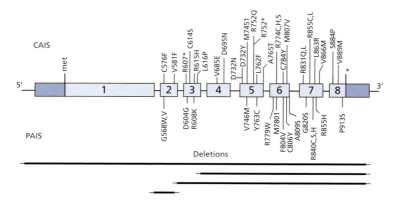

Figure 5.6 Mutations of the androgen receptor gene. Depiction of mutations found in our laboratory of the human AR gene in its eight axons. **Top**: mutations identified with CAIS. **Bottom**: mutations identified with PAIS. Location of mutations is indicated by the wild-type amino acid preceding the codon number, followed by the substituted amino acid. An asterisk indicates a stop codon. Various deletions associated with CAIS are shown at the bottom. Reproduced with permission from reference [58].

4 binding of the AR/androgen complex to the SRE of the promoter of a gene whose transcription is influenced by androgens; a large number of genes are responsive to androgens

5 these transcribed proteins represent the androgen effect.

Deficient androgen effects can be caused at any one of these steps. AIS is defined as an abnormality of the androgen receptor protein.

Multiple mutations of the AR gene have been detected in AIS patients which result in either an abnormal AR protein or complete absence of the AR protein. Examples include a mutation that affects the cysteines needed for the formation of the zinc fingers or the amino acids needed for steroid binding (Fig. 5.6).

It is also clear that the androgen receptor may be entirely normal but a mutation of the SRE of the androgen-responsive gene can result in a lack of androgen effects. A few CAIS patients have been reported to have a normal AR gene.

Genetics of CAIS

As the AR gene is located on Xq11-12, it is an X-linked trait which affects 46,XY subjects, their 46,XX mothers being hemizygotes (Fig. 5.7). In almost all cases the carriers are not affected. On occasion, such a woman reports decreased pubic hair, probably related to cloning of cells expressing the X chromosome carrying the AR mutation.

As expected, hemizygous mothers carrying a 46,XY fetus have a 50% chance of having an affected child, whereas with 46,XX fetuses there is a 50% chance of having a hemizygote daughter.

Psychosexual development in CAIS

Sex dimorphism of central nervous system (CNS)

Studies have shown sex differences in the CNS of human subjects and other mammals. Whether the differences are associated with specific behavior is still not clear in the human species.

CNS function in CAIS

Insensitivity to androgen effects is clear in AIS, as shown by the lack of masculinization of the external genitalia and absence of male secondary sex characteristics at puberty. LH levels are above normal and testosterone concentration tends to be above the adult male range. As for estrogen levels, they are higher than in normal males, resulting in breast development.

Gender identity and gender role (as defined by Money and Ehrhardt [49,50])

These are totally feminine in CAIS. The patients view themselves as entirely female and are regarded by others

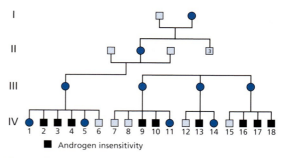

Figure 5.7 Pedigree of a family afflicted with androgen insensitivity. Reproduced with permission from reference [59].

Table 5.3 Marriage, parenthood and sex life of patients with androgen insensitivity syndrome

	CAIS	PAIS	
	Females n = 15	Females n = 10	Males n = 6
Married	53%	44%	33%
Parent by adoption	47%	10%	17%
Heterosexual	93%	70%	83%
Libido (average or strong)	73%	40%	66%
Experience orgasm	80%	80%	100%

as women. Studies have shown that these women readily accept their feminine status and have a positive attitude toward marriage and infant care (Table 5.3).

Sex life

CAIS subjects appear to experience a sex life similar to average women. We have interviewed 15 adult subjects with CAIS; eight of them were married and six had adopted 2–3 children each. Fourteen of the subjects reported being heterosexual. Only one CAIS woman who had refused surgical elongation of her short vagina decided a homosexual relationship was "sweeter" than a heterosexual one. It is of interest that 12 of the 15 women stated that they experienced orgasm. This suggests that androgen effects are not required for female orgasm (see Table 5.1).

Management of CAIS

Diagnosis

The possibility of androgen insensitivity will come to mind in a newborn who, at amniocentesis, was reported 46,XY but appeared with female genitalia at birth. Bilateral inguinal herniae in the neonatal period can also attract medical attention. Later in life, in childhood or adolescence, the presence of testicular gonads in a girl with bilateral herniae will bring up consideration of a possible diagnosis of CAIS.

Some CAIS patients are diagnosed because of an unusual puberty: breasts have developed well but there is little or no body hair and absence of menses. As the abdominal testes enlarge at puberty, they attempt to descend into the labia and might cause some inguinal pain.

The first step in diagnosis will be a karyotype. In newborns up to 3–4 months of age and at puberty,

it will be important to determine levels of androgens and their precursors (17-hydroprogesterone, androstenedione, testosterone, dihydrotestosterone), gonadotropins (LH and FSH), and MIF.

DNA sequencing is now commercially available, which permits identification of the mutation of the AR gene, with the understanding that a lack of mutation in the gene itself can occur in perhaps 10–15% of CAIS patients.

The clinical diagnosis is based on the female genitalia, a genitogram which shows a blind vagina, and an ultrasound/MRI which shows absence of Müllerian ducts (no uterus, no fallopian tubes) with presence of gonads resembling testes.

Sex assignment

The female appearance of the external genitalia at birth in CAIS results in female gender assignment and sex of rearing prior to definite diagnosis.

At this time, medical experts in the field of human sex differentiation, and patients, agree that female gender assignment is definitely appropriate in CAIS.

Counseling of patients and their parents

First, parents of a CAIS newborn must be fully informed by expert counselors and medical professionals. This includes an explanation of normal sexual differentiation and of the specific abnormality of the AR gene. The information presently available on the long-range physical and psychologic development of adult CAIS subjects must be presented. Help from a volunteer patient may be useful.

Two important questions are usually brought up: the future sex life of CAIS women and their reproductive possibility. Our present information permits total reassurance for a normal sex life. As to reproduction, we introduce the notion of "family by adoption" suggested by Money.

For CAIS patients themselves, information should be offered and adjusted to their chronologic age. The issues of "family by adoption" and "abnormal gonads" can be introduced fairly early in childhood. In the past, the nature of karyotype was brought up in adolescence. However, it has been suggested that it could be discussed at 8–12 years of age [51]. Although the patient may not completely comprehend the significance of the karyotype, it is thought that they will reflect on this information with time and be less disturbed than they would be in adolescence.

Surgical treatment

Gonadectomy is advised in CAIS because of an increase in gonadal tumors (most often gonadoblastoma, rarely malignant). The risk is extremely low before puberty and we usually recommend postponing gonadectomy until puberty. The advantage of this delay is that the gonads of CAIS permit estrogen secretion and breast development. This spontaneous breast formation is a major contribution to a positive female body image.

About one-half of CAIS women are able to participate in normal intercourse. However, the others need lengthening of their vagina. The timing for this surgery is usually when the patient shows interest in sexual intercourse.

Endocrine treatment

After gonadectomy, the patient requires estrogen replacement therapy. The choice will be either estrogenic skin patches or oral preparations, particularly contraceptive pills which have the advantage of giving the CAIS subjects a sense of normalcy.

Estrogen therapy will be continued until the expected age of menopause. Bone monitoring by DEXA checks is important. The patients must also follow the routine prevention rules for breast cancer.

Partial androgen insensitivity syndrome (PAIS)

History and clinical appearance

A series of familial cases who presented with ambiguous external genitalia including perineoscrotal hypospadias, very short phallus, testes descending in labioscrotal folds, and gynecomastia, were reported in 1947 by Reifenstein [52]. Other patients were described later by Lubs et al, Rosewater et al, and Gilbert-Dreyfus et al [53–55].

Amhein et al demonstrated in 1977 that some of the patients previously described presented mutations of their AR gene, their mutation resulting in partial masculinization both during fetal life (ambiguous genitalia) and at puberty (poor virilizing and gynecomastia) [56].

Gonads and ducts

The adult gonads appear as small testes with marked tubular sclerosis, large patches of Leydig cells but no spermatogenesis because of maturation arrest. The ducts are often mixed, with limited fallopian tubes and vas deferens.

Hormones

In PAIS, as in CAIS, the karyotype is 46,XY. Studies of the Y chromosome show a normal SRY gene – the gene needed for development of the gonads into testes.

As in the complete form, subjects with PAIS have elevated levels of plasma androgens, particularly androstenedione and testosterone. However, dihydrotestosterone values are similar to normal young adult males.

Regarding the gonadotropins, the LH levels are in most cases well above the normal range and FSH is also elevated. MIF is expected to be in the range of normal males.

Pathophysiology and genetics

Multiple mutations of the AR gene have been reported in PAIS, as for the complete form (see Fig. 5.6). The mutations are distributed throughout the gene but are particularly concentrated in the ligand-binding domain and to a lesser extent in the DNA-binding domain (see http://androgendb.mcgill.ca).

The variable clinical expressions of PAIS are related not only to the multiple AR mutations but also to a different expression of the same mutation. Hence, members of the same family can be masculinized to various degrees.

Like CAIS, PAIS is an X-linked trait, the hemizygote mother usually showing no abnormality.

Management

Diagnosis

At birth, PAIS will be considered in an infant with ambiguous genitalia and 46,XY karyotype. In this condition, the plasma androgen values will be the same as or slightly higher than those of normal adult males. In addition, MIF should also be similar to normal males. Unfortunately, it is often difficult to obtain a complete hormone panel in small infants or premature babies.

The detection of an AR gene mutation will be diagnostic. DNA studies can be obtained commercially, but they tend to be expensive.

It is of interest that the PAIS diagnosis is often made without determination of an AR mutation. In The Netherlands, Boehmer et al studied a number of cases considered as PAIS; however, molecular studies found that almost all cases had no mutation of the AR gene [57]. Instead, they were found to present a mutation of the 17β-hydroxysteroid dehydrogenase gene. Our experience with several subjects considered as PAIS showed that most of them had no mutations of either the AR gene or 17β-hydroxysteroid dehydrogenase gene and no etiologic diagnosis could be made.

Sex assignment

Whereas female sex assignment is quite obvious and generally accepted in CAIS, decisions are more controversial and difficult in PAIS. The problems are the same as for all infants born with ambiguous external genitalia and 46,XY karyotype. Several factors must be considered.

The degree of masculinization of the genitalia is related to the degree of androgen effect which occurred in the fetus. Poor masculinization indicates low androgen effect; high masculinization reflects good androgen effect. Low androgen effect is the result of either low androgen secretion with normal AR activity or normal androgen secretion with low AR activity. In the first case, androgen therapy will be effective but not in the second case.

Correction of genitalia along female lines is easier than along male lines and requires fewer surgeries (see Table 5.2).

Fertility is not a question as none of the patients will be able to reproduce. In abnormalities of 46,XY sex differentiation, only subjects with 5α-reductase deficiency can produce sperm while subjects with complete gonadal dysgenesis and the presence of a uterus can carry a pregnancy by obtaining an egg fertilized by their spouse's sperm.

Experience has shown that, at puberty, PAIS subjects develop breasts and there is little enlargement of the phallus, even though body hair may be normal and male in distribution.

Sex assignment must be made in the first few weeks of life of the infant. The parents should be fully educated about the intricacies of sex differentiation. They should be made aware of the possible life problems related to a specific diagnosis and the special circumstances of a case. We have come to the conclusion that after receiving all available information, the decision about the sex of rearing should be made by the parents. The decision process may take time, two to six weeks, as there is need of full understanding and sometime reconciliation of various opinions. Indeed, the parents must feel that their decision

is the best possible under the special set of conditions of their child. The firm conviction of the parents about the sex of rearing will play an important role in the future development of the gender identity of the patient.

Surgical treatment

For PAIS subjects reared in the female gender, gonadectomy is advised before puberty and usually before two years of age. Experience has shown that the gonads in PAIS secrete large amounts of both androgens and estrogens. Although the latter would be helpful in girls, the masculinizing effects are unpredictable and sometimes rather marked. PAIS babies assigned to the female gender will also require partial recession of their clitoris as well as appropriate revision of their vagina and correction of labial folds.

For PAIS children reared in the male gender, repair of the hypospadias with construction of a penile urethra must be carried out. These patients will also need formation of a scrotum which will permit the descent of the testes. At puberty, gynecomastia, sometimes quite extensive, appears and will require mastectomy.

Endocrine treatment

If the gonads are still in place at the time of puberty, the secretion of estradiol results in very normal breast development. However, the risk of gonadal tumor increases at puberty. Following gonadectomy, patients raised in the female gender will require estrogen replacement therapy as described for CAIS.

For subjects raised in the male gender, testes may be kept in place if they are easily palpable for careful observation to rule out tumors. Although these testes produce usually average male virilization, they also produce gynecomastia.

Psychologic treatment

Some aspects of therapy in the postnatal period have been discussed in the section on management. Later, parents and patients will need additional care, once a year or more often if necessary. Questions from parents require answers and progressive information should be imparted to the patient. Some patients will profit from support groups while others wish to maintain their privacy. Websites about sex differentiation might be helpful (www.hopkinschildrens.org/specialties/categorypages/intersex/index.html).

	Average number of surgeries	Satisfaction with sex of rearing	Satisfaction with sexual function
CAIS women $n = 14$	0 in 8 subjects 1 in 6 subject	14 (100%)	11 (78%)
Ambiguous women $n = 18$	2.1	14 (78%)	8 (44%)
Ambiguous men $n = 21$	5.8	16 (76%)	14 (66%)

Table 5.4 Average number of surgeries and satisfaction in patients with CAIS and 46,XY ambiguous genitalia

Long-range follow-up of subjects presenting with androgen insensitivity

Our clinic has followed a number of 46,XY patients who presented with abnormalities of sex differentiation at birth or in childhood and who are now adults: 16 women with CAIS [58] and 41 born with ambiguous genitalia. Among the latter group, 19 were reared as female and 22 as male. The group of 41 with ambiguous genitalia included 16 patients with AR mutations. Among the others, 11 presented partial gonadal dysgenesis while 14 had no specifically characterized etiology.

As shown in Table 5.4, all CAIS women had a gonadectomy but only one-third of them required vaginal lengthening. In the group with ambiguous genitalia, the women had an average of 2.1 surgeries compared with an average of 5.8 surgeries in men.

Table 5.4 also shows that the majority of subjects born with ambiguous genitalia (79% of women and 77% of men) were satisfied with their sex of rearing given at birth. However, one subject raised as male changed to female gender in adulthood, whereas another subject raised as female changed to male.

Most CAIS women (81%) were satisfied with their sexual function. However, the group of subjects born with ambiguous genitalia had a much lower percentage of satisfied patients: 50% of the women and 68% of the men.

Sexual preference in androgen insensitivity (see Table 5.3) was mainly heterosexual: 94% in CAIS, 70% and 83% in females and males with PAIS, respectively.

As expected, there was no reproduction in subjects reared female but this was also true in subjects reared male.

References

1. Kavoussi SK, Christman GM, Smith YR. Healthcare for adolescents with Turner syndrome. *J Pediatr Adolesc Gynecol* 2006;**19**:257–265.

2. Turner HH. A syndrome of infantilism, congenital webbed neck, and cubitus valgus. *Endocrinology* 1938;**23**:556.

3. Albright F, Smith PH, Fraser R. A syndrome characterized by primary ovarian insufficiency and decreased stature: report of 11 cases with digression on hormonal control of axillary and pubic hair. *Am J Med Sci* 1942;**204**:625–648.

4. Ford CE, Jones KW, Polani PE, De Almeida JC, Briggs JH. A sex-chromosome anomaly in a case of gonadal dysgenesis (Turner's syndrome). *Lancet* 1959;**1**(7075):711–713.

5. Migeon CJ, Berkovitz GD, Brown TR. Sexual differentiation and ambiguity. In: Blizzard R, Kappy M, Migeon C (eds) *Wilkins: The Diagnosis and Treatment of Endocrine Disorders in Childhood and Adolescence*, 4th edn. Springfield, IL: Thomas Books, 1994: 573–715.

6. Gravholt CH. Epidemiological, endocrine and metabolic features in Turner syndrome. *Euro J Endocrinol* 2004;**151**:657–687.

7. Neely EK, Rosenfeld RG. Turner syndrome. In: Lifshitz F (ed) *Pediatric Endocrinology*, 4th edn. New York: Marcel Dekker, 2003: 239–2568.

8. Doswell BJ, Visootsak J, Brady AN, Graham J Jr. Turner syndrome: an update and review for the primary pediatrician. *Clin Pediatr* 2006;**45**(4):301–313.

9. Kim JY, Rosenfeld SR, Keyak JH. Increased prevalence of scoliosis in Turner syndrome. *J Pediatr Orthopaedics* 2001;**21**:765–766.

10. Landin-Wilhelmsen K, Bryman I, Windh M, Wilhemsen L. Osteoporosis and fractures in Turner syndrome – importance of growth promoting and oestrogen therapy. *Clin Endocrinol* 1999;**51**:497–502.

11. Lippe B, Geffner ME, Dietrich RB, Boechat MI, Karngarloo H. Renal malformations in patients with Turner syndrome: imaging in 141 patients. *Pediatrics* 1988;**82**:852–856.

12. Modi D, Sane S, Bhartiya D. Accelerated germ cell apoptosis in sex chromosome aneuploid fetal human gonads. *Mol Hum Reprod* 2003;**9**(4):219–225.

13. Bodri D, Vernaeve V, Figueras F, Vidal R, Guillén JJ, Coll O. Oocyte donation in patients with Turner's syndrome: a successful technique but with accompanying high risk of hypertensive disorders during pregnancy. *Hum Reprod* 2006;**21**(3):829–832.

14. Germain EL, Plotnick LP. Age-related anti-thyroid antibodies and thyroid abnormalities in Turner syndrome. *Acta Paediatr Scand* 1986;**75**(5):750–755.

15. Elsheikh M, Wass JAH, Conoway GS. Autoimmune thyroid syndrome in women with Turner's syndrome – the association with karyotype. *Clin Endocrinol* 2001;**55**:223–226.

16. Mederios CC, Marini SH, Baptista MT, Guerra G Jr, Maciel-Guerra AT. Turner's syndrome and thyroid disease: a transverse study of pediatric patients in Brazil. *J Pediatr Endocrinol Metab* 2000;**13**(4):357–362.

17. Lowenstein EJ, Kim KH, Glick SA. Turner's syndrome in dermatology. *J Am Acad Dermatol* 2004;**50**(5):767–776.

18. Barrenäs ML, Linden-Wilhelmsen K, Hanson C. Ear and hearing in relation to genotype and growth in Turner syndrome. *Hearing Res* 2000;**144**:21–28.

19. Alexander D, Ehrhardt AA, Money J. Defective figure drawing, geometric and human, in Turner's syndrome. *J Nerv Ment Dis* 1966;**142**(2):161–167.

20. Migeon BR, Luo S, Jani M, Jeppensen P. The severe phenotype of females with tiny ring X chromosome is associated with inability of these chromosomes to undergo X inactivation. *Am J Hum Genet* 1994;**55**(3):497–504.

21. Ross J, Roeltgen D, Zinn A. Cognition and the sex chromosomes: studies in Turner syndrome. *Horm Res* 2006;**65**:47–56.

22. Russell HF, Wallis D, Mazzocco MM et al. Increased prevalence of ADHD in Turner syndrome with no evidence of imprinting effects. *J Pediatr Psychol* 2006;**31**(9):945–955.

23. Zinn AR, Ross JL. Molecular analysis of genes on Xp controlling Turner syndrome and premature ovarian failure (POF). *Semin Reprod Med* 2001;**19**:141–146.

24. Rosenwaks Z, Wentz AC, Jones GS et al. Endometrial pathology and estrogens. *J Am Coll Obstet Gynecol* 1979;**52**(4):403–410.

25. Chang HG, Clark RD, Bachman H. The phenotype of 45,X/46,XY mosaicism: an analysis of 92 prenatally diagnosed cases. *Am J Hum Genet* 1990;**46**:156–167.

26. Medleg R, Lobaccaro JM, Berta P et al. Screening for Y-derived sex determining gene SRY in 40 patients with Turner syndrome. *J Clin Endocrinol Metab* 1992;**75**(5):1289–1292.

27. Fernández-García R, García-Doval S, Costoya S, Pásaro E. Analysis of sex chromosome aneuploidy in 4 patients with Turner syndrome: a study of "hidden" mosaicism. *Clin Genet* 2000;**58**:201–208.

28. Coto E, Toral J, Menéndez MJ et al. PCR-based study of the presence of Y-chromosome sequences in patients with Ullrich–Turner syndrome. *Am J Med Genet* 1995;**57**:393–396.

29. Sarafoglou K, Ostrer H. Familial sex reversal: a review. *J Clin Endocrinol Metab* 2000;**85**(2):483–493.

30. Hoepffner W, Horn L-C, Simon E et al. Gonadoblastomas in 5 patients with 46,XY gonadal dysgenesis. *Exp Clin Endocrinol Diabetes* 2005;**113**:231–235.

31. Page DC. Hypothesis: a Y-chromosomal gene causes gonadoblastoma in dysgenetic gonads. *Development* 1987;**101**(suppl):151–155.

32. Uehara S, Hashiyada M, Sato K, Nata M, Funato T, Okamura K. Complete XY gonadal dysgenesis and aspects of the SRY genotype and gonadal tumor formation. *J Hum Genet* 2002;**47**:279–284.

33. Mitchell CL, Harley VR. Biochemical defects in eight SRY missense mutations causing XY gonadal dysgenesis. *Mol Gen Metab* 2002;**77**:217–225.

34. Canto P, Söderlund D, Reyes E, Méndez JP. Mutations in the desert hedgehog (DHH) gene in patients with 46,XY complete pure gonadal dysgenesis. *J Clin Endocrinol Metab* 2004;**89**(9):4480–4483.

35. Le Caignec C, Baron S, McElreavey K et al. 46,XY gonadal dysgenesis: evidence for autosomal dominant transmission in a large kindred. *Am J Med Genet* 2003;**116A**:37–43.

36. Fechner PY, Marcantonio SM, Ogata T et al. Report of a kindred with X-linked (or autosomal dominant sex limited) 46,XY partial gonadal dysgenesis. *J Clin Endocrinol Metab* 1993;**76**:1248–1253.

37. Meyers CM, Boughman JA, Rivas MR, Wilroy RS, Simpson JL. Gonadal (ovarian) dysgenesis in 46,XX individuals: frequency of the autosomal recessive form. *Am J Med Genet* 1996;**63**:518–524.

38. Aittomäki K. The genetics of XX gonadal dysgenesis. *Am J Hum Genet* 1994;**54**(5):844–851.

39. Conn J, Gillam L, Conway GS. Revealing the diagnosis of androgen insensitivity in adulthood. *BMJ* 2005;**331**:628–630.

40. Morris JM. The syndrome of testicular feminization in male pseudohermaphrodites. *Am J Obstet Gynecol* 1953;**65**(6):1192–1211.

41. Jacobs PA, Baikie AG, Court Brown WN, Forrest H. Chromosomal sex in the syndrome of testicular feminization. *Lancet* 1959;**2**(7103):591–592.

42. Lyon MF, Hawkes SG. X-linked gene for testicular feminization in the mouse. *Nature* 1970;**227**(5256):1217–1219.

43. Meyer WJ III, Migeon BR, Migeon CJ. Locus on human X chromosome for dihydrotestosterone receptor and androgen insensitivity. *Proc Natl Acad Sci USA* 1975;**72**(4):1469–1472.

44. French FS. Baggett B, VanWyk JJ et al. Testicular feminization: clinical, morphological, and biochemical studies. *J Clin Endocrinol Metab* 1965;**25**:661–667.

45. Keenan BS, Meyer WJ, Hadjian AJ, Migeon CJ. Androgen receptor in human skin fibroblasts. Characterization of a specific 17beta-hydroxy-5alpha-androstan-3-one-protein complex in cell sonicates and nuclei. *Steroids* 1975;**4**:535–552.

46. Lubahn DB, Joseph DR, Sar M et al. The human androgen receptor: complementary deoxyribonucleic acid cloning, sequence analysis and gene expression in prostate. *Mol Endocrinol* 1988;**2**:1265–1275.

47. Chang C, Kokontis J, Liaos S. Structural analysis of complementary DNA and amino acid cequences of human and rat androgen receptors. *Proc Natl Acad Sci USA* 1988;**85**:7211–7215.

48. Gehrig U, Tomkins GM, Ohno S. Effect of the androgen-insensitivity mutation on a cytoplasmic receptor for dihydrotestosterone. *Nature* 1971;**232**:106–107.

49. Money J, Ehrhardt AA. *Man and Woman, Boy and Girl.* Baltimore: Johns Hopkins University Press, 1972.

50. Money J, Lewis VG. Gender-identity/role: G-I/R part A: XY (androgen-insensitivity) syndrome and XX (Rokitansky) syndrome of vaginal atresia compared. In: Dennerstein L, Burrows G (eds) *Handbook of Psychosomatic Obstetrics and Gynecology.* New York: Elsevier, 1983: 51–60.

51. Warne GL, Zajac JD. Disorders of sexual differentiation. *Endocrinol Metab Clin North Am* 1998;**27**(4):945–967.

52. Reifenstein EC. Hereditary familial hypogonadism. *Proc Am Fed Clin Res* 1947;**3**:86.

53. Lubs HA Jr, Vilar O, Bergenstal DM. Familial male pseudohermaphroditism with labial testes and partial feminization: endocrine studies and genetic aspects. *J Clin Endocrinol Metab* 1959;**19**:1110–1120.

54. Rosewater S, Gwinup G, Hamwi GJ. Familial gynecomastia. *Ann Intern Med* 1965;**63**:377–385.

55. Gilbert-Dreyfus S, Sébaoun CA, Belaïsh J. Etude d'un cas familial d'androgynoïdism avec hypospadias grave, gynécomastia et hyperoestrogénie. *Ann Endocrinol* 1975;**18**: 93–101.

56. Amhein JA, Klingensmith GJ, Walsh PC, McKusick VA, Migeon CJ. Partial androgen insensitivity: the Reifenstein syndrome revisited. *N Engl J Med* 1977;**297**:350–356.

57. Boehmer AL, Brinkmann AO, Sandkuijl LA et al. 17β-Hydroxysteroid dehydrogenase-3 deficiency: diagnosis, phenotypic variability, population genetics, and worldwide distribution of ancient and de novo mutations. *J Clin Endocrinol Metab* 1999;**84**(12):4712–4713.

58. Wisniewski AB, Migeon CJ, Meyer-Bahlburgh HFL et al. Complete androgen insensitivity syndrome: long-term medical, surgical, and psychosexual outcome. *J Clin Endocrinol Metab* 2000;**85**(8):2264–2269.

59. Migeon CJ, Wisniewski AB, Brown TR. Androgen insensitivity syndrome. In: Charousos GP, Olefsky JM, Samols E (eds) *Hormone Resistance and Hypersensitivity.* Philadelphia: Lippincott Williams and Wilkins, 2002: 409–439.

60. Migeon CJ, Brown TR, Fichman KR. Androgen insensitivity syndrome. In: Josso N (ed) *The Intersex Child.* Basel: Karger, 1981: 171–202.

61. Migeon CJ, Berkovitz GD. Congenital defects of the external genitalia. In: Carpenter SEK, Rock JA (eds) *Pediatric and Adolescent Gynecology.* Philadelphia: Lippincott Williams and Wilkins, 2000: 85.

62. Migeon CJ, Pappas K. Sex chromosome anomalies. In: *Encyclopedia of Life Sciences.* Chichester, UK: John Wiley, 2006. www.els.net/

The Gynecologic Approach to the Child, Adolescent, and Young Adult

Albert Altchek

Mount Sinai School of Medicine and Hospital, New York, NY, USA

The child

If the reason for the visit is sexual assault it may be wise to refer the patient to the special emergency room of a large hospital which has an organized team for evaluation, emergency treatment of trauma, prevention of pregnancy and sexually transmitted disease, psychologic help, legal aspects, collection of evidence, follow-up, and careful records for possible later court testimony. Potential problems include criminal aspects, lengthy trials, in separated marriages the suspicion of molestation during visits to the other parent, and dermatologic disease masquerading as molestation.

The physician can only testify to physical findings. Some molested children, especially adolescents, might have had coitus without physical evidence. Molestation is decided by the court since simple touching of the vulva is molestation which does not have physical signs.

For the office visit, have an experienced office assistant welcome the patient, ask the purpose of the visit, reduce anxiety and alert the physician in case any special equipment is needed. Many children fear the possibility of injections. Mothers fear "pelvic examinations," loss of virginity, and pain.

Preliminary preparations

- Environment to help communication: a quiet examining room is preferably to a busy, noisy clinic. A trained female nurse or aide who is sympathetic to the child should be available rather than the usual gynecologic nurse oriented for the adult patient, rapid history taking, examination, and instructions. Ideally, prior reports and old hospital records should be available.
- Appropriate facilities: examining light (I find that a good headlight is ideal – it always lights the proper spot and keeps the hands free); disposable nonlatex gloves (latex sensitivity) for general examination, and sterile gloves. Consider facilities for:
  - testing for gonorrhea, chlamydia, streptococcus group A, *Staphylococcus aureus*, *E. coli*, bacterial vaginosis, candida, *Trichomonas vaginalis*, fungi, and for special situations such as for anaerobes or shigella
  - vaginal cytology for maturation index (percent parabasal, intermediate and superficial) and for Papanicolaou (Pap) cytology. The maturation index can be estimated by an immediate unstained microscopic wet smear at 100x or 400x magnification. A wet smear may show motile trichomonads, candida, and bacterial vaginosis
  - Gram stain of air-dried glass slide swab to approximate the number of bacteria, predominant organism, and number of WBC (Quick Take 6.1)
  - for the experienced physician, a device to visualize the upper vagina such as a pediatric vaginoscope (Fig 6.1), hysteroscope, nonspecific short endoscope used for pediatric sinus inspection, and different sizes of the traditional vaginal bivalve speculum (Fig. 6.2).

The adult accompanying the child is usually the mother, occasionally the mother and father and infrequently the nanny or other caretaker. Written permission is required

Pediatric, Adolescent, & Young Adult Gynecology. Edited by A. Altchek and L. Deligdisch. © 2009 Blackwell Publishing, ISBN: 978-1-4051-5347-8.

for examination and treatment from the mother or father if they are not present.

On opening the door to the examining room, I usually introduce myself and my aide to the mother and to the child. I have a broad smile, as does the aide. The physician should be calm, relaxed, and not rushed. For the first few minutes it may be helpful to calm the child and make her feel part of the team by informal chatting to her about who combed her hair and fixed her beret, where she bought her shoes, her age, and then her symptoms. If the child holds onto the mother, try to do some of the general examination while she is held for reassurance. Sometimes the child clings to the mother and stays in a far corner

of the room. If the child has had an unhappy experience with other professionals she may scream, cry and refuse to be examined. The child is reassured that we do not have injections or "shots." The child may be so terrified it becomes a judgment call on how to proceed. It may be wise to have her return for a second visit at which time she may be calmer. If, however, there seems to be some potentially urgent or dangerous situation, the mother should be informed. If it is not feasible to examine the child in the office, consider examination under general anesthesia if needed, or referral (Quick Take 6.2).

The child is told in front of the mother that only the mother, the doctor or the doctor's nurse is allowed to examine the child or touch her "private parts." She is also told that children gossip so that when other children in the class ask how she is, she should simply say "fine."

The child and mother are informed that after the history there will be a preliminary general examination for precocious development and for signs of systemic skin disease. The minimal gynecologic examination should be inspection of the vulva with a good light. The mother is informed that the child will remain a virgin.

History

Why is the child here? Is there a note from the referring physician, when was the onset, was there another problem at the time, did she take some unusual medicine, is the problem mild, medium or severe, does it occur daily, does it occur in episodes, and are the symptoms worse during the day or during the night? Usually the problem refers to the vulva where there may be itching, burning or pain. Is there a vaginal discharge or vaginal bleeding, does the child scratch which will further irritate the area and might provoke bleeding, does she rub the vulva against furniture edges, does she scratch the skin of the body generally, is there dysuria, is there frequency of urination which would

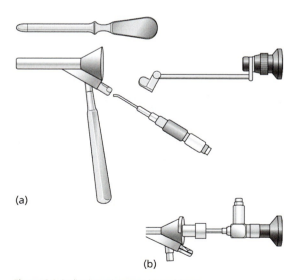

(a)

(b)

Figure 6.1 Pediatric vaginoscope by Karl Storz.

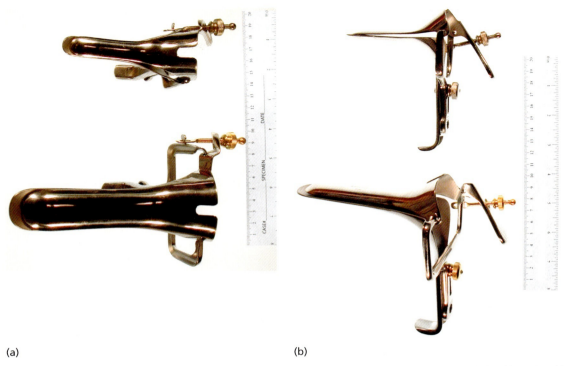

(a)   (b)

Figure 6.2 Traditional Graves (duckbill) bivalve vaginal speculums: the child's miniature speculum is short with narrow blades. (a) Top view. (b) Side view. The adolescent speculum is the same length as the adult's but has narrower blades. The narrow speculum is referred to as a Pedersen's or virginal speculum.

suggest cystitis or urethritis? Is it vulvar dysuria, which occurs as the acid urine touches the inflamed vulva and therefore the child holds the urine in for many hours before voiding? Is the child on any medication, is she allergic to any food or medicine?

• Past history – any allergies, eczema, skin patches or cradle cap?

• Family history – any allergy, asthma, hay fever, eczema patches, or sensitive skin, health of siblings and parents, any family history of diabetes or cancer?

Observe the child's actions. Is she calm, frightened, does she fidget, is she nervous, restless, does she scratch or rub the skin generally, is she talkative, is she able to volunteer a history, does she appear sociable and verbal and of appropriate intellectual and physical development?

Examination

Usually the child wants the mother to be present during the examination. A female nurse or aide is always present. Before examining the child, it is wise to inspect soiled underwear. If there is any suspicion of bleeding, test the discharge on the underwear for occult blood (Quick Take 6.3).

The entire skin of the child should be inspected before the vulva. This is done for two reasons: the vulva

---

Quick Take 6.3

Examination

• Inspect underwear, test discharge for blood, inspection of general body skin (are there signs of atopic dermatitis, psoriasis?)

• Observe – does she scratch other parts of the body? Is she jumpy? Is she socially, physically and intellectually of appropriate development?

• Perform a general physical examination from head, to chest, to general skin inspection, sexual development

• Lastly inspect the vulva

• This mimics the usual well-child examination routine

problem may be related to a general skin problem, and the child will accept this more readily than a direct inspection of vulva since it simulates the usual routine pediatric check-up. Look behind the ears for erythematous fissures, particularly under the ear lobes, look for keratosis pilaris (keratin spicules) on the external surfaces of the arms and thighs, look at the lower eyelid skinfolds to see if they are prominent or if there is any edema and darkening of the skin under the eyelids. Is there perioral pallor? Inspect the nasolabial folds for evidence of seborrheic dermatitis. All these findings may suggest atopic dermatitis.

Examine the skin for signs of psoriasis, especially flakes in the scalp, on the elbows, and on the knees. Look at the antecubical fossa of the elbows and behind the knees for patches of eczema and erythema fissures (Chapter 7). Examine the buttocks for micropustules. Palpate the abdomen. Are there inguinal masses, adenopathy, hernia? Does she have abdominal pain? Examine the vulva to determine the size of the hymen, the external urethral meatus, the size of the clitoris and foreskin prepuce, the labia majora with signs of maturation or hair growth, as well as in the pubic area and axillary area, inspect the vestibule just external to the hymen for erythema and discharge and signs of laceration of the hymen. There may be confusing bilateral paraurethral fossae. Also inspect the perineum between the vagina and rectum. Look at the anus. With atopic dermatitis there may be a small edematous papule at 12 o'clock which is a marker for an anterior anal fissure (Chapter 7). Check for urethral prolapse or protrusion of a polyp or mass from the vagina. If there is a polyp, where is the base of the polyp – is it from the hymen or higher in the vagina (Chapter 26)?

Most children object to rectal examination. It may be helpful for questions of acute appendicitis and acute pelvic pain.

For vaginal bleeding, visualization of the vagina may be attempted by holding the labia apart and/or examination in the knee–chest position. For the suspicion of vaginal foreign body (usually wads of toilet tissue and a foul, dark bloody discharge), vaginal irrigation using a urethral catheter may be considered (Chapter 7).

Assessment and plan

After the history and examination the physician has to make an assessment and plan. Is this a chronic, not dangerous condition or could it be suggestive of a potentially dangerous situation which might require relatively urgent action such as a prompt abdominal and pelvic sonogram, blood tests, urine analysis and culture, or consultation and referral, or examination under anesthesia and surgery?

The adolescent

Preparation

If the mother wishes to come into the examining room with the patient then this is usually permitted in order to get a complete medical history which the patient may not be completely aware of. If the mother does not want the patient to hear the medical details she should speak to the physician separately privately. In general, when the patient is actually examined it is preferable for the mother to leave the room. This is part of the adolescent being responsible for her own healthcare. A female aide or nurse is always present when the doctor is in the room with the patient. If the mother is present the patient may be too embarrassed to reveal a problem and to ask urgent questions. For example, she may be sexually active or planning to become sexually active and wants advice on contraception. The examining room should be quiet. Privacy is extremely important otherwise the patient will not feel free to talk. Another problem is the cost of medical care. In the USA, the patient is usually covered by the mother's or parents' health insurance up to the age of 18 or 20. If the parents do not have private medical insurance and are unable to pay, in many cases the individual state might pay.

The ideal set-up includes a good light source or headlight, a narrow, adult-length vaginal speculum (the short speculum for prepubertal children will not reach the cervix) (see Figs 6.1, 6.2) and available facilities to test for gonorrhea, chlamydia, streptococcus A, *Staphylococcus aureus*, yeast, bacterial vaginosis, microscopic wet smear, Gram stain, and perhaps urine testing for chlamydia and gonorrhea. There is a new test using liquid-based cytology for the latter two.

The permission of the patient is required for the physician to report to the mother despite the fact that the mother is paying for the care. Medical insurance claims should have a mechanism which will not reveal the diagnosis, perhaps by using code numbers rather than words.

The adolescent patient may come for medical care alone, with or without the permission or knowledge of her parents. Each state has different regulations. Generally,

Quick Take 6.4

Some acute problems of the adolescent

Bleeding problems

- Heavy dysfunctional uterine bleeding
- Menorrhagia due to congenital coagulation defect
- Complications of pregnancy

Acute pain

- Complications of pregnancy
- Torsion of ovarian cyst or tumor
- Pelvic inflammatory disease
- Herpes simplex type 2 vulva ulcer; if near the urethra these may lead to urinary retention
- Acute appendicitis and other general surgical problems

emergency care is given at once. In New York State, sexually transmitted disease may be treated and contraceptive advice may be given without the parents' knowledge (Chapter 44).

Some urgent problems include heavy vaginal bleeding, prolonged menses (menorrhagia), acute surface vulva pain, vulvovaginitis and acute pelvic pain from salpingitis, adnexal torsion, ectopic pregnancy, and appendicitis (Quick Take 6.4).

In preparation for the visit of the pubertal child, the physician should be aware of disorders of puberty. One of the most urgent is anovulatory dysfunctional uterine bleeding (ADUB) with severe vaginal bleeding which may last for 3–4 weeks (Chapter 22). Other related problems include precocious puberty, delayed puberty, and abnormal decreased or missed periods (oligomenorrhea), polycystic ovarian syndrome, congenital adrenal hyperplasia (present at birth and late onset atypical), hypothalamic amenorrhea, primary or secondary amenorrhea, possibly related to marked changes in weight, thyroid dysfunction, exercise for marathon races, change of lifestyle and stress at school, living in an out-of-town school and at summer camps. The physician should have a general understanding of sexuality and its associated problems: education for life, sex education, and avoiding unwanted pregnancy, and sexually transmitted disease.

Other problems include dysmenorrhea (primary or secondary), vaginitis (candida, bacterial vaginosis, trichomonad vaginitis, endocervicitis, gonorrhea and chlamydia), foul bloody vaginal discharge due to a tampon or other foreign body, and herpes simplex type 2. The AIDS virus may be present and asymptomatic (Chapter 40).

The most common ovarian neoplasm is the benign dermoid cyst (mature cystic teratoma). Rarely, there is a malignancy which grows rapidly, causes pain, and presents as a large mass. Very rarely, a small ovarian neoplasm might produce estrogen or testosterone with its clinical effects (Chapter 47). For good practice and continuity of care, the adolescent and young adult should be aware of the desirability of appropriate routine vaccinations.

Social and lifestyle concerns and problems that may first become manifest in the adolescent include obesity (now a worldwide problem for developed countries), lack of exercise, substance abuse, gender identification, depression, inability to be responsible, and lack of interest in education.

The patient is reassured that whatever is discussed in the examining room will not be discussed with anyone else unless the patient wishes it. The patient is asked without the mother present why she has come to the office (the real reason): for a routine check-up or is there some special problem, or both? Common problems include vaginal itching, burning, and vaginal discharge. Detailed questions are asked regarding the onset, severity, amount and description of discharge, and whether there is any abnormal bleeding. Is there scratching, dysuria or pain on bowel movements and is the patient sexually active?

History

If the problem is related to menstrual disturbances, a history is taken regarding the onset of menarche (menstrual periods), regularity of menses from the first day of one period to the first day of the next, duration of each menstrual flow, premenstrual molimina (breast swelling, bloating, etc., which suggests ovulation), pain at the time of menses or prior to the menses, and the amount of bleeding as estimated by numbers of tampons or number of external pads. The patient is asked to keep a menstrual calendar recording her menses and any dysmenorrhea. She is asked when the breasts developed. Usually there is an average of 2.5 years from the time of breast enlargement to menarche (menses). The onset of menses is very variable depending on family history, geography, weight, nutrition and whether there are any disturbances of the general health. Questions are also asked about pain separate from the time of menses which might be caused by ovarian cysts or a gastrointestinal problem. A basic understanding of all these problems is important so the physician can be comfortable in managing them.

Sometimes the patient is already sexually active and may deny this, thinking that since she had sex only a few times she could not possibly be pregnant. With the possibility of pregnancy, one has to consider ectopic pregnancy, miscarriage, and hydatidiform mole (Chapters 33, 48).

General examination

Examination includes height, weight, any hirsutism, particularly on the side of the face or under the chin, any hair loss from the scalp, lower abdominal male escutcheon, any signs of metabolic syndrome including an increased abdominal girth compared to the hips. The skin behind the neck is inspected for acanthosis nigricans which may indicate impending diabetes mellitus. Evidence of acne is sought on the face, chest, and upper back. Signs of atopic dermatitis are sought; in the adolescent the lesions are usually drier and itchy as contrasted to the moist lesions of the younger child. After explanation, unless the patient is apprehensive, the breasts are examined, searching for masses or fibrocystic changes, as well as the axilla for lymph node enlargement and the development of axillary hair. The size of the breasts and pubertal development are estimated according to the Tanner system. The abdomen is palpated for any masses or tenderness. Note any body piercing, often with a ring on the umbilicus which may become infected.

Gynecologic examination

The vulva is inspected for hair growth on the mons pubis and labia majora. The size of the clitoris is estimated. The external urethral meatus is inspected as well as the hymen and hymen orifice. Any sign of discharge is observed. A narrow vaginal speculum examination of the vagina and cervix may or may not be necessary. If there is unusual bleeding or discharge from the vagina, examination would be appropriate after explaining this to the patient and being very gentle. If the patient refuses vaginal exam then it is not performed. In some patient groups vaginal examination is equated with loss of virginity. Usually examination can be done without any damage to the hymen in most cases where the hymen is relatively open and relatively pliable.

The speculum should be at room temperature. I have found that disposable plastic bivalve speculums are not as precise or as easy to maneuver as the traditional stainless steel which I autoclave in the office. The patient must be relaxed otherwise examination is futile. Gently place some lubricating jelly (or anesthetic jelly) at the introitus. Despite the fact that the opening of the vagina (introitus) is vertical, the speculum is introduced slowly obliquely to avoid rubbing the sensitive urethra and then gently rotated to the horizontal position to conform with the transverse vaginal space. These small details can make a great difference in successful visualization. Rectal examination is considered if there is pelvic pain to palpate for ovarian masses or signs of endometriosis or appendicitis. Endometriosis may be suggested by a fixed retroverted uterus with tender thickening or nodularity of the sacrouterine ligaments or in the cul-de-sac.

Following this examination, the physician may summarize their thoughts by reviewing the patient's Subjective complaints, Objective findings, evaluation and Assessment and Plan ("SOAP") for further care. The latter might be a repeat visit or specific tests such as pelvic or renal ultrasound, cultures for sexually transmitted disease or, if there is a question of unusual congenital anomaly, then an MRI of the pelvis.

As with the child, the physician has to make a decision – is this a chronic condition, is it an urgent situation or is it an emergency? Does the patient require close supervision? Is she reliable? Should there be a consultation?

The young adult

The young adult blends with the later stages of puberty with continuation of very similar gynecologic problems. The young adult is often concerned with vulvovaginitis, pelvic pain, dysuria, tenderness of the vestibule when attempting sexual relations, sexually transmitted disease, contraception, abortion, pregnancy complications, and recurrent urinary tract infections. Ectopic ureter often is not discovered until young adulthood (Quick Take 6.5).

The patient usually knows her history so that the physician may have the patient fill out a form about her past medical history even before she comes into the office. She might also write down her concerns and the reason for the visit. Until recently, Pap cytology of the cervix was performed routinely. Some physicians do not undertake

Quick Take 6.5

Common reasons for visits by young adults

- Vaginal itching, burning, and discharge
- Contraceptive advice
- Is she pregnant?
- The "morning after" pill
- Forgot to take OC
- Breakthrough bleeding while on OC
- Fear of STD (STI)
- Pap cytology, HPV testing
- Pelvic pain or discomfort
- Dyspareunia

cytology and high-risk papilloma virus (hrHPV) testing until the patient has been sexually active for more than a year or two (or until age 21) because although as many as 80% of young adults and college women are found to have papilloma virus, about 80–90% apparently spontaneously cure themselves after 1–3 years. Delay in testing for HPV is done to avoid anxiety and for fear that it might cause the physician to do excessive surgery such as conization or the leep procedure which might remove a large cone of the cervix. This might cause future problems with premature delivery in pregnancy.

The usual adult visit takes less time than the visit of a younger patient. Sometimes the young adult needs extensive information on various types of contraception in which case it is often helpful to give her printed material about the subject after a brief discussion. The most common gynecologic problem of the young adult is vulvovaginitis.

At present it is recommended as routine that women age 30 and over should have Pap cytology and a simultaneous hrHPV test. If the latter is positive the patient requires careful observation because it suggests that the HPV virus may have been present for several years and may persist which may provoke cervical dysplasia.

CHAPTER 7
Vulvovaginitis in the Child

Albert Altchek

Mount Sinai School of Medicine and Hospital, New York, NY, USA

Introduction

Vulvovaginitis is the most common gynecologic problem of the child. Almost all will develop an episode of vulvo-vaginitis at one time or another.

The child is susceptible because (Quick Take 7.1):

• the vulva is exposed to the environment. It lacks the protective thick labial pads and pubic hair of the adult. In addition, vulva skin is delicate and sensitive (Fig. 7.1)

• the anus is nearby. No matter how carefully the child cleans herself, there is always a high bacterial count on the skin near the anus

• the lack of estrogen results in the vaginal wall being thin (about 6 versus 30–40 cells thick), without glycogen and lactobacilli (Döderlein bacilli), and with a neutral pH (rather than a protective acid pH). It is also warm and moist. Thus the vagina is an excellent bacterial culture medium (Fig. 7.2)

• poor local hygiene is common. Playing in sand lots results in contaminated abrasions. Tights and leotards rub, bind, and chafe. Incorrect and inadequate cleaning after the toilet, especially with coarse toilet tissue, occurs frequently when children are in a rush. During summer vacations children wear wet, often sandy swimsuits for many hours.

Most vulvovaginitis is a primary nonspecific vulvitis triggered by a episode of poor hygiene and in turn setting off a secondary vaginitis (Figs 7.3–7.6; Box 7.1; Quick Take 7.2).

Pediatric, Adolescent, & Young Adult Gynecology. Edited by
A. Altchek and L. Deligdisch. © 2009 Blackwell Publishing,
ISBN: 978-1-4051-5347-8.

> ### Quick Take 7.1
>
> **Why the child is susceptible to vulvovaginitis**
>
> • The vulva is exposed
> • The vulva skin is thin and sensitive
> • It is near the anus
> • The vaginal wall is thin, lacks protective acid pH and is a good bacterial culture medium
> • Poor local hygiene

Primary vulvitis

Vulvitis causes erythema, itching, burning and pain, resulting in rubbing, scratching and an awkward gait. Sometimes the situation is discovered when the teacher reports that the child is "masturbating" in school. There is also vulvar dysuria – pain while voiding as the acid urine wets the irritated skin of the vestibule and vulva. Characteristically, the child is fearful of voiding, holds in the urine and voids infrequently with a large volume. Dysuria caused by cystitis results in frequent voiding with pyuria and bacteriuria. Dripping of vaginal discharge into the voided urine may cause false positives. A bacterial culture colony count may be helpful (Quick Take 7.3).

Acute deep unilateral labium majus abscess

Whereas most vulvitis is superficial skin irritation, in recent years, worldwide there has been an increase in rapidly developing, unilateral labium majus abscesses due to a virulent *Staphylococcus aureus* or streptococcus group A β-hemolytic infection. Although the source of entry is

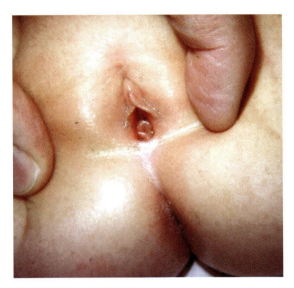

Figure 7.1 Vulva of child. Lacks protective pubic hairs and labial pads (gloves should be worn).

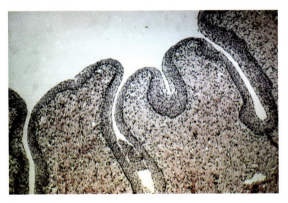

Figure 7.2 Prepubertal thin anestrogenic vaginal wall. Wrinkled surface due to autopsy fixative.

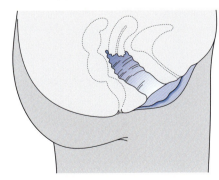

Figure 7.3 Primary vulvitis.

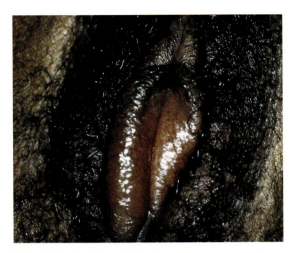

Figure 7.4 Acute edema of labia minora.

often unrecognized it is usually a puncture by a thorn, large insect, pin or sharp pencil. Within hours the abscess develops and the child becomes toxic (Figs 7.7, 7.8). Urgent surgery is usually necessary because antibiotics are ineffective. In order to insure adequate postoperative drainage of the abscess, it is marsupialized with excision of a liberal amount of the wall (Fig. 7.9). This avoids the need for painful changing of drains. The routine culture of the frank pus is often negative. The mother is alerted to the problem and needs to understand that the area will take several weeks of secondary healing from below. Warm sitz baths are used.

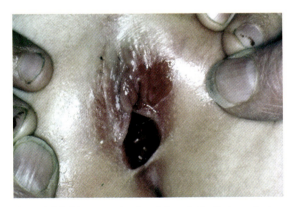

Figure 7.5 Left inner anterior denudation of skin. Having patient holding labia apart may reduce anxiety (gloves should be worn).

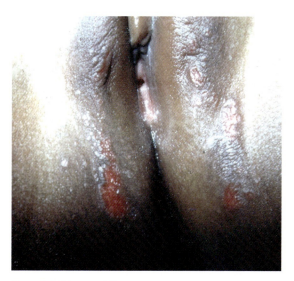

Figure 7.6 Vulva excoriation.

Less often than primary vulvitis, there is primary vaginitis (and often a secondary vulvitis) which is more deserving of investigation since it may be associated with a foreign body or a specific infection (streptococcus group A, gonorrhea) (Fig. 7.10).

Vaginitis causes a vaginal discharge which may have a malodor, blood, and various colors (gray, mucous, greenish, yellow tinted), consistency, and volume. The various colors may be related to varying predominant organisms originating in the anal area (no matter how clean it seems to be). With certain skin conditions there may be vulva and perianal fissures which allow access to the anestrogenic (atrophic) vagina which is an excellent bacteria culture medium. The discharge is often irritating and may cause a secondary vulvitis, especially if the underwear is not changed frequently (Quick Take 7.4).

There may be a rare congenital ectopic ureter exiting on the anterolateral wall of the vagina. The ectopic ureter arises from the upper renal pole where the urine is not concentrated. The distal ectopic ureter often is dilated and tortuous. The characteristic presentation is morning passage of a large amount of watery, purulent fluid which does not look or smell like urine. The vagina continues dribbling during the day. Most cases are not discovered until young adulthood (Chapter 26). There is also a normal ureter on the affected side.

Box 7.1 Causes of prepubertal vulvovaginitis

Nonspecific primary vulvitis
Specific vaginal infections

A. Usual colon organisms – *Escherichia coli*, *Proteus vulgaris*
B. Unusual colon organisms – typhoid, shigella
C. Hemolytic streptococcus group A
D. Gonorrhea
E. Chlamydia
F. Bacterial vaginosis
G. Pneumococcus
H. *Staphylococcus aureus*

Infections with other microorganisms

A. Candida – vaginitis, vulvitis (prefers estrogenic vagina)
B. Trichomonad (prefers estrogenic vagina)

Pinworm infestation
Local physical factors

A. Foreign body in vagina
B. Trauma
C. Gynecologic neoplasms, labial agglutination
D. Urologic: urethral prolapse, ectopic ureter
E. Rectal: anal fissure, pruritus, ectopic anus
F. Covering: diapers, tights
G. "Ballet dancer's bottom"

Allergic – irritant contact
Systemic illness with vulvovaginal manifestations

A. Measles
B. Chicken pox
C. Scarlet fever. hemolytic streptococcus
D. Typhoid, dysentery
E. Draining pelvic abscess (inflammatory bowel disease)
F. Blood dyscrasias
G. Behçet syndrome

General skin disease with vulvar manifestations

A. Atopic dermatitis
B. Seborrheic dermatitis
C. Psoriasis
D. Lichen sclerosus
E. Condylomata acuminata
F. Molluscum contagiosum
G. Herpes simplex
H. Herpes zoster
I. Pediculosis pubis
J. Scabies
K. Bacterial infection: impetigo, erysipelas, cellulitis, boils
L. Tinea, fungi
M. Intertrigo

Other sexually transmitted disease – syphilis, chancroid, lymphogranuloma venereum
Psychosomatic

Quick Take 7.2

Most vulvovaginitis is:

- Primary nonspecific vulvitis
- Triggered by an episode of poor hygiene
- Associated with mixed nonspecific bacterial culture from the anus
- Corrected by improved local hygiene

Quick Take 7.3

Vulvitis causes:

- Itching, scratching, burning, pain, redness
- Vulvar dysuria
- Unusual gait
- Secondary vaginitis

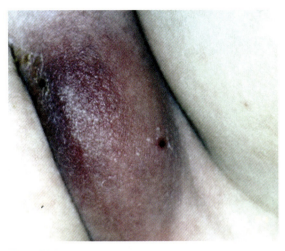

Figure 7.8 Puncture site on left lateral margin – site of entrance of virulent streptococcus or staphylococcus.

Vaginal discharge

With vulvovaginitis, the child may be irritable, cranky, and restless. She may be uncomfortable sitting in the class room and unable to concentrate on her studies. Sometimes the situation is discovered because the child has been ostracized. Her classmates and teachers stay away because of the bad smell which she does not appreci-ate since it is with her constantly. This tends to happen particularly with a vaginal foreign body with its chronic, bloody, foul-smelling discharge. Adolescents may have a horrible smell from a forgotten vaginal tampon or some-times from a severe trichomonad vaginitis (foul odor) or a bacterial vaginosis (rotten fish odor) (see Quick Take 7.4).

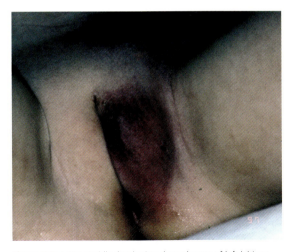

Figure 7.7 Acute rapidly developing deep abscess of left labium majora.

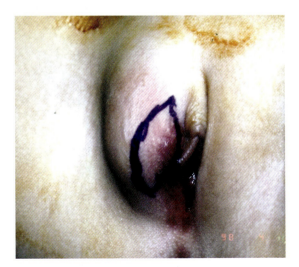

Figure 7.9 Right deep acutely developing abscess of deep labium majus. Outline marking of marsupialization to allow adequate drainage of deep locules of pus.

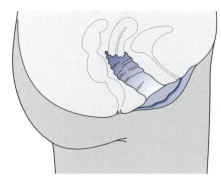

Figure 7.10 Primary vaginitis with secondary vulvitis due to irritating vaginal discharge.

Physiologic discharge

There may be a normal physiologic vaginal discharge in the first two weeks of life due to the maternal estrogen effect stimulating endocervical mucus and vaginal cell desquamation. Less often, there is withdrawal bleeding from the effect on the endometrium. Physiologic discharge may occur several months before menstruation due to estrogen. Physiologic discharge is usually scanty and asymptomatic. Cultures of the vagina often show almost all the bacteria found in the anus; however, Gram stain reveals few bacteria, few white blood cells (WBC), and there is no predominant pathogenic germ. There is no simple test for bacterial quantitation. A Gram-stained vaginal swab is the simplest laboratory test. Therefore culture alone is inadequate in defining etiology.

For vulvovaginitis vaginal cultures are performed if there is a significant or persistent discharge, bleeding, or suspicion of molestation or sexually transmitted disease. Consider streptococcus A, *Staphylococcus aureus*, fungal, and gonorrhea cultures. Rapid testing for chlamydia may yield a presumed result not reliable for legal situations. Purulent discharges may give a false-positive test (see Chapter 41). Vaginal swabs may also be used for vaginal

---

Quick Take 7.4

Vaginitis can cause:

- Vaginal discharge and bleeding
- Malodor, especially with prepubertal foreign body toilet tissue wads causing dark bloody discharge
- Secondary vulvitis

---

cytology, maturation index, Gram stain, and microscopic wet mount.

Voided urine tests for chlamydia and gonorrhea have been developed for apprehensive children.

Clinical judgment

The evaluation, assessment, and action plan are based on overall clinical judgment. Since most cases are nonspecific primary vulvitis triggered by poor hygiene, at least initially, a vaginal swab may not be necessary, especially in an apprehensive child (see Quick Take 7.2).

Visualization of the distal vagina is attempted by gently holding the labia apart while the child is supine in the frog-leg position; this may help to decide whether the problem is primary vulvitis or primary vaginitis. Sometimes with the older child a knee–chest position is helpful (Chapter 6).

The usual vaginal foreign body is wads of toilet tissue. For diagnosis and treatment, there may be urethral catheter irrigation of the upper vagina to wash out the wads. These techniques depend on the emotional status of the individual child and the facilities and preference of the physician. Usually there is more than one wad, inserted at different times. Another approach is examination under anesthesia (Chapters 6, 13).

Indications for vaginoscopy

Vaginoscopy is considered for vaginal bleeding, suspicion of a foreign body, neoplasm or congenital anomaly, or persistent or recurrent vulvovaginitis. For the apprehensive child examination is done under light general anesthesia by a pediatric anesthesiologist. Sedation alone may be unsatisfactory because of unpredictable reactions, including the depth and length of sedation.

Vaginoscopy requires a variable time of observation during and after the procedure. Appropriate instruments should be available for visualization, swabs, alligator forceps for removal of foreign bodies and a microsurgical punch biopsy. There is no standard vaginoscope, hysteroscope, cystoscope or speculum. Veterinary otoscopic speculums have been used. Infusion of saline into the vagina and compression of the vulva distends the vagina to improve visualization of its surface and allow recording with a video camera. For operative procedures a miniature, short narrow Graves bivalve vaginal speculum may be used. It is adjustable to allow for different sizes of foreign bodies, for operating instruments, and for vaginal size (Chapter 6). I use a headlight attached to an optical loop.

Careful evaluation at the initial visit usually gives a presumptive cause of the vulvovaginitis. If it does not respond to conservative management, consider re-evaluation or consultation.

Interpretation of cultures

Persistent or severe vaginitis may be due to a specific infection caused by a predominant organism.

β-Hemolytic group A streptococcus, the cause of "strep throat," is seasonal, matching strep pharyngitis in school children. The organism spreads by contaminated hands, although when the vaginal culture is positive, the throat may be negative. There is a characteristic severe vaginal inflammation with a heavy discharge which is bloody and therefore a frequent cause of vaginal bleeding. It is treated like strep throat with penicillin for 10 days.

Interpretation of vaginal cultures requires an overall view, and is only one factor in clinical diagnosis and management. The laboratory often reports "normal flora" vaginal cultures. There are usually about four organisms. If anaerobic cultures were also done, they would be positive. There may be colonization or contamination by a potentially dangerous organism from the anal area. With a foul-smelling bloody discharge from a foreign body, there are large numbers of nonspecific anaerobic bacteria and white blood cells. The vaginal maturation index (MI) done from a midvaginal swab indicates the percent of parabasal, intermediate, and superficial cells. Different laboratories use different reporting methods and may reverse the cell type sequence. The prepubertal MI is mainly parabasal and in puberty the superficial and intermediate cells increase. Even with the presence of estrogen, a severe vaginitis MI may show fewer superficial cells because of surface desquamation. With experience, cell types can be recognized by wet microscopic smear.

Some traditional reviews of causes of vulvovaginitis simply divide it according to the bacterial culture report.

Clinical judgment of the overall situation is of extreme importance in interpreting the culture report. This is all in addition to the many factors which affect the report such as how the culture was obtained, transportation, and laboratory technology.

Pelvic inflammatory disease (salpingitis) from ascending gonorrhea vaginitis is unusual in the prepubertal child. In the adolescent with endocervical glands, about 1–2 days after menses, there may be an ascending infection into the tube. If acute salpingitis occurs the cervicovaginal culture may become negative in a few days as it is replaced by mixed infection (often from the anus).

Any sexually transmitted disease raises the question of molestation (Chapter 11). Nevertheless, gonorrhea and bacterial vaginosis may sometimes be transferred from mother to daughter by close contact in bed. Trichomonad vaginitis may be transferred by contaminated wet wash cloths. Condyloma (HPV positive) of the vulva and perianal area may be acquired at delivery or from a caretaker's hands changing diapers and wiping the anus.

Sometimes the predominant organism is from the colon, such as a virulent *E. coli* or proteus. In the USA, shigella vaginitis is sometimes seen, especially in the south west. It presents as a heavy persistent white discharge, often bloody, and sometimes resistant to usual antibiotics. It begins as chronic diarrhea which then spreads to the vagina. At the time of diagnosis there may not be diarrhea and the stool culture may be negative.

Causes of vulvovaginitis (Box 7.1)

Different parts of the world may have unique local etiologies, including schistosomiasis and amebiasis.

Candida
Candida infections in the child are unusual despite the higher incidence in adults. It prefers an estrogenic environment. In the adolescent there may be a candida vulvitis causing an agonizing vulva itching, pain, and burning presenting as symmetric red lesions with scalloped edges and satellite pustules. There is no discharge. Diagnosis is visual or by scraping for wet microscopic mount or culture (Fig. 7.11).

Candida vaginitis causes a cottage-cheese white lumpy discharge. Diagnosis is readily made by wet smear showing spores and hyphae (Fig. 7.12).

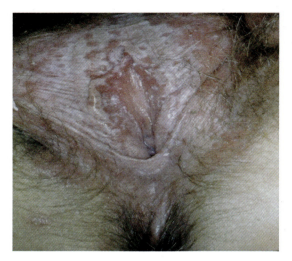

Figure 7.11 Candidiasis of adolescent vulva, with irregular scalloped borders and satellite pustules. Causes agonizing pain and itching without vaginal discharge. May suggest diabetes mellitus or immunosuppression.

Like candida, the trichomonad prefers the estrogenic vagina. If the mother has a clinical vaginal trichomonad infection there is about a 5% chance that the newborn will acquire it at vaginal delivery. It presents as a

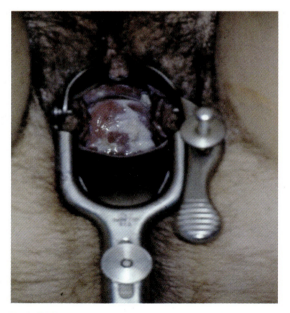

Figure 7.12 "Cottage cheese" white lumpy vaginal discharge from vaginal candidiasis verified by wet smear of hyphae and spores or culture.

neonatal heavy white discharge and sterile pyuria due to vaginitis and urethritis. Immediate microscopic wet smear of the vagina or urine may show the trichomonads. Usually there is spontaneous cure in about two weeks as estrogen decreases. With older girls it may occur after coitus.

Pinworms

If the child has pinworms there is about a 20% chance of vulvovaginitis. The pinworm migrates out of the anus during the night to deposit microscopic eggs on the vulva. Sometimes they lose their way and enter the vagina, where they act like a foreign body. There may be characteristic nightmares, sleep disturbances, and scratching during the night, as well as vaginal discharge with a nonspecific vaginal culture without a predominant organism but with many bacteria. Diagnosis is by having the mother examine the anus with a flashlight during the night or early morning to search for the pin-sized white moving worms. Another method is touching the anus in the morning with transparent sticky clear tape (or plastic spatula), pasting it on a glass slide and taking it to a laboratory for microscopic examination. The pinworm nightmares may be misinterpreted as molestation nightmares. Since the pinworm treatment is simple and safe many pediatricians recommend therapy based on clinical evaluation. Everyone in the household takes one soluble pill (mebendazole 100 mg). The sheets and night clothes are all washed in hot water. The child is instructed to wash the hands before going to bed, and before breakfast. Reinfection is common. It is not rare in the USA and in some parts of the world it is one of the most common causes of vulvovaginitis (Quick Take 7.5).

Quick Take 7.5

Worsening of symptoms at night may be due to:

- Excess heat and humidity from pajama pants, excessive blankets
- Pinworms
- Atopic dermatitis
- Bad dreams, fear of molestation
- Reaction to fabric or dye of pajamas or nightgowns

Atopic dermatitis

Atopic dermatitis (AD) occurs in 17% of children in the USA. There continues to be a steady increase in prevalence which before 1960 was 3%, paralleling the increase in asthma. Nevertheless 25% of cases have no family or personal history or atopic background. Of those who develop AD, 45% have it within the first six months of life, by the end of the first year 60% have it and by five years 85% have it. About 50% of children with AD develop asthma and even more develop allergic rhinitis. The diagnosis revolves around chronic pruritus and age-associated morphology and distribution [1]. Physical and psychologic stress worsens AD.

Pediatric dermatologists believe that AD rarely involves the vulva. In my referred private practice, of those with atopic dermatitis there is 100% involvement of the vulva. Since there is no specific histology the diagnosis is clinical, made by a suggestive personal and family history of allergy, asthma, and eczema and on examination suggestive finding of atopic dermatitis by general and vulva inspection. The acute phase has been called "glistening redness" (in Latin) which simply describes the acute non-specific inflammation. The severe itching causes rubbing and scratching which if continuous can cause lichenification. It often recurs but tends to improve with puberty. AD cannot be cured but it can be controlled by avoiding irritants (Quick Take 7.5).

There is a subacute lesion of atopic dermatitis which I have observed during continuous personal follow-up of the same patients over many years [2]. It has not been reported previously because different physicians see different patients at different times in clinics each with a different focus, such as pediatric, gynecology, and pediatric dermatology. Very often, the skin of the entire body is not examined. Traditional pediatric dermatology teaching is that AD rarely affects the vulva and therefore the physician tends to overlook the vulva. If we do not know what to look for, we do not see it.

Aside from a family and personal history the clinical clues are a past history of cradle cap, eczematous patches on the torso and extremities, allergies, sensitive skin, general body scratching, recurrent sinusitis, bronchitis, and asthma, chronic recurrent vulva itching with rubbing, scratching and awkward gait, usually without vaginal discharge. The vulva itching and discomfort may be worse at night because of local increased heat and humidity from

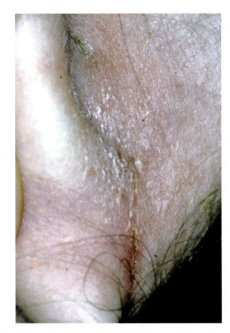

Figure 7.13 Erythematous fissures behind ears with crusting and flaking.

excessive blankets, pajama pants or underwear (see Quick Take 7.5). Patients often have recurrent ear infections, reaction to wool clothing, and recurrent severe agglutination of the labia minora.

Observe the child while the history is taken. There is frequent scratching of the arms and torso. She may look irritable, jumpy, and itchy.

The general body examination starts with the head. Behind the ears are erythematous fissures and possibly crusting and flaking (Fig. 7.13). Less common but more characteristic of AD are deep fissures under the ear lobe (Fig. 7.14). Ear symptoms are not frequent because the area is cool, dry and not near bacteria (unlike the vulva). I often show the ears to the mother so she can be a "medical detective" and keep a record of worsening and possible clue to allergies. Very often shrimps, chocolate, nuts and hot dogs can provoke the skin. I caution the mother and child not to discuss this with others to avoid friends and relatives examining the child and causing embarrassment. When the child looks down, this emphasizes a prominent lower eyelid fold due to edema, giving a swollen and pale look referred to as atopic pleat, Morgan's fold or Dennie's fold. In AD it usually presents at

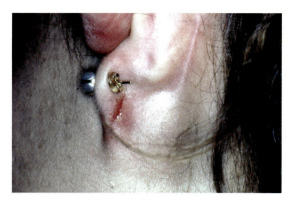

Figure 7.14 Deep fissure under ear lobe characteristic of atopic dermatitis.

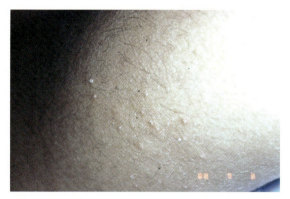

Figure 7.16 Keratosis pilaris on the arm, keratin specules found by gentle stroking or lateral lighting.

birth or in the first week of life and lasts for a lifetime [1]. This is an underappreciated clinical sign which when explained becomes instantly recognizable. Below the fold is a darkening of the skin as if the child was up all night. Increasing skin reaction makes the folds more prominent. The cheeks become chapped, especially when exposed to excess sun or cold wind. There is perioral and perinasal pallor due to edema (Fig. 7.15) [1]. The lateral nose often has a seborrheic type dermatitis.

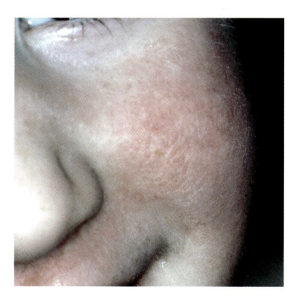

Figure 7.15 Perioral and perinasal pallor, chapped cheeks, lower eyelid fold difficult to see.

There may be keratosis pilaris of the torso and on the lateral surfaces of the arms (Fig. 7.16) and thighs. These keratin spicules are pointed in one direction so that gentle stroking will perceive them going cephalad but might not show them going caudad. They can be visualized by an oblique light. The entire skin is sensitive. In young children the mother's grasp may leave a red mark on the torso, as does a tight belt. Dermatographism is displayed by a firm stroke of a dull pointed instrument on the skin causing an initial red line followed by a wheal and erythematous flare, indicating sensitive skin generally. With AD, in addition the initial red line is replaced in about 10 seconds by a white line called white dermatographism (Fig. 7.17) [1]. There may be characteristic erythematous fissures in the axilla and lesions in the anterior cubital fossa of the elbow and the popliteal fossa behind the knee (Fig. 7.18).

The anterior knees and elbows have rough 1–2 mm small hard papules. Older children may have dry healed scratch marks on the back, dorsum of the hands and adjacent dorsum interdigital skin webs. There may also be active or healed 2 cm patches of eczema on the arms, torso, and legs. As the skin is inspected, the child may be seen scratching her arms.

I have noticed with AD an overlooked occasional dermatitis of the areola of the breast which presents as breast pain.

There is a characteristic syndrome of episodes of acute anxiety, outstretched arms, perspiration, and tachycardia, not previously described. It is associated with clinical signs of AD as well as the vulva lesions, particularly the perineal

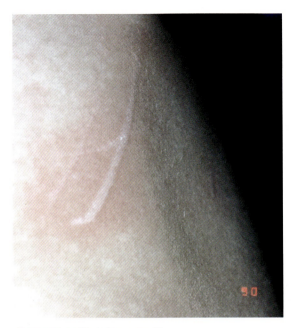

Figure 7.17 "White" dermatographism.

fissure and 12 o'clock anterior anal lesion. Most of these children wear diapers and are frustrated because they cannot rub the thighs together or scratch. When the diaper is off the child can rub. Less often, even without a diaper the child is taught never to touch or rub the vulva and therefore has the same frustration. Fissures behind the ears are asymptomatic, because it is cool, dry and away from the anus. Perineal and interlabial fissure are symptomatic

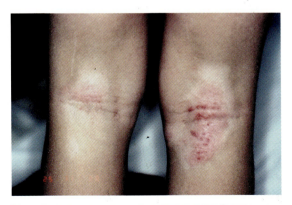

Figure 7.18 Characteristic popliteal fossa irritation of atopic dermatitis.

because of local heat, humidity and the proximity of the anus. A personal unpublished study shows a large number of colon organisms and fungi in the perianal area and perineum which reach the fissures and can cause sudden agonizing discomfort.

The vulva lesions, which have not been described previously, are characteristic. The most common lesion is symmetric erythematous fissures between the labia minora and majora (Fig. 7.19). Figure 7.20 shows a characteristic right interlabial fissure which was deep enough to cause some spontaneous bleeding. The patient complained of a "cut." Note the normal hymen. Figure 7.21 shows another patient with a similar right interlabial fissure but smaller fissure.

Figure 7.22 shows a left interlabial fissure. It is fine and precise as if made by an artist with a scalpel.

The next most common vulvar skin lesion of AD is the midline perineum fissure between the vagina and rectum (Fig. 7.23). The midline fissure may be confused with a rare congenital midline raw surface due to incomplete epithelial surface covering. Rarely the healed perineal fissure may have a "heaped up" appearance.

At the posterior end of the perineal fissure where it reaches the anus at about 12 o'clock, there may be local erythema or an inflamed papule (Fig. 7.24). If the inflammation becomes chronic the papule may swell, persist and resemble an anterior hemorrhoid (Fig. 7.25).

Infrequently with AD the bilateral symmetric interlabial fissures join together in the midline anterior to the clitoris to form a single midline fissure. This is the least common and least severe finding (Fig. 7.26).

The anterior anal fissure can cause pain with a hard bowel movement and cause streaks of bright blood on the stool surface. In addition, there is often a functional bowel disturbance. Despite courses of an oral cathartic, rectal examination may reveal numerous pellets of hard stool. Watery stool from cathartics passes around these pellets. There may also be urinary bladder functional disturbances when the rectal mass is significantly enlarged. Treatment involves digital removal of all the hard stool. Because of pain it may require general anesthesia.

Another aspect of vulvar atopic dermatitis is swelling of skin of the prepuce (foreskin) around the clitoris, giving the false impression of an enlarged clitoris and possible congenital adrenal hyperplasia (Fig. 7.27). The latter incorrect assumption is increased with the presence of agglutination of the labia minora with a single perineal

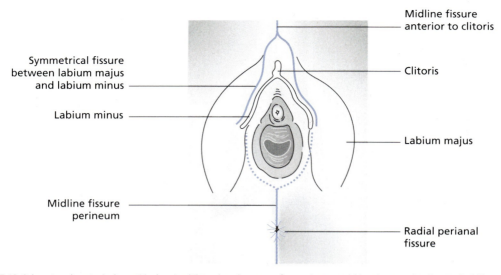

Midline fissure
anterior to clitoris

Symmetrical fissure
between labium majus
and labium minus

Clitoris

Labium minus

Labium majus

Midline fissure
perineum

Radial perianal
fissure

Figure 7.19 Subacute vulva atopic dermatitis showing bilateral erythematous fissures between labia minora and majora and midline perineal fissure between vagina and rectum. Less common is the single midline fissure anterior to the clitoris formed by fusion of the bilateral interlabial fissures.

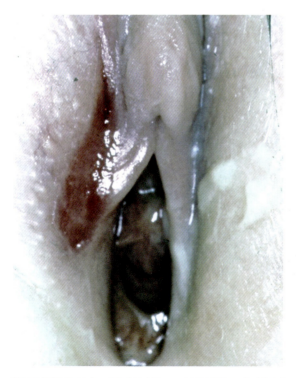

opening, as often happens with atopic dermatitis. Occasionally the foreskin adheres to the clitoris, trapping smegma and causing intense local pain. With lysis of adhesions, the clitoris is cleaned and exposed. This gives instant relief and confirms the diagnosis.

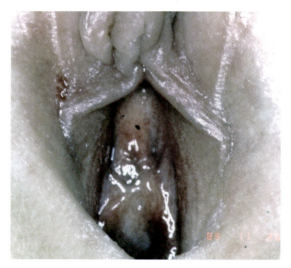

Figure 7.20 Right deep interlabial fissure which felt like a "cut" and caused bleeding. Note intact hymen.

Figure 7.21 Another child with a smaller version of Fig. 7.20 in the same location.

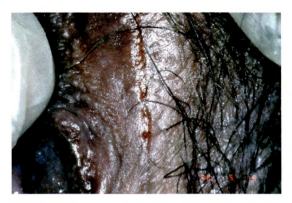

Figure 7.22 Left interlabial fissure atopic dermatitis. These fissures are fine and precise as if made by an artist with a scalpel.

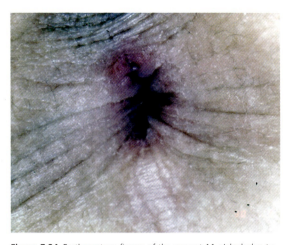

Figure 7.24 Erythematous fissure of the anus at 11 o'clock due to underlying infected fissure.

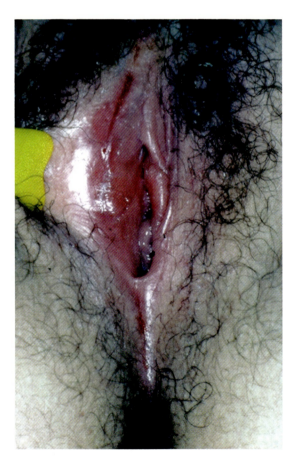

Figure 7.23 Adolescent with right interlabial fissure and midline perineal fissure.

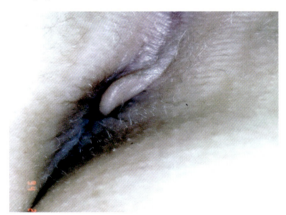

Figure 7.25 Chronic inflamed anterior anal fissure causing a persistent anterior pseudo-hemorrhoid.

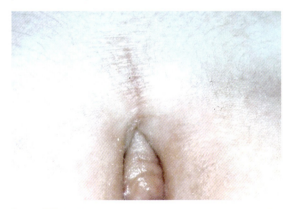

Figure 7.26 Midline fissure anterior to clitoris, less common in AD.

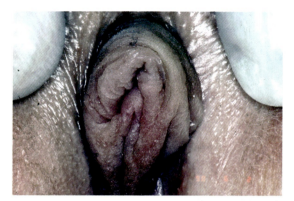

Figure 7.27 Infrequent swollen foreskin due to AD simulating clitoromegaly.

The characteristic vulva lesions of subacute atopic dermatitis may be more reliable in diagnosis than the suggestive multiple general skin lesions. When present, it appears to be the most precise method to diagnose AD. Biopsy reveals nonspecific inflammation.

Recurrence or increased severity of vulva AD symptoms may be due to secondary bacterial (often staphylococcus) infections.

AD is differentiated from sexual molestation by the:
- characteristic family history
- characteristic past history of the patient
- general skin examination of the patient
- characteristic vulva lesions, and normal intact hymen.

Lichen sclerosus of the vulva

Although some think that lichen sclerosus (LS) occurs only in postmenopausal women, about 20% of cases are pediatric. It is usually confined to the vulva. Pediatric LS is not associated with malignancy. In mature and postmenopausal women there is an association with malignancy.

Lichen sclerosus has similar fissure distribution to atopic dermatitis but whereas the latter fissures are sharp and precise, the lichen sclerosus fissures are coarse, irregular, and broad. This condition tends to be confused with sexual molestation and trauma. It bleeds readily, has the suggestion of lacerations and there may be areas of ecchymosis. In addition to characteristic fissures, there is a whitening of the skin resembling delicate cigarette paper.

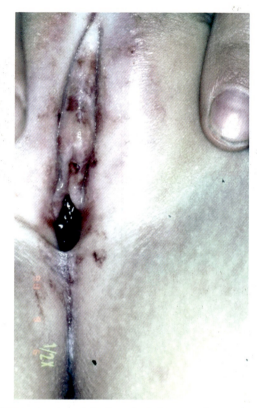

Figure 7.28 Lichen sclerosus, white delicate "cigarette paper" skin with ecchymoses (gloves should be worn).

With experience a clinical diagnosis can be made. The lesion usually remains confined to the vulva (Figs 7.28–7.31). The subcutaneous tissue has a spongy myxoid layer which bleeds with slight trauma to the skin. There are two obvious symptoms: continuous itching for the past year, and "the child was well until she went on a long bike trip" and developed "blood blisters." The trauma of sitting on a bicycle seat bruises the delicate tissue of lichen sclerosus and results in subepithelial bleeding which become dark areas which change with time. The condition is thought to be due to a local autoimmune disease. The pathology is diagnostic (Fig. 7.32) and it stains with immunoglobulin. Atopic dermatitis and lichen sclerosus may coexist. With atopic dermatitis, the biopsy is nonspecific. Usually there are no other lesions of lichen sclerosus in any other parts of the body. Although previously it was treated by excision or laser obliteration, the consensus is that it will recur. Usual treatment is topical steroids (Chapters 35, 36).

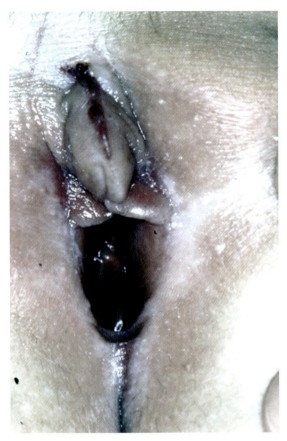

Figure 7.29 Lichen sclerosus. Recurrent ecchymoses may cause dark blue-black color which may come and go. Prominent perineal fissure.

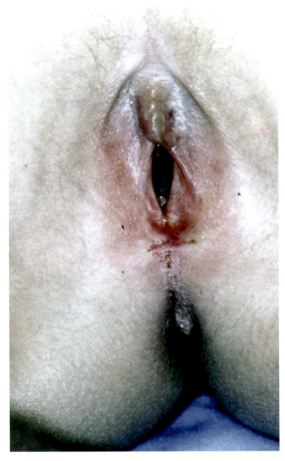

Figure 7.30 Lichen sclerosus. Periclitoral ecchymosis, perineal fissure and anterior anal pseudo-hemorrhoid.

Sometimes at puberty lichen sclerosus improves. If it continues, about the time of menopause the clitoris may become concealed by foreskin adhesions and rarely the vaginal introitus becomes so stenotic that surgical relaxation is required. There is an association with malignancy in the postmenopausal woman.

Lichen planus

Most cases of lichen planus occur in women aged 30–60. About 2–3% of reported cases are under age 20. It is under-reported because of variations in presentation and difficulty in diagnosis.

The classic primary lesion is a small, shiny, flat, reddish or violacious papule which may be extremely pruritic, localized to the flexural surfaces of the wrists, legs, genitalia,

and mucous membranes. There may be pinhead white papules with a lace-like pattern on the inner cheek, and the vestibule of the vulva [1]. There may be a desquamative inflammatory gingivitis or a desquamative inflammatory vaginitis with sharply demarcated areas with a bright red color (vulvovaginal-gingival syndrome). Rarely, it may involve the entire vagina. There is a heavy gray malodorous discharge. The wet smear shows many polymorphonuclear white blood cells and parabasal cells [3].

Condylomata acuminata

Condylomata acuminata, also called venereal warts, used to be very rare in children. In recent years it has become

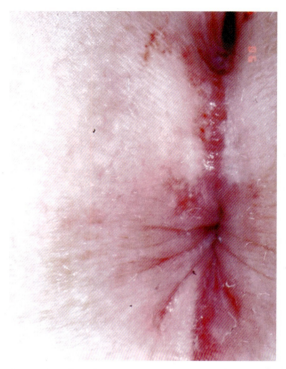

Figure 7.31 Lichen sclerosus. Perineal and perianal fissures. The fissures are in the same area as AD but are much more coarse and irregular.

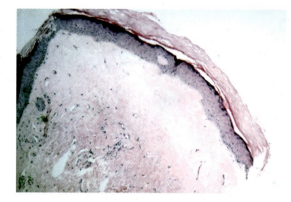

Figure 7.32 Lichen sclerosus. Pathognomonic biopsy: flat rete pegs, subcuticular myxoid tissue which bleeds readily with trauma resulting in ecchymoses.

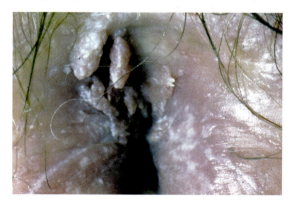

Figure 7.33 Dry warty condyloma acuminata in the perianal area due to HPV.

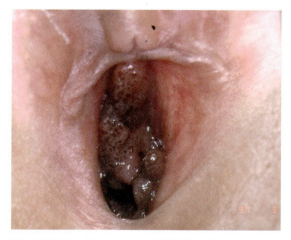

Figure 7.34 Granulomatous, moist condyloma of vaginal mucosa due to HPV.

more common. When the lesion is in the skin it has a characteristic, dry, pointed, warty appearance (Fig. 7.33). It often is present in clusters around the anus. When the lesion forms at the hymen and vaginal mucosal area, it looks completely different to the naked eye, because of a moist, granulomatous appearance like tapioca pudding (Fig. 7.34). HPV causes both conditions. Usually the HPV which causes it is not the high-risk type, which usually causes cervical dysplasia and possibly eventually cervical cancer. The apparent increase in condyloma acuminata in children may be related to increased examination because of concern regarding sexually transmitted disease and molestation. There is recent recognition that HPV in young women is common and with it exposure of the fetus at vaginal delivery with contamination of the vulva, perianal area, and aspiration. The virus prefers mucocutaneous epithelium. This may explain the rare nonmolestation laryngeal papillomatosis in the young child. There are some young children who have never been molested and who develop perianal and vulvar condyloma. Review

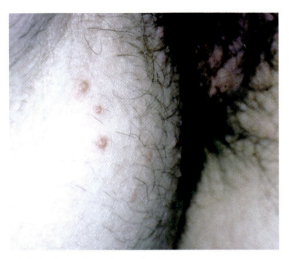

Figure 7.35 Molluscum contagiosum.

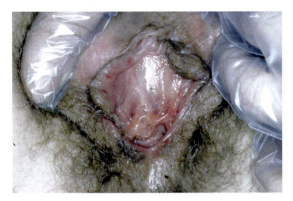

Figure 7.36 Recurrent herpes simplex ulcers of the inner labia minora. Partial immunity results in transient small ulcers. If seen just prior to or just after the ulcer healed the diagnosis is overlooked, despite the history of discomfort.

of the mother's medical records may show HPV during pregnancy. In addition, rubbing the anus when changing diapers may cause microabrasions which may facilitate HPV infection, especially if there is HPV on the caretaker's hands. AD girls have an increased susceptibility to HPV as they do to all skin infections. Imiquimod cream 5% is FDA approved to treat external and perianal warts and condyloma acuminata for children aged 12 and above (Chapters 11, 35, 36, 41).

Molluscum contagiosum

Molluscum contagiosum, despite the fearsome name, is a benign condition which sometimes disappears without treatment after several months. It is caused by a virus and readily infects the young child with sensitive skin, particularly those with atopic dermatitis. There are two ways in which the virus is spread. The first is spread among children at playgrounds with lesions usually on the hands and face. The lesions may appear anywhere on the exposed skin. The other method of spreading is by sexual activity with pubic lesions. The lesion itself is diagnosed with careful inspection and some magnification. It is a hemispherical round projection of the skin with central umbilication (Fig. 7.35). It may be treated by excision, freezing or other methods of destruction. Dermatologists often scrape the lesions away (Chapters 35, 36). The lesions often appear in crops and have pathognomonic histology. Sometimes the lesions spontaneously disappear after several months.

Herpes simplex type 2 (genital)

This sexually transmitted disease is increasing in incidence in humans. About 75% of the population are carriers. In most cases it is asymptomatic. In the young patient, particularly in those with sensitive skin, and in the sexually active adolescent it may produce a primary, very painful ulcer cluster which forms from ruptured vesicles on an erythematous base. If the ulcer is near the urethra the patient may be unable to void because of severe pain from the acid urine touching the ulcer. It may be necessary to place a urethral catheter in order to avoid urinary retention (Chapter 40). When herpes simplex recurs it is always in the same area and on the same side. It is usually unilateral. The diagnosis is established by culture of the ulceration. After a few weeks the blood test for type-specific herpes simplex type 2 antibody develops. Thus if the blood test is negative and the culture is positive it indicates a recent primary infection. Herpes simplex ulcer increases the susceptibility to HIV (AIDS) (Fig. 7.36).

Recurrent herpes of the vulva and perineum may have an atypical fissure appearance.

Herpes zoster

This usually causes a characteristic unilateral chest rash along the costal nerves. It occasionally affects other parts of the body including the vulva, the face, and eyes.

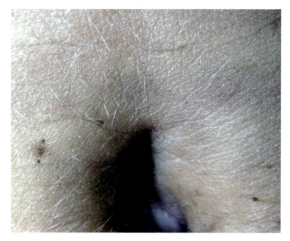

Figure 7.37 Pediculosis pubis in a child. Most cases are seen in the adolescent pubic hair. The body and claws are visible on the patient's right. The nits (eggs) are on the left near the base of the hair.

Pediculosis pubis

Pediculosis pubis (pubic lice, crabs) may be sexually transmitted but in the young patient it can be transmitted in an innocent fashion. If a child goes to camp and has pediculosis pubis (pubic lice) then a week later the whole camp may have it because of interchange of blankets, pajamas, towels, underwear, etc. It has a 90% attack rate after sexual activity or close contact. The diagnosis is made with a good light and some magnification. The louse has prominent claws which look like a dark dot. The nits (very tiny eggs) are attached to the base of hairs (Figs 7.37, 7.38). It causes pruritus.

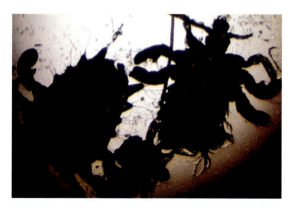

Figure 7.38 Pediculosis pubis, 100x.

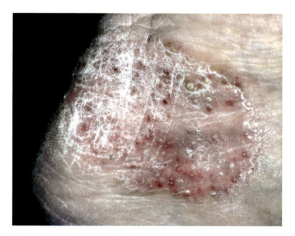

Figure 7.39 Psoriasis on the elbow.

Scabies

Scabies causes intense itching and tends to involve the inner surface of finger web spaces, wrist and pubic areas. It has a tendency to occur in refugee groups where people have been living in a small confined area such as a boat that has been at sea for a long time. The diagnosis is made by scraping the erythematous lines and examining the scrapings under a low-power microscope.

Tinea cruris

Tinea cruris is a dermatophyte infection of the groin promoted by moisture, heat, rubbing of skin surfaces, and obesity.

Psoriasis

Psoriasis is not rare. If it first appears on the general body skin and later appears on the vulva, it is relatively easy to make the diagnosis. The heat, humidity, rubbing of the vulva and exposure to anal area bacteria cause a distortion of the typical lesion which may be seen on the elbows (Fig. 7.39), knees, chest, abdomen (Fig. 7.40), scalp and nails. If psoriasis first appears on the vulva it frustrates the physician because it does not have the characteristic appearance as well as demonstrating resistance to therapy. The biopsy has a characteristic histopathology.

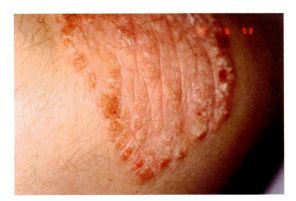

Figure 7.40 Another variant of psoriasis, on the torso.

Behçet syndrome

Although Behçet syndrome is considered rare, it is under-reported because it is not taught. It is not diagnosed, the diagnosis is essentially clinical, and the biopsy is only suggestive of vasculitis. In my select referral practice it is not rare in the adolescent. The diagnosis is suggested by recurrent oral aphthous ulcers, less common vulva ulcers, and inflammatory eye diseases with photophobia and pain. Rarely there are multiple widespread lesions including skin, arthralgias (often only one joint), pericarditis, general vasculitis, immunologic disturbances, neurologic problems, fever, and gastrointestinal complaints.

The acute typical characteristic adolescent picture is frequently a preceding viral infection followed by fever, often up to 102°F. with chills, intense vulva pain, severe swelling of labia minora and majora with acute necrotic, punched-out, deep ulcers with a shaggy necrotic black base, later becoming a necrotic gray purulent color, with sharp, slightly elevated irregular edges (Figs 7.41–7.43). There is often severe vulva dysuria causing

urethral spasm and inability to void. An indwelling catheter is often required. The patient is in agony and screams with pain on walking, sitting or touching the labia. There is a slight dark bloody discharge. Although it has the appearance of severe streptococcus β-hemolytic group A, the cultures are negative, as well as for herpes simplex, other STI and all other diseases. There is usually no inguinal adenopathy and no skin rashes.

The lesions may sometimes recur at intervals of several months, with or without fever. The etiology is unknown. There is no standard therapy for severe cases. Systemic

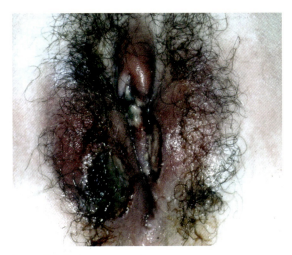

Figure 7.41 Behçet syndrome. Black punched-out ulcer on patient's right labium majus.

cortisone has been used to reduce symptoms. Biopsies are very painful and might require a short general anesthesia. The biopsy should include the edge of the ulcer containing the peripheral normal tissue, as well as the necrotic base,

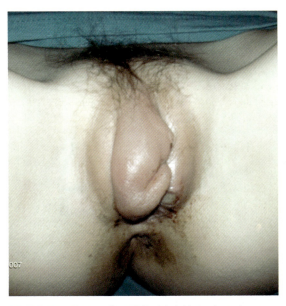

Figure 7.42 Massive swelling of the right labium minora due to underlying medial ulcers. Posterior left labium majus has punched-out gray ulcer seen with raised sharp margins. Courtesy of Dr Chana E. Gelbfish.

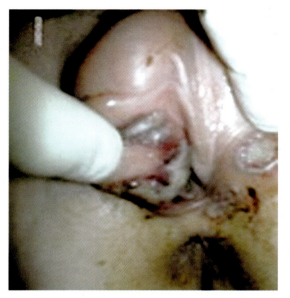

Figure 7.43 Same case as Fig. 7.42. Undersurface of right labium minora with confluent necrotic ulcers; the deepest is anterior near the urethra causing urinary retention. Posterior left labium majus has punched-out ulcer with raised border. Courtesy of Dr Chana E. Gelbfish.

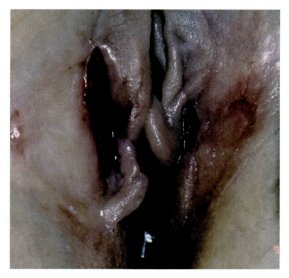

Figure 7.44 Trophic ulcer of the right labium due to congenital spina bifida.

which is least helpful. The biopsy is also studied for various STI or nonspecific infections. There is suggestive vasculitis with round cell perivascular infiltration.

There is usually no preceding trauma, insect bite, sexual activity or viral rash, and no adenopathy.

The patients should be followed up, checking general health, with ophthalmologic examinations at six month intervals or sooner with any symptoms, examination for oral aphthous ulcers (and ruling out confusing herpes simplex virus type 1 which is common in the young patient).

Other factors

Girls born with meningomyelocele of the back resulting in numbness from the waist down may develop trophic ulcer of the vulva (Fig. 7.44).

Vulvodynia (Fig. 7.45) is an extremely sensitive skin reaction, usually at the posterior vestibule just external to the hymen which becomes red and tender to the touch. It develops in late puberty.

Skin infections include impetigo, a superficial infection of staphylococci and/or streptococci, erysipelas, and a superifical cellulitis.

Other sexually transmitted diseases of the vulva include syphilis, chancroid, and lymphogranuloma venereum.

From a psychosomatic viewpoint, the child may discover that by having genital symptoms, people may pay more attention to her (Chapter 13).

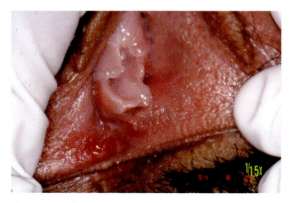

Figure 7.45 Vulvodynia touching posterior vestibule and fourchette causes erythema and irritation.

Quick Take 7.6

Conditions misinterpreted as sexual molestation

- Lichen sclerosus
- Atopic dermatitis
- Trauma from an innocent fall (hymen intact, witnessed, reported immediately)
- Vulva and perianal condyloma (mother had papilloma at birth, caretaker had warts and wiped anal area, negative careful social service investigation).

General principles of management

(Quick Take 7.6, 7.7)

Keep the vulva clean, cool, and dry. Despite what some mothers think, the worst thing which can be done is wash the vulva with hot water and soap.

Stop all topical medications if many have been used in a short time without relief and/or worsening of symptoms. The delicate skin becomes sensitized and they do more harm than good. If needed, prescribe an oral antihistamine to reduce itching and calm the skin, especially with the overactive child with general skin itching. It may be taken at night. Sometimes vulvitis causes sleepiness and disturbs school work.

Although manufacturers praise the disposable diaper as keeping the skin dry, the outer layer is plastic which acts as a barrier for heat and humidity. This irritates the skin, promotes maceration and skin fissures, and increases irritation and infection. Diapers should be frequently examined and changed immediately when soiled. If feasible, let the infant remain without a diaper over a protected mattress for 10–15 minutes after cleaning for aeration and cooling.

Leotards, panty-hose, and tight slacks cause a local increase of heat and humidity as well as binding and chafing. The ideal clothing is loosely fitting white cotton underwear and a dress or skirt. Old-fashioned garter belts can be used to hold up long stockings. In cold weather loose "leggings" can be used when outdoors for warmth but promptly removed when indoors.

Children taking ballet lessons or gymnastics wear tight, nonabsorbent outfits, causing adverse effects. This is compounded by sitting in perspiration-soaked clothing during a rest period which may also trigger recurrent buttock pustules (which I call "ballet dancer's bottom") [4] by exposure to bacteria and by rupturing the pustule and spreading it to adjacent skin.

Wearing wet swimsuits for long periods of time (especially with wet sand) when out of the water because of a later second swim is very irritating. Replace the wet suit immediately.

Avoid pajama pants at night. The child should wear nightgowns without underwear to keep the vulva cool and dry. For the same reason avoid excessive blankets (see Quick Take 5).

Rinse underwear carefully to avoid residue soap and detergents and wash it before the first use.

Avoid bubble bath, soaps, perfumed colognes, shaving, waxing or chemicals to get rid of hair. Avoid skin piercing generally.

Avoid wool sweaters which may sensitize the skin of the entire body. Excessive sunburn on the face and arms may also sensitize the skin.

Sensitive skin may also be a clue to food allergies. Another clue is abdominal discomfort, a tympanic abdomen or a tender palpable ascending or sigmoid colon. Skin tests for allergies are unpleasant and might not always help. Alert the mother to general signs of sensitive skin or simply inspect the vulva for inflammation and have her keep a diary of when the skin or vulva flares up and any unusual food eaten or clothing worn the day before. This should be done after birthday parties when children eat special treats such as shrimps, shellfish, chocolate, nuts, sausages, etc. Sometimes children react to common foods such as wheat, eggs, fruits, milk, and orange juice and may have a perioral rash.

Be cautious about letting the child play in contaminated sand boxes, lie directly on grass or walk through bushes to

Quick Take 7.7

Management of acute vulvitis

- Stop all topical medications especially if many have been used in a short time
- Avoid hot water and soap
- Avoid tights, leotards, panty-hose, pajama pants
- Avoid wool
- Recommend sitz baths with tepid water and colloidal oatmeal

avoid insect bites, irritating plants, exposure to pesticides or animal droppings.

Anything which disturbs the general health or causes severe anxiety will have an adverse effect on skin, including hepatitis or unusual medication.

If feasible, the child should be gently and carefully bathed briefly twice daily with warm water and a minimum of mild unscented soap, "soapless soap" or colloidal oatmeal sitz bath. Even if the child thinks she is able to bathe herself, she should be supervised by the mother for cleansing (from front to back) of the grooves of either side of the labia majora and minora, the perineum (between the rectum and vagina) and the perianal area. The skin is gently blotted dry, rather than rubbed, and allowed to further air dry. With severe irritation, the area may be cleansed with bland vegetable oil on a cotton ball. As the skin is drying, gently apply an emollient cream or ointment to the body skin to keep moisture in the skin, especially for dry skin and atopic dermatitis. For acute inflammation for the first two days, one might consider wet compresses or sitz baths for 5–10 minutes at four-hour intervals using cool water or saline. Primary nonspecific vulvitis is usually mild and usually responds to the above simple regime of good hygiene and avoiding irritation. If the condition is persistent, recurring or severe then re-evaluation or consultation should be considered.

Children with AD are susceptible to many skin infections, especially with staphylococcus and streptococcus, which increase pruritus and may be a cause for failure of therapy. An oral antibiotic may be helpful. Other reasons for failure of therapy are unrecognized diabetes mellitus or immunologic deficiency.

In case of a terrorist emergency vaccination for smallpox, AD patients may develop extensive skin infections from cowpox vaccination.

It may be necessary to prescribe topical corticosteroids for vulvitis. These should be used in small amounts once daily and try to avoid using them for more than two weeks. For intensely acute pruritic lesions try an ointment rather than cream medication which may cause stinging. Creams are used with less acute situations. Lichen sclerosus may require potent corticosteroids (Chapters 35, 36).

The vulval skin may become lichenified from long-term scratching, and biopsy will confuse the diagnosis.

Topical tacrolimus and pimecrolimus have been used with results equal to corticosteroids for AD; however, there is concern about induction of malignancy.

References

1. Paller AS, Mancini AJ. *Hurwitz Clinical Pediatric Dermatology*, 3rd edn. Philadelphia: Elsevier Saunders, 2000.
2. Altchek A. The subacute state of vulva atopic dermatitis. *J Pediatr Adolesc Gynecol* 2007;**20**(2):S131.
3. Ramer MA, Altchek A, Deligdisch L et al. Lichen Planus and the vulvovaginal-gingival syndrome. *J Peridontol* 2003;**74**:1385–1393.
4. Altchek A. Pediatric vulvovaginitis. *Pediatr Clin North Am* 1972;**3**:557–580.

CHAPTER 8

Vaginal Bleeding in the Child

Albert Altchek

Mount Sinai School of Medicine and Hospital, New York, NY, USA

Introduction

Statistics on the incidence and causes of vaginal bleeding depend on patient selection bias, whether it be from the emergency room, referral clinic or private practice. There is a misconception that the leading cause is precocious puberty, based on reports of select referral institutions.

Most prepubertal vaginal bleeding is a result of local causes (Box 8.1) most of which can be discovered by history, examination, and vaginoscopy (Quick Take 8.1). With true central nervous system precocious puberty bleeding, there is the same sequence of normal puberty events including rapid linear growth and sexual development preceding menstruation, but at an earlier age than usual. In addition, there is an estrogenic, midvaginal cytology with increased superficial cells, and elevated serum gonadotropin and estradiol. With nonendocrine local cause vaginal bleeding, there are no physical signs of puberty, the vaginal cytology has mainly parabasal anestrogenic and some intermediate cells, and a local cause is found on examination.

These observations may reduce the need to perform some preliminary, anxiety-provoking investigations for precocious puberty such as brain scans, x-rays for bone age, and hormone tests. Even if the presumed diagnosis is precocious puberty, it is reasonable to do a vaginoscopy to rule out a coexisting local cause of bleeding.

Menstruation has been starting at earlier ages in the past 100 years, but has now leveled off at about age $12^{1}/_{2}$ in the USA. In some families it may begin earlier. At present in

---

Box 8.1 Local nonhormonal causes of bleeding

Trauma

A. Innocent accidents
B. Types of injuries
C. Management
D. Suspicion of molestation
E. Scratching

Severe vaginal infections

A. Group A β-hemolytic streptococcus
B. Rare geographic endemic shigella, schistosomiasis, amebiasis

Vulvar lesions

A. Severe nonspecific vulvitis with scratching and denudation
B. Specific skin lesions
   1. Atopic and seborrheic dermatitis, psoriasis, candidiasis
   2. Rare congenital vaginal and uterine pelvic cavernous venous sinuses
   3. Condylomata acuminata
   4. Lichen sclerosus
   5. Ulcers: herpes, syphilis, chancroid, Behçet syndrome
   6. Polyps of hymen
   7. Rare coagulation defect in association with skin and mucous membrane bleeding
   8. Prolapsed urethra presenting as vaginal bleeding
   9. Rare vaginal and uterine tumors

Foreign bodies in vagina

A. Wads of toilet tissue
B. "Arrowhead" shaped plastic bottle caps
C. Trapped pinworms

---

the USA, menstruation is considered a variation of normal at the age of ten or older. At the onset of menstruation only about half are ovulating and therefore half are at risk for irregular anovulatory dysfunctional bleeding which may present a diagnostic challenge in the young patient (Chapter 23).

Usual local causes of vaginal bleeding

Trauma is the leading cause. An acute situation may require urgent consultation or referral. When the child is first seen with bright red bleeding following trauma there is a tendency to watch and wait in the hope that the bleeding will stop spontaneously. This is not a good policy. It requires expert care. Children do not tolerate blood loss well. If there is active bleeding or if small to medium amounts of bleeding continue after about 5 minutes despite a cold compress to the vulva, consider taking the child to the operating room and using general anesthesia. The anesthetist must be alerted to the possibility of a recent meal. Prior to surgery, if possible have the child void as a test of bladder integrity. It is helpful to have good lighting, such as a combination headlight with an optical loop device, good assistance and appropriate instruments for the narrow child's vagina, including retractors and irrigation. The simplest and most generally available instrument is a miniature Graves bivalve vaginal speculum with a narrow blade of appropriate length (Chapter 6). It gives adjustable exposure with the ability to use a slender alligator grasping forceps. If possible, have a small 1–2 mm cup punch biopsy for suspicious lesions. Suturing high in the vagina may be difficult. Monopolar electrocoagulation may cause injury to adjacent bladder or bowel. Harmonic ultrasound forceps may be used for grasping and coagulation. Visualization of the source of major bleeding is necessary for homeostasis. Catheterize the bladder for residual or bloody urine.

Carefully inspect the entire vagina and do a rectal examination for rectovaginal laceration. Is there a tear through the vaginal vault into the peritoneal cavity? If so, laparoscopy or laparotomy may be needed to inspect and

repair bowel injury. After excising necrotic tissue, fine absorbable sutures are used to repair bladder, vaginal and rectal tissues in layers. Antibiotics and tetanus prevention should be considered (Chapter 10). Rectal tears with contamination usually heal well with irrigation, excision of necrotic tissue, and prompt meticulous surgery.

Occasionally there is severe blunt trauma without external bleeding and a few days later there is a gush of old dark blood from the vagina. Vaginoscopy can reveal spontaneous rupture of a pelvic hematoma through the vaginal wall.

Try to get a careful history of what happened. If there was an accident, was it witnessed? Where did it occur? Running on the wet edge of a slippery swimming pool may cause a fall and straddle injury on the sharp pool edge. There may be vaginal water sport injuries from a water slide, a fall from a water-ski or jet-ski, from a high pressure water jet or a water chute. Children like to climb to reach objects and therefore may fall, resulting in a vulvar hematoma over the pelvic bones and perineal laceration. The hymen remains intact. Sometimes a narrow object such as a broomstick or chair leg may penetrate into the vagina, causing a laceration. Small, nonprogressive vulvar hematomas are best left alone. Surgery is reserved for large expanding hematomas with the hope of finding and ligating a bleeding vessel and removing the clots. Unfortunately such a vessel is not often identified.

Accidental injury is more common than molestation. With the former, there is prompt reporting by the mother and patient, and a clear history. The injury was usually witnessed by the mother or other responsible persons and the findings are consistent with the history.

Severe vaginal infections

Group A β-hemolytic streptococcus is the most frequent cause of a specific bacterial infection causing vaginal bleeding. Vaginoscopy reveals a severe inflammation of the upper vaginal walls and posterior fornix with extensive diffuse petechial hemorrhage in the thin mucosa. There is no specific vessel to treat. It occurs in young children via contaminated hands. Diagnosis is by vaginal culture.

Bleeding may also occur with other severe vaginitis such as acute gonorrhea, and in other geographic areas (shigella, schistosomiasis, and amebiasis), as with foreign body vaginitis.

Vulvar lesions

These may bleed spontaneously, after rubbing or with scratching. They include lichen sclerosus, seborrheic and atopic dermatitis, psoriasis, allergic contact vulvitis, vulva candidiasis, herpes simplex, scabies, bacterial skin infections, and hemangiomas (Chapters 7, 35).

Foreign bodies in the vagina

Foreign bodies cause a persistent, foul-smelling, dark bloody discharge from the vagina and a secondary vulvitis. Most foreign bodies are rolled-up wads of toilet tissue which cannot be discovered by rectal examination, pelvic ultrasound or x-ray. They remain high in the posterior fornix. Soft foreign bodies begin to bleed about two weeks after insertion (Chapters 7, 13). There is always a psychodrama when the diagnosis is made (Chapters 7, 13).

Metallic foreign bodies (hair pins) or hard plastic narrow bottle caps may be felt on rectal examination and may cause bright red bleeding on insertion and when eroding into a vessel. These can be palpated on rectal examination and may be detected by sonography. Try to avoid x-rays. Some plastic objects cause profuse vaginal granulation tissue simulating a malignant neoplasm.

Pinworms searching to return to the rectum may get lost in the vagina and act as foreign bodies. A good headlight with an optical loop is necessary for discovery.

Children in diapers cannot insert foreign bodies into the vagina but older children put small objects in any body openings – ears, nose, mouth, and vagina. Adolescents forget vaginal tampons, resulting in discharge of foul-smelling dark blood.

Polyps of the hymen may hide in the vagina or come out to a length of 2–3 cm over the perineum. They are usually benign and present at birth. When everted, they may be bruised by clothing and bleed. Polyps which originate above the hymen require excision to rule out rhabdomyosarcoma (Chapters 37, 49) (Figs 8.1–8.3).

Prolapsed urethra presenting as vaginal bleeding

In large, inner-city emergency rooms urethral prolapse is a leading cause of pediatric vaginal bleeding. The prolapsed urethra is an acute, painful, swollen, frightening, bleed-

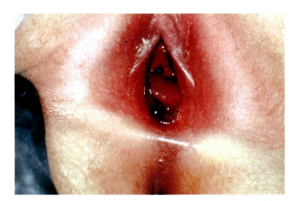

Figure 8.1 Small rhabdomyosarcoma simulating a benign vaginal polyp. The base is above the hymen. The surface is normal vaginal mucosa and a simple superficial surface biopsy is not adequate. The malignancy forms under the mucosa. It had caused vaginal staining for three days in a six-year-old child. The mass moved in and out with coughing.

ing friable mass about 2–3 cm in diameter resembling a malignancy at the introitus (Fig. 8.4). Diagnosis is made by gently passing a urethral catheter through a central umbilicalization into the bladder and elevating the prolapsed urethra to expose and probe the vagina with a wet applicator stick. Most cases are managed by sitz baths and topical estrogen cream with gradual improvement over several weeks. Failure to resolve and/or recurrent pain or bleeding may require surgery. Resection is probably the best surgical procedure but must be done cautiously. The temptation is to pull down and resect too much urethral

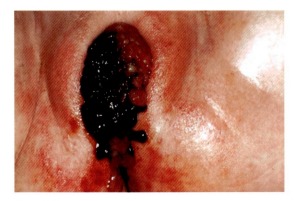

Figure 8.2 Large rhabdomyosarcoma protruding from the vagina. The right side of the tumor is necrotic because of torsion. Age 11 months, sudden protrusion when straining at stool.

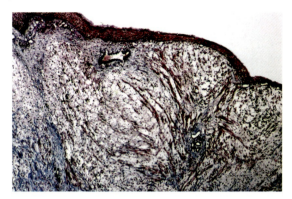

Figure 8.3 Histologic view of Fig. 8.2. The surface is normal vaginal mucosa. The malignancy is submucosal and the entire polyp must be removed for diagnosis.

mucosa which when released moves up into the urethra and leaves a raw surface which becomes stenotic as it heals. Another procedure is a tight ligature over the lesion on an indwelling urethral bladder catheter (Quick Take 8.2).

Vaginal cultures are nonspecific for vaginal trauma, vulva lesions, foreign bodies, and prolapsed urethra. There are many types of organisms, often from the anus, as secondary invaders. When the foreign body is removed the vaginitis will clear even without antibiotics.

Rare causes of vaginal bleeding

There are rare coagulation defects. The most common inherited bleeding disorder is von Willebrand disease

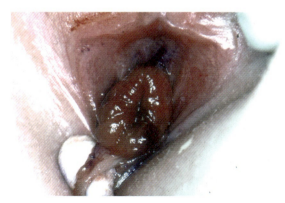

Figure 8.4 Subacute prolapsed urethra, small congenital band at 7 o'clock being held by application stick. The swollen urethra resembles and may conceal the vagina.

> **Quick Take 8.2**
>
> **Common local causes of vaginal bleeding**
>
> - Trauma
> - Severe vaginitis
> - Vulva lesions
> - Vaginal foreign body
> - Urethral prolapse

(vWd). It usually manifests as severe menorrhagia (heavy menses at regular intervals) in adolescence. In the prepubertal child there may be mucocutaneous bleeding (epistaxis, oral, rectal, vaginal), petechiae and prolonged bleeding after trauma. The disease is difficult to diagnose and may require various blood tests, including factor VIII which may have to be repeated (Chapter 23). Estrogen therapy, as with oral contraceptives, can disguise vWd by increasing vW factor. There is often a family history of bleeders. There is a rare acquired vWd.

Other coagulation problems include hemophilia factor XI deficiency and platelet function disorders. The most frequent acquired pediatric bleeding disorder is idiopathic thrombocytopenic purpura (ITP) due to antiplatelet antibodies. Acute lymphoblastic leukemia (ALL) may initially present as lethargy, exhaustion and anorexia, followed by anemia, bleeding tendency, infections, adenopathy, hepatosplenomegaly, and joint pain. The peak incidence is between age two and five. There may be an initial normal complete blood count (CBC), and a blood smear and a bone marrow may be required.

Rhabdomyosarcoma is a rare but aggressive vaginal neoplasm (see Figs 8.1–8.3). It usually presents as a protruding mass and/or vaginal bleeding. Since the neoplasm is submucosal (mesenchymal) initially the surface mucosa is normal vaginal mucosa and resembles a benign vaginal polyp. The clinical clue is the fact that the base is in the vagina (usually high in the anterior wall). Polyps of the hymen are usually benign, although they may bleed if traumatized (Chapter 25).

Rhabdomyosarcoma occurs in the young child about age 11 months. If there is concern about the diagnosis (cytology is not reliable) the child should be examined under general anesthesia with an experienced anesthesiologist by an experienced surgeon and the entire mass should be removed. A shallow biopsy may simply show normal vaginal mucosa.

In addition, the histologic diagnosis requires several types of cells. At the same time, if feasible, there should be a cystoscopy and possible biopsy of the bladder adjacent to the high anterior vaginal wall to detect spread.

Prior to chemotherapy most cases were fatal within two years, unless an early pelvic exenteration was performed. With current chemotherapy there is a reverse prognosis in early cases with the vast majority being cured with only local resection and chemotherapy. These cases are rare and require expert care and follow-up.

Rarely, in the older child there may be rhabdomyosarcoma (Chapters 37, 49).

Vaginal (midline) germ cell tumors in the upper vagina are very rare. We saw an 11-month-old child who had experienced mild vaginal bleeding for about 12 days. Rectal examination and pelvic ultrasound showed a 4 cm tumor which simulated a cervical tumor. MRI showed retroperitoneal abdominal node enlargement. In the operating room we examined the upper vagina and took adequate biopsies for frozen section which confirmed the diagnosis. Then the hematologist did a bone marrow examination for metastasis, a urologist did a cystoscopy (which was negative), and a pediatric surgeon placed a Broviac vascular port catheter for chemotherapy which was started in two days. The vaginal tumor disappeared. The retroperitoneal enlarged nodes persisted on MRI. Later a laparotomy revealed necrotic tumor. The child was apparently cured but is being followed.

A team approach is helpful for select malignancy and anomalies surgery so that multiple procedures can be done with the initial surgery, thereby avoiding several trips to the operating room with repeated general anesthesia.

First case report of xanthogranuloma of the vagina

Our group reported the first case of xanthogranuloma of the vagina [1]. Despite benign histology, this condition requires extremely careful follow-up. Our case was in a 5-year-old who had three brief episodes of dark vaginal bleeding. Vaginoscopy revealed a 1.7 cm granulomatous friable tumor in the left fornix and adjacent left cervix. It was completely removed by multiple biopsies. The pathology report was squamous mucosa with extensive benign chronic xanthogranuloma inflammation, most likely due to a subacute infectious process. The biopsies of the underlining fat, presumably extraperitoneal, were negative. The slides were reviewed at Johns Hopkins and reported as benign fibrous histiocytoma lesion (juvenile xanthogranuloma is an uncommon non-Langerhans cell histiocytosis). There was no further vaginal bleeding and the patient remained asymptomatic. Several months later an MRI showed a 3.8×2.0 solid mass on the left side of the uterus and vagina. At another hospital, preliminary vaginoscopy was negative. Laparotomy revealed a $5 \times 5 \times 2$ cm yellow homogenous retroperitoneal mass at the junction of the uterus and vagina and the ureter had to be dissected out. The pathology was benign fibrous histiocytoma. Short-term follow-up was negative. Such cases must be carefully observed.

The closest case report was in a 30-year-old woman with a 13 cm solid lesion in the rectovaginal septum separate from the vaginal wall which had been slowly growing for 7 years [2].

Rare endocrine bleeding posing as nonendocrine bleeding

Infrequently endocrine bleeding (premature menarche) may begin without physical signs of puberty. The clinical clue is that the midvaginal swab maturation index cytology is estrogenic because the vaginal mucosa is very sensitive to estrogen (superficial and intermediate vaginal cytology increases and can be identified by an immediate unstained wet smear). Parabasal cells indicate lack of estrogen. The mechanism is a sudden, brief, premature spurt of serum estrogen. Isolated premature menarche bleeding may cause one or more episodes of bleeding without physical signs of puberty. It is usually self-limiting and benign but patients should be carefully followed and pelvic ultrasound may be performed.

In McCune-Albright syndrome the first clinical sign may be vaginal bleeding prior to development of breasts, pubic and axillary hair. The diagnosis is made by the characteristic café-au-lait skin pigmentation and polyostotic fibrous dysplasia of bone. Secondary sex development occurs later. The mechanism is an independent functional ovarian cyst producing estrogen. The serum follicle-stimulating hormone is low.

Small estrogen-secreting ovarian neoplasms (granulosa cell tumor) may also cause bleeding before physical signs of puberty. They may be felt on rectal examination and can be imaged by pelvic ultrasound (Chapters 41, 47).

Prepubertal bleeding can be caused by prolonged, untreated hypothyroidism. This causes a marked increase in thyroid-stimulating hormone. Sometimes, the overactive anterior pituitary stimulates prolactin secretion, causing breast enlargement, galactorrhea and an enlarged sella turcica. There may also be an increase of follicle-stimulating hormone stimulating ovarian follicular cysts.

There is no pubertal growth spurt or pubic or axillary hair. The bone age is delayed.

Accidental estrogen ingestion (such as OC) may cause vaginal bleeding without pubertal development (Quick Take 8.3).

References

1. Altchek A, Brovender B, Green I et al. The first case report of xanthogranuloma of the prepubertal vagina. *J Pediatr Adolesc Gynecol* 2006;**19**(2):158–159.
2. Gidwani GP, Ballard LA Jr, Jelden GL, Lavery IC. Xanthogranuloma of the vagina. *Cleve Clin Q* 1979;**46**(4):163–166.

Further reading

Altchek A. Nonendocrine vaginal bleeding. In: Lifshitz F (ed) *Pediatric Endocrinology*, 4th edn. New York: Marcel Dekker, 2003: 257–276.

CHAPTER 9

Ovarian Cysts in the Fetus, Infant, and Child

Robert A. Cusick[1] *& Marc S. Arkovitz*[2]

[1]Children's Hospital of Omaha, University of Nebraska Medical Center, Omaha, NE, USA
[2]Columbia University, New York, NY, USA

Introduction

Ovarian cysts were once thought to be rare during childhood. Historically, an abdominal mass in a female led to the diagnosis of an ovarian cyst. Because symptoms led to the diagnosis, the percentage that required intervention was formerly very high. With the increased use of ultrasound during pregnancy, the documented incidence has greatly increased. With earlier and more frequent diagnosis, the questions of which cysts require intervention and the timing of intervention have been raised.

Fetal ovarian cysts

In utero diagnosis of ovarian cysts has increased with the widespread use of prenatal ultrasonography. Autopsy findings demonstrate an incidence of 32%. Most of these cysts are small (1 cm or less) and not clinically significant. Large ovarian cysts are less common, with an incidence of about 1 in 2500 live births.

Etiology

Ovarian tissue arises from three distinct areas of the embryo: the mesenchyme of the urogenital ridge, the germinal epithelium of the urogenital ridge, and the germ cells of the yolk sac. The germ cells proliferate during the

Pediatric, Adolescent, & Young Adult Gynecology. Edited by
A. Altchek and L. Deligdisch. © 2009 Blackwell Publishing,
ISBN: 978-1-4051-5347-8.

sixth week of gestation. Granulosa cells of the germinal epithelium surround the oocytes from the 20th to the 26th weeks, forming follicles. The theca, arising from the mesenchyme of the urogenital ridge, then surrounds the follicle. These follicles are constantly undergoing maturation and involution from early fetal life until menopause. In the fetus, follicles develop from hormonal stimulation in the setting of an immature hypothalamus-pituitary-ovarian axis. Stimulation is from fetal pituitary gonadotropins (luteinizing hormone (LH) and follicle-stimulating hormone (FSH)), maternal estrogens, and placental human chorionic gonadotropin (hCG). Proof of the role of maternal/placental hormonal stimulation as the etiology of ovarian cysts is suggested by the frequent regression of neonatal cysts soon after delivery.

Fetal ovarian cysts are associated with maternal diabetes, isoimmunization, fetal hypothyroidism, and prematurity. Patients with maternal diabetes and Rh isoimmunization have increased placental chorionic gonadotropins. Fetal hypothyroidism causes increased thyroid-stimulating hormone levels which are thought to cause nonspecific stimulation of the fetal pituitary. Premature infants have an immature hypothalamus-pituitary-ovarian axis which may allow prolonged elevation of LH and FSH. Ovarian cysts do not have a genetic predilection and are not associated with other fetal anomalies.

Diagnosis

Ovarian cysts are most commonly diagnosed by ultrasound during the third trimester of pregnancy. It is rare to identify these cysts prior to 20 weeks gestation. The differential diagnosis of cystic structures in the abdomen

Quick Take 9.1

Fetal ovarian cysts

Ovarian cysts are found in 32% of fetuses but are usually small and do not require intervention. Stimulation of the cysts comes from:

- Fetal pituitary gonadotropins
- Maternal estrogens
- Placental hCG

Risk factors for fetal ovarian cysts

- Maternal diabetes
- Isoimmunization
- Fetal hypothyroidism
- Prematurity

Diagnostic criteria for fetal ovarian cysts

- Female gender
- Cystic structure off midline
- Normal urinary tract
- Normal gastrointestinal tract

Complications of fetal ovarian cysts reported in the literature

- Torsion
- Dystocia
- Hemorrhage
- Bowel obstruction
- Rupture with peritonitis
- Pulmonary hypoplasia
- Polyhydramnios

Some advocate aspiration of all fetal ovarian cysts greater than 5 cm. However, many of these will resolve without intervention and the literature does not support aspiration as the standard of care.

Malignancy is not part of the differential for cystic structures of the ovary in infants. Both cystic and complex cysts should therefore be followed monthly by ultrasound until they resolve.

is lengthy: intestinal duplications, duodenal atresia, hydrometrocolpus, hydronephrosis, bladder distension, cystic meconium peritonitis, intestinal obstruction, lymphangioma, mesenteric cysts, omental cysts, renal cysts, choledochal cysts, liver cysts, anterior meningomyelocele, and urachal cysts. Intestinal duplications can be the most difficult to distinguish from an ovarian cyst. Diagnostic

criteria for an ovarian cyst include: female gender; cystic structure off the midline, identification of a normal urinary tract, identification of a normal gastrointestinal tract. Often, the diagnosis is only confirmed after delivery, with additional imaging studies or surgical intervention. Clinically significant cysts are identified in 1 in 2500 live births. Small ovarian cysts may be found in up to 98% of patients, with only 20% larger than 9 mm. Cysts larger than 2 cm are generally considered pathologic. The appearance and size are the most important factors in determining intervention. Simple cysts are anechoic. Complex cysts may be filled with debris, and have septae or solid components. Complex cysts identified *in utero* indicate torsion.

The question of excluding malignancy is often raised. In the literature, there is only one report of malignancy in a stillborn at 30 weeks. Tapper reported the largest series of immature teratomas at a single institution and found the youngest patient to be 13 months [1]. Concern about malignancy in a prenatally diagnosed ovarian cyst is not an indication for surgical intervention.

Natural history

Most (50–90%) prenatally diagnosed simple ovarian cysts will resolve in the first three months after delivery. FSH and LH increase at birth in response to decreased maternal estrogens and peak at the third month. After the third to fourth month, gonadotropin levels decrease as the hypothalamus-pituitary-ovarian axis matures. This drop in hormonal stimulation leads to resolution of the ovarian cysts.

As mentioned, a significant percentage of fetal ovarian cysts will undergo spontaneous resolution. Heling reported that 28% of 64 ovarian cysts diagnosed *in utero* spontaneously resolved *in utero* [2]. He documented that another 35% resolved soon after delivery. However, a significant percentage of fetal ovarian cysts can also undergo torsion with loss of the ovary. Reported rates of torsion are 20–30%, although some have reported numbers as high as 78%. The principal risk factor for torsion discussed in the literature is size as well as a long pedicle for the ovary. Cyst size is easier to identify and study by ultrasound. Large ovarian cysts have been documented to torse more frequently than small cysts. Following *in utero* torsion, the entire ovary can become disconnected, leaving a free-floating cyst in the abdomen. Bilateral *in utero* torsion with subsequent free-floating cysts has been described. Normal ovaries have also been reported to torse

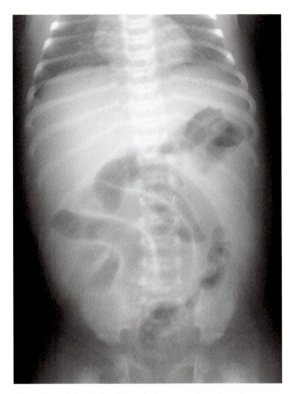

Figure 9.1 Abdominal radiograph demonstrating a bowel obstruction in an infant female presenting with emesis.

in the setting of a long vascular pedicle. Generally, torsion is thought to occur prenatally rather than after birth. Most ovaries that torse are not salvageable. For this reason, some argue that interventions aimed at preserving future fertility should involve *in utero* intervention.

Other complications reported are rare. Dystocia, hemorrhage, rupture with peritonitis, bowel obstruction (Fig. 9.1), and incarceration in a hernia sac have all been reported in isolated cases. Concern has been raised about large cysts causing *in utero* pressure on the diaphragm with resultant pulmonary hypoplasia or polyhydramnios. Polyhydramnios has been described in up to 18% of patients. It is thought to result from partial bowel obstruction secondary to mass effect by the cyst. Obstruction of ureters has also been suggested as a complication from large ovarian cysts.

The long-term sequelae after loss of an ovary in infancy are unknown. Longitudinal studies after oophorectomy document fertility rates similar to those for women with two ovaries. Animal studies suggest some compensation in the contralateral ovary within weeks after oophorectomy. However, fertility clinics demonstrate an increased number of women with one ovary compared to the general population (17% compared to 5.5%). Therefore, the literature is not definitive about decreased fertility after loss of an ovary from *in utero* torsion.

Management

Most recommend following cysts every two weeks with ultrasound as long as they decrease in size. Decisions about intervention primarily are related to future fertility of the fetus. As mentioned, malignancy is virtually unheard of in fetal ovarian cysts. Other complications of ovarian cysts (dystocia, hemorrhage, rupture with peritonitis, and bowel obstruction) are extremely rare. Management therefore is geared toward prevention of torsion. Obviously, this is balanced with the risk of interventions to the mother and the fetus.

Complex cysts are generally straightforward. The majority have already torsed at the time of diagnosis and are not salvageable. They are at low risk for malignancy and for causing other complications. These can be watched until delivery, followed by postnatal ultrasonography. After delivery, most have traditionally recommended resection of complex cysts. The indication for intervention after delivery is to confirm the diagnosis (rule out malignancy or a duplication) and prevent other complications (bowel obstruction from adherence to the inflamed ovary). Further postnatal management of complicated ovarian cysts will be discussed below.

Simple cysts are more controversial. Larger cysts are considered at greater risk of torsion. In general, there are two schools of thought. Some advocate aspiration of all cysts 5 cm or greater *in utero*. *In utero* aspiration has been described as a safe and effective procedure. Those who advocate this approach state it can be done with minimal complications and is associated with higher ovarian salvage compared to controls without intervention. Crombleholme has reported two patients aspirated without any complications to the fetus or the mother [3]. There were no recurrences and he demonstrated preservation of the ovaries. Based on his limited numbers, he recommends the following criteria for prenatal aspiration: ovarian cyst up to 4 cm, rapid cyst enlargement (1 cm/wk), a wandering ovarian cyst (suggesting a long pedicle). Other authors have also suggested sending the cyst fluid for estradiol, progesterone, and testosterone tests to confirm the ovarian origin of the fluid. Giorlandino recommends *in utero* aspiration if the cyst is greater than 5 cm [4]. In a series of 41 fetuses, he demonstrated that cysts which went on to complication (5.7 cm) were significantly larger than cysts that went on to resolve (3.8 cm). In his series, four patients underwent *in utero* aspiration without complication or recurrence. Perrotin has described aspirating cysts <4 cm *in utero* without complication [5]. He points out other studies questioning the 5 cm benchmark as increased risk of torsion, and instead recommends 3 cm. Bagolan reported 14 cases of *in utero* aspiration without complications [6]. Only two of these patients subsequently underwent ovarian torsion with loss of the ovary. Historic controls from the same group showed a torsion rate of 11/13.

Others recommend expectant management with intervention only if there are concerns of hydrops secondary to mass effect or concerns about delivery. As Perrotin points out, if the size is not a clear indicator of torsion risk, what cysts are safe to follow [5]? If the indications broaden, this will increase the number of procedural complications. As Perrotin states: "Aspiration carries a risk of rupture of membranes, bleeding, intrauterine infection, and premature labor" [5]. The benefits of ovarian salvage do not justify such risks. There is also concern about cyst recurrence after aspiration in the setting of ongoing hormonal stimulation, bleeding into the cyst, aspiration of an intestinal duplication, or induction of labor. In Crombleholme's series, one patient thought to have an ovarian cyst was followed and later found to have a cloacal malformation instead [3]. Also, 14% of Bagolan's patients required an operation at birth [6]. In other words, the cyst required two invasive procedures.

In conclusion, the literature is not clear on the role of *in utero* aspiration. Risks and benefits need to be discussed with the family. The experience of the interventionalist must also be factored into the decision. The theoretic decrease in fertility of the fetus must be weighed against the immediate risk to the fetus and mother. A conservative approach is indicated. Intervention should be reserved for bilateral large cysts or polyhydramnios. Intervention based solely on size is not supported in the literature.

Delivery recommendations

The majority of fetal ovarian cysts are small and therefore do not affect delivery considerations. Cysts up to 11 cm

in size have been safely delivered vaginally. If the cyst is large enough to warrant concern about mode of delivery, it is also at risk of affecting pulmonary development and warrants prenatal aspiration. Presence of an ovarian cyst is not an indication for a cesarean section.

Ovarian cysts in infancy

Presentation

Most cysts in this age group are diagnosed by ultrasound *in utero*. Most infants are asymptomatic. If not diagnosed *in utero*, patients most frequently present with a painless abdominal mass. Sometimes, in the setting of autoamputation after torsion, the infant may present with a wandering abdominal mass. Large cysts can cause respiratory distress, emesis or discomfort, although this is unusual. Peritoneal signs are associated with cyst rupture. An inflammatory reaction to the cyst wall can cause a bowel obstruction (Fig. 9.2) or peritonitis. Rarely, there can be a spontaneous bleed into a cyst causing hemorrhagic shock.

Management

The management of ovarian cysts in infancy is controversial, and depends on size, ultrasound characteristics (simple or complex), and whether the cyst is symptomatic. In cases of diagnostic dilemma, laparoscopic exploration is indicated for diagnostic and therapeutic reasons (Fig. 9.3). All symptomatic cysts require intervention.

Most small (<5 cm) ovarian cysts require serial ultrasounds until resolution is demonstrated. Initially these can be every two weeks with decreasing frequency as the cyst resolves. If the cysts persist after six months, enlarge or have ultrasound characteristics of a malignancy (very rare), intervention is indicated. Malignancy is rare in this age group, and rarely influences intervention.

For large ovarian cysts (<5 cm), there is more controversy. The traditional recommendation is surgical intervention. This is based on the belief that larger cysts are more likely to cause torsion, and intervention decreases this risk. In addition to large size, the shallow pelvis and long vascular pedicle in infants predispose to torsion.

Others recommend a conservative approach even if the cyst is >5 cm. There are no clear data correlating size and risk of torsion. Even large ovarian cysts have been shown to resolve in numerous series reports. Brandt

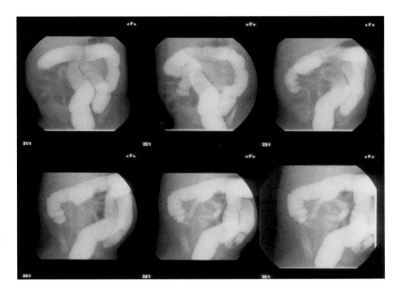

Figure 9.2 Barium enema in the same patient demonstrating a partial obstruction at the terminal ileum. At exploration, the child had adhesions secondary to *in utero* ovarian torsion.

points out that most torsion occurs *in utero* (92%), suggesting that intervention in infancy is less likely to prevent torsion [7]. Also, the most common surgical intervention is oophorectomy, without ovarian preservation. For this reason, if the goal is to preserve the ovary, nonintervention is more likely to be successful. There is no clear

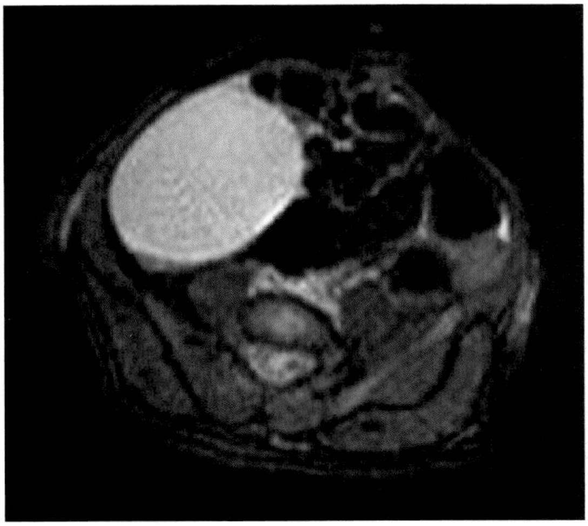

Figure 9.3 MRI performed for an unknown cystic abdominal mass in an infant female. The child was symptomatic (emesis) and the cyst was resected laparoscopically.

evidence that postnatal intervention increases ovarian salvage or, more to the point, increases fertility 20 years in the future.

With regard to complex cysts, historically most authors have recommended resection. Again, malignancy in this age group is not a concern. The youngest reported patient with malignant teratoma was a 14-month infant, although benign teratomas have been described at a younger age.

Recently, some have advocated following even complex cysts. On ultrasound, complex cysts have fluid debris, retracting clot, septae or solid components. These likely represent *in utero* torsion, but could represent hemorrhage into the cyst which will be self-limiting. Luzzatto reported following 27 neonates after a prenatal diagnosis of an ovarian cyst [8]. Two were aspirated and three were operated on by surgeon choice. The remaining 20 were followed, including 13 complex cysts. Three complex cysts which did not resolve required surgery. During long-term follow-up, all nine patients with simple cysts and two of ten with complex cysts demonstrated two normal ovaries on long-term follow-up. Similar success, in terms of both safety and survival of the ovary, has been reported by others.

Complex cysts can therefore be followed if they fulfill the following criteria: the cyst is clearly ovarian in origin, there is no solid component, the α-fetoprotein (AFP) and

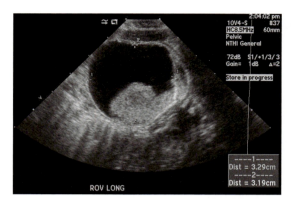

Figure 9.4 Ultrasound with the typical findings of a complex ovarian cyst in infancy. This was followed but never resolved and required resection.

bhCG are normal, and the patient is asymptomatic. If they fail to resolve, intervention is required (Fig. 9.4). Again, every effort should be made to preserve ovarian tissue.

Ovarian cysts in childhood

Ovarian cysts are less common in prepubertal girls compared with newborns, but the differential diagnosis is more extensive. Malignancies become a real consideration, although these make up only a small percentage of ovarian masses in childhood (less than 10%). The differential diagnosis of a cystic ovarian mass includes simple (follicular) cyst, corpus luteal cysts, paraovarian cysts, mature teratoma, immature teratoma, cystadenoma, and cystic lymphangioma. Cysts (follicular and luteal) and mature teratomas account for 70% of these patients. Malignancy in this age group tends to present as a solid mass, and includes immature teratoma, yolk sac tumor, juvenile granulose cell tumor, Sertoli-Leydig cell tumor, and dysgerminomas.

Childhood levels of gonadotropins reach a nadir at six months of age. Estradiol and gonadotropin levels remain low in prepubertal girls. These low levels prevent full follicular development, although activity remains in the ovary. In order to determine the incidence of childhood ovarian cysts, Qublan used ultrasound to study 108 healthy girls from two to nine years of age; 35% of asymptomatic patients were found to have ovarian cysts [9]. The majority (83%) were less than 1 cm in size and most (89%) resolved in six months. The conclusion was that the majority of childhood ovarian cysts are not clinically significant (<1 cm) and therefore do not require intervention. Cysts larger than 2 cm require an evaluation for hormonal stimulation.

Presentation

In general, ovarian cysts in children are asymptomatic. They may be diagnosed by ultrasonography for other indications. Symptoms may be related to mass effect, hormonal activity or torsion (pain). A palpable mass may be associated with ovarian torsion, or not. Patients may have a low-grade temperature and a mild leukocytosis, even without torsion. Because two-thirds of torsions occur on the right side, presumably from the presence of the sigmoid colon on the left, the presentation may be identical to acute appendicitis. Torsion can be confused with urinary tract infection, gastroenteritis, renal calculi, and mesenteric adenitis. Some report an accurate prenatal diagnosis in only 50%. Sometimes these symptoms are intermittent, consistent with chronic torsion.

Diagnosis

The diagnosis of an ovarian cyst is suggested by a mass on physical exam. The mass is generally smooth and in the lower abdomen. Physical exam focuses on signs of precocious puberty: axillary or pubic hair, breast development, hyperpigmentation of the labia. LH, FSH, and estradiol levels should be obtained.

A plain abdominal film may show calcifications in the setting of a teratoma. Ultrasound is generally the

Quick Take 9.3

Diagnostic studies of ovarian cystic masses

- CBC
- AFP
- bhCG
- Abdominal radiograph
- Ultrasound

diagnostic test of choice. The most important information to be determined is whether the mass is ovarian in origin, and determining cystic from solid. Cystic masses can represent simple or complex cysts. Both mature and immature teratomas can be mainly cystic on ultrasound. All other malignancies of the ovary primarily appear solid on ultrasound. Once the diagnosis of an ovarian mass is confirmed, serum is sent to determine AFP and bhCG. Malignant teratomas tend to have an elevated AFP, while an embryonal carcinoma causes an elevated bhCG.

Management

The majority of ovarian cysts in childhood are benign, follicular cysts. They are thought to result from low circulating levels of gonadotropins. The majority of these cysts will resolve without intervention. Qublan followed 65 cysts in asymptomatic girls aged 2–9 years, and demonstrated that 89% resolved by six months [9]. Millar et al reviewed 1818 ultrasounds peformed at their institution in prepubertal girls, and found an incidence of 2–5% [10]. Most of the cysts were small and did not require intervention. This incidence was constant from infancy through childhood (eight years in this study). Brandt recommends conservative management if:

- the cyst is clearly ovarian
- the cyst is simple
- the patient is asymptomatic
- the AFP and bHCG are normal [7].

Quick Take 9.4

Surgical techniques

- Laparoscopic approach for diagnosis and treatment
- Detorsion if indicated
- Preservation of ovarian tissue even if necrotic

As with infants, the relationship of cyst size and torsion risk is controversial. However, no clear correlation of size and torsion risk has been documented. Warner has documented resolution of large cysts in childhood [11]. In his series of 92 children, including both complex and simple cysts, 90% of cysts 5 cm or greater resolved spontaneously. Warner recommends intervention if:

- the cyst is symptomatic
- there are signs of a large mass with complications (hydronephrosis)
- there is evidence of a neoplasm
- the ovarian origin is in question
- there is failure to resolve.

Millar also documented resolution of large ovarian cysts in her series without intervention. Monthly ultrasounds with intervention for failure to resolve at 3–6 months seems reasonable, although the literature has not clearly defined the endpoint. Simple cystectomy is indicated for simple cysts, and this can usually be performed laparoscopically. Hormonally active cysts and benign cystic teratomas can also be simply resected with preservation of the ovary.

Complex cysts in this age group should be resected rather than followed. Complex cysts generally indicate torsion, but could also indicate a malignancy. Interestingly, malignancy and torsion almost never coexist. Beaunoyer reported 76 children with torsion, the largest series reported, and without any cases of malignancy [12]. In other words, benign disease causes torsion more often than malignant disease. Beaunoyer reports torsion is most likely on the right side (74%), and can be asynchronous in 11% of patients, causing loss of both ovaries. He recommends resection of the necrotic portion of the ovary with preservation of the rest, followed by consideration of oophoropexy of the remnant. The contralateral ovary should also be pexed in the setting of simple tubo-ovarian torsion with an elongated ligament. Torsion can also occur in the setting of a normal ovary but long adnexal attachments. In this setting, one should also consider oophoropexy in the contralateral side.

Complex cysts may also represent a teratoma. These represent 50% of ovarian neoplasms in children (Fig. 9.5). In Tapper's series, the average age at diagnosis was 13 years [1]. He reported that these are rare under six years, and especially under 24 months. Teratomas are generally well circumscribed, and contain at least two germ cell layers. They may be mature (benign; Fig. 9.6) or immature

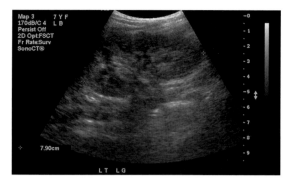

Figure 9.5 Ultrasound of a cystic teratoma in a 7-year-old girl who presented with pain.

(malignant). Presentation of a teratoma is typically abdominal pain with an adnexal mass. Ultrasound is very accurate for cystic teratomas. Treatment is complete surgical resection of the cyst with ovarian preservation. Laparoscopic cystectomy is accepted and frequently performed in adults. In children with mature teratomas, the safety of laparoscopic resection has been reported. Simple cystectomy is reasonable if the preoperative AFP is normal, the cyst is not primarily solid, and there is no evidence of spread beyond the ovary. A return to the operating room is indicated if yolk sac elements are identified. Contralateral ovarian biopsy is unnecessary if the gross and ultra-

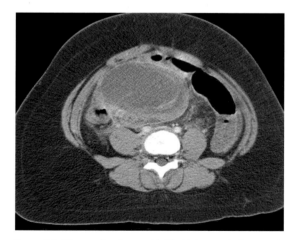

Figure 9.6 CT scan of an 8-year-old girl with low-grade fevers and right lower quadrant pain. This was initially diagnosed as a perforated appendicitis with an abscess and was percutaneously drained. The child was later explored secondary to persistent symptoms and was found to have a mature teratoma.

sound appearances are normal. There were no recurrences reported in Templeman's series [13]. Yearly ultrasounds until puberty are recommended followed by annual pelvic examinations after puberty. Adjuvant therapy is only required in the setting of malignancy.

In the setting of ovarian cysts with evidence of hormonal activity, several entities must be considered. High estradiol levels along with LH and FSH levels that do not respond to LH-releasing hormone (LHRH) stimulation suggest autonomous secretion of estrogens by the cyst, resulting in precocious pseudopuberty. An autonomously acting ovarian cyst can occur in isolation. In Millar's series, five patients were reported presenting with precocious sexual development [10]. Two patients' cysts resolved spontaneously (2.7 and 5.5 cm), as well as the symptoms. Three patients underwent cyst excision (4.5–5 cm), which demonstrated a follicular cyst with luteinization. One improved, the other two had recurrent symptoms of increased estrogen secretion and multiple recurrences of cysts requiring intervention. Both had increased bone age from the estrogen stimulation. Both received gonadotropin-releasing hormone (GnRH) agonist therapy, with a poor response.

True precocious puberty is central in origin. Millar reported seven of these patients [10]. One had a 2 cm ovarian cyst which resolved, while the other patients had smaller cysts. None required intervention. In the McCune-Albright syndrome, children aged 2–5 present with metrorrhagia and other signs of precocious puberty. The syndrome is also associated with café-au-lait spots and polyostotic fibrous dysplasia, although these can develop later. McCune-Albright syndrome is diagnosed by mutations in the Gsα proteins. Increased secretion of gonadotropins causing true precocious puberty is associated with multiple, small ovarian cysts. Surgical intervention is generally not indicated.

Surgical techniques in the management of ovarian cysts

The ideal surgical approach for an ovarian cyst is laparoscopy which allows confirmation of the diagnosis and therapeutic intervention. Generally three trocars are required: an umbilical port for a 30° scope and ports in the left and right upper quadrants. In neonates, 3 mm instruments are used; 5 mm instruments can be used in

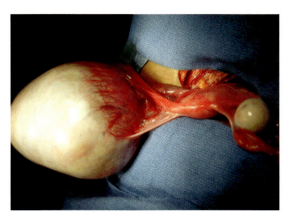

Figure 9.7 Operative picture of a mature teratoma resected through a Pfannenstiel approach.

older children. Pressures can be limited to 10 mmHg in infants, with flow rates initially at 1 L/min. Once within the abdomen, the ovarian origin of the cyst can be confirmed. The cyst can then be aspirated by passing a needle directly through the anterior abdominal wall. This facilitates resection as well as removal through the umbilical port. Unless there are obvious signs of malignancy, the cyst can be resected using a combination of cautery, harmonic scalpel, and endoshears. The cyst wall should be sent for pathology. Frozen sections rarely add to the management of ovarian cysts. The contralateral ovary should be visualized, with cyst resection if necessary.

In the setting of malignancy or a necrotic mass, the procedure can be converted to an open procedure through the Pfannenstiel approach (Fig. 9.7). In the setting of torsion, detorsion and preservation of the ovary is the standard of care. Previous concerns about detorsion, venous emboli, and malignancy have not been supported in the literature. Malignant masses rarely torse. A biopsy at the time of detorsion can be sent with a return to the operating room at a later date in the setting of malignancy. Tumor markers can also be sent postoperatively and worrisome masses can be followed with serial ultrasounds. Every effort should be made to preserve a portion of the ovary, even if it is grossly necrotic. Viability can be very difficult to determine grossly or even with fluorescein. Cohen used ultrasound to document activity within the ovary that was preserved despite a necrotic appearance in 54 of 58 patients at three months [14]. Torsed ovaries should undergo detorsion, resection of the cyst with biopsies,

and preservation. In the setting of a long pedicle which seems likely to torse again, the ovary can be pexed to the pelvic side wall with interrupted, nonabsorbable suture. The data for oophoropexy are not compelling, and this procedure probably should be decided on a case-by-case basis.

Some have advocated simple percutaneous aspiration with ultrasound guidance. This is an inferior approach for the following reasons:
- it does not confirm the diagnosis
- the needle can roll off the cyst, causing injury to other structures
- simple aspiration can allow recurrence compared with resection of the cyst wall
- laparoscopy allows examination of the rest of the abdomen.

With the increasing use of laparoscopy, even in the neonatal period, and the advancement of instrumentation, this has become the standard of care.

Conclusion

Ovarian cysts, both *in utero* and in childhood, are increasingly diagnosed. Malignancy is rarely found in childhood and therefore management is geared to prevent the other rare complications and promote future fertility. The literature increasingly supports conservative management of ovarian cysts, even in the setting of large cysts or cysts with evidence of a previous torsion. Ovarian preservation should be the basic tenet of the surgical approach except for malignancies. As Way said in 1946, referring to oophorectomy for ovarian cysts in *The Lancet*, "If a conservative operation can achieve the same results as a radical one it is obviously better, and the choice of the radical operation to save time is a prostitution of the art of surgery" [15].

References

1. Tapper D, Lack EE. Teratomas in infancy and childhood. A 54-year experience at the Children's Hospital Medical Center. *Ann Surg* 1983;**198**:398–410.
2. Heling KS, Chaoui R, Kirchmair F et al. Fetal ovarian cysts: prenatal diagnosis, management and postnatal outcome. *Ultrasound Obstet Gynecol* 2002;**20**:47–50.

3. Crombleholme TM, Craigo SD, Garmel S et al. Fetal ovarian cyst decompression to prevent torsion. *J Pediatr Surg* 1997;**32**:1447–1449.

4. Giorlandino C, Bilancioni E, Bagolan P et al. Antenatal ultrasonographic diagnosis and management of fetal ovarian cysts. *Int J Gynecol Obstet* 1993;**44**:27–31.

5. Perrotin F, Potin J, Haddad G. Fetal ovarian cysts: a report of three cases managed by intrauterine aspiration. *Ultrasound Obstet Gynecol* 2000;**16**:655–659.

6. Bagolan P, Giorlandino C, Nahom A. The management of fetal ovarian cysts. *J Pediatr Surg* 2002;**37**(1):25–30.

7. Brandt ML, Helmrath MA. Ovarian cysts in infants and children. *Semin Pediatr Surg* 2005;**14**(2):78–85.

8. Luzzatto C, Midrio P, Toffolutti T et al. Neonatal ovarian cysts: management and follow-up. *Pediatr Surg Int* 2000;**16**:56–59.

9. Qublan HST, Abdel-hadi J. Simple ovarian cysts: frequency and outcome in girls aged 2–9 years. *Clin Exp Obstet Gynecol* 1993;**27**:51–53.

10. Millar DM, Blake JM, Stringer DA et al. Prepubertal ovarian cyst formation: 5 years' experience. *Obstet Gynecol* 1993;**81**:434–438.

11. Warner B, Kuhn JC, Barr LL et al. Conservative management of large ovarian cysts in children: the value of serial pelvic ultrasonography. *Surgery* 1992;**112**:749–755.

12. Beaunoyer M, Chapdelaine J, Bouchard S et al. Asynchronous bilateral ovarian torsion. *J Pediatr Surg* 2004;**39**(5):746–749.

13. Templeman CL, Hertweck SP, Scheetz JP et al. The management of mature cystic teratomas in children and adolescents: a retrospective analysis. *Hum Reprod* 2000;**15**(12):2669–2672.

14. Cohen SB, Oelsner G, Seidman DS et al. Laparoscopic detorsion allows sparing of the twisted ischemic adnexa. *J Am Assoc Gynecol Laparosc* 1999;**6**(2):139–143.

15. Way S. Ovarian cystectomy of twisted cysts. *Lancet* 1946;**July 13**:47–48.

Further reading

Bryant AE, Laufer MR. Fetal ovarian cysts. *J Reprod Med* 2004;**49**:329–337.

Cass DL. Ovarian torsion. *Semin Pediatr Surg* 2005;**14**(2):86–92.

Cass DL, Hawkins E, Brandt ML et al. Surgery for ovarian masses in infants, children, and adolescents: 102 consecutive patients treated in a 15-year period. *J Pediatr Surg* 2001;**36**:693–699.

Esposito C, Garipoli V, Di Matteo G et al. Laparoscopic management of ovarian cyst in newborns. *Surg Endosc* 1998;**12**:1152–1154.

Garel L, Filitrault D, Brandt M et al. Antenatal diagnosis of ovarian cysts: natural history and therapeutic implications. *Pediatr Radiol* 1991;**21**:182–184.

Kokoska ER, Keller MS, Weber TR. Acute ovarian torsion in children. *Am J Surg* 2000;**180**:462–465.

Lass A. The fertility potential of women with a single ovary. *Hum Reprod Update* 1999;**5**:546–550.

Lass A, Paul M, Margara R et al. Women with one ovary have decreased response to GnRHa/HMG ovulation induction protocol in IVH but the same pregnancy rate as women with two ovaries. *Hum Reprod* 1997;**12**(2):298–300.

CHAPTER 10

Genital Trauma

Diane F. Merritt

Washington University School of Medicine, Washington, DC, USA

Introduction

Genital injuries produce much psychologic anxiety and concerns about future reproductive potential and psychosexual development. The goal for the healthcare provider is to evaluate and treat the injury without creating additional trauma for the victim, determine the cause of the injury (accidental or sexual abuse), and address and prevent long-term physical or psychologic damage.

Every obstetrician-gynecologist in general practice should have the ability to evaluate and manage genital injuries. Most injuries are minor and do not require surgical attention or hospitalization; however, some coitally related injuries and some accidental injuries result in significant trauma which requires expertise. Worldwide, the most common cause of genital injuries in young women is childbirth, as a result of difficult or unattended deliveries and from prolonged obstructed labors. Rape of women and children as victims of violence or child prostitution will also result in trauma to the genitals, and management of these injuries will be addressed.

The World Health Organization's (WHO) Department of Injuries and Violence Prevention (VIP) has spearheaded efforts to improve and standardize injury surveillance systems, promote injury control policy, and provide low-cost improvements in injury care. The Essential Trauma Care Project promotes improvements in trauma care and has published guidelines for trauma care before admission to hospital. The goal is to seek a certain minimal level of care for virtually every injured person worldwide. The guidelines for essential trauma care seek to establish achievable and affordable standards for injury care worldwide [1].

Impact of age on the genital tissues

Newborn infants will demonstrate the effects of maternal and placental estrogen on the genital tissues at birth. Transient estradiol secretion equivalent to the level of the midfollicular phase of the menstrual cycle occurs along with follicular development and atresia. The hymen of a newborn female infant is prominent, thick, redundant, edematous, and pink in color. The vaginal tissues are moist and mucus is often present. The clitoris is prominent and slightly swollen. As the effects of maternal estrogen dissipate, ovarian steroid and gonadotropins levels fall and remain at very low levels until 6–8 years of age [2]. The prepubertal child's hymen is thin, flat, and red with a clearly defined edge; blood vessels are clearly visible (Fig. 10.1). Thin overlying skin bleeds profusely from relatively minor trauma. Blunt forceful penetrating trauma to the vagina may result in noticeable injuries. The hymen is more likely to tear than tolerate any stretching or distension.

At puberty, with the onset of endogenous estrogen production, the genital tissues undergo another change. The labia minora elongate and become fuller; the hymenal tissues become plump, pink, and may have a redundant petal-like appearance (Fig. 10.2). The vaginal tissues also become pink and moist, and rugae develop. Clear mucus-like vaginal secretions are a hallmark of estrogen effect in early puberty. Once an adolescent begins to ovulate, proliferative-phase clear secretions give way to thicker white secretions of the secretory phase of the menstrual cycle. This physiologic leukorrhea is not a sign of infection but the normal biologic effect of estrogen and progesterone on the cervical and vaginal tissues.

Pediatric, Adolescent, & Young Adult Gynecology. Edited by A. Altchek and L. Deligdisch. © 2009 Blackwell Publishing, ISBN: 978-1-4051-5347-8.

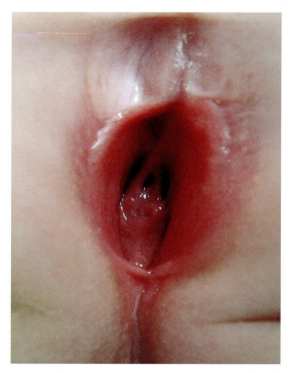

Figure 10.1 Impact of age on genital tissues. A prepubertal child with a thin, flat hymen, clearly defined edge, blood vessels clearly visible. Labia minora small.

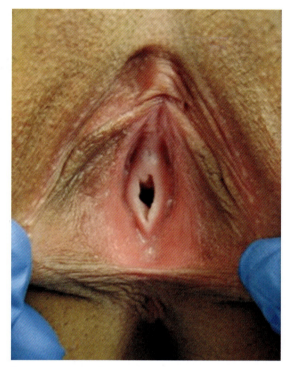

Figure 10.2 Impact of age on genital tissues. Estrogen production at puberty brings changes to the introital tissues. The labia minora elongate and become fuller, and the hymenal tissues become redundant with a petal-like appearance. Clear mucus secretion signals estrogen stimulation.

Menstruating adolescents can often place a small tampon without difficulty. Initial attempts at consensual intercourse may be painful or result in tears to the hymen and bleeding, but this is not always the case. Blunt forceful penetrating trauma in the estrogenized adolescent may result in tears of the hymen or vagina, with abrasions and ecchymoses, or may result in no or minimal superficial trauma changes which may heal rapidly in a matter of days.

The size of the vaginal (hymenal) opening in a virginal patient depends on the age, stage of development, position examined (supine or knee-to-chest) and method of examination (labial separation or traction), level of relaxation of the patient, and degree of obesity. A healthcare professional cannot tell with certainty, by examination, if a young woman has or has not had intercourse [3,4].

The genital examination of children can be modified to reassure the child and enhance co-operation. Children may be examined in their mother's lap. If the child is co-operative she may be examined supine in a frog-legged position (Fig. 10.3), supine with feet in stirrups or prone in the knee–chest position. To adequately visualize the introitus, both labial separation and lateral traction will allow the examiner to see the urethra and hymen, and document any findings.

Mechanisms and categories of female genital injury

Children and adolescents may sustain accidental genital injuries by falling onto an object, which result in straddle injuries or impalement. Blunt trauma or crush injuries to the pelvis resulting in pelvis fractures (as in motor vehicle accidents or collapse of buildings) may result in trauma to the bladder, vagina, and urethra. Chemical or thermal

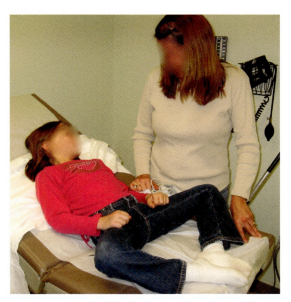

Figure 10.3 This child is demonstrating the "frog leg" or "diamond" leg position as her mother stands nearby.

burns and insufflation injuries have been reported and will be discussed. Finally, children and adolescents may be victims of rape, sexual abuse, and female genital mutilation. Obstetrically related birth injuries are outside the scope of this chapter but vulvar hematomas and vaginal lacerations will be discussed.

Straddle injuries

Vulvar trauma usually occurs as the result of straddle injuries. Examples of accidental straddle injury include falling onto the frame of a bicycle, playground equipment or piece of furniture, entering or exiting a swimming pool (especially above-ground pools) (Fig. 10.4) or bathtub, being thrown from a sled against a tree or other obstacle, or being kicked in the groin. The soft tissues of the vulva are compressed between the object and the pubic symphysis and pubic rami. Nonpenetrating injuries usually involve the mons, clitoris, and labia, and result in linear lacerations, ecchymoses, and abrasions. Blood vessels torn by trauma can bleed into the loose areolar tissue in the labia or along the vagina and overlying the clitoris and pubic symphysis; mild bruising or hematomas may form.

Vulvar hematomas

Vulvar hematomas can be very painful and may prevent a child or adolescent from urinating because of pain and swelling. If the hematoma is not large, the perineal anatomy is not distorted, and the patient has no difficulty emptying her bladder, she can be managed with immediate application of ice packs and bedrest (Fig. 10.5). As the hematoma resolves, the blood will track along the fascial planes. The ecchymotic discoloration may take weeks to resolve.

If the patient has a large vulvar hematoma and is unable to void, place an indwelling urinary catheter and continue bladder drainage until the swelling resolves. Very large vulvar hematomas that distort the vulvar anatomy may dissect into the loose areolar tissue along the vaginal wall and along the fascial planes overlying the symphysis pubis and lower abdominal wall. Pressure from an expanding hematoma can cause necrosis of the skin overlying the hematoma (Fig. 10.6). Evacuate the hematoma to reduce pain, hasten recovery, and prevent necrosis, tissue loss, and secondary infection (Fig. 10.7). Incise large vulvar hematomas at the medial mucosal surface near the vaginal orifice. In order to shorten the patient's convalescence, debride the wound of all devitalized tissue, ligate bleeding vessels and place absorbable sutures to control bleeding. Place a closed system drain, which prevents reaccumulation of blood to reduce pain and the risk of bacterial growth [5].

The periclitoral area has a rich blood supply. Hematomas in this area require careful isolation of the bleeding vessels and hemostasis (Fig. 10.8). If adequate hemostasis is not attained, the patient will be at risk for bleeding and formation of recurrent hematoma.

Accidental penetrating injuries of the vagina

These injuries occur if the victim falls upon a sharp or pointed object and impales herself. Examples of household and common objects which can cause impalement include in-lawn sprinkling systems, pipes, fenceposts, furniture (chairtops, bedposts, legs of stools), handles of brooms, tree branches, and tent stakes. The vulva may display no signs of injury but the vagina, urethra and bladder, anus, rectum and peritoneal cavity can be pierced by sharp or pointed objects. Generally there is a clear history of the impalement incident. The physical findings closely mimic penetration by blunt forceful trauma so sexual

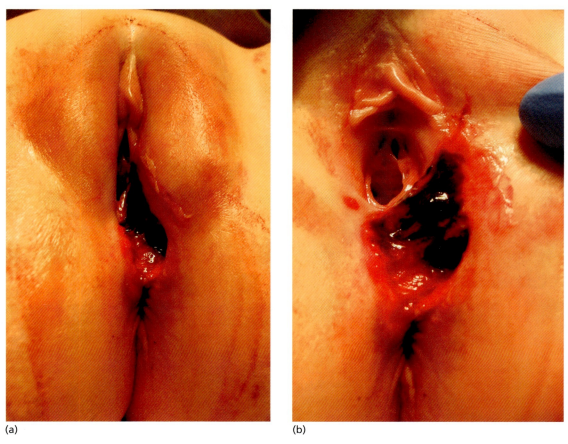

(a)　　　　　　　　　　　　　　　　　　　　(b)

Figure 10.4 A patient jumped off a diving board at a swimming pool and sustained this laceration. Note that the hymen and vagina are spared. A careful examination under anesthesia determined that there was no rectal or vaginal injury. The injury was closed in layers.

assault must be ruled out by history or corroboration by an eye witness. The family can be asked to bring the object to the hospital for assessment by the trauma team.

Generally these patients require an examination under anesthesia to fully assess the extent of the penetrating injury. If the rectum or peritoneal cavities are entered, an exploratory laparotomy is indicated to determine the full extent of injuries and initiate repairs. Rectal injuries above the sphincter may require a diverting colostomy.

There have been reports of high-pressure insufflation injuries that result when girls fall off jet skis and water skis, slide down water chutes, and come in direct contact with pool or spa jets [6–8]. As pressurized water enters the vagina, the walls may overdistend and tear. These patients will present with vaginal bleeding. Such injuries may pro-

duce no sign of external trauma and only careful vaginal examination (often under anesthesia) will reveal the true extent of injury and cause of bleeding. Patients who participate in water sports can prevent vaginal insufflation injuries by using protective clothing such as wet suits or cut-off jeans while water or jet skiing, and by keeping their feet together when entering the water on a slide.

Coitally related vaginal injuries

Although the vagina can be injured accidentally, clinicians should suspect consensual intercourse or sexual assault when an adolescent presents with vaginal trauma (Figs. 10.9, 10.10). Predisposing factors for coital injury include initial coitus, resumption of intercourse after a long abstinence, congenital anomalies of the vagina,

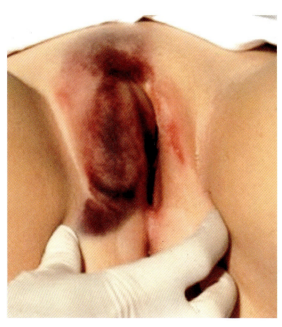

Figure 10.5 Nonexpanding hematoma in a child who fell onto a metal bar while climbing at the playground. The child was able to void and was treated with ice packs and bedrest.

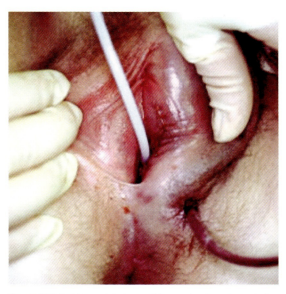

Figure 10.7 Incision and drainage of large vulvar hematoma. Incise over the hematoma on the inner surface of the labia and evacuate the hematoma. A drain has been placed in this patient.

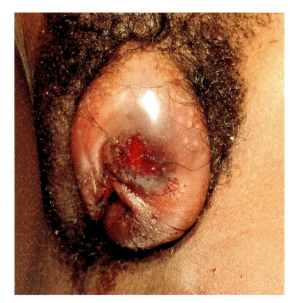

Figure 10.6 Expanding vulvar hematoma with marked distortion of the anatomy.

unusual coital positions that permit deep penetration, concomitant inebriation or drug use by either partner, brutality, violence, and use of a foreign object [5]. The patient may be distressed or too embarrassed to explain her injuries, and initially she may offer a misleading clinical history. Failure to perform a proper pelvic examination to evaluate vaginal bleeding will compound the error and lead to a delay in diagnosis and treatment. Minor lacerations of the introitus and lower vagina can occur with initial coitus. Adolescents who sustain deep vaginal lacerations from coitus may present with intense vaginal pain, profuse or prolonged vaginal bleeding, and shock. Because digital vaginal examination is inadequate to assess injuries of this nature, a patient with profuse vaginal bleeding should be inspected with a speculum.

The most frequent types and sites of injury in rape victims include tears and abrasions of the posterior fourchette, tears and abrasions of the labia minora, tears of the fossa navicularis, and lacerations and ecchymosis of the hymen. Patients with vaginal agenesis may sustain deep lacerations from failed attempts at penetration. Urethral intercourse may occur in patients who have vaginal agenesis.

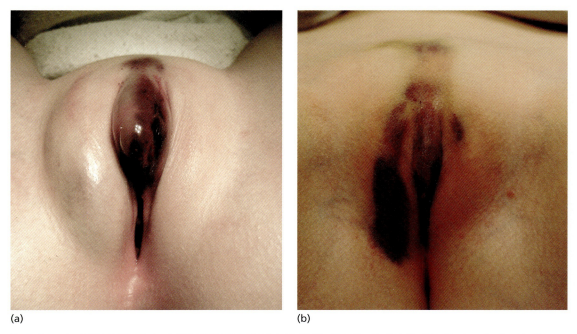

(a)   (b)

Figure 10.8 Periclitoral hematoma. This girl fell on the edge of a chair at school. Note the vagina and hymen are not involved. Since the hematoma was nonexpanding, the child was observed. The second photo was taken five days later. The hematoma is beginning to resolve and the blood is tracking along tissue planes.

Genital injuries from motor vehicle accidents or crush injuries

Crush injuries resulting from motor vehicle accidents, falls, and collapsed buildings can produce pelvic fractures. As a result, sharp spicules of the pelvic bone may penetrate the vagina and lower urinary tract. This may lead to lacerations o f the bladder, urethra or vagina.

Urethral injuries

Urethral injuries in girls are uncommon. Most occur as a result of straddle-type injuries or secondary to pelvic fractures where sharp bony spicules tear the urethra, bladder or vagina. Rarely urethral injuries can be self-inflicted when a girl inserts a foreign object directly into the urethra. The most common indicator of urethral disruption in females is blood at the introitus, vagina or urethral meatus, hematuria, the inability to void or labial edema. Imaging of the female urethra in the case of suspected disruption is challenging. McAninch suggested that females with suspected urethral injuries should undergo diagnos-

tic urethroscopy [9]. Problems arise if a urethral injury is unrecognized and the urethra is further damaged by attempts at blind catheterization, although this has been recently challenged [10].

The treatment depends on the severity and location of the injury. Urethral contusions can be managed by placement of a catheter into the bladder for several days to allow the bladder to drain while the urethra heals. Suprapubic bladder drainage is also an acceptable option for urinary diversion, but stenting of an injured or repaired urethra is usually performed over a catheter. There is controversy in the literature over whether urethral injuries should be repaired initially or delayed until the swelling, hemorrhage, and inflammation resolve. Expertise in the repair of urethral transection or bladder disruption is needed to prevent complications from these injuries. Failure to properly diagnose and treat a urethral injury may result in urinary incontinence, urethral stricture, and vesicovaginal or urethrovaginal fistulas. These patients often have multiple injuries, so the management approach must reflect this [11].

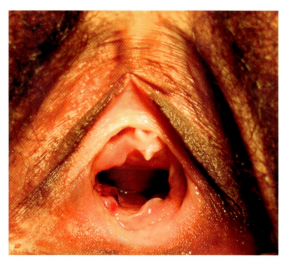

Figure 10.9 This teen sustained a laceration of the hymen at 8 o'clock from consensual intercourse.

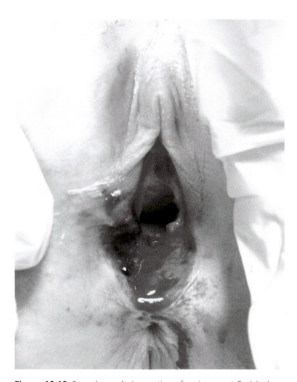

Figure 10.10 Sexual assault. Laceration of perineum at 6 o'clock, transection of hymen at 5 o'clock, with associated anal penetration of prepubertal child.

Bladder injuries

The female bladder may be injured by blunt trauma secondary to a motor vehicle accident, a fall from a significant height or by a heavy object falling on an individual, or penetrating wounds (bullet or stab wounds). The nature of the injury depends on whether the bladder is empty or full at the time of the injury as well as the mechanism of the injury. The hallmark of bladder injury is gross hematuria which is present 95% of the time [12]. Palpation over the bladder may show tenderness or a distended bladder. Leakage of urine into the abdomen may cause infection and peritonitis. In women, blood and urine may come from the vagina if the vagina is also injured. A speculum examination is mandatory in these cases and radiographic imaging for pelvic fractures and genitourinary trauma should be done before suturing any vaginal lacerations. A retrograde cystogram can be done to diagnose a ruptured bladder. Fill the bladder with contrast through a urethral catheter. Imaging the bladder by use of excreted contrast material is not adequate and may result in a false-negative study [12].

A 2002 consensus panel agreed upon four categories of urinary bladder injury: contusion, intraperitoneal rupture, extraperitoneal rupture, and combined intra- and extraperitoneal rupture [13]. Bladder contusions are treated with bladder drainage. Extraperitoneal bladder ruptures are treated nonoperatively by catheter drainage. Surgical repair is mandatory if there is a concomitant vaginal or rectal injury or injury to the bladder neck. Intraperitoneal bladder ruptures require immediate surgical repair. Usually a two-layer watertight closure with absorbable sutures is performed. The bladder is then drained by catheter for two weeks. Penetrating injuries of the bladder are handled by surgical exploration. These patients may have other organ injuries, so careful examination of the trajectory tract is necessary.

Genital burns

Because the perineum is hidden between the thighs, it is generally protected from burn injuries. When they occur, burns of the female genitalia and perineum are most likely to be associated with extensive burns involving one-third to one-half of the total body surface area, which carry a 30–70% mortality rate. The most common burn in adults is by flame, whereas children usually are scalded by liquids or immersion [14,15]. Chemical burns have been reported from self-induced abortions [16] and from placement of batteries in the vagina [5,17]. Genital burns can occur from use of medications intended to treat genital warts such as podophyllin or trichloroacetic acid. Such chemical burns should be treated immediately by irrigation to neutralize the chemicals and prevent further damage [18].

The management of genital and perineal burns includes topical application of antimicrobials (1% silver sulfadiazine) and in serious cases, short-term urinary diversion for comfort and hygiene. A mixture of silver sulfadiazine and estrogen cream has been helpful for minimizing scarring from mucosal burns of the genital tract [5]. In cases of perineal burns, contractures can be prevented with use of thigh abduction, hip exercises, early ambulation, and pressure garments. Scarring as a result of perineal burns affects skin texture, pigmentation, and pliability. A burn victim's ability to maintain hygiene with micturition and defecation may be compromised, which can have a devastating impact on sexuality and body image.

Vaginal foreign objects

While tampons, vaginal suppositories, and medications have been designed to be placed into a woman's vagina, other objects placed accidentally or intentionally are referred to as vaginal foreign bodies. Children will frequently present with foreign bodies in the vagina. The most common objects are wads of toilet paper or fibrous material from clothing, carpets, and bedding. Other common household objects that we have removed from the vagina include pen or marker caps, crayons, hair barrettes, bobby pins, safety pins, buttons, and batteries. These objects are small enough to be inserted without causing pain from distension of the hymen. Children generally will not place objects larger than the vaginal opening due to discomfort. Once inserted into the vagina, the objects tend to be retained. Children may not be able to provide the history of placing a foreign object or they may be quite straightforward in explaining to their caregiver precisely what they placed in their vagina. Adolescents may place a tampon and forget to remove it, or place a second tampon and wedge the previous one deep into the fornix. The retained tampon becomes overgrown with bacteria, creating an offensive odor. Condoms may slip off or break and these may be found in the vaginal vault. Foreign objects may be inserted into the vagina as part of a sexual experience, out of curiosity or by patients with a psychi-

atric disorder. Occasionally the foreign object becomes wedged and cannot be removed, resulting in a visit to the gynecologist or emergency department.

Symptoms of a retained vaginal foreign body include vaginal discharge, often foul smelling and associated with pink, red or brown vaginal bleeding, dysuria, and a rash or swelling and erythema of the perineum. Treatment of the vaginal discharge will not result in improvement until the foreign object is removed. Examination of the vulva and vagina, utilizing lateral traction of the labia minora, may allow the examiner to see into the vagina and glimpse the foreign body. Small items like wads of toilet tissue may be lavaged from the vagina using a pediatric feeding tube, syringe, and warm tap water. Small solid objects in the vagina can be milked out by placing a finger in the rectum. Forgotten tampons can be removed with vaginal forceps pierced through the finger of an examining glove, and the glove can be pulled around the tampon to reduce the odor before discarding it in a sealed plastic bag or another exam glove.

Other objects may be wedged up in the vagina or be too large to remove without instillation of lidocaine jelly, sedation or examination under anesthesia. The object may be grasped with a tenaculum, sponge forceps, clamp or tonsil snare under direct visualization with a vaginal speculum. If the object is difficult to remove, techniques borrowed from retrieval of rectal foreign bodies can be implemented [19]. A large Foley catheter with a 30 cc balloon can be placed past the object, the balloon inflated and traction applied to the catheter to remove the wedged object. A wedged-in hollow object like a jar or bottle can be filled with wet plaster, into which a tongue blade can be inserted like a Popsicle stick. When the plaster hardens, traction can be applied on the tongue blade. Forceps or spoons can be used to deliver a round object. Sharp, jagged objects like broken glass should not be removed without adequate anesthesia in the operating room to allow for atraumatic removal. Foreign objects may erode into the wall of the vagina or perforate through the vagina. Once an object has been removed, antibiotics are not usually required. Topical vaginal estrogen cream may facilitate healing if the walls of the vagina are traumatized or abraded.

Female genital mutilation

It is estimated that 100–140 million girls and women in the world have undergone some form of female genital

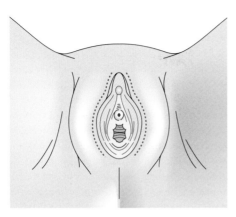

Figure 10.11 Female genital mutilation. In type II the clitoris and labia minora are removed (blue) and in type III the external genitalia are stitched (infibulated) to narrow the vaginal opening (dotted lines).

---

mutilation (FGM), and two million girls are at risk from the practice each year. Most of these women live in sub-Saharan Africa, and some live in the Middle East and Asia. Due to immigration of women from countries where FGM is practiced to other lands, medical staff all over the world are now caring for these women. FGM may be carried out in infancy or childhood, at adolescence or at marriage. In some cultures where FGM is practiced, women who give birth are re-infibulated following vaginal deliveries. A designated elder, village barber or traditional birth attendant usually performs FGM. The WHO, the International Council of Nurses (ICN), the International Confederation of Midwives (OCM), and the International Federation of Gynecologists and Obstetricians (FIGO) have openly condemned this practice of willful damage to healthy organs for nontherapeutic reasons. FGM is considered to be a form of violence against girls and women.

Types of FGM

Female genital mutilation, often referred to as "female circumcision," refers to all procedures involving partial or total removal of the external female genitalia or other injury to the female genital organs whether for cultural, religious or other nontherapeutic reasons. The different types of female genital mutilation known to be practiced today include the following.

- Type I – excision of the prepuce, with or without excision of part of or the entire clitoris

Box 10.1 Reasons for FGM [20]

- Sociologic reasons
  - Identification with cultural heritage
  - Initiation of girls into womanhood
  - Social integration
  - Maintenance of social cohesion
- Psychosexual reasons
  - Reduction or elimination of the sensitive tissues of the outer genitalia, particularly the clitoris, in order to attenuate sexual desire in the female
  - Maintain chastity and virginity before marriage
  - Increase male sexual pleasure
- Hygiene and esthetic reasons
  - In certain cultures the female genitalia are considered dirty and unsightly and are removed to promote hygiene and esthetic appeal
- Myths
  - Enhancement of fertility
  - Promotion of child survival
- Religious reasons
  - Belief that it is demanded by the Islamic faith. The practice actually predates Islam

---

- Type II – excision of the clitoris with partial or total excision of the labia minora
- Type III – excision of part or all of the external genitalia and stitching/narrowing of the vaginal opening (infibulation)
- Type IV – pricking, piercing or incising of the clitoris and/or labia; stretching of the clitoris and/or labia; cauterization by burning of the clitoris and surrounding tissue; scraping of tissue surrounding the vaginal orifice (angurya cuts) or cutting of the vagina (gishiri cuts); introduction of corrosive substances or herbs into the vagina to cause bleeding or for the purpose of tightening or narrowing it; and any other procedure that falls under the definition given above [20].

The most common type of female genital mutilation is excision of the clitoris and the labia minora, accounting for up to 80% of all cases; the most extreme form is infibulation, which constitutes about 15% of all procedures (Fig. 10.11, Box 10.1).

Health consequences of FGM

The immediate consequences include severe pain, shock, hemorrhage, urinary retention, ulceration of the genital region and injury to adjacent tissue. Long-term complications include cysts and abscesses, keloid scar formation, damage to the urethra resulting in urinary incontinence, dyspareunia, sexual dysfunction, and difficulties with childbirth. During vaginal deliveries, the infibulated woman has to be opened to allow passage of the baby. De-infibulation is also neccessary to prevent formation of vesicovaginal and rectovaginal fistulas, as well as undue suffering of the mother and baby, including increased risk of stillbirth and maternal death. After opening an infibulated vulva to allow for childbirth or to treat urinary retention, hematocolpos or infection, the healthcare worker should refuse requests to re-infibulate. This can result in professional and ethical dilemmas for the healthcare worker. Increased awareness of the harmful effects of FGM and greater access to healthcare services have resulted in requests to "medicalize" FGM and have the operation performed by healthcare professionals in clinical settings. The WHO policy forbids performing this procedure in a medical setting [21].

Management of external genital and vaginal injuries

Initial first aid at the scene

Initial first aid for a vulvar injury or vaginal laceration is compression of the bleeding. A clean dressing (wash cloth, sanitary pad, towel) can be held in place over the vulva by the victim or caregiver. Compression of the vascular plexus requires firm pressure of the soft tissues against the underlying bony pelvis. Expansion of a hematoma can be prevented by such pressure and minimize the blood loss and injury sustained. A vaginal injury in an older adolescent can be packed using tampons until a professional examination can take place. In the emergency department setting, the vagina can be packed with sterile gauze until gynecologic expertise is available. Ice packs can be held in position over minor hematomas and lacerations until expertise can be arranged for assessment. The ice packs will slow the bleeding and decrease the swelling.

Minor injuries of the external genitalia and vagina

After initial assessment, an apparently bloody injury may be quite superficial or minor. With the patient on an examination table, gently rinse or wipe away blood. Place the patient on a bedpan or fracture pan and pour warm water over the perineum to find the source of the bleeding. Direct inspection of a laceration will then allow the examiner to determine if there is active bleeding or if the bleeding has stopped. If the injury is very superficial and no longer bleeding actively, application of triple antibiotic ointment and good hygiene is all that is needed. A small sanitary pad can be worn in the underwear as a dressing. Avoid trying to tape dressings to the skin of the vulva, as they will quickly become soiled by urine and feces. Minor lacerations can be repaired under local anesthesia or with conscious sedation. Superficial abrasions of the hymen do not require suturing. If there is an injury to the mucosal genital surfaces, application of an estrogen cream can benefit the healing process and decrease scarring. A pea-sized amount can be massaged into the tissues once or twice a day for 3–7 days. Superficial vaginal lacerations that are oozing but not bleeding may be managed with vaginal packing. The packing should be moistened with estrogen cream or saline to allow for easier removal. Vaginal lacerations that are actively bleeding should be sutured by someone with expertise to avoid injury to the urethra, bladder, and rectum.

Major injuries of the external genitalia and vagina

Patients who are subjected to blunt, penetrating forceful trauma usually sustain lacerations in the posterior aspect of the hymen. Deep lacerations must be evaluated; if necessary, examine these patients and repair their injuries under general anesthesia. Lateral vaginal wall and posterior fornix lacerations can occur. In serious cases, the cervix may be avulsed from its attachment to the vagina, and the tear may extend along the vagina and enter the peritoneal cavity. The bowel, omentum or fallopian tubes may eviscerate through the laceration. These patients present with vaginal bleeding and may be at risk of morbidity or death from exsanguination, unless properly diagnosed and managed. If you suspect that a child's or adolescent's injury extends above the hymen but you cannot assess the true extent of the injury or repair it, you must perform a complete examination under general anesthesia.

Every hospital should have a defined protocol for collection of forensic evidence in cases of alleged or possible sexual assault. It is important to provide a clear description of the injuries with accompanying photo documentation if available. If it is deemed necessary to inspect the

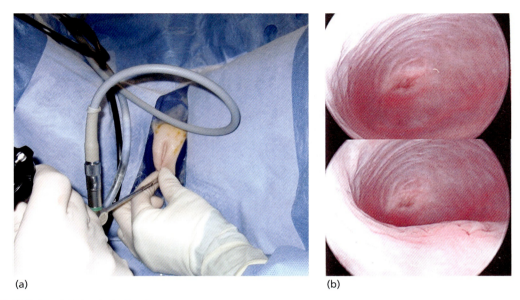

(a)   (b)

Figure 10.12 Prepubertal vaginal cystoscopy.

vagina of a trauma victim and if a Huffman or Pederson vaginal speculum is too large for a prepubertal child or young adolescent, use a pediatric cystoscope and saline irrigation to visualize the vagina and determine the extent of vaginal injuries (Fig. 10.12). Gently hold the labia together, allowing the fluid to distend the vagina and facilitate careful inspection of the vaginal walls and cervix. This technique is also very useful to determine whether there is a foreign body present in the vagina of a child. The importance of using a suitable light source and proper positioning, and obtaining complete co-operation (which may require sedation or anesthesia), cannot be overemphasized when attempting to repair vaginal injuries.

Perforations into the peritoneal cavity mandate an exploratory laparotomy or laparoscopy to determine if other structures, such as the bowel or blood vessels, have been injured. In the child or young adolescent who has a small-caliber vagina, begin repair of lacerations with the deepest (most distal from the introitus) vaginal injuries first, and end with introital lacerations to allow for maximum working space and visualization. Postoperative application of topical estrogen cream to injuries of the mucosal surfaces of the vagina and introitus may decrease formation of granulation tissue and promote healing without stricture [5].

Sexual abuse of children

Sexual abuse of girls includes penetrative, intercrural, oral-genital intercourse, and fondling. This problem can occur in any segment of society, in developed and undeveloped countries, and crosses all socio-economic lines [22].

The essential components of medical care after a rape include collection of a medical history and forensic evidence, evaluation for sexually transmitted infections and preventive care, evaluation for risk of pregnancy and prevention, repair of injuries, counseling and follow-up. Obtain consent for examination from the legal guardian unless the guardian is the alleged accused. When a child alleges sex assault, forensic tests may prove positive. Vaginal, rectal and skin swabs are ideally done within hours of the assault. It is now known that healing of physical signs of genital trauma is rapid, and children underestimate rather than exaggerate the extent of their abuse. The combination of these factors means that delayed examination may result in negative findings even when there has been penetration [23,24]. Bruising (bite marks), grip marks, scratches, and lacerations should be documented as soon as possible (preferably within 24 hours, as by 72 hours healing may have occurred).

A normal hymenal orifice does not exclude child sexual abuse, and a minor abnormality alone does not prove child sexual abuse. Minor bumps in the hymen margins associated with intravaginal ridges are normal variants. Marked hymenal asymmetry, sharp or square angles, and healed transections of the hymen should be considered signs of previous trauma. Most hymenal transections caused by forceful or attempted penetration are found in the posterior hymen between 5 and 7 o'clock. These transections may extend to the posterior vaginal wall or fourchette. Hymenal lacerations may heal rapidly in prepubertal girls if the abuse stops. If the hymen is acutely stretched without loss of tissue, it may recover and even in cases of penetration, there may be normal findings at the time of the exam. Attenuation of the hymen due to chronic abuse does not usually recover, and in such cases, the vaginal orifice will appear to be enlarged and the hymenal tissues will appear deficient. Even after puberty, the hymen will be deficient and will not change even with the effects of endogenous estrogen. Acute genital trauma, which causes swelling, erythema, abrasions and bruising, may resolve in a few days. When there is tissue damage, wound healing may occur in 48–72 hours and regeneration of new surface epithelium may be complete in 5–7 days [24].

In a published study of 2384 children referred for possible sexual abuse, 96.3% had a normal examination. In this series, even in children with a history of anal or vaginal penetration, only 5.5% had abnormal medical findings [25]. There is no association between hymenal changes and participation in gymnastics, cycling, horseback riding or other sports. Tampon use has little effect in postpubertal girls [26]. Anal injuries may occur in cases of sodomy. Perianal redness may be due to poor hygiene, diaper rash, pinworms, eczema, seborrheic dermatitis, lichen sclerosus, and streptococcal infections. Intercrural intercourse may be associated with erythema of the perianal and labial regions [26]. On rare occasions, penetration of the vagina in a child will result in vaginal tears that may extend to the fornices or into the peritoneal cavity. Referral to an experienced sexual assault or trauma center is recommended when there is severe vaginal or anal injury.

The primary purpose of conducting a forensic examination is to collect evidence that may help prove or disprove allegations of child abuse. Strict adherence to the principles for forensic collection, listed in Box 10.2, is necessary.

Box 10.2 Principles of forensic examination

- Collect specimens as soon as possible
- Avoid contamination of the specimen by use of uncontaminated gloves
- Label all specimens accurately
- Dry all wet specimens; refrigerate liquid specimens
- Ensure that all specimens are secure and tamper proof
- Maintain continuity of evidence
- Document all collection and handling procedures, including examiner, list of specimens

---

The clinical management of survivors of rape is detailed in the 2001 WHO guide to development of protocols for use in refugee and internally displaced person situations [27].

When preparing a child for an examination, encourage her to ask questions about anything she is concerned about or does not understand at any time during the examination (Box 10.3). Explain what will happen in terms the child can understand. If the child is in pain or cannot relax consider giving medication. Never restrain or force a frightened or resistant child to complete an exam. If there are injuries to be repaired, perform the examination under general anesthesia. Supportive counseling should be provided through the examination process. The victim and her family may be referred for social support and psychologic counseling services.

Psychologic factors associated with genital injuries

The ability to bear children and have sexual relations in the future is a topic that should specifically be addressed with adolescent victims of genital injuries and their families. When appropriate, offer reassurance of reproductive capacity, as these concerns will not always be verbalized by a patient or her family members. Appropriate medical care and family support will help the patient to recover emotionally as well as physically. Children and teens who are recovering from an isolated genital injury seldom have long-standing psychologic trauma from the event. The exception would be an isolated injury which leaves lasting scarring or vaginal stenosis, such as extensive genital burns. Victims of sexual assault may suffer from sleep

Box 10.3 Examination of a child or young teen who has been sexually assaulted

- Small children can be examined on the mother's lap. Older children can be given the choice of being examined lying on an exam table or on the mother's lap

- Check the hymen using separation and lateral traction, looking for any fresh or healing tears in the hymen and vaginal mucosa

- Digital examination of the vagina should not be performed

- Look for vaginal discharge and if present, collect specimens with a cotton swab

- Do not use a speculum to examine prepubertal girls; it is extremely painful and may cause serious injury. A vaginal examination of a prepubertal child is usually performed under general anesthesia

- A speculum may be used in an older teen if there is suspicion of penetrating vaginal injury and internal bleeding, and to collect cervical specimens. Depending on the setting, the child may need to be referred to a higher level of healthcare

- Conduct an examination of the anus, noting anal fissures and tears. Do not perform a digital anal exam

- Follow the local protocol for obtaining specimens for forensic testing and sexually transmitted infections

disturbances, nightmares, flashbacks, anxiety, and anger. Depression is common in these victims, and often is compounded by feelings of guilt and shame. Offer specific referrals for professional counseling to all victims of sexual assault. Counsel the family so that they can be supportive of the young victim. In cases where the abuser is a member of the family or was allowed access to the child, establish that the child will be safe when returned to the home environment and arrange for long-term follow-up with the child and her family.

References

1. Mock C. *Guidelines for Essential Trauma Care.* Geneva: World Health Organization, 2004.
2. Speroff L, Fritz MA. *Clinical Endocrinology and Infertility*, 7th edn. Philadelphia, PA: Lippincott, Williams and Wilkins, 2005:362.
3. Underhill RA, Dewhurst J. The doctor cannot always tell. *Lancet* 1978;**1**(8060):175–176.
4. Kellogg ND, Menard SW, Santos A. Genital anatomy in pregnant adolescents: "normal" does not mean "nothing happened." *Pediatrics* 2004;**113**:e67–69.
5. Merritt DF, Rimsza ME, Muram D. Genital injuries in pediatric and adolescent girls. In: Sanfilippo JS, Muram D, Dewhurst J, Lee P (eds) *Pediatric and Adolescent Gynecology*, 2nd edn. Philadelphia, PA: WB Saunders, 2001.
6. Niv J, Lessing JB, Hartuv J et al. Vaginal injury resulting from sliding down a water chute. *Am J Obstet Gynecol* 1992;**166**(3):930–931.
7. Perlman SE, Hertweck SP, Wolfe WM. Water-ski douche injury in a premenarcheal female. *Pediatrics* 1995;**96**:782–783.
8. Haefner HK, Anderson F, Johnson MP. Vaginal laceration following a jet-ski accident. *Obstet Gynecol* 1991;**78**:986–988.
9. McAninch JW, Urethral injuries in female subjects following pelvic fractures (editorial comment). *J Urol* 1992;**147**:144.
10. Shlamovitz GZ, McCullough L. Blind urethral catheterization in trauma patient suffering from lower urinary tract injuries. *J Trauma* 2007;**62**(2):330–335.
11. Cummings JM, Boullier J. Urethral trauma. Available online at: emedicine.com/med/topi3083.htm.
12. Corriere JN, Sandler CM. Diagnosis and management of bladder injuries. *Urol Clin North Am* 2006;**33**:67–71.
13. Gomez R, Ceballos L, Coburn M et al. Consensus statement on bladder injuries. *BJU Int* 2004;**94**(1):27–32.
14. Weiler-Mithoff EM, Hassal ME, Burd DA. Burns of the female genitalia and perineum. *Burns* 1996;**22**(5):390–395.
15. Michielsen D, Van Hee R, Neetens C et al. Burns of the genitals and perineum in children. *Br J Urol* 1996;**78**:940–941.
16. Tipton PF. Nightmare from the sixties. *Ann Intern Med* 2000;**132**:1002–1003.
17. Yanoh K, Yonemura Y. Severe vaginal ulcerations secondary to insertion of an alkaline battery. *J Trauma* 2005;**58**(2):410–412.
18. Waguespack RL, Thompson IM Jr, McManua WF et al. Genital and perineal burns. *AUA Update Series* 1995;**14**:31–34.
19. Couch CH, Tan EGC, Watt AG. Rectal foreign bodies. *Med J Aust* 1986;**144**:512–513.
20. Female genital mutilation. World Health Organization fact sheet #241. Available online at: www.who.int/mediacentre/factsheets.
21. World Health Organization. *Female Genital Mutilation. The Prevention and Management of the Health Complications. Policy Guidelines for Nurses and Midwives.* Geneva: World Health Organization, 2001.
22. World Health Organization. *Managing Child Abuse. A Handbook for Medical Officers.* Geneva: World Health Organization, 2004.

23. McCann J, Kerns D. *The anatomy of child and adolescent sexual abuse: a CD-ROM atlas/reference.* St Louis, MO: Inter Corp, 1999.

24. World Health Organization. *Guidelines for medicolegal care for victims of sexual violence.* Geneva: World Health Organization, 2003.

25. Heger A, Ticson L, Velasquez O et al. Evaluation of sexual abuse in children and adolescents. *Child Abuse Neglect* 2002;**26**(6–7):645–659.

26. Hobbs CJ, Hanks HGI, Wynne JM. *Child Abuse and Neglect. A Clinician's Handbook,* 2nd edn. Philadelphia, PA: Harcourt, 2000.

27. World Health Organization. *Clinical Management of Survivors of Rape. A Guide to the Development of Protocols for Use in Refugee and Internally Displaced Person Situations.* Geneva: World Health Organization, 2001.

11

CHAPTER 11
Sexual Abuse

Nancy D. Kellogg
University of Texas Health Science Center at San Antonio, TX, USA

Introduction

Sexual abuse is a clinical diagnosis with legal, cultural, and health implications. The definition of sexual abuse is variable and encompasses a spectrum of circumstances including "date rape," incest, sexual activity involving a minor, sexual contact involving a child and adult, pornography, sexual harassment, and online solicitation of a minor for sex. The diagnosis of sexual abuse in a clinical setting relies upon a comprehensive and sensitively conducted medical history; the examination approach, photodocumentation, diagnostic procedures, and forensic evidence collection vary considerably, depending on the type and circumstances of sexual abuse, as well as the resources and expertise available in the community. Medical and mental health concerns should be adequately addressed since sexual abuse can result in long-term disabling effects on the patient's well-being, relationships, and health.

Definitions

There are several aspects for the clinician to consider in defining sexual abuse or assault. It is first important to be familiar with the legal definitions of sexual assault and reporting mandates within one's state or country. All states require reporting of suspected child abuse and generally provide immunity from liability as long as the report is made in good faith. The legal definition of child/adolescent sexual abuse, however, varies somewhat from state to state. Most states provide age parameters that

define a "minor" and most states clearly indicate that any sexual activity between a minor and an adult is abusive and reportable. With regard to sexual activity between two consenting adolescents, some states require the clinician to report if it is deemed abusive (lack of consent, drug-facilitated sexual assault, etc.) while other states require reporting based only on age criteria. Still other states provide age criteria for reporting sexual assault but modify the age criteria for a subset of adolescents. For example, in one state, any sexual contact involving at least one minor may be illegal and reportable, but if the adolescents are mutually consenting and both are between 14 and 17 years old, these conditions could be claimed as a defense during criminal proceedings.

In states where sexual acts involving two consenting adolescents are reportable because of age-defined criteria, such cases are generally not prosecuted. Recently, some states are attempting to reinterpret or reinstate child abuse reporting laws to require that clinicians report sexual abuse based on age criteria only. Proponents of this approach reason that minors do not have the knowledge necessary to consent to health risky behavior such as sexual activity, and opine that mandated reporting will deter adolescents from engaging in sexual activity because of the threat of parental notification and criminal prosecution. It is not clear, however, which of the two consenting adolescents would be prosecuted. With such laws, the potential for deleterious effects on adolescent health is significant. Reporting all sexual activity that involves a minor would breach the adolescent's right to confidential healthcare and likely produce reluctance to seek or maintain healthcare among those who are sexually active. There are no current data to support the contention that age-based reporting laws would deter sexual activity among adolescents. The long-term effects of such laws

Pediatric, Adolescent, & Young Adult Gynecology. Edited by A. Altchek and L. Deligdisch. © 2009 Blackwell Publishing, ISBN: 978-1-4051-5347-8.

could be devastating if adolescents do not seek healthcare, causing sexually transmitted infections and pregnancies to be undetected and untreated. In states such as Kansas, physicians have filed suit against the state attorney general to oppose reinterpretation of child abuse laws based solely on age criteria.

In a clinical setting, sexual abuse may encompass contact and noncontact types of sexual encounters that affect the health and well-being of the patient. For example, sexual harassment may result in significant anxiety and school refusal in some children. Such children may fabricate symptoms to avoid going to school. Sexual harassment now extends to the Internet as students may receive sexually explicit or insulting material from others. In one study, 20% of adolescents were solicited for sex by strangers through the Internet.

While many studies have supported the association of child/adolescent sexual abuse with deleterious medical and mental health consequences, symptoms may not be evident in all victims initially. The clinician should be aware of the effective and often long-term coping strategies of children who are victims of sexual abuse and realize that an apparently well-adapted patient should not evoke incredulity in the clinician. Each patient is different in the nature and degree of their response to abuse.

The victim's perception of the abuse comprises yet another way in which abuse is defined. Many adolescents feel that the sexual assault must involve beating or bodily injury to be considered a "rape." Many do not realize that a verbal refusal is sufficient to establish the parameters of a rape. About one-third of all sexual abuse victims blame themselves to some degree for the assault or abuse. Self-blame can, in turn, influence whether a victim labels a sexual assault as abuse. Self-blame can derive from illogical ideas such as "If I wasn't there, it would not have happened." Clinicians can play a key role in helping victims to appropriately define their sexual experiences.

Clinical presentations

Up to 90% of sexual assault or abuse presents to a clinical setting because the victim tells someone they were abused. Other indicators, such as acute or healed findings of anogenital trauma, are rare among victims and even rarer as initial clinical presentations of sexual assault. In addition, anogenital trauma can result from consensual

---

Box 11.1 Definitions of sexual abuse

Legal: varies from state to state; usually based on age definition of a "minor" with or without provisions for "consent" for cases involving adolescents. All states require reporting of suspected abuse

Clinical: contact and noncontact types of sexual encounters that adversely affect the health or well-being of the patient. Includes sexual harassment and Internet solicitation for sex

Victim's perspective: some adolescents and children may not label their sexual experience as "abusive" unless they receive bodily injury or experience self-blame

---

sexual contact but is less common than trauma resulting from sexual assault. The severity or number of anogenital injuries does not correlate with the likelihood that the assault was nonconsensual. Bodily injury, however, such as ligature marks or bruises on the forearm sustained during the victim's attempt to protect their face while being hit, may provide more specific evidence of assault. In addition, adolescents who present to clinical settings with signs of alcohol and/or drug toxicity should be questioned carefully about the possibility of sexual assault. Many state laws include provisions for drug-facilitated sexual assault when a person is unable to consent due to impairment from such substances. The clinician should be especially concerned about sexual assault if the patient gives a history of drinking small amounts of alcohol or another drink followed by rapid onset of altered mental status and/or brief alternating periods of impairment and lucidity; such symptoms suggest drink spiking with drugs that incapacitate the victim.

Victims may also present with sexually transmitted infections (STIs); STIs are rare in children, but common among sexually active adolescents and young adults. The presence of an STI in a patient who is sexually active and also sexually assaulted has no forensic significance since the origin of the STI cannot be determined. However, sexual abuse in childhood is correlated with earlier and unprotected sexual activity in adolescence. The presence of an STI should prompt the clinician to ask the adolescent about the type and nature of all sexual contact, including nonconsensual and abusive encounters. As discussed in detail under "Testing for STIs," the presence of a "sexually transmitted infection" does not always imply sexual contact. Familiarity with different modes of transmission will assist the clinician in the appropriate interpretation of tests for STIs.

While many victims of sexual abuse or assault may have behavioral symptoms, it is not known how many victims initially present to clinical settings with such symptoms. Victims often learn to accommodate the abuse and are adept at hiding their symptoms of anxiety, depression, and post-traumatic dissociation. Mood swings typical of adolescence may mask or obfuscate symptoms attributable to victimization. As with detection of an STI, behavioral changes and problems should prompt the clinician to ask further questions regarding abuse and violence, including sexual assault.

If a patient presents with a history of sexual abuse or assault or reveals sexual abuse during the course of a medical assessment, the clinician should be aware of the options and resources available in deciding the best course of action. When the assault has occurred within the previous 72 hours, the patient should be referred urgently for forensic evidence collection. These examinations are usually conducted at regional hospitals by sexual assault nurses or physicians. Very rarely, a victim may present with genital injuries that require hemostasis and laceration repair; these patients should also be referred urgently to a hospital setting, preferably one with an established sexual assault program.

Most adolescent and child victims of sexual assault, however, do not require emergency medical attention and present beyond the interval when forensic evidence collection is indicated. The urgency of the medical assessment for these patients depends primarily upon emotional and physical symptoms, as well as the need for establishing a safety plan to protect the victim from further abuse. Many areas of the US have well-established programs that provide medical evaluations, victim assistance and crisis counseling for victims of sexual abuse. In the US, medical evaluations of children and adolescents are usually conducted by experienced and trained pediatricians or nurses as well as gynecologists, emergency medicine physicians, and family practitioners. Where such programs are available, the clinician should refer the patient for complete medical assessment and treatment. A report to child protective services and/or law enforcement should be made immediately; referral to a specialty program does not obviate the clinician's legal obligation to report.

Child/adolescent specialty programs can provide other valuable guidance to clinicians. Many parents present to clinicians with the concern that their child has been sexually abused based on an observed physical or behavioral symptom. Table 11.1 provides examples of presenting complaints and possible diagnoses for some of the more common clinical presentations. Some of these concerns may present within the context of a custody dispute or parental strife. The parent's underlying fears or anxieties can influence the perceived symptoms in their child. It is important to recognize such situations and conduct an unbiased medical assessment, acknowledging the potential for incongruence between the presenting complaint and medical findings. If the medical assessment reveals a benign or normal condition and the parent appears more frustrated or angry than relieved by your diagnosis, parental motivation should be assessed carefully.

Clinical evaluation

Since most victims of sexual abuse or assault do not have examination findings, forensic evidence or an STI that provide specific evidence of sexual assault or abuse, the history from the victim is often the most important evidence for legal proceedings and the most important consideration in the clinical diagnosis of sexual abuse or assault. The extent to which a medical history is gathered depends on clinician expertise and comfort, the local investigative procedures for interviewing victims, the victim's willingness to talk, and the context within which the victim first discloses. For example, if a child or adolescent discloses sexual abuse for the first time within a clinical setting, the clinician may encourage and support the patient by allowing them to share any information they wish, but deferring the complete assessment to an experienced sexual abuse unit. The clinician still needs to gather information necessary to assess the patient's immediate medical, psychologic, and safety needs. Such information is best gathered from the patient directly, out of the presence of family members. Family members may be supportive but also distraught, unsupportive or disbelieving; either situation can impact the victim's willingness to disclose information to the clinician.

While certain components of the medical history may be more reliably gathered from a parent (past medical and surgical history, chronic medical conditions, medications), asking the patient such questions allows for rapport building and prepares the child for the types of questions you will ask and details required. Beginning with past medical history enables the clinician to assess the language skills of the child and provides a familiar doctor–patient

Table 11.1 Presenting symptoms and differential diagnoses

Presenting symptoms/signs	Differential diagnoses
Genital/anal bleeding or bruising	Trauma: sexual abuse or accidental
	Superficial excoriations due to local irritants, hygiene issues, obesity, infections
	Anal fissures
	Dehisced labial adhesions
	Lichen sclerosus et atrophicus*
	Urethral prolapse
	Group A β streptococcus infection
	Shigella vaginitis
Genital discharge	STIs: gonorrhea, chlamydia, trichomonas
	Infections that are not STIs: bacterial vaginosis, group B streptococcus, candida, "usual or normal genital flora"
	Noninfectious causes: leukorrhea (physiologic vaginal discharge associated with pubarche), smegma, foreign body
Genital/anal erythema	Nontraumatic irritants: sensitivity to soaps, bleach, insect bites, diaper dermatitis
	Trauma: accidental or nonaccidental**
	Normal physiologic appearance*
	Irritation due to diarrhea/constipation or hygiene issues*
"No hymen" or "opening too big"	Normal variations in anatomy
	Lack of knowledge regarding anatomy
	Anal dilation due to presence of stool, encopresis, neurologic deficit or examination position
	If verified, healed penetrative trauma (usually abusive)***
Genital or anal scar	If verified (thickened, usually raised lesion sometimes with contraction of surrounding tissue), healed trauma, abusive and nonabusive causes possible***
	Labial adhesion*
	Congenital anomalies: linea vestibularis (flat, midvestibule white line), diastasis ani (defect in external anal sphincter appearing as a fan-like smooth white area usually at 12 o'clock in the anal folds), partial or complete failure of midline fusion (smooth, depressed white area appearing between the posterior commissure and the anal verge)

*More common in preadolescents.
**Erythema, in the absence of any other findings, is nonspecific for trauma or abuse.
***Rare.

milieu, re-establishing the goal of the doctor-patient encounter as a co-operative venture towards healing.

History

The components of the medical history that are pertinent to sexual assault include the following.

- Past medical history: chronic medical conditions that may impact anogenital examination findings, such as encopresis, Crohn disease (rectal prolapse, anal skin tags/fistulas), Behçet disease (genital and oral ulcers)
- Menstrual history: menarche (years of menstruation correlated with regularity of cycles), last menstrual period

---

Box 11.2 Resources

Reporting: child protective services hotline; local police or sheriff department

Medical evaluations: children's advocacy centers, regional hospitals

Victim assistance: children's advocacy centers, rape crisis centers, Office of the Attorney General

---

Box 11.3 Sexual assault emergencies

Medical: significant pain/bleeding; assault within 72 hours; acute intoxication

Psychologic: acute anxiety/panic attacks, shock, suicidal ideation

Safety: perpetrator access to victim, nonbelieving parent, victim fearful of parental repercussions

(need for pregnancy testing), regularity of cycles and menstrual volume (need for pregnancy testing), prior gynecologic exam/tampon use (may be better prepared to tolerate sexual abuse/assault examination)

- Sexual history: prior encounters with male and/or female partners, last contact (STI risk; interpretation of exam findings with regard to abuse/assault – acute findings may be specific to assault only if consensual contact is remote), types of sexual contact with consensual partners (STI risk, sites that need to be tested for STIs), use of barrier contraception (STI risk)
- Past abuse history: prior sexual abuse/assault (may modify interpretation of exam findings and treatment plan for therapy), prior or present physical abuse (some teens fear repercussions from parents if sexual abuse revealed)

Physical symptoms/concerns

Conditions that may obscure exam findings include encopresis, obesity (more difficult to visualize hymen and vestibule), folliculitis (pustules caused primarily by shaving pubic hair).

Conditions that may be sequelae of abuse include dysuria after genital contact, pain and/or bleeding after penetration, vaginal discharge (may be STI).

Symptoms reported by patients that may reflect anxiety/concerns stemming from abuse include genital pain, discharge, enlarging stomach, nausea (pregnancy concerns). Note that exam findings often do not reflect reported symptoms, but the clinician needs to provide appropriate reassurance.

Behavioral symptoms

More commonly reported symptoms include the following.

- Sleeping difficulties: nightmares, trouble falling or staying asleep (symptoms of anxiety, intrusive memories)
- School or work difficulties: trouble concentrating or staying on task due to intrusive thoughts of abuse
- Eating difficulties: significant changes in weight (may be reflective of an eating disorder or depression)
- Self-injurious behaviors or thoughts: cutting, overdosing, wishing they were dead
- Delinquency: truancy, crime, runaway, drug/alcohol use

History of abuse

Recommended only for experienced/trained clinicians functioning within the parameters of a child abuse multidisciplinary program; this information should be available to the clinician performing the examination.

- Type of sexual contact: will guide the clinician to target sites for forensic evidence collection and STIs.
- Last abusive sexual contact: guides the clinician in determining schedule for STI testing taking into consideration various incubation periods; if last contact is within 72 hours, exam and evidence collection are urgent.
- Threat/accessibility of abuser to child or adolescent victim: determines urgency of child protective services or law enforcement referral.
- Ingestion of drugs or alcohol, or changes in level of consciousness: toxicology screen (urine and/or blood) to document drug-facilitated sexual assault.
- Frequency of abuse: greater frequency increases risk of STI transmission.
- Abuser risk factors, if known: IV drug abuser, multiple sexual partners of same or different genders, gang member; more extensive STI testing recommended if risk factors present.
- Child or adolescent's feelings/reactions to abuse: many children are ambivalent about getting the abuser into trouble and prefer not to report. Such patients may be reluctant to disclose all details of abuse. If victims appear protective of their abuser and disclose only low-risk types of sexual contact, the clinician may wish to test for STIs anyway on the assumption that not all abuse details have been disclosed.
- Child's perception of adult reactions to abuse: the child may fear repercussions by the abuser or parental disbelief. Approximately one-third of the mothers of children abused by the mother's partner or husband do not believe their child's disclosure of abuse. Clinicians should explicitly ask if victims are afraid of their parents or of going home.

Examination

If the clinician determines that sexual assault likely occurred within the previous 72 hours, a prompt referral to a specialized program with trained sexual assault examiners is strongly urged. Evidence collection requires not only adherence to state protocols and expert examiners, but also specialized equipment and space requirements to ensure appropriate processing and maintenance of a chain of custody for forensic materials. If sexual assault is likely but the last contact occurred more than three days prior, then the clinician may want to refer to pediatricians with expertise and knowledge in the field. The examination may not need to be conducted immediately, but the clinician should contact the specialist promptly to determine the best time to schedule the examination, depending on the needs of the child, family, and the investigative agencies involved. In areas where no specialists are available or in cases where it is not clear whether there is a sufficient suspicion of abuse that warrants reporting, the clinician may opt to examine the child in their office or other clinical setting.

There are three components of the medical examination for suspected sexual abuse or assault: collection of forensic evidence from bodily surfaces, orifices and clothing/linens, visual inspection for bodily, anogenital, and/or oral injury(s), and testing for STIs. The extent to which each component is utilized depends primarily on the history from the victim, as well as examination findings. For example, if a preverbal child presents with a "vaginal discharge" and the parent is concerned about sexual abuse but the exam reveals that smegma is the discharge and there are no injuries, then the clinician may opt not to collect forensic evidence or test for STIs. If the same child has hymenal bruising and scant vaginal secretions, then the clinician will likely opt for forensic evidence collection and testing for sexually transmitted diseases, with a follow-up exam for further testing for STIs in two weeks.

Collection of forensic evidence from bodily surfaces

Detailed instructions are included with each evidence collection kit, and collection protocols are established by state agencies. In general, evidence collection should be done prior to other exam procedures. Most protocols require the victim to unclothe over paper or a sheet which is submitted for debris analysis. Then, samples are taken from the oral cavity, head hair, pubic hair, fingernails, genitals, genital orifices, and anus, and any areas suspicious for dried secretions or bitemarks are swabbed. The areas sampled depend upon the specific protocol instructions, the history of assault, and examination findings.

Samples are air-dried, sealed, and signed in accordance with chain of custody procedures. Typically, the sealed kit is retained in a locked, secured freezer and law enforcement picks the kit up. State forensic labs process the contents for DNA and genetic markers; some labs process the samples with less sensitive or specific tests such as acid phosphatase and P30 protein. Forensic analysis of samples continues to evolve and improve, and will likely affect the procedures and time frame for forensic evidence collection in the future.

Judicious use of forensic evidence collection procedures is advised. The process is somewhat intrusive and may be traumatic to younger patients. In one study of prepubertal children who underwent sexual assault examinations, including forensic evidence collection, approximately two-thirds of the evidence was found on clothing or linens, and no body swabs were positive for forensic materials after 13 hours. Overall, about 25% of kits collected in prepubertal children will be positive for forensically important information. Such studies suggest that forensic evidence collection in prepubertal children should be conducted only in select cases beyond 24 hours. Forensic evidence collection in adolescents and adults is still warranted when such victims present within 72 hours of sexual assault; in select cases, samples may be submitted beyond 72 hours, depending on the examination findings and circumstances.

Visual inspection for bodily and oral, genital, and anal injuries

Victims of acute assault should be examined carefully for bruises, especially involving the face, neck, and head (more common sites for blows) as well as the forearms and lower extremities (more common sites for defensive injuries). While areas of tenderness may be noted, the clinician should be cautious in attributing such findings to trauma without accompanying erythema, ecchymoses or edema; muscle strain and anxiety are other possible causes. Forced oral-penile penetration may result in intraoral injuries, possibly accompanied by grasp marks or bruises to the cheeks or neck. Petechial hemorrhages associated with forced penetration generally occur at the junction of the soft and hard palate, near the uvula. Male genital injuries from sexual assault are rarely seen. Violent pulling of the penis may result in a degloving pattern, with the skin separating circumferentially at the base of the penis; such injuries are far more common within a context of physical, not sexual, abuse.

Female genital injuries from sexual assault are uncommon. While erythema and superficial excoriations of the vestibule and vulva are frequently noted, such findings are nonspecific for trauma. Most acute injuries of sexual assault occur in the posterior vestibule, between the posterior attachment of the hymen and the posterior commissure. Other acute injuries include lacerations and/or bruising of the hymen, and abrasions and bruising of the vestibule or inner labia minora folds. Findings that indicate healed penetrative trauma of the hymen include posterior clefts (defects in the hymen between 3 and 9 o'clock position that extend the entire width of the hymen at a discrete point), and scarring in the posterior vestibule (palpable or causes contraction of surrounding tissue). Deep notches extending more than 50% of the width of the hymen located in the posterior half of the hymen are concerning findings for healed penetrative trauma. The majority of acute injuries heal without sequelae or scarring, in a matter of a few days. In one large patient series of children and adolescents who were examined for acute and nonacute sexual assault, 96% had normal or nonspecific findings of penetrative trauma. While "it's normal to be normal," "normal" does not mean "nothing happened"; in a study of 36 adolescents undergoing sexual abuse examinations while pregnant, 82% had normal "intact" hymens and no scarring.

Anal findings of acute or healed penetrative trauma are rarer than genital findings. Acute findings include deep anal tears, usually in a stellate pattern close to the midline, and hematomas, which should not be confused with hemorrhoids. Healed penetrative trauma of the anus is exceedingly rare; any scarring should be confirmed by palpation or observed contraction of the tissue. Anal dilation, once thought to be an indicator of acute or chronic penetration, is a nonspecific finding for sexual abuse and can be attributable to a number of nontraumatic and physiologic causes.

Examination techniques

There are several examination techniques that can be utilized in the assessment of anogenital trauma. There is also significant potential for examiners to artifactually create abnormalities that may inappropriately be interpreted as scars, hymenal clefts or notches. For this reason, it is essential for examiners to be well trained in techniques and to photodocument findings so that more experienced examiners can review the techniques and interpretation of findings.

Examination techniques utilized in all females are labial separation and labial traction. With the former, the labia majora are parted with the ventral surfaces of fingers of both (gloved) hands, to allow visualization of the labia minora, periurethral tissues, and part of the vestibule and hymen. While this technique usually yields little information, it does allow for the patient to become accustomed to the positioning of the examiner's hands. The second technique, labial traction, is accomplished by grasping the labia majora with the thumb and mid/lateral aspects of the index finger and pulling the labia outwards without too much traction sideways (which could result in iatrogenic tears at the posterior commissure). With this technique, the vestibule is usually well visualized and the hymenal opening becomes evident, allowing for visualization of bruises, tears, notches, and clefts in these structures.

Because the adolescent hymen tends to be redundant and findings can be concealed with the folds of the hymen, the examiner may opt for any of the following techniques to more adequately evaluate the hymen: cotton-tipped applicator probe, Foley catheter, and/or visualization in prone knee–chest position. Utilizing a Q-tip or Foley catheter requires expertise and a gentle touch, as these techniques can cause significant discomfort in a victim. The cotton-tipped applicator can be placed along the internal base of the hymen sequentially at 3, 6, and 9 o'clock, exerting gentle pressure outwards to "stretch" the rim at these points; this technique is sometimes difficult because the hymenal and vaginal tissue may be contiguous in some patients. The Foley catheter technique involves inserting the tip of the catheter into the vaginal vault, inflating the balloon with 15 cc of water, and then gently retracting the catheter until the hymen is "splayed" upon the inflated balloon. The caveat with this technique is that the retracted balloon may simply flatten the hymen against the vestibule, creating the appearance of an "absent" hymen.

The prone knee–chest examination is perhaps the most reliable alternative technique since there is no direct manipulation of hymenal tissue, but it is a difficult position for the patient as it can be embarrassing and technically difficult to master. The patient gets on her knees on the exam table, knees near the end of the table, in line with the hips; she then lays her hips and shoulders on the exam table with a "sway-back" or lordotic curve to the small of her back. The examiner then places their thumbs at the level of the posterior commissure, and lifts the buttocks superiorly until the posterior rim of the hymen is visible. This technique is necessary to confirm any clefts that are seen in the supine position; in addition, hymenal hemorrhages are sometimes better visualized in this position. The prone knee–chest position is the best position for evaluating anal trauma; after several seconds, the anus sometimes dilates and the stellate pattern of tears becomes visible in some victims.

The male genitalia should be examined carefully for bite marks, bruises, and excoriations while the victim is in the supine position; males should be placed in the prone knee–chest position whenever anal trauma, acute or nonacute, is suspected. In general, specimens for forensic evidence and STIs should be gathered when the victim is in the supine position.

Colposcopes and photodocumentation

As mentioned above, photodocumentation is critical to sexual abuse or assault examinations for several reasons. First, examiners may misinterpret findings and images allow for review by experts without requiring the victim to be re-examined. Also, images provide ample opportunity for expert examiners to train others in the correct examination techniques, written documentation, and accurate assessment of findings. Photocolposcopes provide every aspect required for appropriate documentation: a patient record attached to the photographs, electronic storage of patient files, a mechanism for sending images to others through secure encryption, and, most importantly, high-quality images. Most companies that make photocolposcopes also provide technical assistance to ensure continuous operation of equipment. Photocolposcopes are, however, expensive. Digital cameras can be used, with photographs taken by an exam assistant, and are preferable to no photographs at all. The optimal magnification for most anogenital photographs is 3–10×, a factor sometimes difficult to control with digital cameras.

Testing for STIs

There are several testing modalities available for STIs. Table 11.2 summarizes some of these tests, as well as the advantages and disadvantages of each. The clinician should select the test based on their assessment priorities: to ensure that all information gathered is forensically sound and will hold up unequivocally in court, or to ensure that the victim is tested optimally to make certain that all potential adverse outcomes of the abuse are addressed. This choice is most difficult when testing for chlamydia.

While the culture is considered the legal "gold standard," the sensitivity of the culture is low, averaging 60–70%. Nucleic acid amplification tests are more sensitive, but the Centers for Disease Control and Prevention requires two of these tests, targeting different genomes of the organism, to equate the result to a gold standard, an approach which is costly and requires that the child be retested. In a significant majority of cases, the diagnosis of sexual abuse is based on the victim's history, not the exam findings.

If the clinician feels confident in their diagnosis prior to conducting the exam, then they may wish to use the STI tests to optimize their *management* of the patient rather than to *diagnose* sexual abuse; in which case, the clinician should become familiar with the test they are using so that the rationale for using the test can be adequately explained if court testimony is required. If the clinician wishes to legally confirm the diagnosis of sexual abuse, then the gold standard may be the appropriate test. In victims with prior sexual contact with another abuser or with a partner, testing for STIs no longer has forensic significance to the abuse, so the most sensitive and specific test is appropriate.

Other diagnostic tests

The clinician should evaluate the need for pregnancy and drug testing, depending on the history and clinical presentation of the victim. If the victim of an acute assault is menarcheal, a pregnancy test should be conducted and confirmed as negative prior to giving postcoital contraception. Since adolescents do not always report their menstrual history with accuracy, the clinician should test for pregnancy whenever there is a concern. A drug test (urine and/or serum, depending on the time frame and symptoms) and/or electrolytes should be conducted whenever the victim reports ingestion of a substance that altered their mental status or there are signs of intoxication on examination. Drug-facilitated sexual assault is a recognized entity, and drugs such as Xanax, ketamine, Rohypnol, γ-hydroxybutyric acid, and even insulin have been used.

Management

Comprehensive management of the sexual abuse or assault survivor must encompass the medical, mental health, and safety needs of the victim.

Table 11.2 Tests for STIs

STI test	Technique	Tests	Advantages	Disadvantages
Gonorrhea/ chlamydia	Dacron cotton-tipped applicator: vaginal, cervical, urethral*	Culture NAATs**	Legal "gold standard" High sensitivity and specificity; urine samples may be submitted	Low sensitivity for chlamydia "Gold standard" requires two positive results with NAATs
		DNA probes DFA***	No refrigeration No refrigeration; oral/rectal samples acceptable	Low sensitivity Low specificity; available for chlamydia only
Trichomonas	Cotton-tipped applicator or spun urine	Wet mount	Quick results, low cost	Low sensitivity, depending on examiner expertise
		Culture: InPouch TV, Trichosel, Diamond's media	More sensitive depending on examiner expertise	? Some examiners may be better at detection
Human papillomavirus	Clinical diagnosis	N/A	Noninvasive	Small and atypical lesions may not be detected
	Biopsy	Biopsy	May clarify diagnosis; subtyping may be done (?useful)	Painful; low sensitivity if examiner not expert
	HPV DNA tests	Tissue sample: dot blot hybridization, Southern blotting, PCR	Southern blotting considered by some to be "gold standard"	High cost, labor intensive, interpretation of subtypes uncertain
Herpes simplex: type 1 and 2	Cotton-tipped applicator: swab vesicle or ulcer or serum	Culture NAAT: PCR	"Gold standard"; good sensitivity/specificity "Gold standard"; may be better than culture as viral shedding decreases; good sensitivity/specificity	May be less sensitive as viral shedding decreases ?
		Glycoprotein G type-specific assay	Used to detect past disease in suspects when victim is positive; high sensitivity/specificity	5% of population with HSV do not have glycoprotein G
Syphilis	Serum	RPR†, followed by specific antitreponemal test	Cost-effective	RPR may eventually become negative in some individuals
		ELISA screen, followed by RPR	More specific than RPR, less labor intensive	?
Hepatitis A/B/C	Serum	Hep A: IgM antibody Acute Hep B: IgM antibody to core antigen Acute Hep C: total antibody	None	None
HIV	Serum	HIV antibody	None	None

*Only cultures should be used for oral and anal samples
**NAATs: nucleic acid amplification tests: polymerase chain reaction (PCR), ligase chain reaction (LCR), transcription-mediated assay (TMA or APTIMA), strand displacement analysis (Becton-Dickinson Probe)
***Direct fluorescent antibody
†Rapid plasma reagin

Table 11.3 STI treatment and prophylaxis (first-line drugs)

STI	Prophylaxis	Treatment
Gonorrhea	Ceftriaxone 125 mg IM or cefixime 8 mg/kg (max of 400 mg) po x1	Same as prophylaxis; prepubertal children should get ceftriaxone IM
Chlamydia	Azithromycin 20 mg/kg (max 1.0 g) po ×1	Same as prophylaxis or doxycycline 100 mg po bid ×7 days
Trichomonas	Metronidazole 2.0 g po ×1	Same as prophylaxis
Human papillomavirus	? HPV vaccine	Cryotherapy, laser, surgical excision, clinician-applied podophyllum resin 10–25% or trichloracetic acid, patient-applied imiquimod 5% cream ×3d/week, up to 16 weeks
Herpes simplex virus	None currently recommended	Children: aciclovir 80 mg/kg/d po tid ×7–10 days Others: aciclovir 1.2 g/day po tid ×7–10 days
Syphilis	None currently recommended	Benzathine penicillin G 50,000 u/kg IM ×1 (max 2.4 million units, adult dose)
Hepatitis, HIV	None currently recommended	

Medical

Immediate medical needs include surgical or medical management of acute injuries, STI prophylaxis (Table 11.3), and postcoital contraception in cases where the sexual assault involves penile contact or penetration occurring within five days of the examination and the pregnancy test is negative. Plan B, Ovral, and LoOvral are currently approved options and may be available over the counter in some regions. Victims of acute sexual assault may also be candidates for STI prophylaxis against chlamydia, gonorrhea and, in some cases, trichomonas and HIV. Prophylaxis for HIV is costly and requires several weeks of antiviral medication with significant side effects; the efficacy of this prophylaxis is currently unknown.

Fortunately, most victims of sexual abuse or assault do not sustain injuries that require urgent medical or surgical intervention. If an anogenital injury is bleeding profusely, surgical repair may be necessary. All victims of acute sexual assault should be examined carefully for fractures, intra-abdominal injuries, and intracranial injuries.

Mental health

It is important to provide appropriate medical follow-up, especially for victims of acute sexual assault, considering the prolonged incubation period of some STIs, especially human papillomavirus (HPV). Since HPV is one of the more prevalent STIs, a follow-up exam 2–3 weeks after the initial evaluation and, in some cases, several months later is recommended to optimize detection of this disease which carries the risk of cancer later in life. Follow-up examinations also provide opportunities for the clinician to reassure the victim of injury resolution as well as encouraging the victim and their families to enroll in or continue with mental health services.

Any victim of sexual abuse or assault should be screened carefully for self-injurious behaviors and suicide risk. Forearms should be examined carefully for evidence of cutting, a behavior often concealed from parents. Every sexual abuse or assault victim, school age and older, should be queried about self-injurious thoughts and behaviors; sample questions include "Have you ever felt so bad about yourself that you wanted to hurt yourself or die?" Affirmative responses need to be further clarified to determine suicide risk; for example, many adolescents feel like hurting themselves when they are angry but do not wish or intend to die. Inquiry as to the nature (was there a plan for self-injury that they intended to carry out), frequency, evidence of prior injury, and associated symptoms of depression will help the clinician differentiate between those in need of immediate crisis assessment and intervention and those with less urgent mental health needs.

The clinician can play a key role in initiating the emotional recovery of the victim. Victims and family members may have a number of fears and anxieties, some of which can be alleviated by the clinician. For example, victims and family members may be wondering whether the victim "is still a virgin" or may believe the abuse did not occur when they are told the exam is "normal." Clinicians may clarify such terms and provide reassurance that "normal" does not mean "nothing happened." Some victims feel guilty because they delayed their disclosure; the clinician can reassure them that most victims delay their disclosure due to a variety of valid fears. The clinician can also provide encouragement that recovery from sexual assault and return to normalcy is possible. The victim's fears can sometimes be revealed by asking "What would you like to see happen?" or "Are you afraid of anything or anybody?"

Documentation

To the extent that it is possible, the clinician should document their questions, and the patient's answers, in quotes. This is particularly important if the victim is disclosing abuse for the first time, since the circumstances of the "first outcry" are critical to the investigation and legal proceedings that follow. Examination findings should be carefully documented, with extensive details of any visible injury(s). Location, size, color, and characteristics such as bleeding and abrasions should be noted on bodily and/or anogenital findings. As discussed above, photodocumentation is strongly urged, and should support the written documentation of injuries.

The clinician should provide a meaningful interpretation of the findings for nonmedical professionals involved in investigation. The following is one example.

- Normal examination findings
  - Can be consistent with history provided. Note that the majority of exams in sexually abused children are normal or nonspecific, regardless of the type of sexual acts.
  - No specific concerns for sexual contact/abuse identified from medical history
- Nonspecific examination findings (findings can be attributed to both traumatic and nontraumatic causes)
  - Can be consistent with history provided. Note that the majority of exams in sexually abused children are normal or nonspecific, regardless of the type of sexual acts.
  - No specific concerns for sexual contact/abuse identified from medical history

- Abnormal examination findings related to penetrative injury/sexual contact
  - Consistent with type(s) of sexual acts described
  - Consistent with time lapse since last incident of abuse
  - Inconsistent with type of acts described (or no acts described); suggests more penetrative acts of trauma
- Abnormal examination findings not related to penetrative injury/sexual contact
- Other

The summary documentation of the clinician's findings should reflect the extent of their evaluation; for example, if the clinician did not ask questions regarding abuse details, then the summary should only address the exam findings and appropriate interpretation.

Role of the physician in the investigation

Excepting forensic evidence collection, the physician should prioritize the clinical needs of the patient over the needs of the investigation. For example, some investigators may request STI testing in a young child when the history and clinical parameters do not indicate such testing is needed; this decision should be left to the clinician. The clinician should not be required to evaluate investigative information provided by child protective services or the police unless they feel competent to do so; certainly the physician may assist investigative agencies in the interpretation of medical records. The physician should clearly document the injury(s), the relevance of the injury to the assault, the history from the patient, and the medical diagnosis and treatment, including a statement as to the interpretation of a "normal" examination as it relates to sexual assault, and be available for questions that may arise during the investigation.

In some cases, the clinician may encounter a parent who is disbelieving or unsupportive of their child victim. In such cases, the physician should immediately contact child protective services since this is a safety emergency for the child. If a child is afraid to go home or leave with a parent, child protective services should be notified immediately. Families that feel threatened by the suspected abuser may be advised to contact law enforcement and seek a protective order. In some cases, the family can be referred to domestic violence service agencies if the sexual offender is also a batterer; such agencies may be able to offer interim safe housing for these families.

Role of the physician in testimony

The physician may be required to provide testimony in a variety of different legal settings. Most commonly, the physician may testify in a civil child protective services hearing to establish whether the child is safe in their home, or in criminal proceedings where the guilt or innocence of the suspected abuser is established. In civil proceedings the burden of proof is usually "preponderance of the evidence" and witnesses are generally given more liberty in the nature and extent of their testimony. In child protective services hearings, there may be three or more attorneys representing the state, the child or children, and the parents; these proceedings take place in the days to weeks following the investigation of a case. In criminal proceedings, physician testimony is more narrowly defined and determined by the judge and attorneys; the burden of proof is usually "beyond a reasonable doubt." In criminal trials, if the physician's clinical approach is based on the goals of establishing medical diagnosis and treatment, the information gathered and opinions rendered are generally admissible in court under a hearsay exception. Criminal proceedings generally take place months to years after the investigation.

Other less common legal proceedings that may require physician testimony are custody hearings, in which the parameters of child visitation with separated parents is determined, and civil lawsuits, where a child's parent may file suit for monetary compensation of emotional or physical damage to the child resulting from the abuse.

Prevention strategies

The prevention of sexual abuse and assault entails a multidimensional approach. The goal of primary prevention is to prevent sexual abuse before it occurs and the target audience is everyone. Current primary prevention approaches include anonymous helplines for individuals who are sexually attracted to children and self-esteem programs for children and teens. Secondary prevention targets victims and focuses on promoting disclosure to stop abuse that is occurring; harsh penalties for convicted offenders is another approach. Tertiary programs provide services to both victims and perpetrators to reduce the likelihood of revictimization and address the long-term adverse effects of abuse.

The physician has the opportunity to implement prevention strategies in a number of ways. During well-child check-ups the physician may encourage the parent to educate their children to be verbal in situations that are uncomfortable for any reason; in addition, parental monitoring of computer activities is advisable to reduce the child's likelihood of exploring sexually explicit sites that might be accidentally or intentionally encountered by the child, in addition to preventing online solicitation for sex. Physicians can serve as community role models by openly discussing sexual violence, dispelling the shameful stigma that promotes secrecy of this widespread problem. Finally, the physician can ensure that identified victims and perpetrators in their practice seek and follow through with the appropriate therapy and treatment.

Further reading

Adams JA. Evolution of a classification scale: medical evaluation of suspected child sexual abuse. *Child Maltreat* 2001;**6**:31–36.

Adams JA, Girardin B, Faugno D. Adolescent sexual assault: documentation of acute injuries using photo-colposcopy. *J Pediatr Adolesc Gynecol* 2001;**14**:175–180.

American Academy of Pediatrics, Committee on Adolescence. Care of the adolescent sexual assault victim. *Pediatrics* 2001;**107**:1476–1479.

American Academy of Pediatrics. Sexually transmitted diseases. In: Pickering LK (ed) *Red Book: 2006 Report of the Committee on Infectious Diseases*, 26th edn. Elk Grove Village, IL: American Academy of Pediatrics, 2006:166–177.

Berenson AB, Chacko MR, Wiemann CM, Mishaw CO, Friedrich WN, Grady JJ. A case-control study of anatomic changes resulting from sexual abuse. *Am J Obstet Gynecol* 2000;**182**:820–834.

Centers for Disease Control and Prevention. Sexually transmitted diseases treatment guidelines 2002. *MMWR Recomm Rep* 2002;**51**(RR-6):1–78.

Christian CW, Lavelle JM, DeJong AR, Loiselle J, Brenner L, Joffe M. Forensic evidence findings in prepubertal victims of sexual assault. *Pediatrics* 2000;**106**:100–104.

Friedrich WN, Fisher JL, Dittner CA et al. Child Sexual Behavior Inventory: normative, psychiatric, and sexual abuse comparisons. *Child Maltreat* 2001;**6**:37–49.

Heger AH, Ticson L, Guerra L et al. Appearance of the genitalia in girls selected for nonabuse: review of hymenal morphology and nonspecific findings. *J Pediatr Adolesc Gynecol* 2002;**15**:27–35.

Heger A, Ticson L, Velasquez O, Bernier R. Children referred for possible sexual abuse: medical findings in 2384 children. *Child Abuse Neglect* 2002;**26**:645–659.

Heppenstall-Heger A, McConnell G, Ticson L, Guerra L, Lister J, Zaragoza T. Healing patterns in anogenital injuries: a longitudinal study of injuries associated with sexual abuse, accidental injuries, or genital surgery in the preadolescent child. *Pediatrics* 2003;**112**:829–837.

Kellogg ND, American Academy of Pediatrics Committee on Child Abuse and Neglect. The evaluation of sexual abuse in children. *Pediatrics* 2005;**116**:506–512.

Kellogg ND, Parra JM, Menard S. Children with anogenital symptoms and signs referred for sexual abuse evaluations. *Arch Pediatr Adolesc Med* 1998;**152**:634–641.

Kellogg ND, Menard SW, Santos A. Genital anatomy in pregnant adolescents: "normal" does not mean "nothing happened." *Pediatrics* 2004;**113**(1). Available online at: www.pediatrics.org/cgi/content/full/113/1/e67.

Kellogg ND, Baillargeon J, Lukefahr JL, Lawless K, Menard SW. Comparison of nucleic acid amplification tests and culture techniques in the detection of *Neisseria gonorrhoeae* and *Chlamydia trachomatis* in victims of suspected child sexual abuse. *J Pediatr Adolesc Gynecol* 2004;**17**:331–339.

Leder MR, Emans SJ, Hafler JP, Rappaport LA. Addressing sexual abuse in the primary care setting. *Pediatrics* 1999;**104**:270–275.

CHAPTER 12

Adolescent Sexuality

Don Sloan
New York Medical College, New York, NY, USA

Introduction

Every medical specialty has its unique challenges. In dermatology, it is that rash never seen before. In cardiology, the heart rate with a first time heard rhythm. In general surgery, a pain pattern that does not fit into a known scheme. In gynecology, it is the treating of the adolescent patient, especially the first time.

One of the greatest diagnostic and therapeutic tools of the gynecologist as a primary care physician for women is the quality of identifying with the patient. By age and socio-economics. To understand the home environment, the workplace, the marital and sexual foibles. That acronym, HATAH? (How Are Things At Home?), has stood many a clinician in good stead. The answer opens the door to what you need to know. As to adults, to think like the patient comes easier from having been there before and having gone down that same road. HATAH does the rest. However, that advantage is lost somewhat when dealing with the youngster. The age gap alone can do you in.

Whether the doctor is male or female, those same challenges are there. It has been more than enough years since the doctor was an adolescent and changes in modern computer technology, school curricula, exposure to the arts such as the cinema and TV and the speed and ease of travel have exposed today's youngsters to avenues of life that were never available in the older clinician's youth.

It potentially gets worse. If you do not gain the trust and confidence of that teenage female patient sitting across your desk, you have committed two clinical crimes: one,

you have failed her in her needs and two, that may put her off seeking out help in the future. That young patient is judging you as you are judging her. You might never get a second chance to make up for whatever mistakes occurred the first time around.

The embryology of sexuality

One of the rare occasions when researchers can transfer lower animal data to *Homo sapiens* is in the work done on the laboratory rat. The 48-hour window at birth when the newborn rat pup has differentiated gonads but an undifferentiated brainstem allows for its stimulation with various sex hormones. The subsequent changes in rat behavior located a CNS point, now labeled the sex center, at the base of the hypothalamus. Intensive neurodissections of the human brainstem and positron emission tomography (PET) computer models have revealed a near identical area. Human gonadotropin-releasing factor (GnRF) messages from its stimulation to the pituitary and eventually the gonads have given us consistent data.

Female and male sexual anlages

By laboratory study and evidence-based medicine research, it has been accepted that the female human animal is slightly advanced over her male counterpart for the first decade or so of extrauterine life and this starts from the moment of conception.

How is it that human female offspring are developmentally just ahead of their male counterparts, until puberty and early adolescence when both intellect and physical prowess match up? It is because the human conceptus starts out in an undifferentiated manner, and for the first

Pediatric, Adolescent, & Young Adult Gynecology. Edited by A. Altchek and L. Deligdisch. © 2009 Blackwell Publishing, ISBN: 978-1-4051-5347-8.

several (6–9) weeks of intrauterine life, the X chromosome is in control so that the conceptus at that point is a female. When the Y chromosome is passed on by the sperm in around 51% of conceptions, it makes its presence felt at that point. GnRF, estrogen, progesterone and even prolactin have already been isolated in the conceptus.

For the next two to three weeks, the Y chromosome acts on the hypothalamus to release the Müllerian duct inhibiting system (MDIS) protein that suppresses ovarian maturation and by the 14th intrauterine week, full converson to the male hormones has been achieved. The ovaries formed at the level of the metanephros transform into testicles and descend into the labia majora, which become the scrotal sac to achieve the necessary cooler 34°C to allow future sperm to form and survive.

Types of sex and sex assignment

There are six clear forms of sexuality: genetic, chromosomal, hormonal, gonadal, anatomic, all self-explanatory, and social. The first five are predetermined by the passing of the X or Y sex chromosome from the sperm. Turner's (XO) and Kleinfelter's syndrome (XXY) are examples of gross mistransfers. Most others are not seen clinically because they are not compatible with life. In about 2% of cases, there are vague aberrations among the sexes, rarely detected because they usually do not functionally affect the human being.

A delivery room attendant notes the external genitalia and then assigns a sex to the neonate and indelibly marks the birth certificate. The newborn is automatically raised in that social sex environment. Studies have shown that as early as in the hospital newborn nursery, that social sex is operative. Blue blankets are placed on male cribs, pink on female. Friends and family visitors describe the activity of the male child as robust, hearty and manly; the female is called sweet, dainty and lady-like. One experiment deliberately switched two one-day-old infants, male and female, and their blankets. The adjectives stayed true to the sex that had been assigned. The visitors were obviously depicting the actions of the assigned sex, not the actual behavior. Many theories have suggested that such incompatibility could account for adult sexual orientation, transsexuality or when adults insist that assignment was faulty. Some go to great lengths to make corrective hormonal and surgical changes.

It has been further suggested that the time lost in development to make this conversion accounts for the male inferiority in intellect and even physical ability until the beginning of adolescence. Both young boys and girls then go through the normal chronologic sequence of pubarche (the onset of pubic development and hair growth), thelarche (the development of the breasts to full growth according to the Tanner scale), adrenarche (the onset of the sex hormones from the third layer of the adrenal gland) and finally, in the female, menarche (the onset of menses).

It is at that point that the social sex takes full command. The young female at menarche is traditionally passed on by her pediatrician and now faces the gynecologist for the first time. The gynecologic clinician is facing an adolescent who has enjoyed a certain superiority over her male counterpart, albeit subtle, but is about to reach parity, surpassed in physique due to the anabolic power of the androgens.

The physiology of adolescent female sexuality

The period between childhood and sexual maturity's onset at adolescence has been called "the long inch." It is so short but so much is happening in the young woman's development. The young patient's chronologic age seems to matter little. She has already passed through her pubarche, thelarche, adrenarche, and menarche. That sixth form of sexuality is now taking hold and the clinician must be prepared to face any of her functional conflicts.

Over a variable period of several months to a few years, starting with the onset of the teens, three stages of female sexuality take place. They are a sexual interest followed by a period of time of sexual activity and finally, a form of sexual intercourse (coitarche). The stage at which the gynecologist first sees the patient is dependent on many factors, such as familial influences, home living conditions, socio-economics and the extent of education and peer exposure. More advanced lifestyles take over, via computer technology and the internet, media and literature laxities, and ease of travel.

Interviews and surveys taken at various medical centers with sexuality services have reported that key roles are played by home influences, the structure of the patient's church and school communities, and then by the family physician or gynecologist.

The first gynecologic encounter

The ACOG recommends that the initial gynecologic visit occur at age 13–15. This should be focused on preventative measures and education, one of the clinician's chief roles. The doctor must cover such topics as the girl's adolescent development, those six forms of sexuality, the menarche, sexual orientation, family planning where applicable, sexually transmitted diseases (STDs), nutrition, and injury prevention. The goal is clear: the establishment of a mutually respectful inter-relationship that could last the lifetime of either.

As with all clinical office consultations, the intake starts with a handshake, an eye-to-eye contact and the establishment of some form of mutual address. William Masters, of the Masters and Johnson sex therapy team, always insisted that his patients address him as "Doctor" despite his optional use of first names based on the patients' ages, marital status, and comportment. He urged the establishment of a level of respectful authority that would be necessary to act as an accepted teacher. On the other hand, many clinicians have credibly suggested that first name usage may indicate a sense of warmth and friendship rather than disrespect. Since so much depends on the personalities of both parties, this is best left up to the individual situation and usually finds its own level.

The clinician must always be aware, however, of any inappropriate behavior on the part of the patient, such as any form of patient–doctor seduction with subtle sexual moves that are intended to control the exchanges. It must be made clear that their professional relationship is based on exactly that – professionalism – and that the patient will take away valued advice only when that is established. Patient–doctor seduction, regardless of how subliminal or stemming from either side, distorts the doctor's care and professional intent.

The sexual history

The problems presented by the patient, of whatever quality and severity, must be clearly understood. Any language barrier must be overcome. The physician should remember that in front of the desk is a possibly troubled youngster with very likely a totally different set of lexicon innuendos and aphorisms.

A good practice is for the gynecologist to develop a set of terms and language that is clearly identified with the adolescent. This can sound crude and outside the doctor's usual vocabulary. But the doctor will develop a better rapport with the patient if they are more or less on the same page. Sexuality is so misrepresented in our culture that young girls need as much valid information as possible and from someone they trust who is knowledgeable and communicative.

The clinician needs to find ways of letting the patient know their exchanges will be mutual. Rather than "What are you talking about?," "Tell me more about that" is a way of getting the patient to explain her problems in more neutral terms instead of her vernacular, without telling her blatantly you just do not understand. Unless she feels comfortable, the youngster will feel she is not getting through, the clinician is insensitive and the generation gap between them is too wide.

It cannot be overstressed that the patient must get the message that her privacy and confidentiality are being protected. This is likely the first trait she is seeking in someone who could become her trusted doctor and friend for a lifetime of need. However, she should be reminded that, as a teenager, she is a part of a family complex and certain things might have to be shared with her guardians, only with an assurance that her health is primary. The message to be conveyed is that they all have the same shared goals.

Medical details

The patient's organic history follows. This starts with a recap of her childhood diseases and infirmities and any hospitalizations and exposures to domestic and foreign syndromes and endemics. Then any advent of prior sexual involvement, female or male, and any past pregnancy history and its outcome. That will lead to the need for family planning, now or eventually.

Also to be discussed are the teenage issues of date rape, mood swings of note, school performance, seatbelt and possible bicycle helmet use, safe driving, alcohol, street drug and tobacco use, and any eating disorders. HATAH is a nice way to start it all off.

Parental involvement

One or more parent(s) will perhaps have accompanied the patient, especially the first time. It should be stated at the outset and reconfirmed that despite what might eventually occur because of the patient's youth, her complaints and the legal framework of the community, her confidentiality will be protected. The patient and parents are always to be offered an initial few private moments with the doctor to set those ground rules.

One of the well-accepted Freudian tenets is the role the father plays in his daughter's concerns. Studies have clearly shown that father separation from the children of either sex by death, divorce, work pattern, economics, alcohol, etc. by the age of 14 is high on the list as a background for those who are sexually or maritally dysfunctional as adults.

First physical and breast examination

The first visit with the young lady does not have to include her first pelvic exploration or even a physical exam of any sort. It is exactly that portion of the visit that is most feared by the young woman. Although her pediatrician might have been a male, this is likely the first time she feels she will be exposed to a "strange" male as an "adult." This first visit can be just to get acquainted and then the physical and pelvic exams can be rescheduled, depending on the urgency of the situation.

The eventual pelvic exam warrants more common sense than didactic instruction. Whether to have a third party present, such as a parent/guardian or office aide, has been debated since Hippocrates wrote his oath. With some staff always within the general office/clinic, the patient should be allowed to set that rule, assuming that patient–doctor seduction is not an issue. For the actual exam, the hands of the physician should always be gloved to further instill the imprimatur of professionalism, using a bare-hand exam only when the pathology indicates.

The girl's first breast exam will be most significant. This could be the first opportunity to remind the patient that what is happening that day will continue regularly for the rest of her life. Your instructions should include self-examination of the breast, adding a clinical aura to the meeting, and a good add-on here is to teach her that by far most meaningful future breast lumps are patient detected.

Tanner scale

In the mid-20th century, University of London Emeritus Professor of Pediatrics, James Mourilyan Tanner devel-

oped a classification of sexual development that has become the standard for the gynecologic evaluation of the adolescent. Every first visit chart note should include a Tanner scale designation for future adrenarche and thelarche references. The Tanner scale is as follows.

Pubic hair (adrenarche/female)

- I none (prepuberty)
- II long, downy hair growth with slight pigmentation
- III more coarse and curly, with some lateral extension
- IV coarse and curly adult quality, across entire pubis
- V hair extends to medial surface of the thighs

Breasts (thelarche/female)

- I no glandular tissue; pale areola follows skin contour
- II breast bud forms; areola distinctly noticed
- III noted elevation of bud; areola at skin contour
- IV areola and nipple papilla form own mound above skin
- V breast full size; areola returns to skin contour

First pelvic examination

Whenever the first genital exam takes place, always based on an individual response to that first exchange and history, its necessity must be fully explained, no matter how obvious. The message from the clinician is how important this step is in her development as an adult woman and how a satisfactory experience will be passed on to her own future offspring with equal rewards.

It is most helpful if the office has a supply of accurate sketches and models to fully explain the next steps in the exam. The patient should be reminded that if she is virginal, the exam will in no way interfere with any moral or religious concerns, that there are all sizes of specula for the Pap smear and cultures, when indicated, and that at first, the rectal exam may suffice to get an adequate idea as to her pelvic status. It is wise to add that eventually, a full vaginal bimanual examination will be needed to reassure all involved that she is ready to take on a full female life. A dental metaphor sometimes helps, reminding the patient that many, including the doctor, cringe when hearing the dentist say "Open wide," but that both exams are necessary for good health.

In order to help overcome this initial anxiety, it may be useful to demonstrate how tension will cause muscle contraction and make the pelvic exam painful from a involuntary contraction of the bulbous and ischiocavernosus muscles. Have the patient make a tight fist and then gently touch the dorsalis muscle between the thumb and the index finger with any sharp object, such as an open safety pin. Next, have her relax her fist and then apply the pin in an identical fashion. The difference in pain perception will be dramatic and it will be an indelible lesson in the need to relax.

Patient evaluation and discussion

The first rule for the clinician is to remember that the patient in front of you, regardless of her age, is a sexual being. Barring the unexpected and rare disorders such as sexual identification dysfunctions, infections, anomalies, palpable pelvic masses, various endocrinopathies or pregnancy and its ramifications, she is a normal and healthy sexual female human being.

That word "normal" should be explained, for as a doctor, your principal function is to make the abnormal into normal. Whatever the patient might disclose about her own sexuality is most likely a variant of that norm. Concerns are addressable only when the patient herself asks for such help.

The adolescent's own childhood

Over her first two years of life, the female toddler became aware of her body parts, with oral and then genital exploration that proved to be occasionally gratifying. Then came the elimination functions up to the third year. Over the next preschool years came genital interest that was characterized by self-exploration and romantic attachment to any of her guardians or close significant others, all normal beginnings. This is true whether the youngster will ultimately determine for herself if she is hetero- or homosexual.

At around seven to nine years old, she became intensely curious about others, with information obtained from peers, the media, and teachers. Then she entered adolescence when she became more aware of her own genital anatomy and casual contacts with others of either sex. She will have started reading and got all sorts of media exposure. There was playful sexual exploration that was considered clandestine and avoided consciously.

Masturbation

By the mid to later teens, now in need of gynecologic scrutiny, she might have had some inadvertent or deliberate masturbation experience. An inquiry must be gentle and designed to avoid accusation as an aberrant activity. Instead of "Do you masturbate or play with yourself?" it is better to ask an assumption question, such as "How old were you when you first touched yourself?" The reply will be in a form of a denial or a relieved admission that might have been concerning her. This is then explained to the patient as a normal event in her sexual development and not as a mark of shame.

The patient is then taught that there are three forms of sexuality – heterosexual, homosexual and autosexual – and that all three are normal and healthy expressions of her creativity and within the bounds of proper social behavior. The adolescent will have had a first inadvertent masturbatory episode but may deny it, sometimes vigorously. This may be a signal that she is having difficulty addressing that urge and is wrapped up in the myths of guilt and shame. It is then that the messages from a trusted doctor will do the most good. Because masturbation is so loaded an issue in our culture, it is reasonable that the doctor should mention it at the first visit, and possibly return to it when or if the patient attends for continuing care.

Now in your care

The adolescent has reached a time of turmoil, upheaval and confusion in her early teens. Trusted teaching is needed for her to face the inevitable – that her sexual interest and activity will lead to her coitarche and she will need understanding parents, significant others in her life and her doctor to be prepared. She has reached a time in her life when sexual exploration and experimentation are normal patterns in her development. But subliminal anxiety remains as well. There is a constant rate of suicide and self-harm in the adolescent group because of unsettled conflicts, out of concerns that center about her answers to HATAH and/or her sexuality. There may be hidden issues such as masturbation, multiple sex partners or sexual experimentation. Denial is a frequent defense mechanism and the clinician must be careful not to harshly expose it in a patient. The last thing she needs is a prosecutor or judge and jury.

Just about the biggest crime committed by the intake physician is to be judgmental in any way. To any partner or masturbatory active patient, do not preach abstinence. To a partner or masturbatory virgin, do not preach such involvement. Ideally, do not preach at all. Stay objective. Ask the right question; then listen and hear.

One good rule to keep in mind – haste makes waste. Proceed slowly. The patient is likely in great fear, despite her outer appearance, and needs time to ask and react.

Sexually transmitted diseases

Adolescents are disproportionately affected by STDs due to unprotected sexual encounters and poor access to healthcare, or healthcare they will accept. The taller columnar epithelium of the ectocervix leaves them open to a higher rate of such infections. Barrier contraception use, one study showed, dropped from 75% in the ninth grade to a low of 50% by the time they were seniors. The leaning to be more daring and experimental is higher at that point. A 2006 Centers for Disease Control (CDC) survey reported that one-third of US girls are coitally active by age fifteen and they tend to have multiple partners.

Confidentiality and staying within legal bounds

The Health Insurance Portability and Accountability Act of 1996 (HIPAA) that went into full effect in 2004 has not drastically changed the gynecologist and adolescent scene. The HIPAA has generally allowed for state regulations and considers that if a minor is being treated for a condition that renders her emancipated, she also has the right to exert HIPAA confidentiality regulations when parental needs and rights come into play. Protected Health Information (PHI) rules are under the aegis of the states and it is up to the doctor's discretion whether the exposure of the patient would negatively affect her well-being. Some states have such legal PHI entities as "anonymous" testing and "confidential" testing that differentiate between

types of patient records and how they are labeled. The courts have often been protective of doctors in cases when controversy has arisen.

Emancipation

The independent status of the adolescent also plays a role in her care. The states have overwhelmingly protected the minor's right to confidentiality. Proof of maintaining separate living quarters, with or without a significant partner, and having given birth are among the ways emancipation is determined. Such allowed conditions include contraception prescribing, pregnancy-related issues, STDs, substance abuse, mental health disorders, pelvic exam needs and any condition that requires a report to the local health authorities.

When the state does not have it specifically spelled out, the consenting adolescent, not the parent(s), controls the healthcare decisions. This is the best opportunity to relate to the parent(s) the same message as was given to the young patient – that all medical decisions made by the gynecologist are a part of their shared goal, which is the well-being and health of the youngster. All parties involved often yield quietly when this is realized.

Keys to dealing with adolescent sexuality

The gynecologist cannot move into adolescent sexuality as a discipline without encountering the concept of the "friends with benefits" phenomenon that characterizes adolescent sexual behavior. Much of our present social order penalizes the young woman instead of supporting her. The clinician must bear in mind that despite progress made since women gained their suffrage, sexual issues retain a more controlling factor when it comes to young girls. We may be becoming less misogynist but we remain somewhat androcentric. Girls are often considered lewd or loose when they have multiple sex partners, for example, but boys are proudly thought of as "macho" and manly.

Coitarche

The techniques of coital connection may be discussed by the adolescent gynecologist. Oral sex is often spoke of by the female adolescent as not being "real sex" and "I am still a virgin." Nevertheless, it is real sex to the partners and often the girls yield just to gain peer approval or to "get a date to the movies on Saturday night." Sex must be taught to the patient as a whole-person experience, and the principal sex organ, the brain, functions as such whether it is penile-vaginal insertion or not. This myth was expanded during the 1998 Oval Office fracas over whether "sex" had occurred when there was only oral participation.

A subtle but key problem is that many young women who present to the gynecologist for education about their sexuality are physically mature but perhaps not so emotionally. Adolescence is an time of action and restraint. Schools, churches, and parents often teach repression of urges in order to concentrate on study and careers. But those exciting forces that are normally blossoming in the youngster must be allowed to surface and be expressed in a healthy format. Nature will not be denied.

The gynecologist's challenge

The onus is on the doctor for the clinician usually has the advantage of knowing what has already taken place at home, school, church, and playground. Knowing that the patient is sexually interested and wants to move forward, the doctor's role is clear.

The counseling must display a sense of confidence, knowledge and ability to listen and hear in an objective manner and give the message that the doctor appreciates the age/cultural difference. It must be clear that confidentiality will be honored. Humor, even if well-meant, must not be allowed to diminish the seriousness of the session and it must be stressed that the doctor is acting as a clinician, scientist and teacher, not as judge and jury.

Finally, the clinician must "know thyself." The physician should feel comfortable in this setting or recrimination

can creep into the relationship. If that is the case, a wise and honest gynecologist will accept those self-limitations and refer the patient on to someone who will accept the young patient without those barriers. We must remember what Hippocrates decreed: *primum non nocere* – first, do no harm.

Acknowledgments

The author would like to thank the following individuals for data personally communicated to him used in this chapter: Hara Marano, Editor-at-Large, *Psychology Today*, New York, NY; Luci Fernandes PhD, University of Connecticut, Department of Anthropology, Storrs, CT; Allison Sloan DaSilva, Librarian, Reading, MA; Justin Frank MD, Department of Psychiatry, George Washington University Medical Center, Washington, DC; and Helen Miller, Counsellor, Kensington High School, Philadelphia, PA.

Further reading

ACOG. Recommendations in ages 13–15 ObGyn Visit. *ObGyn News* 2006.

Anderson S, Schaechter J, Brisci J. Adolescent patients and their confidentiality: staying within legal bounds. *Contemporary Obstet Gynecol* 2006.

Hewitt GD. The young woman's initial gynecologic visit. *Female Patient* 2006;31.

Masters W, Johnson V. *Human Sexual Response*. Boston, MA: Little, Brown, 1966.

Rivlin ME, Martin RW. *Manual of Clinical Problems in Obstetrics and Gynecology*, 5th edn. Philadelphia, PA: Lippincott, Williams and Wilkins, 2000.

Wikipedia. The Tanner stages. Available online at: en.wikipedia.org/wiki/Tanner_stage

CHAPTER 13

Psychologic Aspects of Gynecologic Problems

Albert Altchek

Mount Sinai School of Medicine and Hospital, New York, NY, USA

Introduction

Almost every gynecologic problem of the young patient has a psychologic counterpart.

If the child has had several unpleasant examinations, when she arrives at the office she may be terrified, cling to the mother and refuse to remove her clothing or be examined. This is not unusual (Chapter 6).

Rarely there may be the opposite reaction. With an almost seductive approach, she may volunteer "I have something interesting down there." Some children who need attention discover that reporting genital complaints creates immediate concern.

With separation of parents and divorce, there may be suspicion, real or planned, regarding legal aspects of visitation and alimony. One parent may repeatedly ask the child about inappropriate touching or molestation which sometimes makes the child think it did happen.

Specific gynecologic problems

Vulvovaginitis

The most common gynecologic problem of the child is vulvovaginitis. Sometimes the child thinks it is punishment for self-exploration of her "private parts" and she is afraid to tell the mother. Sometimes the mother is slow in taking the child to the office through concern that it might be due to someone in the family, or she is worried

Pediatric, Adolescent, & Young Adult Gynecology. Edited by A. Altchek and L. Deligdisch. © 2009 Blackwell Publishing, ISBN: 978-1-4051-5347-8.

about creating suspicion that the child has a gynecologic anomaly which might reduce future fertility, or from simple embarrassment.

Vaginal foreign body

Vaginal foreign body causes a persistent, foul-smelling profuse, bloody vaginal discharge and is often not diagnosed for months. Sometimes the presenting problem is psychologic because the child is avoided by friends and teachers because of the malodor which the child herself may not appreciate.

Most foreign bodies are wads of toilet tissue which cannot be detected by pelvic ultrasound or rectal examination. The usual sequence of events occurs when the child rubs the itchy vulva with a finger covered by toilet tissue after voiding. By accident the finger enters the vagina and then is withdrawn. The toilet tissue remains in the vagina and due to levator muscle reaction, it is pulled up and remains high in the posterior fornix. Muscle action causes the sheet of toilet tissue to roll up into a ball or wad which develops a dark gray-black appearance. Less frequently, the foreign body is a narrow plastic bottle cap resembling an arrowhead which may provoke a severe midvaginal granulomatous reaction resembling a malignancy. The diagnosis is made by discovery and removal of the foreign body usually by irrigation or vaginoscopy, depending on the individual child.

Then comes the psychodrama. The mother wants to know the cause. When it is explained she may thrash the child, screaming "Who did this to you?" The child always denies all knowledge of how it got there. The child may understand that it is not proper to put a finger there. It is also possible that she may have forgotten or did not want to remember that she herself did it. With toilet tissue the symptomatic discharge may not begin until after several weeks. Almost inevitably, there is more than one wad and careful examination shows they were inserted at different times. The mother and child may cry hysterically.

Management requires a calm explanation to the mother, emphasizing that the child is not evil, that it will not affect her health or reproductive ability, that the mother should not discuss it with anyone else (except medical professionals) and that the mother should not berate the child further. Reaccumulation of the wads is not rare. The best prevention is to let the child know that if it recurs she will not be able to go to summer camp or some other event. Another approach is a reward.

To avoid temptation, keep the child away from toilet tissue. Supply bulky soft witch hazel pads to use after voiding and give the child a packet to take to school. These pads are used to treat hemorrhoids and are too bulky to insert into the vagina and cannot be torn into smaller pieces. Thus the child learns that she has to assume responsibility for her health. Of course, the child should also be evaluated regarding the cause of itching (Chapter 7).

Normal development

When children are about age 10 they become aware and sometimes alarmed by body change. The breasts ("boobs") start to develop, and pubic and vulva hair appear. Axillary odor and hair may cause concern. The girl may react with sensitivity, shyness, modesty, and a concern for privacy.

With these changes comes anxiety and almost all girls wonder "Am I developing normally?" Movie stars have no axillary or arm and leg hair, and are slender. Their breasts are symmetric. In addition, girls become taller and sometimes awkward compared to boys of the same age who are usually less socially oriented. The patient needs reassurance that no one in the world is exactly symmetric and that she is developing normally.

She must be prepared for menarche. If she is not prepared and the first menses occurs when she is away at summer camp, she may be frightened and think that she has injured herself.

Anovulatory dysfunctional uterine bleeding

Only half of adolescents ovulate when menstruation begins and therefore half are at risk for usually painless anovulatory dysfunctional uterine bleeding (ADUB). This may cause complete irregularity of menstrual flow regarding amount and timing. Less common is the characteristic pattern of three months of amenorrhea followed by continuous bleeding for a month. The latter causes a dramatic psychodrama. The mother drags the daughter to the office, claiming that she is hemorrhaging. Unless the physician is prepared, there is chaos (Chapter 22). The physician has to make an immediate clinical decision regarding hospitalization, ruling out dangerous blood loss, incomplete abortion, coagulation defect, trauma, rigid foreign body, and rare vaginal tumor. Most cases are ADUB which is best managed by high doses of oral contraceptive (OC) pills, even if tests are still pending, and observation. The important thing is that the bleeding usually stops in one or two days with OC if the diagnosis is correct (Chapter 22).

Rokitansky syndrome

A more stressful and prolonged psychodrama occurs when the diagnosis of Rokitansky syndrome (congenital absence of the uterus and vagina) is made. The usual situation is a healthy adolescent, physically and emotionally perfectly normal, with normal growth and development, who does not menstruate. The mother may state that the primary care doctor reassured her daughter, saying "Don't worry – you are on the curve" (of estrogen-directed development). Later x-rays for bone age, chromosomes, and hormone tests are done, which are normal. Eventually she is referred for examination which should have been done at birth. With careful inspection of the dimple where the vagina should be and rectal examination revealing an absence of the uterus, the clinical diagnosis can usually be made in a few minutes by someone with experience.

Both mother and daughter want to know the diagnosis at once. The mother immediately cries "It must be my fault, I should have taken more vitamins or rested more." The patient wails "Why is God torturing me?" Both are unable to process any new information because of the severe reaction of depression which may persist for about six weeks. I always advise psychiatric consultation but the patient refuses, saying "I am not crazy." I explain that she is correct but I am giving her difficult news and I do not want her to discuss the situation with anyone other than a discreet professional person.

Quick Take 13.1

Possible psychologic management of Rokitansky syndrome

- No one in the world is perfect.

- The cause is unknown and it is no one's fault.

- You are fortunate not to have a life-threatening congenital anomaly.

- You are blessed to have a supportive family, good intelligence, good general health and you are attractive. Unless you tell someone about the matter, no one will know.

- About 15–20% of all married couples with a uterus are infertile.

- You will find satisfaction from achievement in school, arts, helping others, etc.

- This will enhance your self-image and self-worth and cause others to want to be your friend or be associated with you.

- One way or another, a functioning vagina will be made. Normal orgasm for yourself and your husband/partner will occur.

- Go out socially.

- I expect that sooner or later you will find someone and develop a mutual close emotional relationship. If a permanent relationship is planned and the partner desires children, consider explaining that it would be necessary to adopt children, or consider a surrogate mother to carry the child created by *in vitro* fertilization of the patient's egg and husband's sperm.

Conclusion

I find that I am nearly always forced to be a practical psychiatrist. I am always concerned about suicide, which has not happened with my patients, and about patient self-esteem. The physician has to emphasize the positive (Quick Take 13.1).

Further reading

Altchek A. Congenital absence of the uterus and vagina. In: Altchek A, Deligdisch L (eds) *The Uterus: Pathology, Diagnosis and Management.* New York: Springer-Verlag, 1991:272–293.

Altchek A. Psychologic aspects of adolescent obstetric and gynecologic conditions. In: Heacock DR (ed) *A Psychodynamic Approach to Adolescent Psychiatry: the Mount Sinai Experience.* New York: Marcel Dekker, 1980:239–278.

Altchek A. What to do when there is no vagina. *Contemp Obstet Gynecol* 1988;**32**:50–68.

Altchek A. Pediatric and adolescent gynecology. In: Nichols DH, Evard JR (eds) *Ambulatory Gynecology.* Philadelphia, PA: Harper and Row, 1985:20–62.

CHAPTER 14

Approach to and Evaluation of the Adolescent Female

Anne Nucci-Sack, Mary Rojas, Ivanya L Alpert, Elizabeth Lorde-Rollins, Mara Minguez, & Angela Diaz

Mount Sinai Adolescent Health Center, New York, NY, USA

Introduction

Adolescents have drive, curiosity, and desire for autonomy, all counterpoised with normal insecurities and uncertainties about themselves and what lies ahead. Life is filled with new challenges that require guidance to navigate. Without direction, these challenges result in risk-taking behaviors and poor outcomes. Relationships are crucial and can happen, or not, in an instant. As an adolescent health provider, you will greatly impact future experiences by helping your patients to make healthy choices and by identifying resources in addition to managing any medical issues they may bring to the clinical encounter. This chapter will concentrate on reproductive health services in the adolescent female, a crucial component in integrated care.

Adolescent-friendly services

Staff and practice competencies are signaled in the behaviors and skills of staff, the physical environment, the written and visual materials, and programming. Evening, weekend, and summer hours are critical so as not to interfere with other important activities such as school or work. Physical environment creates a "feeling." Posters, literature, videos, and artwork with positive messages about personal identity, sexual, and cultural diversity and pride

Pediatric, Adolescent, & Young Adult Gynecology. Edited by A. Altchek and L. Deligdisch. © 2009 Blackwell Publishing, ISBN: 978-1-4051-5347-8.

further this goal. Create a safe place to talk about negative experiences such as violence, sexual coercion, sexually transmitted infections (STIs), and other sensitive topics.

Communication should be sincere, direct, and clear. It should be respectful, nonjudgmental, age and developmental stage appropriate. Be aware of the way culture and sexual orientation affect an adolescent's reproductive health. Examine your own preconceptions. Some clinicians may find it challenging to assess patient populations with whom they've had little experience, such as poor or homosexual patients. Showing interest demonstrates caring and quickly builds the relationship which is as important in the long term as the actual services provided during that visit.

Confidentiality is the first cornerstone of adolescent health. Know the confidentiality laws for your state, and get comfortable talking about them with adolescents and their families. Inform patients which services will be provided confidentially (e.g. STI screening) as well as instances when confidentiality will be breached (e.g. ongoing abuse). This discussion should occur with both the adolescent and the parent (if present), before taking a history.

Developmental stages

There are considerable differences between a young adolescent and an older one (Table 14.1). Their developmental stage will affect how you communicate and what to expect.

An adolescent's cognitive development affects her ability to make decisions. In the early stages, thinking is

Table 14.1 Developmental tasks across adolescence

Task	Early (10–13 years)	Middle (14–17 years)	Late (18–21 years)
Physical	Body changes begin Menses and sexual maturation	Body changes almost complete	Changes complete
Cognitive	Concrete – very literal	Increased capacity for abstraction	Abstract
Body image	Concern with body changes	Becoming comfortable with "new body"; concerns with "looking good"	Acceptance
Emotional	Concerned with peer acceptance	Sense of invulnerability	Understanding of behavioral consequences
Peer relationships	Mostly with same-sex peer groups	Begins to have special and/or sexual relationship	Individual relationships more important than peer groups

concrete, health information or advice is taken literally. For example, discussion with an early adolescent about a chlamydia infection and the increased risk of infertility will likely be interpreted literally, i.e. she is infertile and does not need to use birth control. When giving information or advice, target your language to the adolescent's cognitive and emotional stage of development.

The medical interview

General considerations

Adolescents want to talk about sensitive issues, behaviors, and risks; however, providers fail to ask about these issues. Ask directly about all aspects of their lives, including areas of strength and struggle. A provider who does this demonstrates interest, competence and willingness to handle their disclosures. Evaluate the adolescent in the context of her social circumstances and "culture." Best outcomes are achieved when expectations are clear and concrete, and the patient is treated with respect in a nonjudgmental and gender-neutral manner. Partnering with the adolescent will maximize your "data-gathering ability" and will open opportunities for education and motivation. Demonstrating empathy through legitimizing, validating, and supporting the adolescent patient will enhance the development of rapport. If clinicians are hesitant in their questioning and information exchanges, the adolescent's response will be limited.

The first visit

The introduction

If a parent accompanies the adolescent, the provider should introduce themselves to the adolescent first and then to the parent. Another option is to allow the adolescent to introduce the adult with her. This sends a message that the adolescent is your patient. Before the actual interview begins, take the time to clearly explain how the visit will be structured, beginning the interview with the adolescent and the parent together. This allows for parental concerns to be voiced early. Obtain the chief complaint from the parent and the patient individually, as they are likely to diverge. Parents are particularly helpful around family medical history. However, for the remainder of the interview, the parent should not be present, since the adolescent may not feel comfortable disclosing sensitive information. Ask the parent to have a seat in the waiting room and assure her that she will be brought back into the room for a final "wrap-up." If the adolescent requests the parent be present then the parent should be asked to return for the examination portion. The adolescent usually appreciates some time alone with the physician, as long as the physician's body language and tone remain open, friendly, and nonthreatening.

The medical and psychosocial interview

The components of the conventional medical interview apply to the adolescent patient: chief complaints, history of present illness, past medical history, family medical history, allergies, medications/immunizations, and review of systems. The psychosocial assessment is of equal importance and may be supplemented with information obtained through a self-administered report questionnaire such as the AMA's Guidelines for Adolescent Preventative Services (GAPS) [1]. However, we recommend a face-to-face psychosocial interview which allows the clinician to quickly yet comprehensively explore the "culture" and "context" of an adolescent's life. The "HEEADSSS Interview" (Home, Education, Employment, Eating, Activities, Drugs, Sexuality, Suicide, Depression, and Safety) [2] is a well-established tool originally created by Henry Berman and later modified by Erick Cohen. The information gleaned from such an interview helps build rapport.

Pay close attention not just to the content of the responses, but to facial expression and body language. The importance of nonverbal communication cannot be overemphasized. Likewise, if you are making poor eye contact or have an "avoidant" body posture, your interview will be unproductive.

The gynecologic and sexual history

Menstrual irregularities are common among adolescent females. Always ask for the last menstrual period (LMP) and if it was a typical period for her. The LMP should be considered a vital sign when working with adolescents. In the event of a missed menses, all female patients (including those who report being sexually naïve) should have a pregnancy test, as the consequences of missing a pregnancy are severe.

Interviewing around sexual activity is essential. Prepare the adolescent for the next set of questions. "I ask all my patients about sensitive subjects, like sex and drug use, and I want to let you know upfront that I don't discuss this information with anyone, unless your or someone else's life is in danger. Are you comfortable with that?" Ask about touching, kissing, digital penetration, as well as vaginal, oral, and anal intercourse. Ask about her first sexual encounter, the total number of partners, same-sex partners, number of sexual partners over the past three months, alcohol or drug use, condom use and how well she feels she can communicate with partners. Ask whether sex is consensual. "A lot of my patients feel pressured to have sex. Has that ever happened to you?" Inquire about last sexual intercourse, whether it was protected and how, and age of her partner. If sexual activity is reported as unprotected and within 120 hours of the patient's visit, offer emergency contraception.

Over 20% of adolescents have experienced nonconsensual sex [3] and it is imperative to screen for abuse at every visit. If you do not ask about forced sexual activity, it is unlikely that she will volunteer this information; however, asking does not guarantee that your patient will disclose, as she may not feel comfortable enough to discuss this at the first visit. Especially in patients who are very fearful

or tense during a pelvic exam, you may suspect past or current sexual abuse and should gently revisit this inquiry at the end of the exam after the patient is dressed. Do not press your patient, as trust and rapport are important for disclosure. A pressured adolescent is less likely to continue care. If your patient discloses that she has been sexually abused, first establish that she is safe now, and ask her if she feels comfortable sharing with you what happened to her.

Familiarize yourself with local resources and reporting requirements. If there is a past history of abuse but none currently, it is useful to have resources such as adolescent survivor groups to which you may refer your patient. Let her know that the abuse was not her fault and that it may take time to heal from this experience. Social work referral is imperative and should be reinforced at future visits if the patient will not accept referral at the first visit.

If she is abstinent, positively reinforce the adolescent's behavior and review strategies for sexual decision making. When counseling abstinence to a sexually active adolescent, do so in a nonjudgmental fashion. Let her talk freely. If sexually active ask about her reasons for engaging in sexual activity and whether she is protecting herself from unintended pregnancy and STIs. At every visit a thorough discussion of safer sex, including condom and/or dental dam use, and contraceptive counseling is indicated.

Pregnancy history and contraceptive history are equally important. If the adolescent has used previous methods of contraception and has discontinued them, ask why, for future prescribing guidance. Any information that can guide you to a better understanding of the patient's abilities or obstacles to adherence will improve outcomes.

Collect a detailed history of STIs; ask specifically about chlamydia, gonorrhea, syphilis, herpes, human papillomavirus, abnormal Pap smears, HIV, and pelvic inflammatory disease. If she has had a previous gynecologic exam, then the date and results of her last Pap test should be ascertained.

Initial gynecology exam

The American College of Obstetricians and Gynecologists recommends that the first gynecologic visit take place between the ages of 13 and 15. A pelvic exam is not necessarily indicated: the purpose is often to educate both the patient and parent regarding developmental changes. Often, there are concerns about whether the changes they are observing are normal. In many cases, these concerns center on menarche, characteristics of the patient's menstrual cycle, and breast asymmetry. The provider should inform and guide on a variety of emerging concerns. For early adolescents, concerns may center on the timing of pubertal changes while for older adolescents, concerns regarding STIs and sexuality may be at the forefront.

Visual aids can facilitate the adolescent's understanding of her anatomy, diminish anxiety, and promote questioning. It is important to explain that a gynecologic exam may involve a combination of cervical screening, STI screening, and evaluation of gynecologic complaints such as pelvic pain or vaginitis. Adolescents often have the misconception that they are being tested "for everything." Explanations should be made simple but clear with ample opportunity for questions. The provider should frequently assess understanding by asking the patient "Was that clear? Did you understand? Is there anything you would like me to go over again?"

It is helpful to let her handle speculums, Ayre spatulas, cytobrushes, and cotton-tipped applicators prior to a pelvic exam. Offer the option of seeing the pelvic exam performed with a hand-held mirror. She should always feel in control and choices should be presented often. Asking her questions can relieve some concerns. "Are you worried this procedure will hurt?" Explain that while the pelvic exam does not often hurt, "it does feel strange to have something in the vagina, as the vault is being opened so that the cervix may be seen." A cut-away picture that demonstrates the position of the speculum in the vagina may be especially helpful. Suggest relaxation techniques that will lessen the pressure she will feel against her vaginal walls, like deep breaths and conscious relaxation of the muscles that stop urine flow.

Reassure your patient that she may stop the exam at any time. During the exam, a calm and steady flow of conversation on a topic the patient finds interesting is often relaxing to the patient. Be sure to break that line of discussion, when indicated, to gently narrate what your next move is going to be so she can anticipate and connect what she is experiencing with the stepwise illustrations discussed earlier.

Meet with the adolescent after the exam, while she is dressed, in order to communicate your findings, give her an opportunity to ask questions privately, and to ask what she wants shared with her parent. The parent can then be invited to join the discussion.

Sexually transmitted infections

When discussing sexually transmitted infections, use a clear definition. "STIs are a group of over 20 diseases that can be spread by having unprotected sex with someone who is infected." A middle adolescent may not be able to understand consequences of STIs and would benefit most from focusing on symptoms and manifestations. The late adolescent will want to discuss how STIs can affect fertility. Ask about any concerns and assess the patient's knowledge and attitudes. Adolescents often have specific questions such as, What is it? How can she get it? How could she tell if she had it before? How can she get tested? What treatments are available? How can it be prevented? A priority for the adolescent is often to find out who infected her; therefore, it is imperative to explain that symptoms may appear right away or they may not show up for weeks, months or even years. Review the symptoms and use visual aids to demonstrate examples of discharges or skin lesions. Make it clear that many STIs can be asymptomatic yet still infect partners. In addition, be direct and explain that not all STIs are curable, but several can be easily cured with a cream, a pill or a shot. Differentiate between early and late effects of an STI; for example, do not assume that they know that while chlamydia is easily treated in its early stages, tubal damage resulting from protracted chlamydia infection may not be reversible.

Many adolescents lack the skills to negotiate condom use, leading to inconsistent and incorrect use. Teach effective condom use with a demonstration and also provide samples. Inform her that condoms should also be used with any sexual toys if they are going to be shared. Stress the importance of getting to know each partner well before having sex since several difficult questions (such as a past history of having an STI, willingness to get tested again, and prior unsafe sexual encounters) should precede sexual activity with any new partner. Use scenarios to demonstrate how to ask her partner such difficult questions and how to negotiate condom use. "What do you think you would do if you felt ready to have sex with your partner, but he said he didn't like condoms?" Include alcohol and drug use in your conversation, and explain that the use of these substances can impair judgment and make it harder to negotiate the use of condoms. Finally, be sure to obtain multiple contact sources for follow-up and provide the patient with resources such as clinics to go to for care, pamphlets or website addresses for further information (see below).

Contraception

Individual circumstances are important when counseling about reproductive health. Assess internal barriers to contraception such as attitudes, knowledge, motivation, and chronic illnesses, along with external barriers such as insurance, cost of method, access, side effects, cultural influences, pertinent family history, and partner support. These factors can directly affect choice of method and compliance.

Address any particular concerns; specifically, if the adolescent has used any method in the past and the reasons why she either discontinued or failed to be compliant. Adolescents often use peers as a source of information and, as a result, tend to have misconceptions about risks and side effects. Discuss the different contraceptive methods and their advantages and disadvantages. The adolescent must understand that the ultimate decision is hers and that you are there to offer information and help her. "Choosing the correct contraceptive method can be confusing, but I am here to help you through." The ideal contraceptive method is inexpensive, widely accessible, convenient and with minimal side effects. Be upfront: "There is no perfect method, but you and I will work together to figure out which one is best for you." Reiterate that all methods are safer than pregnancy. Discuss possible side effects. In addition, let her know that the hormonal methods may delay fertility, but are completely reversible once stopped. Adolescents are often preoccupied with future fertility and addressing this issue can increase compliance. To assure compliance, investigate what the adolescent's social environment is like and ask how the contraceptive will be integrated into her life. Make a plan with her: where it will be stored, what is her best time for administration, how she can remember administration, what to do if she experiences any side effects, where she should go for follow-up visits, and how to access it. Be sure to review best practices in case of missed doses. Encourage her to get the support of her partner and/or her parent whenever possible.

Pregnancy

Adolescents are often reluctant to disclose concerns about pregnancy; they may present with nonspecific complaints such as fatigue, headaches, abdominal pain, nausea or dizziness. The visit goals for pregnant patients are multifaceted, encompassing both emotional and medical needs.

Providers should confirm the pregnancy, perform a gynecologic exam to screen for infections, determine gestational age, identify possible complications, and discuss all options. Consider the patient's developmental level. Early adolescents may have difficulty imagining hypothetical situations. Ask direct questions to help focus on future goals and how these would be affected by various pregnancy alternatives. Vague questions such as "How do you plan to take care of a baby, if you decide to carry this pregnancy to term?" may be misinterpreted by a young adolescent. Be direct and clear. "Where will you live? What will happen with school? How will you pay for all the things that the baby will need?" Late adolescents are usually able to weigh options rationally if they are given time to explore their feelings. They respond well to general questions such as "What would be the advantages of continuing the pregnancy? Of terminating?" or "How do you think you would feel if you chose to continue the pregnancy? To terminate?" However, they may forget their problem-solving skills in a crisis situation and the provider will need to help them to recall these skills. The patient may be tempted to make decisions in order to please her friends or displease her parents or be tempted to make a quick decision to "get this over with." Refocus her on her needs and concerns when deciding what to do with a pregnancy. Remind her that pregnancy can have a lifetime impact.

Take time to counsel the adolescent about her options and discuss her feelings about the pregnancy. Present all options, including abortion and adoption as well as continuing the pregnancy and keeping the child. Remember to refer to the "pregnancy" rather than the "baby," even with those patients who state a desire to go to term. After speaking alone with the patient, it is appropriate to ask her if she would like to involve a parent, partner or other concerned adult in the decision-making process. Every effort should be made to encourage her to draw on existing sources of support. However, if she chooses not to involve her family, her confidentiality should be maintained.

Box 14.1 Recommendations

- Know the confidentiality laws in your state as well as adolescent health resources.
- Avoid taking notes while the patient is answering questions.
- Tailor education to the patient's developmental stage and psychosocial circumstances.
- Provide clear and simple explanations of signs, symptoms, testing, and treatment.
- Encourage treatment responsibility by encouraging self-management techniques such as a medication log or symptoms diary.
- Encourage communication with parents, but discourage parents from taking control.
- Use praise liberally when the patient complies with treatment management, and avoid criticism or confrontation over noncompliance.
- Perform risk prevention counseling at every visit.
- Regularly screen for STIs.
- Emphasize the necessity of condom usage for protection against STIs at every visit.
- Reiterate that abstinence is the only method that is 100% effective for pregnancy prevention.
- Carefully discuss advantages and disadvantages of the available contraceptive methods.
- Recognize and address internal barriers to using contraception. Consider knowledge, attitudes, motivation, and chronic illnesses.
- Address cultural beliefs, method availability, insurance/cost, side effects and partner support.
- Discuss back-up methods, including emergency contraception.
- Encourage partner's involvement when deciding on birth control.

For patients who are terminating the pregnancy, contraceptive methods should be discussed at the initial pregnancy visit and a two-week postabortion follow-up appointment should be scheduled. At the follow-up visit, screen for complications of the procedure as well as depression or other mental health concerns and to make sure that she has initiated contraception if planned. Even patients who go forward should be made aware that fertility is increased after delivery, and contraceptive options can be explored during pregnancy.

Laws regarding pregnancy termination for adolescents are state specific. Adolescents may be able to petition the court for exemptions to parental notification, especially in cases where there are concerns about physical abuse in response to disclosure of the pregnancy. Financial constraints may also make it difficult for an adolescent to obtain an abortion or prenatal care; however, some states provide free or low-cost health insurance that covers these services. Providers need to be aware of the specific laws in their state, as well as potential resources, so that they can effectively counsel and advocate for their patients.

Conclusion

Adolescence is the only time in our lives when we face parallel psychologic and physical growth; a time when we build the foundation of who we become as adults. As providers, we have the unique opportunity to positively influence our patients as they navigate through these challenging years. In order to offer our patients the best care, we must take the time to equip ourselves with the information necessary to efficiently accomplish this goal. Caring for an adolescent can be a challenge in itself, but there are lifetime rewards for our patients and ourselves.

References

1. American Medical Association. *Guidelines for Adolescent Preventive Services (GAPS): Recommendations Monograph.* Washington, DC: American Medical Association, 1997.
2. Goldenring J, Rosen, D. Getting into adolescent heads: an essential update. *Contemp Pediatr* 2004;**21**:64–90.
3. Rickert VI, Wiemann CM. Date rape among adolescents and young adults. *J Pediatr Adolesc Gynecol* 1998;**11**(4):167–175.

Further reading

American College of Obstetricians and Gynecologists. Primary and preventive health care for female adolescents. In: *Health Care for Adolescents.* Washington, DC: American College of Obstetricians and Gynecologists, 2003: 1–24.
Breech L, Holland-Hall C, Hewitt G. The "well girl" exam. *J Pediatr Adolesc Gynecol* 2005;**18**:289–291.
Emans SJ, Laufer MR, Goldstein DP. *Pediatric and Adolescent Gynecology.* Philadelphia, PA: Lippincott, Williams and Wilkins, 2005.

Greydanus D. *Caring for Your Adolescent: Ages 12 to 18*. Oxford, UK: Oxford University Press, 1998.

Peake K, Epstein I, Medeiros D (eds). *Clinical and Research Uses of an Adolescent Mental Health Intake Questionnaire: What Kids Need to Talk About, Part I. Social Work in Mental Health*. Philadelphia, PA: Haworth Social Work Press, 2004.

Websites

- AMA's Guidelines for Adolescent Preventative Services (GAPS): www.ama-assn.org/ama/upload/mm/39/gapsmono.pdf

- Center for Young Women's Health: www.youngwomenshealth.org

- Go Ask Alice!: www.goaskalice.columbia.edu

- Guttmacher Institute: www.guttmacher.com/sections/adolescents.php

- National Women's Health Information Center: www.4woman.gov and www.4girls.gov

- Society for Adolescent Medicine: www.adolescenthealth.org/

- HEEADSSS psychosocial interview for adolescents: www.sh.lsuhsc.edu/pediatrics/Junior%20Clerkship/Forms/HEEADSSS.pdf

Puberty in Girls

Frank M. Biro

Cincinnati Children's Hospital Medical Center, Cincinnati, OH, USA

Puberty is one of the many changes experienced by the preteen and early teen; pubertal changes occur in context of changes in cognitive (development of formal operational thought) and social (the process of "adolescence") development. With attainment of formal operational thought, also called abstract thought, the adolescent becomes more aware of the thinking process. This may lead to "overthinking" (attributing more complex causation to certain situations) and a sense of egocentrism ("all the world is thinking about the same things that I am").

This may lead to a clinical encounter in which the adolescent believes that she has imparted true and adequate information to a question from the provider, but the provider arrives at erroneous conclusions. For example, a teen reporting with abdominal pain may believe that this is adequate information for the clinician to deduce that she is concerned she is pregnant. The clinician should also be aware that adolescents perceive many encounters with healthcare providers to be very stressful, leading to a state of "hot cognition." That is, in nonstressful situations, the adolescent may be practicing "cool cognition" and be able to calmly and coolly evaluate the situation. However, during "hot cognition," the same adolescent may not be utilizing all her cognitive skills. This is not unique to the adolescent; the healthcare provider may reflect on the last situation in which they felt under a great deal of stress, and whether they were able to utilize the most sophisticated cognitive abilities.

Puberty consists of a series of biologic changes, including maturation of the hypothalamic-pituitary-gonadal (HPG) axis, pubertal growth spurt, changes in body com-

position, development of secondary sexual characteristics, and attainment of fertility. Puberty may be considered in terms of sequence, tempo, and timing. Although many recognize "puberty" as the onset of secondary sexual characteristics, there are several other changes that precede breast and pubic hair development. The fetus in the third trimester has a functioning luteinizing hormone-releasing hormone (LHRH) pulse generator and HPG axis, which becomes inactivated during the first year of life. There appear to be two major mechanisms for this: negative feedback from the small concentration of sex steroids, which appears to be the major mechanism until age two, and direct inhibition of the central nervous system (CNS), hypothesized to be through γ-aminobutyric acid (GABA), the mechanism from age three until the reactivation of the LHRH pulse generator during later childhood. During the late prepubertal period there is increased amplitude and frequency of LHRH pulses, initially at night; ultimately this leads to increased sensitivity to LHRH, increased secretion of follicle-stimulating hormone (FSH) and luteinizing hormone (LH). Other changes that occur prior to the appearance of breast or pubic hair include rising levels of sex hormones and the onset of the pubertal growth spurt. Indeed, a longitudinal study of acne in girls noted that many girls had the appearance of comedonal acne prior to the development of secondary sexual characteristics [1].

The stages of pubertal development that are used commonly are called Tanner stages, published by Marshall and Tanner. A similar series was published shortly after Dr Tanner's important work, by von Wieringen and colleagues [2]. Figures 15.1 and 15.2 demonstrate the Tanner stages, using van Wieringen's photographs.

Stage 1 breast development is prepubertal and stage 2 is defined by the appearance of a breast bud. In stage 3

Pediatric, Adolescent, & Young Adult Gynecology. Edited by A. Altchek and L. Deligdisch. © 2009 Blackwell Publishing, ISBN: 978-1-4051-5347-8.

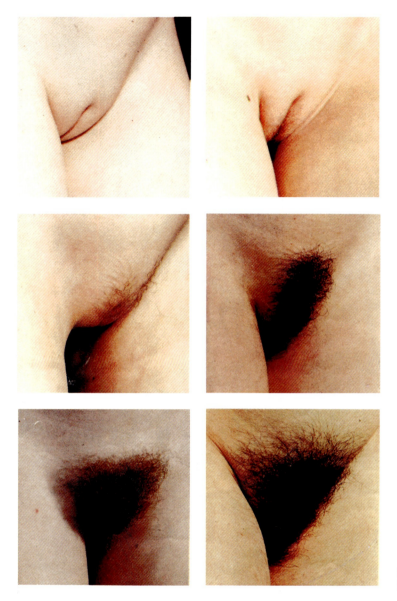

Figure 15.1 Stages in development of pubic hair, girls.

breast development, the breast forms a mound above the chest, and in stage 4, there is a separation of the areola and papilla from the surrounding breast tissue. In stage 5, adult breast development (although some women do not attain stage 5), the areola regresses to the breast contour and there is elevation only of the papilla.

Stage 1 pubic hair development is also prepubertal and stage 2 is defined by a few straight hairs, generally along the vulva. In stage 3, the hair is darker, coarser, and curlier, and extends over the mons. Stage 4 pubic hair is adult in character but does not extend to the thighs, while Stage 5 does extend to the thighs.

The definitions of various manifestations of puberty include adrenarche (activation of the adrenal medulla for production of adrenal androgens), pubarche (appearance of pubic hair), thelarche (appearance of breast tissue), and

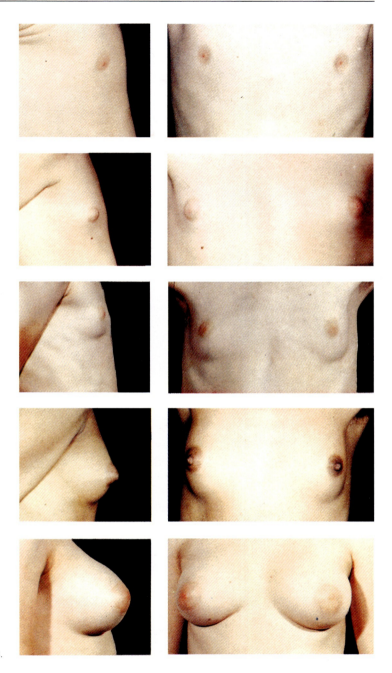

Figure 15.2 Stages in breast development, girls.

menarche (age of first menstrual period). There has been an increasing awareness of the differences in girls who have pubic hair development, as contrasted to breast development, as the initial presentation of secondary sexual char-

acteristics. A longitudinal study demonstrated that the age of onset of puberty was the same between the two pathways (breast development initially, as contrasted to pubic hair development initially). However, age of menarche was earlier in those with initial breast development (12.6 years as contrasted to 13.1 years), and those with initial breast development had greater adiposity and body mass index both at the onset of puberty and 1–2 years prior to onset of puberty [3].

Several contemporary researchers have examined secular trends in the age of onset of puberty. The data from Herman-Giddens, noting many more girls entering puberty at younger ages [4], have been corroborated by several other authors, although some have noted these changes occurring only in select ethnic and racial groups [5], and others have noted minimal longitudinal decreases in age of menarche over the late 1980s to the early 21st century (2.3 months), reflecting in part the racial and ethnic changes in the US population [6]. The age of onset of breast development in the US, when comparing data from several different studies, is 9.96–10.44 years in white non-Hispanic girls, and 8.87–9.78 in black non-Hispanic girls; for pubic hair development, it is 10.4–10.6 in white non-Hispanic girls and 8.78–9.68 in black non-Hispanic girls [7,8]. The age of menarche is 12.5 in non-Hispanic white, 12.0 in non-Hispanic black, and 12.1 in Mexican American girls [6,8]. The interval between onset of puberty to age of menarche is 2–2.5 years, and the 95th percentile is four years; that is, any girl who does not have menarche within four years of onset of puberty has experienced a stall in pubertal maturation.

The biologic changes associated with puberty can lead to issues for the adolescent girl. The areas that could be affected include musculoskeletal, mental health, and gynecologic. Adolescent girls are at risk for several types of musculoskeletal problems. Rates of knee injuries are four times greater in teen women when compared to teen men [9], and all teens are at risk for Osgood–Schlatter disease, a constellation of findings that include swelling and pain at the tibial tuberosity. Additionally, all teens are at increased risk for strains and sprains.

There are several issues from a mental health perspective. Self-esteem changes during the teen years; whereas teen males overall experience an increase in self-esteem, white teen females experience a decrease in self-esteem through midadolescence, which recovers during the late teen years [10]. Rates of depression are twice as great in teen females, when contrasted to males [11].

Gynecologic problems that may present during the teen years include irregular menstrual cycles, dysfunctional uterine bleeding, and propensity to sexually transmitted infections. Although these issues are covered in other chapters of the text, one could reflect that the relative immaturity of the hypothalamic-pituitary-ovarian axis would contribute to irregular menses and dysfunctional uterine bleeding, whereas partner factors and immaturity of the cervix and persistence of the ectropion increase the risk of sexually transmitted infections.

References

1. Lucky AW, Biro FM, Huster GA, Leach AD, Morrison JA, Ratterman J. Acne vulgaris in premenarchal girls. An early sign of puberty associated with rising levels of dehydroepiandrosterone. *Arch Dermatol* 1994;**130**:308–314.

2. Roede MJ, van Wieringen JC. Growth diagrams 1980: Netherlands third nation-wide survey. *Tijdschr Soc Gezondheids* 1985;63(suppl):1–34.

3. Biro FM, Lucky AW, Simbartl LA et al. Pubertal maturation in girls and the relationship to anthropometric changes: pathways through puberty. *J Pediatr* 2003;**142**:643–646.

4. Herman-Giddens ME, Slora EJ, Wasserman RC et al. Secondary sexual characteristics and menses in young girls seen in office practice: a study from the Pediatric Research in Office Settings Network. *Pediatrics* 1997;**99**:505–512.

5. Sun SS, Schubert CM, Liang R et al. Is sexual maturity occurring earlier among US children? *J Adolesc Health* 2005;**37**:345–355.

6. Anderson SE, Must A. Interpreting the continued decline in the average age at menarche: results from two nationally representative surveys of US girls studied 10 years apart. *J Pediatr* 2005;**147**:753–760.

7. Herman-Giddens ME, Kaplowitz PB, Wasserman R. Navigating the recent articles on girls' puberty in *Pediatrics*: what do we know and where do we go from here? *Pediatrics* 2004;**113**:911–917.

8. Biro FM, Huang B, Crawford PB et al. Pubertal correlates in black and white girls. *J Pediatr* 2006;**148**:234–240.

9. Hewett TE, Lindenfeld TN, Riccobene JV, Noyes FR. The effect of neuromuscular training on the incidence of knee injury in female athletes. A prospective study. *Am J Sports Med* 1999;**27**:699–706.

10. Biro FM, Striegel-Moore RH, Franko DL, Padgett J, Bean JA. Self-esteem in adolescent females. *J Adolesc Health* 2006;**39**:501–507.

11. Angold A, Costello EJ, Erkani A, Worthman CM. Pubertal changes in hormone levels and depression in girls. *Psychol Med* 1999;**29**:1043–1053.

CHAPTER 16

Delayed Puberty

Janice L. Bacon
University of South Carolina School of Medicine, Columbia, SC, USA

Introduction

Failure to develop a timely onset and normal progression of puberty is of great concern to patients and their families. Although the term "delayed puberty" is frequently applied to a delay of the onset of puberty, it may also be appropriately utilized when progression through puberty is delayed or arrested. In addition, the lay population may use the term "delayed puberty" for describing primary amenorrhea or delayed menarche.

A thorough review of the development of the gonads and embryogenesis of the female reproductive system may enhance education about the clinical scenarios of delayed puberty.

The differential diagnosis of the causes of delayed puberty may be generally grouped into those originating from central etiologies, such as the hypothalamus and pituitary, and those of specific organ systems, including the thyroid, adrenal, and ovary. In addition, there is often temptation to attribute delayed pubertal onset or progression to physiologic constitutional causes. This diagnosis, however, should be reached only after other disorders have been excluded [1]. Box 16.1 lists a more comprehensive differential diagnosis of delayed puberty.

In order to determine a delayed progression of puberty, understanding of the normal pubertal process and timing must be considered. Many factors contribute to normal pubertal development, including family history and familial disorders, body mass index and body fat, athletic endeavors, medical diseases, race and geographic considerations. Box 16.2 contains a list of factors

Pediatric, Adolescent, & Young Adult Gynecology. Edited by A. Altchek and L. Deligdisch. © 2009 Blackwell Publishing, ISBN: 978-1-4051-5347-8.

Box 16.1 Differential diagnosis of delayed puberty

Central causes
Hypothalamus
  Eating disorders
  Competitive athletics, ballet
  GnRH deficiency
Pituitary
  Neoplasm (prolactinoma)
  Secondary to
    Sarcoidosis
    Tuberculosis
    Histiocytosis X
    Hemochromocytosis
Systemic diseases
  Cystic fibrosis
  Crohn disease
  Celiac disease
  HIV disease
  Sickle cell disease
  Renal failure
Endocrinopathies
  Hypothyroidism
  Cushing syndrome
  Addison disease
  Ovarian failure
  Androgen excess disorders
  FSH/LH resistance
  Aromatase deficiency

Genetic syndromes/disorders
  Lawrence–Moon–Biedl
  Prader–Willi
  Turner
  Kallmann (Kal-1 gene,
    FGFR-1 gene)
  Receptor mutations/Leptin
    mutations
Malignancy
  Chemotherapy
  Radiation therapy
Other causes
  Autoimmune oophoritis
  Depression
  Medications associated with
    elevated prolactin or
    treatment of malignancy
  Head trauma
  Prior surgery (gonadectomy)
  Substance abuse (marijuana)
  Physiologic delay

---

which may influence the onset and progression of normal puberty.

Summary of events in normal pubertal maturation

Maturational changes in the control of the gonadotropin-releasing hormone (GnRH) neuron trigger the onset of

Box 16.2 Factors influencing the onset and progression of normal puberty

Family history
Familial disorders
   Genetic syndromes
   Medical diseases
   Endocrine disorders
Race
Geographic location
Body mass index
Percent body fat
Athletic endeavors

Box 16.3 Physical milestones of puberty in girls

Adolescent growth spurt
   Girls: average height gain 25 cm
   Boys: average height gain 28 cm
   Peak pubertal growth velocity 2 yrs earlier in girls than boys
Thelarche
   Breast budding 8–13 yrs, mean 11.2 yrs
   (some healthy Caucasian girls start at 7 yrs; some healthy African-American girls start at 6 yrs)
Menarche
   12.9 yrs Caucasian girls
   12.2 yrs African-American girls
   Average time from breast budding to menarche 2–8 yrs, but may be shorter if adolescence delayed
Ovarian volume
   Baseline 0.2–1.6 mL
   Completion of sexual maturation 2.8–15 mL with follicles noted
Uterine size
   Baseline 2–3 cm length
   Full maturation 3–15 cm length with endometrial stripe noted

puberty and constitute its "central drive." This event enhances GnRH pulsatile secretion and pulse amplitude. Many growth factors, including transforming growth factor α and β, epidermal growth factor, insulin-like growth factor (IGF-1), basic fibroblast growth factor, neuron cell adhesion molecules, cytokines and nitrous oxide, further mediate and contribute to this response [2].

GnRH induces secretion of follicle-stimulating hormone (FSH) and luteinizing hormone (LH), which in turn are associated with gonadal stimulation. Concurrent increases in estrogen levels in girls stimulate growth hormone and IGF-1 secretion, which are responsible for the pubertal growth spurt.

The physical milestones of puberty are summarized in Box 16.3.

In the United States, obesity and increased body mass index are increasingly prevalent during childhood and promote an earlier onset of puberty.

Estrogen is the main stimulator of growth hormone production during puberty in boys and girls. The aromatase enzyme mediates the conversion of testosterone to estradiol in both sexes. Estrogen has a biphasic effect on bone epiphyseal growth – low doses (producing a serum level of 4 pg/mL) increase growth rate in girls and boys, while high estrogen doses inhibit growth. Prepubertal girls have faster epiphyseal maturation than boys, due to their eightfold higher levels of estradiol. Estrogen also is important for appropriate bone mineralization, bone turnover and gonadotropin regulation, serum insulin levels and lipid homeostasis [2].

Treatment regimens to stimulate puberty must address the etiology of the delayed puberty. Before plunging into ordering blood work, laboratory testing or imaging modalities, clues to determine the etiology of delayed puberty can often be obtained from a thorough history and physical examination.

Delayed puberty is often identified when there has been no development of secondary sexual characteristics by age 13. Failure to reach this landmark by age 13 is greater than two standard deviations from the normal population and further evaluation is warranted. In some situations, if an etiology for the delay is highly suspected or previously anticipated, further evaluation may be postponed for another year until age 14. When discussing puberty, the documentation of normal progression must also be determined.

Clues to determinants of pubertal timing and progression may be obtained through family history and inheritance patterns. Box 16.4 lists a number of familial factors that contribute to pubertal timing and progression. In addition, pregnancy and neonatal findings may also affect developmental milestones in childhood and adolescence. Neonatal events which may be contributing factors include birth weight and gestational age at delivery, maternal substance exposure (androgen exposure), and congenital anomalies, particularly those involving the craniofacial system, which may result in hypothalamic-pituitary

Box 16.4 Familial factors contributing to pubertal timing and progression

Parental heights
Age of menarche and puberty in first-degree relatives
Fertility of first- and second-degree relatives
Endocrine disorders
Congenital adrenal hyperplasia
Dysmetabolic syndrome
Gonadal dysgenesis
Genetic disorders
  Fragile X permutation carriers
  Autosomal dominant Kallmann syndrome (FGFR1 gene)
Autoimmune disorders
  Thyroid, Addison
  Diabetes
  Premature ovarian failure

dysfunction. In addition, a history of neonatal hernias, lymphedema or other medical history that may indicate hypopituitarism should be considered. A history of prior surgery is important, as occasionally a bilateral oophorectomy may have been performed. Radiation therapy and chemotherapy for infant or childhood malignancy may also produce an adverse effect on puberty.

A careful review of symptoms should be oriented towards chronic medical disorders which may influence subsequent growth and development, including the gastrointestinal and neurologic systems, galactorrhea, medication use and substance abuse, stress or eating disorders, level of athletic participation and other indicators of potential hormone imbalance such as acne and hirsutism.

It is important to review late childhood milestones and those associated with pubertal development, including growth spurts, and events heralding the onset of adrenarche and thelarche.

A review of growth charts during childhood may be very informative when applied to the above historical information. Although adolescents may not seek medical care as routinely as younger children, the continued plotting of height and weight may reveal important information about pubertal progression. The charts may be obtained from the pediatrician. Blank charts kept in the office may be used to plot subsequent growth and development.

A careful history and physical exam should begin with accurate documentation of the patient's height and weight without relying on historical recollection. The exam should carefully note the Tanner staging (see Chapter 15). This may also be compared with pediatric records. When performing a physical exam, attention should be paid to those organ systems which have specific contributions to pubertal delay, including the thyroid and skeleton. In addition, a general survey for congenital anomalies and appraisal of body proportion should be carried out.

Determination of the arm span (middle finger to middle finger) and the ratio of upper to lower body development may provide clues for further investigation. The lower body ratio is determined by measuring the distance from the pubic symphysis to the bottom of the feet (or floor when standing). The upper body ratio is calculated by determination of the total height minus the lower body ratio. In general, a patient's arm span is relatively proportional to her height and an upper to lower body ratio is approximately 0.95.

The neurologic exam can also be helpful, including a determination of smell, fundoscopic visualization, and visual field testing. Though many young women are not candidates for a complete pelvic exam (including speculum and bimanual exam), close inspection of the external genitalia should include determination of clitoral size, patency of the introitus and evidence of estrogenization. The separation of primary amenorrhea from pubertal delay requires visualization of intact genital structures. If needed, a rectoabdominal exam may be better tolerated by younger patients. The availability of transabdominal, transvaginal or even transperineal ultrasound may greatly aid acquisition of necessary information without discomfiting the patient.

During puberty, the rate of growth in height accelerates. Normal approximates 2–2.5 inches per year. The use of a bone age on the nondominant hand and wrist may assist in determining the status of epiphysis closure. A number of medical disorders, including Crohn disease and other acquired endocrine disorders, may affect the final acquisition of stature. Severe nutritional deficiency generally affects the patient's weight rather than height. Otherwise, patients who appear grossly overweight for height associated with pubertal delay may be suffering from growth hormone deficiencies, Turner syndrome, acquired hypothyroidism, Cushing syndrome or even iatrogenic cortisol excess.

Box 16.5 Common causes of delayed puberty categorized by FSH findings

Hypogonadotropic	Hypergonadotropic (elevated FSH)
Hypogonadism (low or NI FSH)	Turner syndrome
Hypopituitarism	Gonadal dysgenesis
Congenital or acquired	Gonadal radiation
Gene mutations	Chemotherapy
Prop-1	Gonadal failure/torsion
Dex-1	Idiopathic
GnRH-R	FSH/LH resistance
Syndromes: Prader–Willi	Gonadectomy (for tumor)
Malnutrition/Chronic disease	Aromatase deficiency
Eating disorders	Autoimmune oophoritis
CNS disorders	
Tumors	
Radiation	
Hypophysitis	
Histiocytosis	
Infections	
Trauma	
Isolated FSH/LSH deficiency	
Excessive physical activity	

Laboratory evaluation

The laboratory and imaging evaluation of patients with delayed pubertal onset or progression may be tailored to suspected etiologies. However, the initial work-up for multiple disorders may be a complete blood count (CBC), urinalysis, FSH, thyroid-stimulating hormone (TSH) and prolactin.

For young women with delayed onset of puberty, the determination of FSH is key since further evaluation is guided by the diagnostic categories of hypergonadotropic or hypogonadotropic hypogonadism.

We will next consider specific evaluation tips and further laboratory or imaging investigations appropriate for some of the more common causes of delayed pubertal onset or progression.

Hypogonadotropic hypogonadism is categorized by an elevated FSH. Disorders with this finding are generally genetic or originate within the ovary. Common causes include autoimmune oophoritis, ovarian failure following treatment of malignancy by chemotherapy or radiation, and genetic syndromes including Turner syndrome (XO), the most common genetic abnormality associated with premature ovarian failure (Box 16.5). Therefore, young women with an elevated FSH should have a karyotype performed.

Patients with a low or normal FSH comprise the larger group of patients with delayed pubertal onset or progression. The etiology may include genetic syndromes, hypothalamic disorders such as eating disorders or excessive athletic participation and disorders associated with hypopituitarism or neoplasms in the CNS. Chronic medical diseases such as renal failure may also be associated with a low to normal FSH value. Due to the more common etiologies exhibited by these findings, a thorough neurologic assessment must be included in the physical exam. Imaging with CT or MRI is prominent in further evaluation, although an MRI may be the most definitive study. (The presence of metal in the patient's mouth, due to orthodontic appliances or braces, may preclude the use of this imaging technique.)

Patients with poor growth may be evaluated by ICF-1 or ICF-1BP3 levels and evaluated by an erythrocyte sedimentation rate (ESR), creatinine, blood chemistries, urinalysis and celiac panel. A celiac panel includes a transglutaminase, an IgA level and detection of antiendomysial antibodies.

The female athletic triad is associated with amenorrhea, disordered eating, and subsequent osteoporosis. This is a variant of chronic disease associated with nutritional abnormalities resulting in delayed pubertal progression, delayed menarche or secondary amenorrhea. Poor nutritional status may be associated with reduced food intake, malabsorption or increased calorie requirements.

Attention to the bone age has been mentioned previously in association with assisting in the determination of the amount of pubertal delay, but bone age can also be useful in estimating the patient's final height. Some chronic medical disorders such as hypothyroidism are associated with delayed bone age versus height age. Constitutional delay, however, is associated with reduced bone age and reduced height age, unless the patient has a genetic predisposition to short stature.

Eating disorders such as anorexia and endocrine disorders, including hypothyroidism, diabetes mellitus and Cushing disease, are associated with developmental delay and poor linear growth. Those renal disorders associated with delayed development include renal tubular acidosis, glomerular diseases requiring chronic steroid use and end-stage renal disease of varying etiologies.

Even if the etiology of developmental delay is strongly suspected, it is prudent to exclude other disorders as well.

Genetic disorders associated with pubertal delay or abnormal delay

Gene mutations involving the endocrine pathways of pubertal development have been identified, including those involving FSH and LH receptors, GnRH receptor mutations and mutations in the regulation of GnRH release (GPR 54 gene). Mutations in leptin and leptin receptor genes as factors affecting normal pubertal development are under investigation, particularly for adolescents classified as "constitutional delay." Receptor mutations involving the hypothalamus, pituitary or adrenal glands have also been proposed.

Therapeutic considerations for pubertal delay

Healthy hypogonadal girls with normal height, weight, and nutrition may begin hormone therapy at an appropriate chronologic age. Many practitioners begin therapy at approximately age 13 with a range of 11–13 years old. Children of short stature may postpone sex hormone replacement to a later age in order to achieve a greater height, taking into consideration bone age and chronologic age. Flexibility is needed in girls with Turner syndrome or active chronic, medical conditions. Care must be taken that the sex hormone therapy is given with appropriate psychologic support and does not hinder the treatment of other medical conditions.

The general principles of hormone therapy include beginning with very low doses and proceeding with gradual incremental increases based on the hormonal pattern of normal puberty. Consideration must also be given to patient tolerance, therapeutic response and appropriate behavioral and psychologic adjustment. Assess growth rate and bone maturation every 6–12 months. Patient and parental feedback should be sought. Deficits in other hormones must likewise be replaced.

Estrogen may be administered by oral, transdermal or systemic depot methods. The transdermal route may be preferred for many patients since it bypasses the liver and may provide more consistent physiologic blood levels. It may also be better for women with a personal or family history of diabetes or insulin resistance, elevated triglycerides, hypertension or increased levels of inflammatory markers.

As girls enter later adolescence, combination oral contraceptive pills (those containing estrogen and progesterone) may be preferred for social reasons.

Examples of pharmacologic preparations for hormone therapy in girls include oral conjugated estrogens (0.3–2.5 mg daily) and transdermal estradiol patches (0.0375–0.1 mg) twice weekly. Once spotting has begun or after 6–12 months of therapy, patients should be started on 5 mg daily of medroxyprogesterone acetate or 100 mg of micronized progesterone nightly increasing to 10 mg of medroxyprogesterone acetate or 200 mg of micronized progesterone when higher estrogen levels are prescribed [3]. Monitoring of the endometrial stripe and the calculation of uterine and ovarian volumes by ultrasound may assist in changing hormone dosages.

Conclusion

A thorough evaluation of the complaint of delayed puberty and comprehensive discussions with patients and families may lead to timely diagnosis of etiology and appropriate therapy to allow adolescents with this presentation to join their peers in anatomic development and social comfort.

References

1. Sedlmeyer IL, Palmert MR. Delayed puberty: analysis of a large case series from an academic center. *J Clin Endocrinol Metab* 2002;**87**(4):1613–1620.
2. MacGillivray MH. Induction of puberty in hypogonadal children. *J Pediatr Endocrinol Metab* 2004;**17**:1277–1287.
3. Drobac S, Rubin K, Rogol AD, Rosenfield RL. A workshop on pubertal hormone replacement options in the United States. *J Pediatr Endocrinol Metab* 2006;**19**:55–64.

CHAPTER 17

Primary and Secondary Amenorrhea

Rachel J. Miller[1] *& Paula J. Adams Hillard*[2]

[1]Children's Hospital and Clinics of Minnesota, Minneapolis, MN, USA
[2]Stanford University School of Medicine, Stanford, CA, USA

Introduction

Amenorrhea is frequently categorized as primary or secondary. Although primary amenorrhea is commonly defined as the absence of menses by age 16, a more appropriate, evidence-based definition is the absence of menses by age 15 years with the presence of breast development, or by age 13 years with no breast development [1]. The American Society of Reproductive Medicine goes further to define primary amenorrhea as the absence of menses greater than or equal to five years after thelarche if thelarche occurs before age 10 [2].

Secondary amenorrhea is frequently defined as the absence of menses for greater than six months after menarche occurs. An evidence-based approach would suggest that the absence of menses for greater than 90 days or three months is a more appropriate marker [3]. Studies suggest that 3–8% of young women aged 13–24 experience secondary amenorrhea [4–6]. Secondary amenorrhea is more common among adolescents and women in their 40s than it is among women in their middle reproductive years, if one excludes pregnancy as a cause. A subset of a large dataset of menstrual records, originally obtained by Dr Alan Treloar and colleagues at the University of Minnesota and comprising records kept by over 1100 women, was subsequently analyzed by a WHO task force. The analysis indicated that amenorrhea (no bleeding in a 90-day reference interval) is rare in all age groups, but particularly among women aged 25–39 years, where the incidence is less than 1%. The incidence of amenorrhea among women less than 20 years was 2–3%, among those 40–44 years, 6–8%, and among those 45–49 years, 3–9% [7].

Amenorrhea, whether primary or secondary, is a sign of a specific condition or disease and not a disease in and of itself. Frequently, treating the underlying condition will also lead to the onset or return of menses. As most causes of secondary amenorrhea can also cause primary amenorrhea if their onset is prior to menarche, the remainder of the chapter will not discriminate between the two types.

Physiologic etiologies

The onset and maintenance of normal menstruation is dependent upon an intact hypothalamic-pituitary-ovarian-uterine axis. Any disruption in one of the four main organs can upset the entire system. However, several etiologies of amenorrhea are actually physiologic. The first is the prepubertal state. The median age of menarche for all girls in the United States is 12.43 years [8]. On average, the interval from thelarche to menarche is two years. Pregnancy and lactation also induce physiologic amenorrhea. The importance of obtaining a pregnancy test on all adolescents and young women with primary or secondary amenorrhea cannot be overemphasized, as the consequences of missing the diagnosis of a pregnancy can be significant. The last physiologic state of amenorrhea in a female's life span is menopause, defined as the cessation of menses for the duration of one year. Obviously, this definition is one that is made in retrospect; an extended time from last menses may represent a physiologic amenorrhea or other pathology. The average age of menopause in the

Pediatric, Adolescent, & Young Adult Gynecology. Edited by
A. Altchek and L. Deligdisch. © 2009 Blackwell Publishing,
ISBN: 978-1-4051-5347-8.

United States is 51 years. However, premature ovarian failure (POF), sometimes termed "premature menopause," can occur in young women or adolescents.

Outflow tract/normogonadotropic

Congenital anatomic etiologies

Menarche is dependent upon the presence of a uterus and patent outflow tract. Two of the most common congenital anatomic conditions associated with amenorrhea due to the absence of a uterus are Müllerian aplasia and complete androgen insensitivity syndrome. Müllerian aplasia (also known as Mayer-Rokitansky-Kuster-Hauser syndrome or Müllerian agenesis) is the absence of the vagina, uterus, and fallopian tubes. It is present in 10% of adolescents presenting with primary amenorrhea [9] and is found in 1 in 5000 females [10]. Patients have a normal female phenotype and genotype with normal secondary sex characteristics. Between 12% and 30% have an associated absent or ectopic kidney and/or skeletal anomaly (most commonly scoliosis); therefore, evaluation of this condition should also include renal and skeletal imaging [11].

Androgen insensitivity syndrome (formerly called testicular feminization) is the diagnosis in 5% of primary amenorrhea with an incidence of 1 in 60,000 [9]. These patients are classically described as having sparse or little pubic hair. These two conditions can also be differentiated by measurement of serum testosterone and/or chromosomal analysis. Girls with Müllerian aplasia have normal female testosterone levels whereas patients with complete androgen insensitivity have very elevated testosterone levels (in the "male" range) and a 46,XY karyotype.

Congenital obstructing anomalies

If the uterus is present, it must have a patent outflow tract for menstrual blood to escape. The most common congenital obstructing anomaly is an imperforate hymen, with an incidence of 1 in 1000 females. A distant second is a transverse vaginal septum with an incidence of 1 in 80,000 females [9]. Differentiating the two obstructing anomalies is important for surgical management, as a septum can be remarkably thick and require specialized surgical expertise. Very rare cases of isolated absence of the vagina or cervix have been described, and must be considered. Imaging with ultrasound is typically the initial diagnostic test, while MRI may be required to further delineate anatomy when complex anomalies (such as a uterine horn with functioning endometrium) are suggested by ultrasound. Patients with an outflow tract obstruction should ideally be identified by an examination in the neonatal period, when the maternal estrogen stimulation allows for an easy examination of the vulvar and hymenal anatomy. Examination during routine well-child care exams is also appropriate. Unfortunately, girls with outflow tract obstruction still typically present with abdominal-pelvic pain once menses has begun and menstrual blood has accumulated in the obstructed uterus (hematometra) and vagina (hematocolpos).

Acquired

In the United States today, acquired causes of amenorrhea are rare in adolescents. Uterine synechiae/Asherman syndrome is less common with modern suction curettage methods compared to older sharp curettage techniques for evacuation of uterine contents following a missed/incomplete or elective abortion. Cervical stenosis due to cervical conization is becoming less common than in the past. This is likely because less aggressive management of cervical dysplasia is becoming the norm, given newer guidelines for the management of HPV-related lesions [1]. Infectious causes of endometrial scarring, such as tuberculosis, are rare in the United States.

Ovary/peripheral/hypergonadotropic hypogonadism

Amenorrhea stemming from POF is characterized by an elevated follicle-stimulating hormone (FSH) level, with a decreased estradiol level. Because the implications of this diagnosis are significant in adolescents and because ovarian function can wax and wane prior to ovarian failure, measurement of these hormone levels on at least two occasions is prudent. Ovarian failure has genetic, autoimmune, and iatrogenic etiologies.

Genetic

Gonadal dysgenesis is the most common cause of primary amenorrhea partly because it includes a broad range of chromosomal anomalies – numeric, structural, presence of Y chromosome or mosaicism [12]. Turner syndrome is the classic and most common form, affecting 1 in 2000 liveborn females [13]. It is characterized by a 45,XO karyotype and stigmata, including short stature, webbed neck, shield chest, and bilateral streak gonads.

Pure gonadal dysgenesis describes all phenotypic females who have streak gonads and a range of sex chromosomal abnormalities but lack the stigmata of Turner syndrome [14]. A prime example is Swyer syndrome. These individuals have a female phenotype but 46,XY karyotype and rudimentary streak gonads. Yet another very rare cause of genetic ovarian dysfunction is luteinizing hormone (LH) receptor mutations. These mutations make the ovaries resistant to luteinizing hormone and thus unable to produce estradiol [15].

Acquired

Premature ovarian failure or POF is defined as ovarian failure with amenorrhea prior to age 40 years. Like normal menopause, there is significantly reduced ovarian estrogen production but few patients experience the typical symptoms of the climacteric. Premature ovarian failure affects 1 in 10,000 by age 20 years and 1 in 1000 by age 30 years [16]. Those cases not due to gonadal dysgenesis are usually (40%) secondary to an autoimmune disorder [9]. The most common disorder is autoimmune thyroiditis but those with type 1 diabetes mellitus and myasthenia gravis, parathyroid and Addison diseases are also at greater risk for developing POF.

Iatrogenic

Chemotherapy, specifically alkylating agents such as cyclophosphamide, is significantly associated with ovarian failure. Cyclophosphamide is commonly used in the treatment of Hodgkin lymphoma and systemic lupus erythematosus (SLE), both of which predominantly affect young women. Ovarian failure was reported in 50% of patients 20–30 years old and 13% of females less than 20 years who underwent cyclophosphamide pulse therapy for SLE [17]. Several studies now suggest that gonadotropin-releasing hormone (GnRH) agonists such as depot leuprolide may be protective to ovaries exposed to chemotherapies [18].

The risk of POF from radiation therapy increases with age and increasing dose received by the ovaries [19]. The average dose required for sterilization is 5–10 Gy or 50–100 rads [20]. Adolescents or young women usually would be exposed to this during spinal or pelvic irradiation for lymphoma, central nervous system tumors, cervical-vaginal or anorectal cancers. Surgical transposition via oophoropexy to move the ovaries from the field of radiation has reduced the ovarian dose by 5–10% [18].

Pituitary

Hyperprolactinemia

Hyperprolactinemia suppresses GnRH secretion, ultimately resulting in amenorrhea. Any persistent fasting morning prolactin elevation greater than 50 ng/dL or single level greater than 200 ng/mL warrants evaluation for the source. Hypothyroidism is the most common cause of hyperprolactinemia and is thought to be caused by thyroid-releasing hormone stimulation of prolactin secretion. Prolactin release by the pituitary is predominantly under inhibitory control by hypothalamic dopamine. Thus, any condition or medication that significantly decreases dopamine will increase prolactin release. Antipsychotic medications are some of the most common culprits, but some antidepressants, opiates, H2 blockers, and illicit drugs can have the same effect (see Box 17.1).

Another important cause of hyperprolactinemia is a prolactin-secreting pituitary tumor or prolactinoma, although these are uncommon in childhood and adolescence. Primary amenorrhea was the presenting complaint in 25.4% of female patients aged 12–19 years in a case series of 59 pituitary prolactinomas [21]. Any prolactin level greater than 200 ng/mL should raise the possibility of a pituitary adenoma. Pituitary microadenomas (defined as <1 cm in size) can cause menstrual irregularities that do not meet the definition of amenorrhea.

Hypopituitarism

Amenorrhea can result from hypopituitarism, although this cause is rare. This can result from trauma, radiation or an infiltrative lesion such as a craniopharyngioma. Empty sella syndrome is the term used to describe a condition in which a mass is removed or infarcts, leaving an empty sella with resultant hypopituitarism. Sheehan syndrome or acute infarction of the pituitary gland secondary to severe hypotension during a postpartum hemorrhage can also result in hypopituitarism and amenorrhea.

Hypothalamus/hypogonadotropic hypogonadism

Hypothalamic dysfunction from a variety of etiologies is the most common cause of amenorrhea. It typically results from decreased pulse frequency of GnRH release and is

Box 17.1 Causes of hyperprolactinemia

Physiologic	Pregnancy, lactation, breast stimulation, stress
Pituitary	Prolactinoma or prolactin-producing adenoma (macroadenoma >1 cm or microadenoma <1 cm), nonfunctional adenoma, acromegaly, Cushing disease, Rathke cyst, lymphocytic hypophysitis, infiltrative diseases, metastatic neoplasms, stalk infarction or compression
Hypothalamus	Hypothyroidism, craniopharyngioma, neoplasms, infiltrative diseases, radiation, encephalitis, pseudo-tumor cerebri
Medication/drugs	• Antipsychotics: phenothiazines, butyrophenones, olanzapine, thioxanthenes, risperidone, molindone, pimozide, haloperidol • Antidepressants – clomipramine, desipramine, pargyline, clorgyline, amitriptyline, fluoxetine • Antihypertensives – verapamil, α-methyldopa, reserpine • Gastrointestinal medications – histamine 2 receptor blockers, metoclopramide, domperidone • Opiates, cocaine and marijuana • Estrogens, antiandrogens and danazol
Other	Chest wall lesions or injury, chronic renal failure, adrenal insufficiency, cirrhosis, PCOS, spinal cord lesions, idiopathic

characterized by laboratory values of decreased FSH and estradiol.

Amenorrhea is one of the four diagnostic criteria for anorexia nervosa [22]. A second criterion is weight: less than 85% of ideal body weight for height. One to 3% of adolescents and young adults are affected by anorexia nervosa in the United States [23]. Even weight loss not meeting criteria for anorexia nervosa can result in a decreased GnRH pulse frequency and amenorrhea. Excessive intense exercise is another important etiology of amenorrhea that frequently is part of the female athlete triad of amenorrhea, disordered eating, and decreased bone mineral density. In this condition, the patients do not necessarily meet the strict DSM-IV criteria for anorexia nervosa or bulimia nervosa but engage in equally harmful behaviors. As eating disorders are typically a diagnosis based on patient history, athletes presenting for preparticipation physical examinations or with menstrual irregularities should be screened for eating-disordered practices, including food restricting or binging and purging, as well as use of laxatives, diuretics, and stimulant medications. They should also be queried as to training intensity, additional exercise outside that required, and any history of fractures or overuse injuries. Individuals with bulimia may be of normal weight, yet have ovulatory dysfunction and menstrual irregularities.

Chronic diseases such as poorly controlled diabetes mellitus, end-stage renal disease, cancers, AIDS or inflammatory bowel disease are commonly associated with amenorrhea. Psychologic stress is another frequently cited culprit. Stress should not be presumed to be the cause of amenorrhea prior to an appropriate evaluation. It has been suggested that tonically elevated levels of cortisol due to stress may play a role [24]. Kallman syndrome or complete gonadotropin deficiency is rare and often associated with anosmia and midline craniofacial abnormalities.

Other infectious or autoimmune disorders, such as tuberculosis and sarcoidosis, can affect the hypothalamus directly, although these causes are rare in adults and particularly rare among adolescents.

Other

Several other common etiologies exist that do not fit well into one of the above categories.

Cushing disease is a rare cause that has classic stigmata of moon facies, buffalo hump, and central obesity with prominent striae. This diagnosis should be considered in the diagnostic evaluation for girls with insulin resistance and hirsutism but is more commonly due to hyperandrogenism and polycystic ovarian syndrome (PCOS).

Hyperandrogenism is perhaps the most common cause of amenorrhea among women, other than pregnancy. It occurs in approximately 7% of adult women, most of whom report that the signs and symptoms began during adolescence [25]. Severe hyperandrogenism can be a result of late-onset congenital adrenal hyperplasia or an androgen-producing ovarian or adrenal tumor. These are both rare when compared to polycystic ovarian syndrome [26]. The current diagnostic criteria for PCOS are those established by the 2003 Rotterdam consensus workshop. They include (after the exclusion of other etiologies for androgen excess) the presence of two of three findings: anovulation, clinical or laboratory evidence of androgen excess, and polycystic ovaries on ultrasound imaging [27].

However, these criteria are controversial in adolescents. Some authors propose instead four of five criteria [28].

1 Amenorrhea or oligomenorrhea two years after menarche
2 Clinical hyperandrogenism
3 Laboratory evidence of hyperandrogenism
4 Clinical or laboratory evidence of insulin resistance
5 Polycystic ovaries

Some of the most commonly prescribed contraceptive medications can also induce amenorrhea, which does *not* have the same diagnostic implications as amenorrhea due to one of the above-noted causes. Combined estrogen-progesterone contraceptives, in the form of pills, patches or intravaginal ring, and depot medroxyprogesterone acetate are frequently used by adolescents, sometimes unbeknownst to their parents or guardians. This history should be elicited in confidence prior to pursuing an expensive evaluation. After ruling out pregnancy, amenorrhea under the influence of hormonal therapies is not pathologic; if an individual who experiences amenorrhea while on a contraceptive method is concerned about the possibility of pregnancy, an alternative formulation should be considered. In particular, because adolescents may find it more difficult to take their contraceptives perfectly than adults may, longer-acting contraceptives should be considered. The levonorgestrol-releasing intrauterine system has a relatively high rate of amenorrhea after the first year of use; reported rates of amenorrhea at the end of one year range from 20% to 50%. Depot leuprolide, used for the treatment of precocious puberty or endometriosis, also induces amenorrhea.

Evaluation

Patient history

The evaluation of primary or secondary amenorrhea begins with a careful patient history. In addition to the routine past medical and surgical history, one will need to include questioning that is more specific to the underlying etiologies of amenorrhea. Pubertal milestones such as thelarche, adrenarche, growth spurt, and menarche

should be elicited. A careful menstrual history should be obtained, including information about average cycle length, longest cycle length, number of days of flow, and the first day of the last menstrual period. In confidence, elicit if the adolescent has ever been sexually active or is currently active, including date of last intercourse. Also, take a confidential pregnancy history including spontaneous and induced abortions and any uterine instrumentation that was required in their management. A complete list of prescription medications and nonprescription supplements should be obtained. Elicit any substances or illicit drugs that the patient is using or abusing. During the routine social history, include a specific and detailed line of questioning about the adolescent's activities and exercise habits and screen for eating-disordered behaviors such as self-induced vomiting, food restrictive behavior, and body image distortion.

Review of systems

After a careful medical history, specific questions should be included in the review of systems. Ask about weight loss or gain as it may relate to an eating disorder or thyroid disease. Screen for an obstructed outflow tract by asking about cyclic abdominal pain. Ask about symptoms including headache, visual field defects, and galactorrhea that could indicate a pituitary lesion. Discreetly question the adolescent about any facial or body hair and its removal via waxing, shaving, plucking or depilatory use. Adolescents with hirsutism frequently may be quite successful in minimizing the appearance of excess hair growth, as it is typically quite embarrassing to them.

Family history

The family history has relevance to a history of amenorrhea. It should include an assessment of first-degree female relatives' pubertal development and age at menarche. If possible, determine biologic parents' adult heights. Ask if other females had congenital anomalies of their reproductive organs or suffered from infertility. Because PCOS is the most common cause of amenorrhea and is frequently not diagnosed as such, a family history of irregular menses, obesity, hirsutism, infertility, diabetes, and early cardiovascular disease suggest undiagnosed PCOS or the metabolic syndrome, which is commonly associated with PCOS. The metabolic syndrome or syndrome X is defined by the World Health Organization as insulin resistance, impaired glucose tolerance or diabetes with hyperinsulinemia and at least two of the following: abdominal obesity, dyslipidemia, and hypertension [29]. Also, elicit any family history of autoimmune or other genetic disorders.

Physical examination

Following the careful past medical, surgical and reproductive history, and a targeted review of systems, a careful but focused physical examination is indicated, with attention to signs that could indicate the etiology of the amenorrhea. Obtain an accurate height and weight for calculation of the body mass index (BMI). Determine the age-based BMI percentile; tables or PDA-based calculators are available to assess adolescent growth percentiles, as adult norms are not appropriate. Note any dysmorphic features or stigmata of Cushing syndrome. Thoroughly examine the thyroid gland. Assess Tanner staging of breasts and pubic hair while simultaneously looking for evidence of androgen excess such as acne and hirsutism. Also, look for acanthosis nigricans usually present in the axilla and posterior neck. Acanthosis nigricans is a sign of insulin resistance, associated with PCOS. A complete pelvic exam is rarely indicated in the young adolescent. However, visualizing the external genitalia for hymenal patency, clitoromegaly, and hirsutism may be indicated. It is usually well tolerated if a complete explanation is given and the adolescent is offered the option of having an accompanying individual of her choice present – typically her mother, for a younger teen – although this option may be declined by an older teen.

Laboratory evaluation

Upon completion of the history and physical examination, consideration should be given to a targeted laboratory evaluation. Every patient presenting with amenorrhea should have a screening urine pregnancy test.

Assuming that the pregnancy test is negative, other initial laboratory testing should include a TSH and prolactin level. Abnormalities in either or both may indicate thyroid disease or a pituitary etiology. To confirm that a medication is the cause for hyperprolactinemia, discontinue the medication for 3–4 days, in consultation with the patient's psychiatrist in the case of psychoactive medications, and perform a repeat prolactin level.

Based on the history and physical examination, other testing may be indicated. If there is concern about a hypothalamic etiology or premature ovarian failure, screening gonadotropins and estradiol levels are indicated; usually an FSH alone is sufficient for screening. Decreased FSH and estradiol levels indicate a hypothalamic etiology that should be correlated with the history and physical. Eating disorders, athletic-induced amenorrhea, and intracranial lesions can all have this laboratory picture. An elevated FSH but decreased estradiol on more than one occasion in the setting of at least four months of amenorrhea is diagnostic of premature ovarian failure. Any patient with initial laboratory values consistent with premature ovarian failure who is less than 30 years old should have a karyotype performed. Further laboratory testing should also include TSH, free T4, thyroid peroxidase antibodies and adrenal, ovarian, islet and parietal cell antibodies, as premature ovarian failure is associated with other autoimmune conditions.

If there is evidence of androgen excess or concern for PCOS, screening 17-hydroxyprogesterone and testosterone and dehydroepiandrosterone sulfate (DHEAS) levels are recommended to rule out other causes of hirsutism, including late-onset congenital adrenal hyperplasia or other adrenal dysfunction. An elevated 17-hydroxyprogesterone should prompt further evaluation for congenital adrenal hyperplasia. Significantly elevated testosterone or DHEAS levels should be further evaluated by imaging for a testosterone-producing ovarian or adrenal tumor, respectively.

Imaging

Imaging in the young adolescent is frequently utilized in lieu of an invasive and potentially traumatizing pelvic exam, but also can be helpful for determining nonreproductive tract etiologies for amenorrhea. A pelvic ultrasound with ovarian imaging can also be used as part of the diagnostic criteria for PCOS or to evaluate a potential hormone-producing adnexal mass. The diagnostic criteria for polycystic ovaries (enlarged ovaries with multiple peripheral follicles) may be present, and if so, can be helpful in the assessment; however, the diagnostic specificity and sensitivity of an abdominal ultrasound for PCOS in adolescents have been questioned. A transabdominal pelvic ultrasound is the imaging modality of choice for screening to confirm the presence of a uterus, but it will also detect any significant outflow tract anomaly. If a uterus is present, measurement of the endometrial stripe provides some evidence of the degree of estrogen stimulation. An MRI may then be used to delineate further whether a distal vaginal obstructive phenomenon is caused by a simple, thin transverse vaginal septum or imperforate hymen, or whether there is a thick septum that would require greater surgical expertise to repair. A bone age may be helpful in determining if constitutional delay may be the diagnosis. An MRI is appropriate for imaging the pituitary gland and investigating a possible lesion and its size.

Diagnostic medications

A progestin challenge is frequently used to determine the presence of an appropriately estrogen-stimulated endometrium with a patent outflow tract. It is performed by administration of 10 mg medroxyprogesterone for 5–10 days. The patient should expect bleeding/spotting within one week of completing the course of progesterone. However, the presence of bleeding does not rule out incipient ovarian failure, and therefore it has been suggested that this test be abandoned [30].

Treatment

As discussed previously, amenorrhea is usually a sign of an underlying condition. Treating the underlying condition will usually result in the onset or return of menses. An example of this is thyroid replacement in patients with hypothyroidism.

Many etiologies such as PCOS and anorexia nervosa can be at least partially treated with lifestyle changes. Discussion about a healthy diet, moderate exercise, and weight maintenance should be a part of any interaction and preventive guidance for an adolescent. However, girls who meet the diagnostic criteria for obesity may need expertise from specialists in their respective fields, including nutrition counseling and psychiatry/psychology. Girls with eating disorders should be managed in conjunction with an eating disorders team that includes the primary physician, a nutritionist, psychologist or other counselor, and may need to include a specialist in eating disorders. Multiple studies have failed to demonstrate the value of adding estrogen to help prevent anorexia-associated osteopenia in the absence of weight recovery [23]. Thus, attention to management of the underlying eating disorder is paramount, rather than a focus on the symptom of amenorrhea.

Premature ovarian failure is treated medically with hormone replacement therapy including estrogens and progestins. Adolescents frequently prefer oral contraceptive pills as hormone replacement rather than estrogen/progestin formulations used to manage menopausal symptoms, as this therapy is typically normative among adolescents. Given the reproductive implications of this diagnosis, counseling is essential when this diagnosis is confirmed.

In the case of medication-induced hyperprolactinemia, consideration should be given to the possibility of switching to an alternative medication that does not have the same side effect; this will need to be co-ordinated with the clinician who is prescribing the offending medication. Dopamine agonists, such as bromocriptine or cabergoline, are the treatment for most patients with hyperprolactinemia caused by a prolactin-secreting microadenoma. Cabergoline is longer acting, more effective, and better tolerated. Consultation with a neurosurgeon is appropriate if a macroadenoma is found.

Polycystic ovarian syndrome is typically treated with combination estrogen and progestin contraceptives – pills, patches or intravaginal ring – unless estrogen is contraindicated by medical or family history. Combined contraceptives increase sex hormone-binding globulin, resulting in lower free or biologically active testosterone and thus benefiting acne and hair growth. They also produce regular withdrawal bleeding, protecting the endometrium while providing simultaneous contraception. Young women with PCOS and insulin resistance may be candidates for the addition of metformin, an insulin-sensitizing agent, although long-term data in adolescents are lacking.

Combination oral contraceptives are frequently the treatment of choice for adolescents with hypoestrogenism that is not a result of an eating disorder. In patients with anorexia nervosa, the return of spontaneous menses as an indicator of recovery will be masked by combination contraceptives. This, however, must be balanced with the patient's need for contraception. Combined contraceptives may mask other underlying conditions such as the others listed above; thus an evaluation of the etiology should be completed prior to beginning therapy.

Surgical therapy is indicated in select etiologies of amenorrhea. An obstructing vaginal septum or imperforate hymen is managed with septum resection or hymenectomy. Uterine synechiae are hysteroscopically lyzed to restore the uterine cavity and efforts made with medications or intrauterine devices such as an intrauterine system or Foley catheter to prevent recurrent adhesions. Testosterone-producing ovarian neoplasms are usually resected because of concern for malignancy. Patients with a Y chromosome should undergo gonadectomy because of the increased risk of malignancy. The timing for this intervention needs to be individualized, balancing pubertal development and the risk of developing a malignancy.

Amenorrhea is frequently divided into the categories of primary and secondary. Both are usually a sign of a specific condition or disease, rather than specific disease entities per se. A complete evaluation, including medical, reproductive, and surgical history, targeted physical examination, and appropriate laboratory testing, is indicated prior to the administration of therapies. The administration of certain medications such as oral contraceptives prior to establishing a diagnosis can lead to the failure to diagnose an underlying condition such as PCOS, with long-term reproductive and general health consequences. Frequently, appropriately treating the underlying condition will result in the onset or return of menses.

References

1. American College of Obstetricians and Gynecologists. ACOG Committee Opinion #300: cervical cancer screening in adolescents. *Obstet Gynecol* 2004;**104**(4):885–889.

2. American Society for Reproductive Medicine Practice Committee. The evaluation and treatment of androgen excess. *Fertil Steril* 2004;**82**(suppl 1):173–180.

3. Popat V, Nelson LM, Calisk A et al. *Amenorrhea, secondary*. Sep 19, 2008. www.emedicine.com.

4. Munster K, Helm P, Schmidt L. Secondary amenorrhoea: prevalence and medical contact – a cross-sectional study from a Danish county. *Br J Obstet Gynaecol* 1992;**99**(5):430–433.

5. Warren MP. Clinical review 77: evaluation of secondary amenorrhea. *J Clin Endocrinol Metab* 1996;**81**(2):437–442.

6. Bachmann GA, Kemmann E. Prevalence of oligomenorrhea and amenorrhea in a college population. *Am J Obstet Gynecol* 1982;**144**(1):98–102.

7. Belsey EM, Pinol AP. Menstrual bleeding patterns in untreated women. Task Force on Long-Acting Systemic Agents for Fertility Regulation. *Contraception* 1997;**55**(2):57–65.

8. Chumlea WC, Schubert CM, Roche AF et al. Age at menarche and racial comparisons in US girls. *Pediatrics* 2003;**111**(1):110–113.

9. American Society for Reproductive Medicine Practice Committee. Current evaluation of amenorrhea. *Fertil Steril* 2006;**86**(suppl 5):S148–155.

10. Pittock ST, Babovic-Vuksanovic D, Lteif A. Mayer-Rokitansky-Kuster-Hauser anomaly and its associated malformations. *Am J Med Genet A* 2005;**135**(3):314–316.

11. Behera M, Couchman G, Walmer D, Price TM. Mullerian agenesis and thrombocytopenia absent radius syndrome: a case report and review of syndromes associated with Mullerian agenesis. *Obstet Gynecol Surv* 2005;**60**(7):453–461.

12. Varner RE, Younger JB, Blackwell RE. Mullerian dysgenesis. *J Reprod Med* 1985;**30**(6):443–450.

13. Gravholt CH. Epidemiological, endocrine and metabolic features in Turner syndrome. *Eur J Endocrinol* 2004;**151**(6):657–687.

14. Felice ME, Feinstein RA, Fisher M et al. American Academy of Pediatrics Committee on Adolescence. Contraception in adolescents. *Pediatrics* 1999;**104**(5 Pt 1):1161–1166.

15. Latronico AC, Anasti J, Arnhold IJ et al. Brief report: testicular and ovarian resistance to luteinizing hormone caused by inactivating mutations of the luteinizing hormone-receptor gene. *N Engl J Med* 1996;**334**(8):507–512.

16. Nelson LM, Popat V. *Ovarian insufficiency*. Jan 15, 2008. www.emedicine.com.

17. Langevitz P, Klein L, Pras M, Many A. The effect of cyclophosphamide pulses on fertility in patients with lupus nephritis. *Am J Reprod Immunol* 1992;**28**(3–4):157–158.

18. Falcone T, Attaran M, Bedaiwy MA, Goldberg JM. Ovarian function preservation in the cancer patient. *Fertil Steril* 2004;**81**(2):243–257.

19. Lo Presti A, Ruvolo G, Gancitano RA, Cittadini E. Ovarian function following radiation and chemotherapy for cancer. *Eur J Obstet Gynecol Reprod Biol* 2004;**113**(suppl 1):S33–40.

20. Hermann T. Radiation reactions in the gonad: importance in patient counseling. *Strahlenther Onkol* 1997;**171**:439.

21. Mindermann T, Wilson CB. Pediatric pituitary adenomas. *Neurosurgery* 1995;**36**(2):259–268; discussion 269.

22. American Psychiatric Association. *Diagnostic and Statistical Manual of Mental Disorders*, 4th edn. Washington, DC: American Psychiatric Association, 2000.

23. Mitan LA. Menstrual dysfunction in anorexia nervosa. *J Pediatr Adolesc Gynecol* 2004;**17**(2):81–85.

24. Berga SL, Daniels TL, Giles DE. Women with functional hypothalamic amenorrhea but not other forms of anovulation display amplified cortisol concentrations. *Fertil Steril* 1997;**67**(6):1024–1030.

25. Azziz R, Sanchez LA, Knochenhauer ES et al. Androgen excess in women: experience with over 1000 consecutive patients. *J Clin Endocrinol Metab* 2004;**89**(2):453–462.

26. Azziz R, Woods KS, Reyna R, Key TJ, Knochenhauer ES, Yildiz BO. The prevalence and features of the polycystic ovary syndrome in an unselected population. *J Clin Endocrinol Metab* 2004;**89**(6):2745–2749.

27. Revised 2003 consensus on diagnostic criteria and long-term health risks related to polycystic ovary syndrome. *Fertil Steril* 2004;**81**(1):19–25.

28. Sultan C, Paris F. Clinical expression of polycystic ovary syndrome in adolescent girls. *Fertil Steril* 2006;**86**(suppl 1): S6.

29. Balkau B, Charles MA. Comment on the provisional report from the WHO consultation. European Group for the Study of Insulin Resistance (EGIR). *Diabet Med* 1999;**16**(5):442–443.

30. Rebar RW, Connolly HV. Clinical features of young women with hypergonadotropic amenorrhea. *Fertil Steril* 1990;**53**(5):804–810.

CHAPTER 18

Precocious Puberty

Peter A. Lee[1] *& Christopher P. Houk*[2]

[1] Indiana University School of Medicine, Indianapolis, IN, USA
[2] Mercer University School of Medicine, Savannah, GA, USA

Normal pubertal development

The features of normally timed and paced female pubertal development are outlined below as a reference for comparison with girls who have evidence of early sexual maturity.

Age of puberty

The lower age limit for onset of puberty in girls, as indicated by onset of breast development (Tanner stage 2), differs by race [1] (Table 18.1); in the United States it is 6.6 years of age (median age is 9.5) in blacks, 6.8 years (median 9.8) in Hispanics (data from Mexican-Americans) and 8.0 years (median 10.4) in whites. The age of menarche (Table 18.1) also differs by race with the lower age limit (median) of 9.7 years (12.1) for blacks, 10.1 years (12.3) for Mexican-American girls years and 10.7 years (12.6) for whites [2].

Physiology of puberty

The hypothalamic-pituitary-ovarian (HPO) axis first becomes active in early infancy during a period that has been referred to as a mini-puberty. Around 6–12 months of age the HPO activity decreases through a central process that dampens the pulsatile release of gonadotropin-releasing hormone (GnRH) from the hypothalamus. This period of relative quiescence remains until the central processes that govern it allow episodic GnRH release to resume. Nonetheless, both the pituitary and the gonads remain capable of full function when stimulated. However, when

Pediatric, Adolescent, & Young Adult Gynecology. Edited by
A. Altchek and L. Deligdisch. © 2009 Blackwell Publishing,
ISBN: 978-1-4051-5347-8.

Table 18.1 Approximate age of onset of pubertal events based upon NHANES III data

	White	Black	Mexican-American
Breast T2			
• 2.5th %ile	8.0	6.6	6.8
• Median age	10.4	9.5	9.8
Pubic hair T2			
• 2.5th %ile	8.0	6.7	7.4
• Median age	10.6	9.4	10.4
Menarche			
• 2.5th %ile	10.7	9.8	10.1
• Median age	12.6	12.1	12.3

GnRH is secreted, gonadotropin release is stimulated and ovarian sex steroids are produced, leading to a centrally mediated, GnRH-dependent puberty. When an increase in serum sex steroids results from exogenous exposure or autonomous ovarian activity, the process is said to be peripheral or GnRH independent.

Puberty involves maturation of the reproductive system as a result of increased gonadotropin, sex steroid and other hormone secretion, resulting in potential for adult sexual and reproductive function. As puberty progresses, the episodic release pattern of the pituitary gonadotropins, luteinizing hormone (LH) and follicle-stimulating hormone (FSH), becomes more pronounced as a result of greater episodic hypothalamic GnRH secretion. In addition, feedback mechanisms on the HPO axis mature. Pubertal onset signals the emergence of a new balance between stimulatory and inhibitory factors/neurotransmitters (including acetylcholine, catecholamines, γ-aminobutyric acid (GABA), opioid peptides, prostaglandins, and serotonin) that

Box 18.1 Glandular hormonal changes at onset of puberty

- Gonadarche
Primary
The activation of the hypothalamic pituitary gonadal axis resulting in sex steroid production and germ cell maturation
- Thelarche
Onset of breast development

- Adrenarche
Secondary
A maturation of the adrenal gland resulting in the production of weak androgens. Typically begins before gonadarche.
- Pubarche
Onset of sexual hair growth, a consequence of adrenarche, gonadarche or both

allows a progressive increase in GnRH, and therefore gonadotropin, release.

Genetic/molecular control of pubertal development

GABA, the LHBβ subunit gene, neuropeptide Y, β-endorphin, leptin and glutamate are involved, as well as recently described components including the kisspeptins, the cognate G-protein coupled receptor (GPR54), and the FGFR-1 (KAL2) gene. A G-protein coupled receptor encoded by the GPR54 gene is required for the pubertal onset of pulsatile LH and FSH secretion [3,4].

The KAL-1 gene encoding the protein anosmin-1 is involved in organogenesis and the KAL-2 gene expressed through fibroblast growth factor receptor 1 (FGFR-1) is necessary for embryonic olfactory bulb and gonadotrope migration.

Terminology used for female pubertal development (Box 18.1)

Gonadarche refers to the onset of the progressive increase in HPO axis activity; *thelarche*, the onset of breast development; *adrenarche* (aka pubarche), the onset of sexual (pubic or axillary) hair growth; and *menarche*, the first menstrual period. Thelarche is the most common initial manifestation of puberty, although a minority of girls (approximately 20%) develop adrenarche first. Adrenarche is a GnRH-independent event that results from an increase in adrenal androgen secretion and does not suggest HPO axis activity.

Physical changes of puberty

Changes include onset and progression of breast growth, genital (particularly labia minora) growth, estrogenization of the vaginal mucosa resulting in pink mucosa with clear secretions, uterine growth with endometrial thickening, accelerated linear growth, and changes in body composition leading to a female-pattern fat distribution. Breast and pubic hair development are commonly divided into one of five Tanner stages, stage 1 being prepubertal and stage 5 being sexually mature. The usual interval from pubertal onset to menarche is 2–2.5 years. Menarche generally occurs during mid-puberty, at Tanner breast stage 4. Ovulation does not necessarily immediately follow menarche. Pubertal development is usually complete 3–4 years after the onset of breast development. Pubic and axillary hair development, apocrine gland maturation with adult-type body odor, and skin changes related to acne are stimulated by adrenal, and to a lesser extent ovarian, androgen synthesis. One indicator of biologic maturity, skeletal age, correlates more closely than actual age with the onset of puberty (bone age = 10.5 years) and menarche (bone age = 12.5 years).

Hormonal changes of puberty

Although mean FSH levels are relatively higher than LH during childhood, levels do not rise dramatically at puberty. In contrast, LH levels are typically undetectable in the prepubertal subject and become detectable during puberty. Accordingly, an LH:FSH ratio of >1 is most useful. While not commonly used for clinical assessment, ovarian hormones such as inhibin A and B both correlate with pubertal ovarian activity and provide evidence of ongoing ovarian follicular activity [5].

A random LH or estradiol value above the prepubertal range verifies puberty. Nonetheless, the dynamic nature of gonadotropin release often makes random measurement of LH (and FSH) insufficient as a screening test in subjects manifesting progressive pubertal development. In these cases, the LH response to GnRH/GnRHa stimulation can be most helpful 30–60 minutes after stimulation. Thus, a random or GnRH/GnRH agonist (GnRHa)-stimulated LH level and an estradiol level above the prepubertal range document puberty.

Levels of adrenal androgens, primarily dehydroepiandrosterone sulfate (DHEAS), above the prepubertal range can be used to document adrenarche.

Box 18.2 Physical changes at onset of puberty

1. Physical characteristics
   a. Breast development – Tanner stage 2 or more
   b. Genital growth with estrogenized vaginal mucosa (pink vs red)
   c. Sexual hair – may not be present at onset
      May be consequence of androgen secretion from the adrenals or ovaries or both; may be preceded by onset of body odor and acne; preceded, accompanied or followed by axillary hair growth
2. Accelerated growth rate
   >6 cm/yr growth rate, for precocious puberty >25%ile increase/yr on growth curve

---

Box 18.3 Categories of early development and precocious puberty

- Premature thelarche
  o No progression, accelerated growth rate, or other changes
- Premature adrenarche
  o Most common cause of premature sexual hair
  o Early onset of adrenal androgen secretion (DHEAS or DHEA)
  o Skeletal maturity is normal for age
  o Should be followed to differentiate from pathologic ovarian/adrenal hyperandrogenism or syndrome X (insulin resistance, hyperlipidemia, ⇑ BP)
- Gonadotropin-independent precocious puberty (peripheral or precocious pseudopuberty) – pubertal changes from hormones produced independently of hypothalamic GnRH
  o McCune-Albright syndrome, ovarian cysts, chronic primary hypothyroidism, sex steroid-secreting adrenal or gonadal tumors, exogenous sex steroids
- GnRH-dependent (central or true) precocious puberty – puberty resulting from GnRH-driven FSH/LH stimulation (HPG axis in normal puberty)

Central nervous system changes of puberty

The activation and remodeling of central neural circuits during puberty lead to changes in cognitive functioning; when combined with sex steroid exposure, these changes often lead to more potent and focused sexual motivation. Together with heightened genital responsiveness, sexual behaviors become more intense during pubertal development.

Early pubertal development

Physical development consistent with changes that may herald the onset of puberty include breast development, sexual hair growth and accelerated linear growth (Box 18.2). If breast development is not accompanied by an increase in growth rate, the diagnosis of precocious puberty should be questioned and the diagnosis of premature thelarche should be considered. When development of sexual hair occurs without a corresponding increase in breast development, the evaluation should be directed toward premature adrenarche or excessive androgen production.

Premature thelarche

Premature thelarche refers to premature breast development without other pubertal changes. It is most commonly seen during the first two years of life and is felt to be due to a greater ovarian hormone production (or increased sensitivity) during early childhood. In fact, the-larche beyond three years of age is associated with increased FSH levels and inhibin B secretion suggestive of enhanced follicular development [6]. Indeed, this is supported by the demonstration of ovarian microcysts [7] that appear to secrete greater amounts of estrogen than average. Premature thelarche is diagnosed when nonprogressive breast development occurs in isolation and is not associated with accelerated linear growth or other evidence of puberty changes. However, because precocious puberty may also manifest isolated breast development as the initial finding, careful monitoring for subsequent changes is mandatory (Box 18.3).

Assessment

History should focus on the age of onset of breast development, progression since onset, the presence of other pubertal changes, growth rate, and family history of pubertal development. Physical examination includes a complete physical examination (including dermatologic inspection) with clear documentation of Tanner staging and the presence or absence of neurologic findings.

In cases where the growth rate is normal and the breast development is minimal and nonprogressive, additional investigation may not be necessary. When evidence suggests more than early static breast development, LH, FSH, and estradiol levels should be measured. Obtaining bone age x-rays, particularly when growth rate is unclear, may also be of benefit. In premature thelarche, skeletal maturation may be normal or slightly advanced for age. While usually not needed, pelvic ultrasound studies may be done. With thelarche, the uterus and ovaries are of normal size, symmetry, and configuration and ovarian follicular microcysts may be visualized.

If studies are consistent with thelarche alone, i.e. prepubertal, and if this condition does not progress, treatment is limited to education and counseling. Regression may occur or breast development may remain static until puberty begins. However, there are variations of normal development during childhood and there is a continuum from premature thelarche, nonprogressive precocious puberty and GnRH-dependent precocious puberty. It may be difficult to differentiate precocious thelarche from precocious puberty, particularly as a minority of those presenting with premature thelarche progress to central precocious puberty. Nevertheless, there is most commonly minimal progression until the usual age of onset of puberty. Without hormonal evidence of pubertal onset, the diagnosis of precocious puberty should not be made.

Premature adrenarche

Clinical findings

Androgen exposure stimulates sexual hair growth (pubarche), both pubic and axillary, as well as acne and adult-type body odor. Thelarche, usually signaling the onset of gonadarche, generally precedes adrenarche in the majority of girls but as many as 20% of girls reach pubarche first. Premature adrenarche uncommonly occurs before the age of six years. In some cases, the skeletal age and height may be slightly more than expected. In children, when androgen production results from a pathologic process there is typically an increase in growth velocity, a significant advance in skeletal maturation and progressive virilization.

Causes

Premature adrenarche is a consequence of premature maturation of the sex steroid-producing zone (zona reticulata) of the adrenal [8]. The onset of physical findings of androgen changes only rarely signals a pathologic state [9]. The hallmark of this adrenal maturation is the identification of the adrenal product, DHEAS, a weak androgen.

In some cases, the development of premature pubarche may be an early manifestation of a subsequent hyperandrogenic state with hirsutism and amenorrhea. Hence, premature pubarche may be seen as a risk factor for the development of polycystic ovarian syndrome (PCOS, ovarian hyperandrogenism). Overweight girls with early sexual hair growth in particular are at risk for development of the metabolic syndrome.

Interestingly, the phosphorylation defect seen in some types of functional hyperandrogenism may also influence insulin sensitivity and metabolism, resulting in hyperinsulinism, which may secondarily amplify LH secretion leading to perpetuation of the hyperandrogenic state. Mild or nonclassic congenital adrenal hyperplasia may also present with similar physical features but tends to show a rapid progression. Androgen-secreting tumors are very rare and usually present with very impressive physical evidence of androgen excess, including very oily skin, severe acne, progressive hirsutism and clitoromegaly.

Assessment

When there are no worrisome physical findings to suggest pathology, such as rapid increase in linear growth, virilization or skeletal maturation, only minimal evaluation and follow-up are necessary. Androgen levels, including DHEAS, DHEA (or androstenedione) and testosterone, may be measured to confirm that levels are consistent with early adrenarche (see Box 18.3). Because of the marked incremental rise of DHEAS that is the signature of adrenarche, measurement of this hormone alone is usually adequate unless there is evidence of virilization. Overweight girls with adrenarche should be monitored for other risk factors of the metabolic syndrome.

Precocious puberty

Diagnosis

The diagnosis of precocious puberty is based on three primary findings:
• development and progression of secondary sexual characteristics
• accelerated linear growth for age
• biochemical documentation of pubertal sex steroid levels (see Box 18.2).
The majority of girls referred for evaluation of precocious puberty have isolated premature thelarche or adrenarche,

which are variants of normal development [10]. However, a girl with early onset of breast development and growth rate acceleration or early breast development followed by progression before 10.6 years of age for whites, 9.7 years for African-Americans and 10.0 years for Hispanics meets the criteria for precocious puberty.

For the girl presenting with precocious puberty, the decision of whether further assessment or observation is indicated is guided by history, physical findings and evidence of progression. Additional diagnostic evaluation employs the measurement of reproductive hormone and imaging (when indicated) to exclude pathologic underlying causes. More than 90% of girls with progressive pubertal changes have central precocious puberty (CPP) and less than 5% of these girls have an underlying abnormality [11]. One demonstrable CNS abnormality results from a hypothalamic hamartoma, an ectopic and redundant collection of GnRH-secreting neurons, whose secretory activity is not dampened by normal inhibitory mechanisms. These hamartomas may be pedunculated or sessile [12]; the sessile variety may be associated with seizures, behavior disturbance, and mental retardation. Hamartomas are usually identified in early childhood and are more frequent in boys than girls. Other CNS abnormalities associated with CPP may not be demonstrable on imaging studies, such as are seen after encephalitis, CNS surgery, brain radiation, and chemotherapy.

Differentiation of categories of precocious puberty

When there is clinical evidence of pubertal progression, an investigation should be undertaken to differentiate CPP from the GnRH-independent type of sexual precocity (Boxes 18.3, 18.4).

• GnRH-independent precocious puberty (also called peripheral precocious puberty or precocious pseudo-puberty): the early physical changes of puberty that occur in this category result from nonhypothalamic stimulated sex steroid production and are pathologic in all circumstances.

• Central precocious puberty (CPP) (also called GnRH-dependent precocious puberty or true precocious puberty): refers to a state of physiologically normal but precocious puberty, resulting from the early activation of the hypothalamic-pituitary-gonadal (HPG) axis leading to ovarian sex steroid production.

Box 18.4 Central (GnRH-driven) precocious puberty

1. Etiologies
   Idiopathic, CNS abnormalities (hypothalamic hamartomas, tumors, congenital abnormalities, post inflammation, post chemotherapy, post radiation), secondary to chronic sex steroid exposure, after dramatic socio-economic/environmental change (adoption from third world countries)
2. Natural history
   • Mature appearance including physical pubertal characteristics
   • Early onset of reproductive capacity
   • Advanced skeletal growth and maturation
     ○ Tall stature in childhood
     ○ If skeletal maturity exceeds concomitant height gain → compromised adult height

---

Central precocious puberty

This form of precocious puberty results from early onset of pubertal hypothalamic GnRH secretion with no demonstrable reason or as a result of CNS abnormalities that are felt to disrupt the balance between the inhibitory and stimulatory factors. While CPP most commonly occurs in the absence of any demonstrable abnormality (idiopathic), brain imaging is often performed as a precaution to exclude CNS lesions and should always be done when other neurologic findings are present. One group of girls seen with CPP making up a disproportionate number are those who have immigrated from underdeveloped countries [13].

GnRH-independent precocious puberty

GnRH-independent precocious puberty results from sex steroid stimulation; however, the production of sex steroids in GnRH-independent puberty does not stem from pituitary gonadotropin secretion, but from exogenous or autonomous endogenous (gonadal or extragonadal) sources. Endogenous sex steroids are autonomously produced, independent of pituitary gonadotropin stimulation or control, or as a consequence of cell surface gonadotropin receptor activation.

History

Pertinent findings on history include growth rates, age of onset, timing of pubertal changes and past medical/family/social/psychologic history. The history should

---

Box 18.5 General physical findings to be noted

1. Height, weight, BMI, relative body proportions
2. Neurologic abnormalities including visual fields
   - may be associated with CNS lesions causing precocious puberty (e.g. hamartomas, optic gliomas)
3. Thyromegaly
   - a form of peripheral precocious puberty rarely occurs with chronic primary hypothyroidism
4. Localized skin hyperpigmentation (café au lait)
   - McCune-Albright syndrome or neurofibromatosis
5. Galactorrhea
   - elevated prolactin levels, may also cause breast development

---

Box 18.6 Hormonal documentation of pubertal onset: either early or normal age

1. Gonadotropins
   - i. Basal levels
       Prepubertal FSH > LH
       Pubertal LH > FSH
   - ii. LH:FSH ratios
       <1 prepubertal
       >1 pubertal
   - iii. GnRH or GnRHa stimulated
       LH at 20, 30 or 40 minutes >7
2. Sex steroids
   Estradiol – because of marked fluctuations and assays with poor sensitivity levels may not be detectible that are above the prepubertal range
   DHEAS – marker of adrenarche

---

assess for possible exposure to exogenous hormones, CNS abnormalities, neurologic symptoms, pubertal history of other family members, and height and growth rates.

Physical findings (Box 18.5)

Physical examination should include careful anthropomorphic measurements including height, weight, arm span (fingertip to fingertip), and upper (sitting height)/lower body (pubic symphysis to floor) segment ratio. Physical examination should document skin findings, thyroid size, Tanner staging, visual inspection of the genitalia, presence of vaginal leukorrhea and appearance of the vaginal mucosa (estrogen effect is pink versus red). Inspection of the vaginal mucosa can be performed by gently spreading the labia while the patient is in the prone position with knees drawn up and legs spread. A bimanual abdominal-rectal examination is usually unnecessary, especially when a transabdominal/pelvic ultrasound is performed.

Diagnostic testing

The assessment of early pubertal development is outlined in Boxes 18.6 and 18.7. The diagnostic work-up is primarily designed to exclude underlying pathology. Initial biochemical evaluation includes measurement of reproductive hormones: LH, FSH, estradiol, and DHEAS (if adrenarche is suspected). If menarche has occurred, a progesterone level may verify ovulation and the luteal phase. Basal LH and FSH levels alone are sufficient to diagnose CPP [14] when they exceed the prepubertal range. Undetectable LH levels (using a third-generation assay) indicate prepubertal status; FSH levels are variable in the

prepubertal state and do not indicate activation of the HPO axis when elevated. However, LH:FSH ratios (using the same assay method) of less than 1.0 support a prepubertal state, while ratios greater than 1.0 suggest puberty. When basal levels are inconclusive or incongruent with other findings, a GnRH or GnRHa stimulation test is indicated. A rise of LH levels after stimulation into the pubertal response range is indicative of CPP. It is important to understand that basal and GnRH-stimulated FSH levels are not sufficiently different between prepubertal and pubertal subjects and thus are often unnecessary during stimulation testing.

A skeletal age radiograph provides information to compare skeletal maturity to chronologic age and height. The

---

Box 18.7 Laboratory evaluation

1. LH and FSH levels
   - (LH < FSH suggests prepubertal; LH > FSH pubertal)
2. Estradiol
   - >5 pg/mL suggestive of puberty
3. Bone age x-ray
   - Advanced greater than 2 SD suggestive of early puberty, bone age greater than height for age on growth curve
4. Pelvic ultrasound
   - ovarian and uterine size and symmetry and endometrial stripe
5. Others based on history and physical examination
   - Thyroid function tests and prolactin
   - Adrenal androgens, e.g. DHEAS
     - documentation of adrenarche

---

normal degree of variation (± 2 SD for age) between skeletal and chronologic age is approximately 20 months. A significantly advanced skeletal age, an accelerated growth rate, and early onset and progression of physical puberty confirm puberty.

Ultrasound estimations of ovarian and uterine volume often provide helpful information in the evaluation of precocious puberty. Bilateral increases in ovarian volume and uterine length to pubertal standards provide additional evidence for CPP. Unilateral asymmetric ovarian enlargement suggests GnRH-independent precocious puberty such as occurs with ovarian cysts or tumor. When other evidence suggests or indicates CPP, magnetic resonance imaging (MRI) of the CNS, focusing on the hypothalamic/pituitary region, is indicated in an attempt to identify lesions associated with increased gonadotropin secretion.

Central precocious puberty

The most common etiology of CPP is idiopathic. However, CPP may occur following CNS trauma, CNS surgery, CNS inflammation or other types of poorly characterized CNS abnormalities such as are seen in cerebral palsy, myelomeningocele or anoxic brain injury. Rarely it occurs with increased intracranial pressure in association with hydrocephalus, brain abscesses or granulomas. Infrequently hypothalamic hamartomas, pineal/subarachnoid cysts, glial and germ cell tumors and rarely astrocytoma or craniopharyngioma are found in association with CPP [15]. An etiology that is becoming more frequent is that associated with successful therapy of leukemia and other solid tumors of childhood. Curiously, CPP may also occur in conjunction with acquired growth hormone deficiency. Because pubertal onset is closely tied to skeletal maturation, any factor, such as prolonged sex steroid exposure, that unduly advances bone age can result in a premature pubertal activation of the hypothalamic-pituitary axis (secondary CPP). This is most commonly seen in patients with congenital adrenal hyperplasia, estrogen-secreting tumors or exogenous sex steroid exposure.

GnRH-independent precocious puberty

GnRH-independent precocious puberty is early puberty resulting from a mechanism other than GnRH-driven gonadotropin-stimulated ovarian sex steroid production. This develops as a consequence of excessive sex steroid stimulation in childhood from gonadal, adrenal cortical, tumor or exogenous sources. The percentage of girls presenting with GnRH-independent precocious puberty is less than 5%. Etiologies include the following.

The McCune–Albright syndrome (MAS)

This syndrome classically involves the triad of localized multicentered osseous lesions known as polyostotic fibrous dysplasia, melanotic cutaneous macules commonly referred to as "cafe au lait" spots, and other endocrinopathies. The presence of any two of these three findings should prompt the practitioner to consider MAS [16]. This unique form of GnRH-independent precocious puberty results from activating mis-sense mutations in the gene for the α subunit of G_s that is involved in signal transduction of many types of tropic hormone signaling. Excessive endocrine function appears to result from autonomous excessive hormone production, a consequence of the G-protein producing stimulation as if tropic hormones were present.

Affected cell lines occur in some but not all of the tissues in involved organs [17]. A mosaic distribution of cells containing this somatic mutation accounts for the unusually variable exacerbations and remissions of affected organs. Endocrinopathies generally involve multiple glands and stem from the constitutive activation of tropic hormone receptors: for example, MSH-like effects in skin, PTH-like effects in bone lesions, and ACTH-like effects on the adrenal gland. GnRH-independent precocious puberty results when the ovaries are involved, glucocorticoid excess with the adrenal cortex, hyperthyroidism with thyroid involvement, pituitary gigantism or acromegaly when the pituitary gland is affected, and hypophosphatemia with parathyroid gland involvement.

GnRH-independent precocious puberty associated with the MAS presents with rapid breast maturation or early onset of vaginal bleeding which results from a rapid rise and subsequent fall of estrogen secretion. Estrogen is secreted spontaneously, without gonadotropin stimulation, and characteristically sporadically from ovarian follicles. These follicles may enlarge into cysts that can be visualized by pelvic ultrasound, creating asymmetrically enlarged ovaries. These ovarian cysts usually spontaneously regress and are followed by a re-emergence of additional cysts or long-standing quiescence. Skeletal age and biologic maturity follow a similar pattern.

Characteristically patients develop early pubertal HPO function (secondary CPP). Unless other illnesses preclude it, those with the MAS can be expected to eventually have normal ovulatory menstrual cycling with fertility.

Chronic primary hypothyroidism

A rare cause of GnRH-independent precocious puberty is associated with chronic primary hypothyroidism. The GnRH-independent precocious puberty occurs even though untreated hypothyroidism typically delays growth and skeletal maturation. Rarely, pubertal changes are associated with primary thyroid gland failure and extremely elevated TSH levels. The principal finding is breast development, which may be accompanied by galactorrhea. While the etiology of this unusual syndrome is poorly understood, factors that appear to contribute to it are excessive prolactin secretion (a consequence of increased TRH secretion) and excessive secretion of the α subunit (common to the FSH and TSH molecule) and TSH, both of which may occupy and activate the FSH receptor.

Estrogen-secreting tumors

Estrogen-secreting tumors of the ovary and adrenal are rare causes of GnRH-independent precocious puberty. Ovarian tumors that secrete estrogen include granulosa cell (which may be associated with Peutz–Jeghers syndrome), lipoid, sex cord or theca cell tumor, carcinoma, cystadenoma, and gonadoblastoma.

Exogenous estrogens

Physical changes of puberty occur after repeated exposure to exogenous estrogens or estrogen-like compounds. These may be present in foods, cosmetics, and medicines.

Ovarian cysts

Ovarian cysts may secrete sufficient estrogen to stimulate breast, genital, and endometrial development. This may be followed by symptoms of diminished estrogen levels, including withdrawal bleeding, when the cyst resolves. Ovarian follicles may form cysts during normal childhood, perhaps secondary to intermittent gonadotropin stimulation, and are also seen in CPP or GnRH-independent precocious puberty (MAS). Such cysts are readily identified by ultrasonography. Since they can be expected to be self-limiting over several months,

serial monitoring with ultrasound and hormonal monitoring is indicated.

Treatment of underlying abnormalities of precocious puberty

When a primary cause for precocious puberty can be identified, treatment should be directed toward that. Examples include thyroxine replacement in primary hypothyroidism as this would result in a reduction in TSH and prolactin, which would allow regression of breast development and cessation of galactorrhea. Tumors including CNS, ovarian or adrenal tumors should be treated. When increased intracranial pressure is identified, this should be corrected, as the CPP may be reversible in these circumstances. Treatment of hypothalamic hamartomas should be medical; the surgical treatment of these lesions may be associated with significant morbidity, especially for nonpedunculated lesions. Obviously, inappropriate exposure to estrogen or gonadotropin should be stopped. Functional ovarian cysts usually require no therapy other than careful monitoring until resolution. Surgery should only be considered if the cyst is at risk of rupture. Surgery otherwise may result in loss of functional ovarian tissue.

In the MAS, agents that reduce sex steroid production or action have met with variable success. Therapies include steroid synthesis inhibitors (ketoconazole) and aromatase inhibitors including testolactone and anastrozole plus limited experience with the newer generation of aromatase inhibitors. This class of drugs is designed to inhibit estrogen production by blocking the synthesis of estrogens from androgen precursors. Treatment with tamoxifen, a mixed estrogen receptor agonist/antagonist, has been reported to reduce vaginal bleeding, growth rates and skeletal maturation [18]. Therapy for primary or secondary CPP using GnRHa therapy is described below.

Rationale for CPP therapy

Therapy for CPP is employed to avoid the consequences of early pubertal progression. These include marked acceleration of physical changes, both pubertal advance and excessive height for age. When the advance in skeletal maturity exceeds the gains made by the linear growth rate, adult height is compromised. Typically children with early puberty share interests with age peers although they are quick to recognize that they are physically different and go to great lengths to avoid incidents of exposure or childhood sex play. While psychosexual development is generally appropriate for age rather than physical maturity, withdrawal behavior, anxiety, depression, and somatic complaints may occur. While libido is increased, inappropriate sexual behavior is seldom a problem. However, in some cases early puberty may be psychologically stressful and may increase the risk for being a victim of sexual predation. Sexual advances by older individuals may be misinterpreted because of a childlike naïve perspective so if sexual behavior or expressed sexual interest is excessive, an external cause should be excluded.

Hence, indications for treating CPP with GnRHa involve a desire to preserve or reclaim lost height potential, cause a regression of pubertal development, and ameliorate psychologic stress/social issues related to tall stature during childhood, advanced pubertal development, early menstruation and dysphoric sexual urges during childhood. Treatment should also include mental health counseling in appropriate patients.

All patients and parents need to understand what is happening, specifically that normal pubertal changes are occurring, albeit at an early age. A simple explanation geared to the child usually provides a great deal of relief, including that it is normal for the body of a girl to change into the body of a woman and that in her situation it is happening too soon and too fast. It is usually appropriate for the parents to be present during such discussions, which may include a general discussion of situationally appropriate sex education.

Therapy for CPP using GnRHa

Indications and criteria for treatment

GnRH agonist (GnRHa) is the treatment of choice [19] for patients with CPP (i.e. having pubertal gonadotropin secretion based on elevated basal LH, an LH:FSH ratio >1 or a pubertal LH response to GnRH stimulation). Therapy should be considered only in patients with pubertal progression, documented accelerated linear growth, and unduly advanced skeletal age (Box 18.8). When there is no accelerated skeletal age for height (that would portend a reduction in adult height prediction), treatment may be withheld as the slowly and intermittently progressive forms of precocious puberty are not associated with di-

---

Box 18.8 GnRHa treatment of precocious puberty

1. Rationale
   - Since pubertal gonadal function is dependent upon stimulation via GnRH receptors on the pituitary gonadotrope cells by episodic secretion of hypothalamic GnRH
   - Since GnRHa therapy results in continued occupation of these receptors, resulting in downregulation of pituitary LH and FSH secretion and release
   - Such therapy stops puberty and associated growth
2. Dosage of GnRHa should be sufficient to:
   - Completely suppress gonadotropin secretion
     - Halt progression of puberty
     - Decelerate growth rate
     - Decelerate rate of bone maturation
   - Adequate suppression may be verified by lack of response to GnRH or GnRHa stimulation testing

---

minished adult height; accordingly, therapy for this reason alone is not indicated [20].

GnRHa dosing must be adequate to suppress episodic gonadotropin secretion by the continual occupation of pituitary gonadotrope GnRH receptors by high levels of GnRHa. GnRHa is available for subcutaneous implantation, as depot injections, short-acting injection, and nasal spray. With adequate dosing, suppression occurs within weeks. Withdrawal bleeding after the onset of therapy should be expected due to the loss of estrogen and the resulting withdrawal bleeding.

Monitoring GnRHa therapy involves confirming lack of pubertal progression (clinically and biochemically), using physical exam, growth measurement, and basal or GnRHa-stimulated LH levels. The latter can be accomplished by the measurement of LH concentration 30–60 minutes after the scheduled depot GnRH injection [21,22].

Changes during therapy

Suppressive GnRHa therapy results in regression of breast size (Tanner stage may not change), a return of the prepubertal appearance of the vaginal mucosa, and cessation of menses, if menarche had been reached before therapy. Documenting a low random LH level or showing a lack of LH response to GnRHa can confirm suppression, which should occur within weeks. With adequate dosing, suppression is demonstrable after the first eight weeks of therapy. Lack of regression of adrenarche-related pubic hair is not expected during GnRHa therapy; therefore this should not be seen as evidence for lack of GnRHa suppression.

GnRHa therapy results in a growth rate deceleration to 5–6 cm/year and in cases with very advanced skeletal age, the rate may well be less than this. If the primary reason for therapy is to increase adult height, growth rates and skeletal maturity should be carefully monitored. Predicted adult height (based on bone age and height) should not diminish while on therapy; unless skeletal age is markedly advanced, predicted adult height is expected to increase. Skeletal maturity (bone age) rate slows to normal until the skeletal age reaches the usual age of puberty, after which skeletal maturation progresses very slowly. Among children with advanced skeletal age in whom GnRHa therapy is inadequate to reclaim lost height potential, the co-administration of growth hormone may be considered. While height gained with combined therapy is statistically greater than with GnRHa therapy alone, this gain may be only a few centimeters [23]. Hence, the benefit should be carefully considered when combined therapy is being considered. Therapy should be discontinued when growth rates become minimal and skeletal age approaches 13.5–14 years.

At presentation, weight is often increased for age since sex steroid stimulates an increase in lean body mass. During GnRH therapy, there is often a disproportionate accumulation of adipose tissue resulting in an increase in BMI. BMI generally falls into the normal range at discontinuation of therapy [24,25]. GnRHa therapy reduces ovarian and uterine volume, while bone mineral density (BMD) (greater than expected for age before therapy) remains relatively constant. Monitoring bone mineral density is not usually indicated during therapy.

Outcome data

Resumption of pubertal HPG activity, as defined by basal or stimulated gonadotropin measurements, begins promptly after discontinuation of therapy. While there is variability in the time to resumption of physical development, this generally proceeds at a rate similar to normal puberty. Among those who experienced menarche prior to therapy, periods resume within months; in those who had not reached menarche before GnRHa therapy, menses usually occur within 18 months, with considerably more time for a minority [26]. Although poorly documented in the literature, ovulatory cycling and menstrual regularity occur appropriately. Pregnancy with birth of normal infants has occurred, and there is no evidence that treatment with GnRHa is associated with future subfertility or disordered sexual function.

Significant psychologic adjustment problems while on GnRHa therapy have not been noted. Although accentuated physical appearance concerns and increased emotional insecurity have been found during therapy [27], there are no recognized long-term detrimental psychologic consequences.

Adult heights after GnRHa therapy are greater than that predicted at onset of therapy and usually fall within the expected (target) genetic height except in cases of severe loss of height potential before the onset of therapy [28–31]. In general, adult heights are greater and closer to target height in those with younger onset of precocity, less advanced skeletal age, no delay in treatment, and longer duration of treatment [32].

While the lack of BMD accrual during therapy may result in low BMD for age, bone accrual resumes after GnRHa therapy is discontinued and by mid-adolescence BMD is normal for age [33,34].

While there is no evidence that ovarian hyperandrogenism is diagnosed more frequently in girls previously diagnosed with precocious puberty or treated with GnRHa, it may be that early ovarian synthesis of androgen may accelerate pubertal onset and therefore increase the risk of future ovarian hyperandrogenism.

References

1. Sun SS, Schubert CM, Chumlea WC et al. National estimates of the timing of sexual maturation and racial differences among US children. *Pediatrics* 2002;**110**:911–919.

2. Chumlea WC, Shubert CM, Roche AF et al. Age at menarche and racial comparisons in US girls. *Pediatrics* 2003;**111**:110–113.

3. Seminara S, Messager S, Chatzidaki E et al. The GPR54 gene as a regulator of puberty. *N Engl J Med* 2003;**349**:1614–1627.

4. Messager S, Chatzidaki EE, Ma D et al. Kisspeptin directly stimulates gonadotropin-releasing hormone release via G protein-coupled receptor 54. *Proc Natl Acad Sci USA* 2005;**102**:1761–1766.

5. Crofton PM, Evans AE, Groome NP, Taylor MR, Holland CV, Kelnar CJ. Dimeric inhibins in girls from birth to adulthood: relationship with age, pubertal stage, FSH and oestradiol. *Clin Endocrinol (Oxf)* 2002;**56**:223–230.

6. Crofton PM, Evans NE, Wardhaugh B, Groome NP, Kelnar CJ. Evidence for increased ovarian follicular activity in girls with premature thelarche. *Clin Endocrinol (Oxf)* 2005;**62**:205–209.

7. Freedman SM, Kreitzer PM, Elkowitz SS, Soberman N, Leonidas JC. Ovarian microcysts in girls with isolated premature thelarche. *J Pediatr* 1993;**122**:246–249.

8. Ghizzoni L, Milani S. The natural history of premature adrenarche. *J Pediatr Endocrinol Metab* 2000;**13**(suppl 5):1247–1251.

9. Ibanez L, Potau N, Dunger D, de Zegher F. Precocious pubarche in girls and the development of androgen excess. *J Pediatr Endocrinol Metab* 2000;**13**:1261–1263.

10. Kaplowitz P. Clinical characteristics of 104 children referred for evaluation of precocious puberty. *J Clin Endocrinol Metab* 2004;**89**:3644–3650.

11. Virdis R, Street M, Zampoli M et al. Precocious puberty in girls adopted from developing countries. *Arch Dis Child* 1998;**78**:152–154.

12. Chemaitilly W, Trivin C, Adan L, Gall V, Sainte-Rose C, Brauner R. Central precocious puberty: clinical and laboratory features. *Clin Endocrinol (Oxf)* 2001;**54**:289–294.

13. Debeneix C, Bourgeois M, Trivin C, Sainte-Rose C, Brauner R. Hypothalamic hamartoma: comparison of clinical presentation and magnetic resonance images. *Horm Res* 2001;**56**:12–18.

14. Brito VN, Batista MC, Borges MF et al. Diagnostic value of fluorometric assays in the evaluation of precocious puberty. *J Clin Endocrinol Metab* 1999;**84**:3539–3544.

15. Rivarola M, Belgorosky A, Mendilaharzu H, Vidal G. Precocious puberty in children with tumours of the suprasellar and pineal areas: organic central precocious puberty. *Acta Paediatr* 2001;**90**:751–756.

16. Lumbroso S, Paris F, Sultan C. Activating Gsalpha mutations: analysis of 113 patients with signs of McCune-Albright syndrome – a European Collaborative Study. *J Clin Endocrinol Metab* 2004;**89**:2107–2113.

17. Shenker A, Weinstein LS, Moran A et al. Severe endocrine and nonendocrine manifestations of the McCune–Albright syndrome associated with activating mutations of stimulatory G protein GS. *J Pediatr* 1993;**123**:509–518.

18. Eugster EA, Rubin SD, Reiter EO et al, for the McCune–Albright Study Group. Tamoxifen treatment for precocious puberty in McCune–Albright syndrome: a multicenter trial. *J Pediatr* 2003;**143**:60–66.

19. Antoniazzi F, Zamboni G. Central precocious puberty: current treatment options. *Paediatr Drugs* 2004;**6**:211–213.

20. Adan L, Chemaitilly W, Trivin C, Brauner R. Factors predicting adult height in girls with idiopathic central precocious puberty: implications for treatment. *Clin Endocrinol (Oxf)* 2002;**56**:297–302.

21. Bhatia S, Neely EK, Wilson DM. Serum luteinizing hormone rises within minutes after depot leuprolide injection: implications for monitoring therapy. *Pediatrics* 2002;**109**: E30.

22. Brito VN, Latronico AC, Arnhold IJ, Mendonca BB. A single luteinizing hormone determination 2 hours after depot leuprolide is useful for therapy monitoring of gonadotropin-dependent precocious puberty in girls. *J Clin Endocrinol Metab* 2004;**89**:4338–4342.

23. Pasquino AM, Pucarelli I, Segni M, Matrunola M, Cerroni F. Adult height in girls with central precocious puberty treated with gonadotropin-releasing hormone analogues and growth hormone. *J Clin Endocrinol Metab* 1999;**84**:449–452.

24. Arrigo T, De Luca F, Antoniazzi F et al. Reduction of baseline body mass index under gonadotropin-suppressive therapy in girls with idiopathic precocious puberty. *Eur J Endocrinol* 2004;**150**:533–537.

25. Palmert MR, Mansfield MJ, Crowley WF Jr, Crigler JF Jr, Crawford JD, Boepple PA. Is obesity an outcome of gonadotropin-releasing hormone agonist administration? Analysis of growth and body composition in 110 patients with central precocious puberty. *J Clin Endocrinol Metab* 1999;**84**:4480–4488.

26. Paterson WF, McNeill E, Young D, Donaldson MD. Auxological outcome and time to menarche following long-acting goserelin therapy in girls with central precocious or early puberty. *Clin Endocrinol (Oxf)* 2004;**61**:626–634.

27. Baumann DA, Landolt MA, Wetterwald R, Dubuis JM, Sizonenko PC, Werder EA. Psychological evaluation of young women after medical treatment for central precocious puberty. *Horm Res* 2001;**56**:45–50.

28. Carel JC, Roger M, Ispas S et al. Final height after long-term treatment with tritorelin slow release for central precocious puberty: importance of statural growth after interruption of treatment. French Study Group of Decapeptyl in Precocious Puberty. *J Clin Endocrinol Metab* 1999;**84**:1973–1978.

29. Couto-Silva AC, Adan L, Trivin C, Brauner R. Adult height in advanced puberty with or without gonadotropin hormone releasing hormone analog treatment. *J Pediatr Endocrinol Metab* 2002;**15**:297–305.

30. Mul D, Bertelloni S, Carel JC, Saggese G, Chaussain JL, Oostdijk W. Effect of gonadotropin-releasing hormone agonist treatment in boys with central precocious puberty: final height results. *Horm Res* 2002;**58**:1–7.

31. Tanaka T, Niimi H, Matsuo N et al. Results of long-term follow-up after treatment of central precocious puberty with

leuprorelin acetate: evaluation of effectiveness of treatment and recovery of gonadal function. The TAP-144-SR Japanese Study Group on Central Precocious Puberty. *J Clin Endocrinol Metab* 2005;**90**:1371–1376.

32. Klein KO, Barnes KM, Jones JV, Feuillan PP, Cutler GB Jr. Increased final height in precocious puberty after long-term treatment with LHRH agonists: the National Institutes of Health experience. *J Clin Endocrinol Metab* 2001;**86**:4711–4716.

33. van der Sluis IM, Boot AM, Krenning EP, Drop SL, de Munick Keizer-Schrama SM. Longitudinal follow-up of bone density and body composition in children with precocious or early puberty before, during and after cessation of GnRH agonist therapy. *J Clin Endocrinol Metab* 2002;**87**:506–512.

34. Antoniazzi F, Zamboni G, Bertoldo F et al. Bone mass at final height in precocious puberty after gonadotropin-releasing hormone agonist with and without calcium supplementation. *J Clin Endocrinol Metab* 2003;**88**:1096–1101.

CHAPTER 19

Dysmenorrhea

Albert Altchek

Mount Sinai School of Medicine and Hospital, New York, NY, USA

Incidence

Reports from reliable institutions give bewildering results of an incidence of dysmenorrhea anywhere from 15% to 85%. The reason for the discrepancy is the method of gathering data. If on enrollment in high school or college all female students are asked the question "Do you have painful periods?" as many as 85% will say yes. However, if there is no such questionnaire, only 15% of girls spontaneously come to the office complaining of painful periods. This suggests that although dysmenorrhea is common and occurs in most young women, apparently it is mild to moderate (tolerable) while 15% have severe dysmenorrhea that disturbs their lifestyle (Quick Take 19.1).

History and pathophysiology

Historically dysmenorrhea was divided into primary "idiopathic" dysmenorrhea, with negative examination and of unknown cause, and dysmenorrhea related to palpable pathology such as tumors or pelvic inflammatory disease. Primary idiopathic dysmenorrhea was thought to be psychologic in origin and psychiatrists had no difficulty in creating explanations such as "rejection of the female role" or "penis envy." Subsequently it was discovered that idiopathic dysmenorrhea is in fact excess prostaglandin PGF_2 formed from menstrual degenerating cell membrane phospholipids of the secretory endometrium of ovulating women. There is a normal physiologic response causing spasm of the uterine muscle wall and of the blood

---

Pediatric, Adolescent, & Young Adult Gynecology. Edited by A. Altchek and L. Deligdisch. © 2009 Blackwell Publishing, ISBN: 978-1-4051-5347-8.

> ### Quick Take 19.1
>
> **Incidence**
>
> - Varies from 15% to 85% depending on method of investigation
> - About 15% have severe dysmenorrhea which disturbs lifestyle

vessels of the endometrium and uterus to reduce bleeding at the time of menstruation when the blood vessels are open and bleeding briskly. We can postulate that there might be an over-reaction to physiologic amounts of prostaglandin so therefore prostaglandin measurements are not always helpful. Spasm of muscle and vessels may cause intense cramping pain (Quick Take 19.2).

Pain is subjective and therefore difficult to measure, making research difficult (Quick Take 19.3). To begin with, expectation has an important effect on pain. If the young girl thinks that when she has her menstrual period, it is "the curse," then obviously it will be painful. If, however, she thinks of the period as her "friend" then it will not seem to be so bad and indeed if the patient is sexually active, it is good news, meaning that she is not pregnant. It is not unusual in certain groups to hear the

> ### Quick Take 19.2
>
> **Primary "idiopathic" dysmenorrhea**
>
> - Results from excessive physiologic production of prostaglandins from degenerating ovulatory endometrium
> - Prostaglandin reduces blood loss by spasm of myometrium and arterioles but may cause severe cramping pain
> - Despite normal amounts of prostaglandin, the uterus may over-react with severe cramps

Quick Take 19.3

Pain is difficult to study

- It is subjective
- It varies with expectation
- It varies with the mood
- There is a normal spectrum of pain sensitivity

expression "I saw my friend last week." Another aspect of pain is the personal threshold. Most people when given a subcutaneous injection will describe a mild needlestick discomfort. A few will say they did not feel anything while some will say it was very painful. Mood also has a strong effect on pain perception. If the patient is happy because of good grades, recognition or achievement then she is on top of the world and nothing could disturb her, including dysmenorrhea. On the other hand, if she is unhappy and sad, it makes pain perception more severe.

Management

The first thing is to be certain of the diagnosis (Quick Take 19.4). Characteristically dysmenorrhea occurs about the time of the bleeding and presents as lower abdominal bilateral cramping sensations. However, with endometriosis sometimes the pain may also be present at times separate from the menstrual period. In addition, certain general medical conditions may cause lower abdominal crampy feelings which may be more severe at the time of menses, as with irritable bowel syndrome. Another factor in differential diagnosis is lactose intolerance.

Quick Take 19.4

Management – what is the diagnosis?

- Careful history and, if feasible, bimanual rectovaginal physical examination
- Consider renal and pelvic ultrasound (sonography)
- For suspicion of congenital anomalies or neoplasm, consider MRI in addition
- Consider intramuscular injections of GnRHa (LH-RH agonist) to cause temporary reversible menopause and cessation of pain as a diagnostic method

Quick Take 19.5

Management of dysmenorrhea

Education

- Ovulation and regular monthly periods may be uncomfortable as opposed to painless bleeding of irregular anovulatory dysfunctional uterine bleeding
- Encourage exercise, healthy lifestyle, good nutrition

NSAIDs relieve 75% of pain
Oral contraceptives relieve 85–90% of pain
Laparoscopy to confirm endometriosis with biopsy and if present, attempt to destroy or excise it. Consider LH-RH agonist-induced temporary menopause after laparoscopy (or as a therapeutic test without laparoscopy). However, there is no consensus regarding long-term LH-RH agonist therapy for the adolescent because of concern about possible reduction of normal bone mass increase

As a diagnostic routine it is reasonable to do a pelvic and renal ultrasound to rule out the possibility of a congenital anomaly. Ultrasound may also reveal an ovarian cyst or a rare tumor of the ovary or the uterus. Ultrasound does not identify superficial peritoneal endometriosis, although it can reveal a deep ovarian endometriosis (endometrioma) causing ovarian enlargement.

The pain of endometriosis is not related to the extent of the disease. Small superficial peritoneal implants may cause severe pain because of production of irritating chemicals, while large hard implants may be quiescent. Physical examination by one-finger vaginal, rectovaginal or rectal examination may be normal, or there may be cul-de-sac tenderness and thick or nodular sacrouterine ligaments. There may only be cul-de-sac tenderness with menstruation.

If the young girl is taught the physiology of menstruation she will understand that with ovulation, there is a certain amount of discomfort which may be accompanied by premenstrual molimina (weight gain, breast fullness, abdominal and breast bloating). There is nothing to fear about a little discomfort and in addition, there is the reassurance that she is ovulating. If she understands that exercise is appropriate, especially at that time, it makes things more normal and therefore less painful.

Mild discomfort is usually treated with acetaminophen or aspirin or more effectively with any of the nonsteroidal anti-inflammatory drugs (NSAIDs) (Quick Take 19.5). These are available over the counter. NSAIDs may cause gastric upset and are best taken with food or milk. In general, the patient is advised to keep the medication with her and take it the moment the pain starts since it works better earlier than after the pains have become severe. With regular menses and severe dysmenorrhea, the NSAID may be started even before the menstrual flow if the patient is not pregnant.

If the pain is severe or not relieved adequately with over-the-counter medications, it is reasonable to try oral contraceptives for several months. In about 90% there is a dramatic reduction in dysmenorrhea because in the anovulatory state there is little prostaglandin formation. If after several months of oral contraceptives there is still no significant relief, then it is appropriate to consider a diagnostic laparoscopy because 50% of such cases will be found to have early endometriosis. Previously, if oral contraceptives (OC) did not relieve the dysmenorrhea pain, it was assumed that the pain was psychologic. It had also been thought that endometriosis did not occur in the adolescent. A less frequent reason of OC failure to reduce pain is congenital anomalies, in particular the syndrome of uterus didelphys, unilateral lower vaginal aplasia and ipsilateral absent kidney where menstrual blood can exit from one uterus but is still blocked in the other "no eponym syndrome" uterus (Chapter 25).

At laparoscopy endometriosis of the adolescent looks different from the traditional endometriosis of mature adult women. With the latter one sees tobacco-stained areas and scarring. Adolescent endometriosis has pink small sprouts with no dark brown areas and no scarring. Diagnosis may be difficult by simple observation and it is desirable to do a biopsy of the cul-de-sac. Without laparoscopy, the diagnosis of endometriosis is presumptive (Chapters 20, 26).

There have been a few case reports of an apparent cure in adolescents with superficial peritoneal endometriosis if discovered early by laparoscopy, treated surgically and/or a predisposing anomaly was corrected. It will reduce symptoms and the tendency for adhesions, but probably not cure the endometriosis. I have noticed that immediate recurrence of pain may be due to adenomyosis (endometriosis in the wall of the uterus) which may be associated with obstructive anomalies.

After discovery by laparoscopy with an attempt to destroy the endometriosis, some follow it with several months (up to six) of monthly intramuscular injec-

tions of gonadotropin-releasing hormone agonist (GnRHa), also known as LH-RH agonist, to cause a reversible menopause. This will scar down residual endometriosis but does not cure it.

Some feel that laparoscopy (or laparotomy) may be avoided by immediate use of LH-RH agonist. If the pain is significantly reduced then it is assumed that endometriosis is probably present.

There is concern about the use of GnRHa for treating adolescents at a time when their bones are accumulating calcium and some advise against its use under 18 years of age. When it is used at any age, dietary supplementation with calcium and vitamin D has been recommended as well as daily oral norethindrone acetate 5 mg "add-back" therapy to reduce bone loss.

There is a paucity of controlled series of adolescent endometriosis. Management of each patient has to be individualized. In adults there is a option of using GnRHa to make a presumptive diagnosis of endometriosis without laparoscopy.

The anomaly of most concern, which is difficult to discover early, is "no eponym". There is a double uterus (didelphys), double cervix, and a double vagina, but the distal vagina on one side does not develop so the menstrual blood accumulates and causes progressive pain with menses despite the fact that there is external bleeding. There is an ipsilateral absent kidney. This anomaly is readily overlooked because there is only one vaginal opening. The easiest method of diagnosis is pelvic ultrasound followed by MRI. Rectal examination will also suggest the diagnosis by palpating a paravaginal mass on the obstructed side. Attempts to cure it by laparotomy do not work. The appropriate corrective surgery is a vaginal approach to open the obstructed vagina, thereby making one vagina and relieving obstruction (Chapter 25).

Obstruction with a single uterus may be due to distal vaginal agenesis, complete transverse septum of the middle vagina or an imperforate hymen. These patients have progressive pain at the time when the menses should be starting but there is no external bleeding (Chapters 20, 21, 24, 25).

Very rarely, there may be a large endometrial polyp or an endocervical fibroid which will cause pain. Infrequently, even without sexual exposure, there may be salpingitis or oophoritis as another cause of pain. In undeveloped areas there may be tuberculosis pelvic inflammatory disease.

CHAPTER 20

Pelvic Pain, Endometriosis, and the Role of the Gynecologist

Farr R. Nezhat[1], Alireza A Shamshirsaz[2], Gazi Yildirim[3], Ceana Nezhat[4], & Camran Nezhat[5]

[1] St Luke's-Roosevelt Hospital Center, University Hospital of Columbia University, New York, NY, USA
[2] University of Iowa Hospital and Clinics, Iowa City, IO, USA
[3] Department of Obstetrics and Gynecology, Yeditepe University Medical Faculty, Istanbul, Turkey
[4] Atlanta Center for Special Minimally Invasive Surgery and Reproductive Medicine, Atlanta, GA, USA
[5] Center for Special Minimally Invasive Surgery, Stanford University Medical Center, Palo Alto, CA, USA

Introduction

Chronic pelvic pain (CPP) is a frequent complaint in adolescent females. It is a complex disorder with multiple causes. The assessment must attempt to differentiate between gynecologic and nongynecologic source of pain. For the young patient with CPP, a multidisciplinary approach may be essential to facilitate diagnosis and management. Endometriosis frequently results in chronic pelvic pain. Historically thought of as a disease that affects adult women, endometriosis is increasingly diagnosed in the adolescent population. Laparoscopy is extremely useful in diagnosis and treatment of endometriosis. The purpose of this chapter is to highlight the chronic pelvic pain, especially endometriosis, in adolescents. Early diagnosis and treatment of endometriosis during adolescence may decrease disease progression and prevent subsequent chronic pelvic pain, adhesive disease, and infertility.

Chronic pelvic pain

Chronic pelvic pain (CPP) is defined, according to the American College of Obstetricians and Gynecologists, as

Pediatric, Adolescent, & Young Adult Gynecology. Edited by A. Altchek and L. Deligdisch. © 2009 Blackwell Publishing, ISBN: 978-1-4051-5347-8.

a noncyclic pain of three months' duration or cyclic pain of six months' duration, either of which interfere with normal activities [1]. Chronic pelvic pain is a common and serious health issue for women and is estimated to have a prevalence of 3.8% in women aged 15–73 [2]. A survey of 70,000 adolescents showed that almost 60% experienced dysmenorrhea and 50% reported school absences because of severe pelvic pain [3].

An accurate assessment of psychosocial issues and impact of the pain on the life of adolescents is essential. Chronic pain can be a significant source of frustration for the patient and her parents, and it is not unusual for them to search for multiple opinions from the medical community. Many of these teenagers will have missed days of school. A definite diagnosis is extremely important because parents and patients are often concerned that cancer or some other life-threatening condition is present. The patient's complaints should be assessed thoroughly so that she feels that her symptoms are taken seriously by the healthcare provider.

Initial evaluation requires a detailed history and physical examination. Chronic pelvic pain may have many different origins, including gastrointestinal, genitourinary, gynecologic, psychologic and musculoskeletal etiologies (Box 20.1).

The nature of the pain must be determined, including its severity, duration, relationship to the menstrual cycle (cyclic or noncyclic), aggravation and relieving factors, and location. The patient can be asked to grade the pain

Box 20.1 Differential diagnosis of chronic pelvic pain

Gastrointestinal
Inflammatory bowel disease
Chronic appendicitis
Obstruction
Constipation
Irritable bowel syndrome
Musculoskeletal
Intervertebral disk herniation
Myofascial pain
Strains/sprains
Fibromyositis
Inguinal hernia
Scoliosis
Gynecologic
Chronic pelvic inflammatory disease
Endometriosis
Adhesions
Leiomyomata
Outflow tract obstruction
Dysmenorrhea
Genitourinary
Interstitial nephritis
Obstruction
Infection
Other
Abuse
Psychosocial stress
Psychiatric disorders
Porphyria
Substance abuse
Heavy metal poisoning

on a scale of 1–10. This can be helpful in deciding on the long-term management of chronic pain.

The history should also include a menstrual history, general health history and family history (endometriosis, inflammatory bowel disease, fibromyalgia, depression, lupus, cancer, interstitial cystitis). A complete history must include questions relating to past or present sexual abuse, as sexual abuse and physical abuse have been noted to be associated with CPP [4].

A complete physical examination, including abdominal palpation, musculoskeletal evaluation, assessment for hernias, and pelvic examination, should be performed. It is helpful to ask the patient during the examination to point with one finger to the location of the pain and then to ask her what factors relieve or exacerbate the pain. For example, those with endometriosis may have a constellation

of symptoms that include cyclic severe dysmenorrhea, dyspareunia, and rectal pressure. The pelvic examination includes an inspection of the external genitalia, hymenal opening, and urethra. If the patient is sexually active, a bimanual examination is performed to assess for uterine size, cervical motion tenderness, adnexal masses or tenderness, and uterosacral nodularity. Evaluation of the cul-de-sac on bimanual examination is an integral part of the assessment, as is performing a careful rectovaginal assessment to rule out any significant pelvic abnormality. Speculum examination is performed to obtain specimens for gonorrhea and chlamydia and a Papanicolaou smear is performed if necessary.

Laboratory tests that should be considered in the evaluation of CPP are complete blood cell count with differential, urinalysis, urine culture and sensitivity, and erythrocyte sedimentation rate.

Radiologic tests may be required during the evaluation. A plain film of the abdomen can be helpful if constipation is suspected. Pelvic ultrasound may be helpful for patients who have a compromised pelvic examination because of body habitus or lack of co-operation, or in patients with a suspected uterine or adnexal abnormality.

Some adolescents with CPP require laparoscopy for further evaluation and treatment. This allows the physician to make or confirm a specific diagnosis, obtain samples for biopsy, lyze adhesions, and perform operative therapeutic procedures [5,6]. Before the procedures, the gynecologist should discuss with the patient and her family the possibilities and limitations of operative surgery during laparoscopy. Diagnostic laparoscopy is usually done under general anesthesia with endotracheal intubation as an outpatient surgical procedure. Patients return home the day of the procedure, rarely missing more than one week of school.

Most adolescents undergoing diagnostic laparoscopy for CCP have pathologic findings at the time of surgery, with endometriosis being the most common finding [5–10]. Other potential findings at the time of laparoscopy include chronic pelvic inflammatory disease (PID), chronic appendicitis, tubo-ovarian abscesses, pelvic adhesive disease, hemoperitoneum, ovarian cysts, pelvic tuberculosis, serositis, and paratubal cysts. The goal of diagnostic laparoscopy is not only to identify pathology, but also to treat it during surgery if necessary. Such surgical interventions may include laser ablation or electrocoagulation of endometriosis, lysis of adhesions, ovarian cystectomy or appendectomy; most procedures are done laparoscopically. Negative findings at laparoscopy can be equally valuable in reassuring the patient and her family and in helping the patient to accept the fact that the pain is likely to respond to medical and psychologic therapy [5,6,11]. Most patients have resolution of pelvic pain after a negative laparoscopy [7].

Role of laparoscopy in chronic pelvic pain

Laparoscopy is a safe procedure in experienced hands [12,13]. We are of the opinion that adolescents with CPP should be referred to experienced laparoscopists able to recognize congenital anomalies, as well as subtle, atypical, and more common appearances of endometriosis. Peritoneal endometriosis can be diagnosed only by direct visualization and confirmed by biopsy. Laufer developed a technique for precise identification of clear vesicles using the three-dimensional effect of lactated Ringer solution introduced into the pelvis. By submerging the laparoscope, clear endometriosis vesicles are readily identified for biopsy, resection or laser vaporization [14]. The advice of Goldstein et al, from nearly a quarter of a century ago, remains valid today: "Laparoscopy is essential for an accurate diagnosis of this condition and provides the means of staging the disease, thus permitting a more rational approach to treatment" [7].

In a series reported by Goldstein et al in which three-fourths of the adolescents with CCP who underwent laparoscopy at Children's Hospital Boston between 1974 and 1983 had intrapelvic pathologic conditions [6], endometriosis was diagnosed most frequently (45%). As expected, the finding of endometriosis increased from 12% in the 11–13 year group to 54% in the 20–21 year group. The next most common finding was postoperative adhesions (13%), usually associated with a history of appendectomy or ovarian cystectomy. Other findings included serositis (5%), ovarian cyst (5%), and uterine malformation (2%). No apparent gynecologic cause of the chronic pain was found in one-fourth of the patients; of those with negative findings, 74% felt that their symptoms were improved at follow-up. Reese et al reported that in 67 adolescent girls who had not responded to analgesia or oral contraceptive for pelvic pain, endometriosis was diagnosed in 73% with laparoscopy/laparotomy [8]. Adhesions were noted in 50.7%, but always in conjunction with other surgical findings. In a more recent

study by Laufer et al, adolescent women aged 13–21 were evaluated for pelvic pain that lasted longer than three months and had not responded to NSAIDs and combined hormone therapy (CHT) [5]; approximately 70% had endometriosis [5].

An association between CPP and bowel to pelvic sidewall adhesions has been debated. The cause of adhesions is unknown, but it is believed to be the result of infection, previous surgery or endometriosis. Nezhat et al showed that adhesiolysis in women with chronic pain causes complete pain relief in approximately half [15].

Advanced operative laparoscopy is a major intra-abdominal procedure. Careful preoperative evaluation optimizes the operative outcome and decreases the incidence of injuries and complications. Most laparoscopic operations are performed under general anesthesia with endotracheal intubation. A Foley catheter is placed in the bladder, as it is unclear how long the surgical procedure will take. An orogastric tube is helpful in emptying the stomach. After the induction of endotracheal anesthesia, the patient's legs are placed in padded Allen stirrups to provide good support and proper position. Although some physicians will perform laparoscopy in the horizontal supine position, our preference is to place the patient in lithotomy stirrups, because of the need for hysteroscopy, cystoscopy or sigmoidoscopy during operation. Padding near the peroneal nerve is essential. To avoid nerve injury, no leg joint is extended more than 60°. The buttocks must protrude a few centimeters from the edge of the table. The patient's arms are placed at the side, padded with foam troughs, and secured by a sheet. This allows the surgeon and assistants to stand unencumbered next to the patient. The anesthesiologist should have easy access to the patient's arm.

Once the patient is positioned, sterile prep and drip is performed in the usual manner. We use either direct trocar insertion or the Veress needle to achieve pneumoperitoneum. The optimal location for the Veress needle and primary trocar is the umbilicus; 12–14 mmHg intra-abdominal gas pressure is usually adequate for adolescent patients. After adequate pressure is achieved, two or three ancillary trocars are placed as described in Chapter 19 [12,13,15].

In thin adolescent patients, there are some risks during abdominal entry. The distance between the anterior abdominal wall and the aorta is often very small. The fascia is thin and offers little resistance. To avoid risk, the Veress needle must be grasped close to its tip, the abdominal wall must be completely elevated and attention must be paid during entry. In thin patients, it is safer to overdistend the abdomen with CO_2 before trocar insertion. Successful insertion depends on an adequate skin incision, trocars in good working condition, proper orientation of trocar, sheath, and surgeon's hand, and control over the instrument's force and depth of insertion.

The initial phase of laparoscopy in adolescents does not differ from that in adults. This is done to assess the extent of disease, document it with photographs or video recording, and identify anatomic landmarks. The characteristics of the bladder, ureters, colon, rectum, uterosacral ligaments, and major blood vessels are noted. The appendix must be inspected for endometriosis. The upper abdomen, including the abdominal walls, liver, gallbladder and diaphragm, is examined for any abnormality. The omentum and intestines are examined to confirm that they were not injured during insertion of the Veress needle and trocar. Surgical procedures and detailed techniques for the treatment of endometriosis will be discussed below.

Endometriosis

In the past, endometriosis (presence of endometrial glands and stroma outside the normal intrauterine endometrial cavity) was not considered a common disorder in teenagers. The etiology of endometriosis has not been definitively determined, but many theories have been proposed.

• Sampson's theory of retrograde menstruation, which proposes that retrograde transport of viable fragments of endometrium through the fallopian tubes at the time of menstruation leads to seeding of the peritoneal cavity with endometrial implants [16].

• Meyer's theory of embryonically totipotent cells that undergo metaplastic transformation into functioning endometrium [17].

• Halban's theory of metastases of endometrial cells through vascular or lymphatic spread [18].

• The theory of deficient cell-mediated immunity with impaired clearing of endometriotic cells from aberrant locations [19].

All these theories explain some aspects of endometriosis, especially when relating to adolescents. Endometriosis is seen predominantly in women of reproductive age but has been described in a wide range of ages from as young as 8.5 years to as old as 76 [20]. Endometriosis affects women from all ethnic and social groups [21]. It has been difficult to establish accurate prevalence rates of endometriosis in adult and adolescent women. Documented rates in adolescent patients undergoing laparoscopy for CPP range from 19% to 75% [5–10,22]. There may be a genetic predisposition to or etiology of endometriosis. Ranney et al first reported the familial occurrence of endometriosis [23]. Simpson and associates reported a 6.9% rate of endometriosis among first-degree relatives of women with the disease, compared with only 1% of control relatives [24]. The most probable mode of inheritance is polygenic and multifactorial. The diagnosis of endometriosis should be strongly suspected in symptomatic adolescents with a family history of endometriosis. It is common for adult women who have endometriosis to bring in their adolescent daughters for evaluation and early diagnosis. Data from the endometriosis study associated indicates that 66% of adult women reported the onset of pelvic pain symptoms before age 20 years. There are, on average, 9.28 years from the onset of symptoms to the diagnosis [21].

Any anomaly that causes obstruction of the genital outflow tract can be associated with the formation of endometriosis, including uterine anomalies, cervical agenesis or stenosis, vaginal septum and imperforate hymen [25]. Adolescents with congenital obstruction, Müllerian malformation and functioning endometrium often have severe endometriosis, even in early adolescence. Unlike endometriosis that is not associated with outflow obstruction, endometriosis in patients with reproductive tract anomalies usually resolves after a patent outflow tract is established [25].

Endometriosis also has been identified in premenarcheal girls who have started puberty and have some breast development [20,26,27]. Yamamoto and co-workers reported a case of endometriosis within one month after menarche [28]. It is not even clear that menarche is required for endometriosis as Whitehouse reported bladder endometriosis in a 22-year-old patient with primary amenorrhea [29]. Reese and colleagues more recently reported on two premenarcheal girls, aged 12 and 13, with endometriosis [8].

Although older teens are more likely to seek gynecologic care than younger adolescents, clinicians must also realize that the disease exists in the preteens and younger adolescents. Endometriosis is believed to be a progressive disease because the prevalence and severity of the stage of the disease significantly increase with age [30,31]. With early diagnosis and treatment, it is hoped that disease progression and infertility can be limited, but this remains to be proved with prospective research.

Clinical presentation of endometriosis

Adolescents' symptoms often differ from those of adults. In adult women endometriosis is suspected in a patient presenting with chronic pelvic pain, dysmenorrhea, dyspareunia, pelvic mass or infertility. The most common symptom noted in adolescents in published reviews is acquired, followed by progressive dysmenorrhea, which is encountered in 64–94% of patients [5,8]. In adults the pain of endometriosis is most often cyclic. In the adolescent endometriosis population, the presenting pelvic pain is often both acyclic and cyclic (62.6%). The presentation of acyclic pain alone is 28.1% and cyclic pain alone is 9.4% [5]. In adolescents with chronic pain not responding to NSAIDs, approximately 90% have endometriosis with acyclic pain [5]. Some patients experience an increase in symptoms at midcycle and again with menses. One significant difference is that adolescents primarily seek medical attention because of pain rather than concern about infertility, which is rarely an issue in teens. Other common symptoms included dyspareunia (14–25%), gastrointestinal complaints (2–46%), urinary symptoms (12.5%), irregular menses (9.4%), and vaginal discharge (6.3%) [5].

Diagnosis of endometriosis

Physical examination findings are also different from those of adults. Due to adhesions, the uterus may be fixed and retroflexed in adults, and ovaries are often tender and enlarged by endometriosis. Nodularity of the cul-de-sac and uterosacral ligaments is another classic finding. In contrast, these findings are uncommon in adolescents, whose pelvic examination findings are often normal, with only mild to moderate tenderness. The adnexa are usually without masses.

Bimanual examination may not be necessary to evaluate pelvic pain, especially in adolescents who are virgins. If a bimanual examination cannot be performed or is declined, a rectoabdominal examination in the dorsal lithotomy position may be helpful. To determine if a pelvic mass is present, a cotton-tipped swab can be inserted into the vagina to evaluate for the presence of a transverse vaginal septum, vaginal agenesis or agenesis of the lower vagina.

A common finding on pelvic exam in the setting of endometriosis is cul-de-sac tenderness [32]. Chatman and Ward reported cul-de-sac tenderness in 78% and cul-de-sac nodularity in 36% of patients [33].

An ultrasound should be utilized to exclude the possible existence of a pelvic mass or structural anomaly, but is not specific for diagnosing endometriosis. Computed tomography (CT) scan with contrast may help in cases of acute pain, but is otherwise not helpful. Magnetic resonance imaging (MRI) is an excellent but expensive modality for evaluation of genital anomalies. CA-125, although very sensitive, is not specific and thus is not helpful in the diagnosis of adolescent endometriosis but may be used to follow the progress of disease. We prefer to rely on reporting of symptoms to follow endometriosis and do not use CA-125 in clinical management.

When the evaluation of pain suggests a chronic gynecologic source, a trial of NSAIDs is recommended. A low-dose oral contraceptive may also improve symptoms of dysmenorrhea by suppressing hormonal stimulation associated with ovulation and by decreasing menstrual flow.

If an adolescent younger than 18 years has persistent pain while taking combination hormone therapy and NSAIDs, a laparoscopic evaluation should be offered [34]. Empiric depot leuprolide has been utilized in adult women with chronic pelvic pain and clinically suspected endometriosis [35,36]. In women older than 18 years, if the pain subsides with the use of a GnRH agonist, a diagnosis of endometriosis can be made. An empiric trial of GnRH agonist is not routinely offered to patients younger than 18 years because the effects of these medications on the bone formation and long-term bone density have not been adequately studied [34–37].

Additionally, some parents are not interested in utilizing empiric therapy due to concerns about using medication with adverse side effects without a definitive diagnosis. We do not routinely recommend empiric GnRH agonist therapy for treatment of presumed endometriosis for young women under age 18. An algorithm for therapy is provided in Figure 20.1.

The definitive diagnosis of endometriosis must be established by laparoscopy, with or without pathologic identification of biopsy specimens. If gynecologists are going

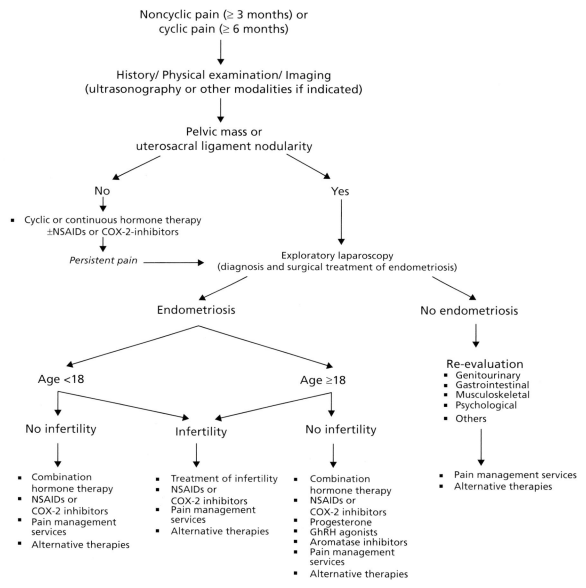

Noncyclic pain (≥ 3 months) or
cyclic pain (≥ 6 months)

History/ Physical examination/ Imaging
(ultrasonography or other modalities if indicated)

Pelvic mass or
uterosacral ligament nodularity

No

Yes

- Cyclic or continuous hormone therapy
  ±NSAIDs or COX-2-inhibitors

Persistent pain

Exploratory laparoscopy
(diagnosis and surgical treatment of endometriosis)

Endometriosis

No endometriosis

Age <18

Age ≥18

Re-evaluation
- Genitourinary
- Gastrointestinal
- Musculoskeletal
- Psychological
- Others

No infertility

Infertility

No infertility

- Combination
  hormone therapy
- NSAIDs or
  COX-2 inhibitors
- Pain management
  services
- Alternative therapies

- Treatment of infertility
- NSAIDs or
  COX-2 inhibitors
- Pain management
  services
- Alternative therapies

- Combination
  hormone therapy
- NSAIDs or
  COX-2 inhibitors
- Progesterone
- GhRH agonists
- Aromatase inhibitors
- Pain management
  services
- Alternative therapies

- Pain management services
- Alternative therapies

Figure 20.1 Evaluation and treatment of adolescent chronic pelvic pain and endometriosis.

to perform the surgical procedure, they must feel comfortable operating on patients in this age range. A diagnostic laparoscopy with subsequent referral to a "specialist" for definitive surgery places the patient at undue risk from two anesthesias.

Endometriosis is staged using the revised criteria of the American Society of Reproductive Medicine

(ASRM) point-based classification system [38]. Classic endometriosis implants have been described as having a blue/brown/gray "powder burn" appearance (Fig. 20.2). Adolescents are more likely to have early or atypical lesions than the classic form (Fig. 20.3). Davis et al found that red flame lesions (Fig. 20.4) are more common in adolescents with endometriosis (84%) than in adult patients

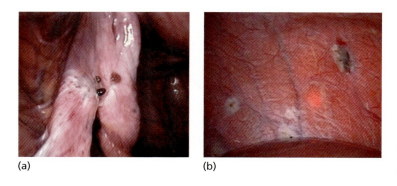

(a)   (b)

Figure 20.2 Different types of endometriotic lesions on the peritoneal surface of (a) the left infundibulopelvic ligament and fallopian tube, (b) the diaphragm.

but white and clear vesicular lesions are also common, as are peritoneal pockets. Peritoneal Allen–Masters windows (Fig. 20.5) are also common in adolescents and should be recognized by the operative gynecologist [39]. Powder

burn lesions are less common in adolescents, consistent with the presumption that these lesions represent older and more advanced implants. Theses findings are supported by Redwine [40] who found that patients with

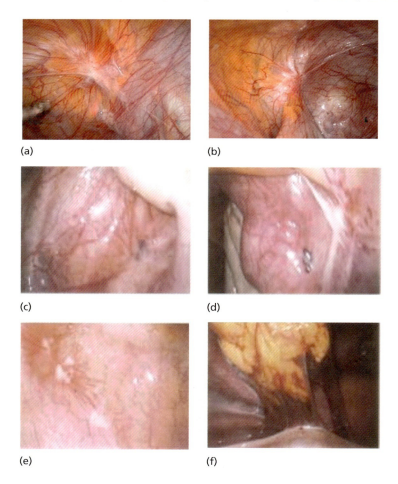

(a)   (b)

(c)   (d)

(e)   (f)

Figure 20.3 A view of typical (c,d) and atypical (a,b,e,f) endometriotic lesions.

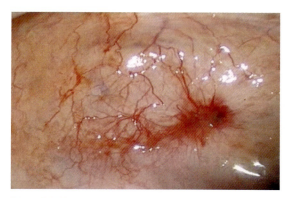

Figure 20.4 Endometriotic red flame lesions.

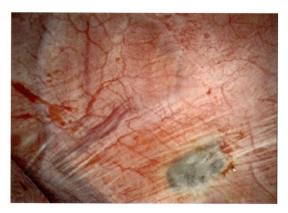

Figure 20.6 A black lesion of the infiltrative endometriosis on the surface of the diaphragm.

atypical endometriosis lesions are, on average, 10 years younger than those who have black lesions (Fig. 20.6) and by Martin et al, who reported evolution of infiltrative lesions from subtle lesions in adolescence to classic lesions 10 years or more later (Fig. 20.7) [41].

It has been suggested that clear and red lesions are the more painful lesions of endometriosis [42]. Clear and vesicular lesions (Fig. 20.8) may be difficult to identify laparoscopically in part because light reflects from the endoscope. Laufer described a technique that assists in the identification of this form of the disease. Filling the pelvis with irrigation fluid and submerging the laparoscope into the fluid-filled pelvis eliminates light reflection, and clear vesicles can be appreciated in three dimensions [14].

If no evidence of endometriosis is identified, a cul-de-sac biopsy to rule out microscopic disease should be performed as endometriosis may be identified without visualization with laparoscopy [32]. Other reports support our finding showing the existence of a significant rate of microscopic endometriosis in adolescents and adults with a visually normal pelvis [5,43].

Staging of endometriosis should follow the revised ASRM classification of endometriosis. Most adolescents have stage I (77–92%) or stage II (8–22%) disease [5,8,44]. The extent of endometriotic implants is not a reliable indicator of the degree of pain or the prognosis with treatment [45]. The severity of dysmenorrhea does not relate to the number of endometrial implants. Only 6.1% and 2% of Reese et al's subjects had stage III and stage IV disease, respectively. None of these patients were younger than 16 at the time of diagnosis, and none of them had an obstructive Müllerian anomaly [8]. Subjects with obstruction of Müllerian anomalies are more likely to present with stage III or IV disease; however, with relief of the obstruction the lesions regress spontaneously [25]. Emmert et al described in one case series of 37 adolescents with endometriosis the types and location of endometriotic implants. All had stage I or II disease, 67% of lesions being pinhead size, 27% rice sized, and 2.7% pea sized. The most common site of lesions was the pouch of Douglas

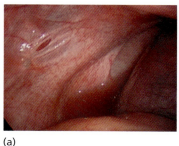

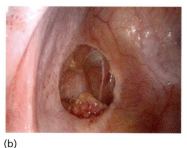

Figure 20.5 Peritoneal Allen–Masters window (a) before, and (b) after excision.

(a)

(b)

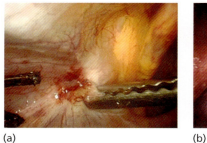

(a)

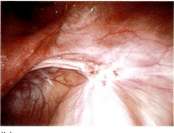

(b)

Figure 20.7 A view of infiltrative endometriotic lesions.

(64.8%) and uterosacral ligaments (37.8%) [44]. However, it is important to remember that endometriosis is a progressive disease (Fig. 20.9).

Treatment of endometriosis

Accurate and early diagnosis is important for the relief of symptoms and for the suppression of possible natural disease progression, which may affect reproductive potential. A physician treating an adolescent with endometriosis should adopt a multidimensional approach and consider

the use of the following components: hormonal manipulation, pain medications, mental health support, complementary and alternative therapies, education, and surgery. The optimal therapy for adolescents and women with

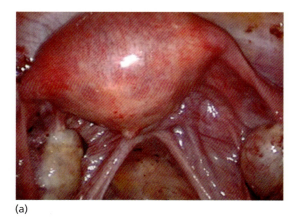

(a)

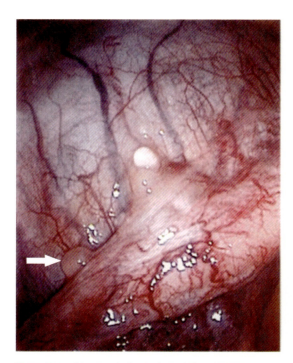

Figure 20.8 White vesicular lesions (arrow) of endometriosis.

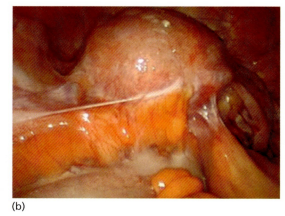

(b)

Figure 20.9 (a) Early and (b) late presentation of pelvic endometriosis.

endometriosis is still being debated. Patients and their parents need to understand the pros and cons of each surgical and medical option and the fact that recurrence of endometriosis is common.

Medical treatment options

Nonsteroidal anti-inflammatory drugs

NSAIDs are an appropriate empiric treatment of dysmenorrhea. Clearly, not all patients with endometriosis find relief from symptoms with NSAIDs alone [46]. NSAIDs may be used in conjunction with hormonal menstrual suppressive therapy to provide sufficient relief.

Hormonal suppression

Because of its low side effect profile and its ability to be taken indefinitely as oral contraceptive pills (OCPs), combination estrogen and progesterone therapy is typically the first line of therapy in adolescents. Taken cyclically, OCPs decrease the endometrial lining and thus decrease the amount of tissue producing prostaglandins, and also suppress ovulation and subsequent luteal-phase symptoms of endometriosis. Continuous combination hormone therapy (OCPs, contraceptive patch or vaginal ring) for menstrual suppression can be used to create a "pseudo-pregnancy." This method has been promoted routinely for adolescents who have endometriosis. Although this method may provide effective relief, the Cochrane Database Review 2003 provided data suggesting that further studies are needed to prove long-term benefit [47]. Breakthrough bleeding is a frequent side effect when active pills are taken continuously. Miller et al compared a 28-day regimen with continuous combination oral contraception and found no increase in spotting days after nine months' therapy, with fewer total bleeding days in the group taking continuous combination oral contraception [48]. Thus, continuous use of combination hormone therapy is believed to be both safe and effective for adolescents with endometriosis-related pain and thus is the first-line hormone therapy for adolescents younger than 16 years.

Because estrogen stimulates endometrial implants and androgens result in atrophy, progestin-dominant pills should be used. In spite of clinical improvement, there is no evidence for regression of endometrial implants with use of OCPs [49]. Progestin-only protocols have been used for the treatment of adult endometriosis with mixed results. Vercellini et al showed that depot medroxyprogesterone acetate (DMPA) was more effective at relieving endometriosis symptoms than were OCPs combined with danazol [50]. Progestin-only regimens consisting of medroxyprogesterone acetate 30–50 mg intramuscularly every 4–12 weeks have been shown to be effective in the treatment of endometriosis symptoms [51]. As with OCP, DMPA provides effective contraception and can be used over the long term, making it a very attractive option for an adolescent with endometriosis. Although mood lability is often cited as a side effect of DMPA, a recent study comparing adolescent DMPA users with control individuals found that adolescents did not show depressive symptoms when using DMPA as a contraceptive agent over a period of 12 months [52]. There was no significant change in negative or positive effect when the adolescents were assessed using a validated questionnaire. However, in a dataset of 3751 women who have endometriosis, treatment with DMPA was the least well tolerated and was the least effective in treating pain compared with combination OCPs, GnRH agonist, and pain medication [53].

One concern, particularly in the adolescent population, is that bone mineral density (BMD) is reportedly lower in patients using DMPA. Cromer et al [54] reported results of a prospective trial comparing the BMD of adolescents using DMPA, Norplant or OCPs. Dual-energy x-ray absorptiometry was performed at baseline, 12 months and 24 months, and findings were compared with those in control individuals. In those using DMPA, BMD had decreased by 1.5% at one year and by 3.1% at two years, whereas in the control group BMD had increased by 2.9% and 9.5% at one and two years, respectively. Scholes et al [55] also observed an adverse relationship between DMPA and BMD in a cross-sectional study, the most significant decrease in BMD being noted in the youngest age groups (18–21 years). The US Food and Drug Administration (FDA) has warned against the long-term use of DMPA because of adverse affects on bone density [56]. This treatment modality is usually reserved for individuals who cannot tolerate continuous combined hormonal therapy or who have a contraindication for their use.

Danazol

Danazol is a derivative of 17α-ethinyltestosterone that induces endometrial atrophy by creating a low-estrogen, high-androgen environment. The standard dosage is 800 mg per day in divided doses for six months followed by continuous OCP use for maintenance suppression of the hypothalamic-pituitary-ovarian axis, which appears to be very effective in the treatment of pelvic pain associated with endometriosis. Dmowski et al reported relief of pain from endometriosis treated with danazol in 85–90% of patients [57]. In the same study, pain returned to the majority of treated patients within one year after therapy discontinuation. We do not prescribe it for adolescents because of its unacceptable side effects, which include weight gain, edema, irregular menses, acne, oily skin, hirsutism, and voice change. Some side effects, such as hirsutism and voice deepening, are not always reversible with discontinuation.

Gonadrotropin-relasing hormone agonist (GnRHa)

GnRHa has been shown to be effective in managing the symptoms and extent of endometriosis. GnRHa creates a "pseudo-menopause" state by downregulating gonadotropin release from the pituitary glands and establishing a hypoestrogenic environment [58]. This acyclic, low-estrogen environment suppresses growth and bleeding in endometriotic implants as well as preventing additional seeding of the pelvis from retrograde menstruation.

GnRHas are available in many formulations: nasal spray, subcutaneous injection, and intramuscular injection. In the adolescent population, compliance is a major issue, so the decision whether to use a twice-daily nasal spray or an intramuscular injection every three months is important. The nasal spray, if selected, is given as one puff twice daily in alternating nostrils. If depot leuprolide is used a dosage of 3.75 mg every four weeks will induce amenorrhea and hypoestrogenism in over 90% of women. Depot leuprolide is also available in an 11.25 mg dosage given every three months. If irregular bleeding occurs and the induction of amenorrhea is not achieved with this dosage, then estradiol levels should be checked and, if not suppressed, the dosage can be increased to 7.5 mg every four weeks or 22.5 mg every three months [59]. It is important to make sure that patients understand that when taking a GnRHa, there will be a stimulatory phase prior to the downregulation. Thus patients will experience a final withdrawal bleed 21–28 days after the initiation of the GnRHa. They will most likely experience a deterioration of symptoms with the initial withdrawal bleed prior to the suppression of pain and bleeding. Dlugi et al showed that monthly injection of 3.75 mg of depot leuprolide for six months resulted in significant reduction

in endometriosis-associated pain [60]. Henzel et al established on second-look laparoscopy that nafarelin was as effective as danazol in reducing pain and endometriosis scores [61].

The side effects of GnRHa therapy include hypoestrogenic symptoms such as hot flashes, vaginal dryness, and decreased libido [58,61].

Because of the long-term hypoestrogenic effects associated with decrease in bone density, the FDA has not approved prescription for courses of therapy lasting longer than six consecutive months [62,63]. This is a major issue for an adolescent who is accruing peak bone mineral density. Therefore, it has been suggested that this therapy should not be offered as a first-line treatment for adolescents younger than 16 years [26]. At six months, GnRHa induces a 5% loss in trabecular bone mineral density and a 2% loss in femoral neck bone mineral density in adult women. Matkovic et al reported that the majority of bone mass growth is achieved by age 20 and after the age of 18 no significant differences in bone mass or bone mineral density were noted at most skeletal sites [64]. This emphasizes that a drug-induced hypoestrogenic state could significantly affect peak bone mineralization that occurs during adolescence, particularly in females younger than 16 years. To minimize bone loss and other hypoestrogenic side effects, "add-back" therapy has been advocated: norethindrone acetate (5 mg per day) conjugated estrogen/medroxyprogesterone acetate (0.625/2.5 mg per day) [65,66]. Barbier has proposed an "estrogen threshold hypothesis" in the treatment of women with endometriosis [65] which suggests that there is an estrogen threshold for the reduction of endometriosis that is lower than the degree of hypoestrogenism resulting in bone resorption.

Add-back therapy has been shown not to influence the primary effect, resulting in less bone loss 12 months after cessation of therapy in adult women. There is some evidence in adults to suggest that immediate add-back therapy may result in even less bone loss [67]. Studies are needed to determined if long-term GnRHa with add-back therapy is safe for adolescents [68]. There is no reason to avoid the utilization of add-back therapy, as studies have not shown increased return of pain with the initiation of add-back therapy [66].

Lifestyle modifications, such as adequate physical exercise and calcium and vitamin D intake, also are essential to maintaining proper bone health when taking GnRHa.

Aromatase inhibitors (AIs)

Endometriosis is an estrogen-dependent disorder. Thus standard medical treatments aim either at inducing hypoestrogenism or at antagonizing estrogen action. Aromatase (estrogen synthetase) is the key enzyme in the synthesis of estrogens mediating the conversion of androstenedione and testosterone to estrone and estradiol (E_2). The aromatase enzyme has been demonstrated locally in endometriotic implants, and a molecular etiology of endometriosis has been proposed [69]. Aromatase is an excellent target for inhibition of the E_2 synthesis as it is the last step in steroid biosynthesis.

In 1996, the third generations of AIs, anastrozole (Arimidex; AstraZeneca, Wilmington, DE), letrozole (Femara; Novartis, East Hanover, NJ), and exemestane (Aromasin; Pfizer, New London, CT), were approved by the US Food and Drug Administration to treat advanced breast carcinoma in postmenopausal women [70].

Aromatase inhibitors inhibit estrogen production in at least four critical body sites: brain, ovary, endometriosis, and periphery (e.g. adipose tissue and skin). The rationale was that continued local estrogen production in endometriotic implants during other medical treatments (e.g. GnRHa) was, in part, responsible for resistance to these treatments. Anastrozole and letrozole have been used successfully to treat endometriosis. The compensatory response to E_2 depletion in the hypothalamus results in higher serum follicle-stimulating hormone (FSH) secretion and ovarian stimulation. Therefore, AIs increase follicular recruitment and may lead to ovarian stimulation and cyst formation. To protect young patients from this, there are several modalities such as adding progestin to AI or using AI with a combination of OCP or GnRHa.

In a pilot trial, 10 premenopausal patients resistant to existing medical and surgical treatments of endometriosis were given an AI (letrozole 2.5 mg) and a progestin (norethindrone acetate 2.5 mg) daily for six months. Endometriosis was evaluated by pretreatment and post-treatment laparoscopies. Both pelvic pain scores and ASRM laparoscopic scores decreased significantly [71]. In another study, each patient was started on a daily regimen of anastrozole plus an OCP to be taken continuously for six months. The pain score was lowered over time with the combination of AI and OCPs [72], and the authors concluded that using AI plus OCP appears to be effective in controlling pain in premenopausal women with endometriosis.

In summary, the use of AI therapy for adolescents with endometriosis is still being debated. However, AIs appear to be the first breakthrough in the medical treatment of endometriosis since the introduction of GnRHa in the 1980s. AI regimens are fairly simple, consisting of taking one or two tablets a day. Finally, the side-effect profiles of AI regimens (including a progestin or OCP add-back) are more favorable compared with treatments using GnRHa or danazol. But prospective randomized trials studies are still needed to clarify the effect of AI on the treatment of endometriosis among adolescent patients.

Surgical treatment of endometriosis

The goals of operative treatment of an adolescent patient with endometriosis are to remove all implants, resect adhesions, reduce the risk of recurrence and postoperative adhesions, and restore the involved organs to a normal anatomic and physiologic condition. These goals may be achieved by using various surgical instruments (scissors, harmonic scalpel, lasers) and a variety of techniques (laparoscopy, laparotomy, combined endoscopy and mini-laparotomy).

Laparoscopy should be preferred as a first-line surgical therapy. It has many advantages compared to laparotomy: less pain, faster recovery, better cosmetic results, and reduced cost. It has been proved that laparoscopy causes less postoperative adhesion formation [73]. Data from animal and clinical studies suggest that laparoscopic operations are more effective for adhesiolysis, cause fewer new adhesions than does laparotomy, and reduce impairment of tubo-ovarian function [74].

Various methods and instruments are used to treat isolated endometriotic implants. The techniques include electrical coagulation, and laser or surgical excision. No single technique or instrument has been shown to be superior to any other. Therefore the instrument should be chosen on the basis of the surgeon's experience. Other considerations include risks, benefits, and expense.

Coagulation is the simplest way to destroy endometriosis. Coagulation is accomplished by touching the implants with care to avoid contact with the bowel, bladder, ureters, and vessels. However, unipolar or bipolar coagulation is not effective for deep endometriosis because of the risk of deep thermal injury.

We prefer a combination of vaporization and excision using CO_2 laser or monopolar electrosurgery for the treatment of endometriotic lesions. The CO_2 laser combined

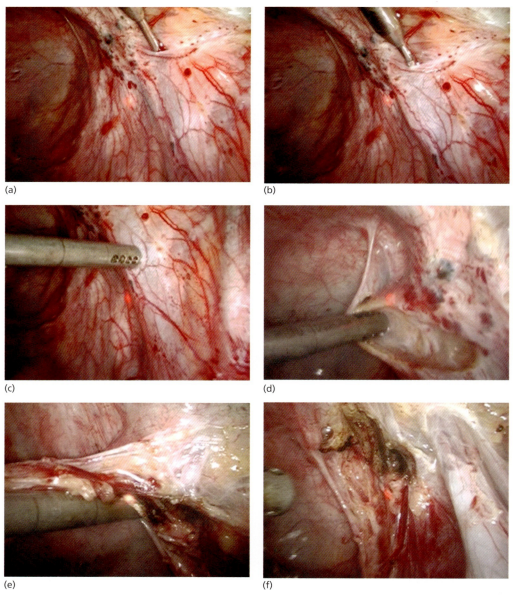

Figure 20.10 Surgical excision of ureteral endometriotic implants. (a,b) Injection of saline. Hydrodissection. (c,d,e) Removal of pathologic areas using CO_2 laser. (f) Final appearance.

with hydrodissection gives excellent vaporization of endometriotic implants [75]. It also offers the advantage of allowing superficial coagulation, deep excision, and a cutting ability. Laser surgery allows destruction of endometriosis with great precision.

Surgical excision of endometriotic implants is safe and effective (Fig. 20.10). Injection of saline into the retroperitoneal space aids identification of tissue planes. Scissors or laser can be used for excision. Surgical excision is a useful method of confirming the diagnosis, especially when

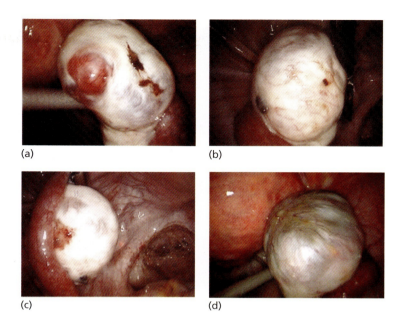

(a)

(b)

(c)

(d)

Figure 20.11 (a–c) Superficial endometriotic lesions on the surface of the ovary. (d) Right ovarian endometrioma type I.

there is an atypical appearance of the implants. When the CO_2 laser was used as an adjuvant option, the results were better, especially in patients with advanced endometriosis [76].

Complete removal of endometriotic implants is difficult because of their variability in appearance and visibility. Powder burn lesions represent foci of inactive disease besides atypical and nonpigmented lesions, which are seen as clear vesicles, ink vascular patterns, white scarred lesions, red lesions, yellow brown patches, and peritoneal windows represent active endometriosis [77]. The peritoneum must be examined from different angles and at different degrees of illumination to see vesicles or whitish lesions. The peritoneal fold must be stretched and searched for small, atypical lesions. Near contact laparoscopy magnifies the peritoneal area.

In treating peritoneal endometriosis, all the implants should be destroyed in the most effective and least traumatic manner to minimize postoperative adhesions. Although different modalities have been used, hydrodissection and a high-power superpulse or ultrapulse CO_2 laser is the best choice for treatment [75]. The CO_2 laser does not penetrate water and hydrodissection gives the surgeon a good fluid backstop. Superficial peritoneal endometriosis is vaporized with the CO_2 laser, coagulated

with monopolar or bipolar current, or excised. Implants less than 2 mm are coagulated, vaporized or excised. When lesions exceed 3 mm, vaporization or excision is needed. For lesions greater than 5 mm, deep vaporization or excisional techniques are used.

The ovaries are a common site of endometriosis (Fig. 20.11). Even normal-appearing ovaries can contain endometriosis under an apparently normal cortex. In adolescent patients it is essential to protect the reproductive organs as much as possible. Endometrial implants or endometriomas less than 2 cm in diameter are coagulated, laser ablated or excised using scissors, biopsy forceps, laser or electrodes. For successful eradication, all visible lesions and scars must be removed from the ovarian surface. For endometriomas over 2 cm in diameter, the cyst is punctured and aspirated. After irrigation and suction, the cyst wall should separate from the surrounding stroma. The cyst wall is removed by grasping its base with laparoscopic forceps and peeling it from the ovarian stroma (Fig. 20.12). Another method involves hydrodissection of the plane between the cyst wall and the ovarian stroma (Fig. 20.13) [78]. Cyst wall closure is not necessary [79], but for large defects, a suture or fibrin sealant can be used.

In a prospective trial, 64 patients with advanced endometriosis underwent either cystectomy or drainage

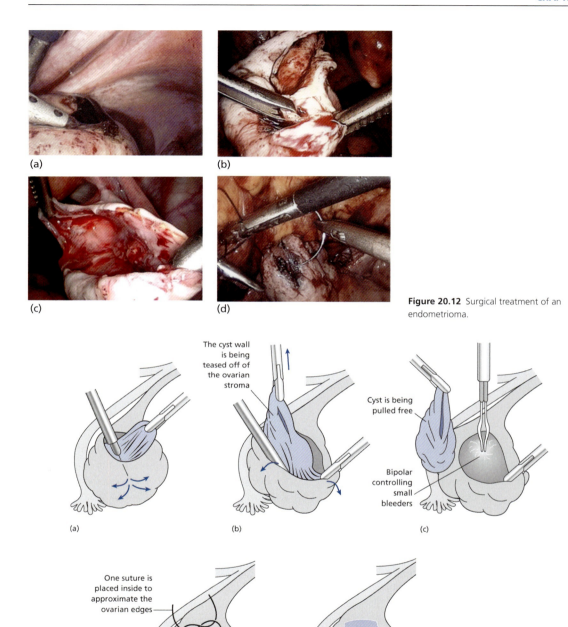

Figure 20.12 Surgical treatment of an endometrioma.

Figure 20.13 Complete excision of an endometriotic cyst from the ovary with hydrodissection.

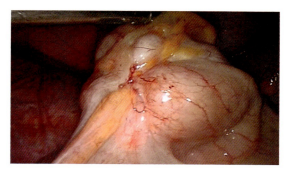

Figure 20.14 Endometriotic lesions on the bowel.

and bipolar coagulation. The 24-month cumulative recurrence rates of dysmenorrhea, deep dyspareunia, and nonmenstrual pelvic pain were lower in the patients who underwent cystectomy than in those who did not [80].

Genitourinary and gastrointestinal endometriosis fortunately is not common in adolescent patients (Figs 20.14, 20.15) but, if endometriosis is seen, it must be treated meticulously. Bowel resection should be performed if necessary and laparoscopy is a safe method [81]. Ureterolysis or enterolysis and adhesiolysis must be performed if necessary (Fig. 20.16).

Finally, the surgical treatment of endometriosis involves destroying endometrial implants (coagulation, vaporization, resection) and associated adhesions, and restoring normal anatomy. The anatomic, physiologic, and genetic factors that predispose each patient to develop endometriosis are not altered by the treatment. Therefore, recurrence is unavoidable unless endometrial proliferation, menstruation or the predominantly estrogenic environment of the patient is altered. Postoperative hormonal suppression treatments are more effective than surgery

plus placebo to obtain relief of pain associated with endometriosis stage III–IV and improvement of quality of life [82]. Second-look laparoscopy may be necessary to treat recurrent or persistent endometriosis.

Conclusion

Endometriosis is one of the most important causes of chronic pelvic pain in both adolescent and adult women. The definitive diagnosis of endometriosis must be established by laparoscopy with pathologic confirmation. The decision about medical or surgical treatment at the time of diagnosis depends on several factors including patient choice, availability of a laparoscopic surgeon familiar with endometriosis, and concerns about long-term medical therapy. If endometriosis is diagnosed at the time of laparoscopy, laparoscopic surgery should be the first choice for treatment.

Adolescents are more likely to have early or atypical than the classic typical lesions. Over the last decade, advances in endoscopic technology have enabled gynecologic surgeons to recognize many atypical appearances of the endometriotic implants not known to exist before, thus allowing their complete excision or destruction. Although cases with advanced endometriosis seem to benefit the most, we also recommend surgical treatment in patients with early endometriosis diagnosed using laparoscopy. Laparoscopic surgery may offer relief or improvement in the majority of patients with endometriosis and chronic pelvic pain. However, the combination of surgical treatment and pre- and postoperative hormonal manipulation with psychologic support will provide the best long-term results.

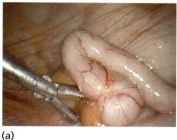
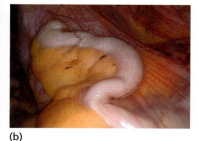

Figure 20.15 Endometriotic lesions on the appendix and mesoappendix.

(a)

(b)

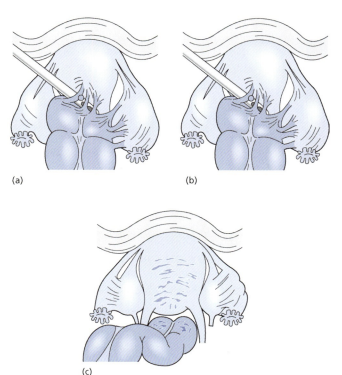

(a)   (b)

(c)

Figure 20.16 Lysis of severe adhesions and enterolysis and posterior dissection.

References

1. Scialli A, Barbiere R, Glasser M et al. *Chronic Pelvic Pain: an Integrated Approach.* APGO Educational Series on Women Health, 2000.

2. Zondervan KT, Yudkin PL, Vessey MP et al. Prevalence and incidence in primary care of chronic pelvic pain in women: evidence from a national general practice database. *Br J Obstet Gynaecol* 1999;**106**:1149.

3. Klein JR, Litt IF. Epidemiology of adolescent dysmenorrheal. *Pediatrics* 1981;**68**:661.

4. Harrop-Griffiths J, Katon W, Walker E et al. The association between chronic pelvic pain, psychiatric diagnosis, and childhood sexual abuse. *Obstet Gynecol* 1988;**71**: 589.

5. Laufer M, Goitein L, Bush M et al. Prevalence of endometriosis in adolescent women with chronic pelvic pain not responding to conventional therapy. *J Pediatr Adolesc Gynecol* 1997;**10**:199.

6. Goldstein DP. Acute and chronic pelvic pain. *Pediatr Clin North Am* 1989;**356**:573.

7. Goldstein DP, de Cholnoky C, Emans SJ et al. Laparoscopy in the diagnosis and management of pelvic pain in the adolescent. *J Reprod Med* 1980;**24**:251.

8. Reese KA, Reddy S, Rock JA. Endometriosis in an adolescent population: Emory experience. *J Pediatr Adolesc Gynecol* 1996;**9**:125.

9. Vercellini P, Fedel L, Arcaini L, Bianchi S, Rognoni MT, Candiani GB. Laparoscopy in the diagnosis of chronic pelvic pain in adolescent women. *J Reprod Med* 1989;**34**:827–830.

10. Kontoravdis A, Hassan E, Hassiakos D, Botsis D, Kontoravdis N, Creatsas G. Laparoscopic evaluation and management of chronic pelvic pain during adolescence. *Clin Exp Obstet Gynecol* 1999;**26**:76–77.

11. Goldstein DP, de Cholnoky C, Leventhal JM et al. New insight into problem of chronic pelvic pain. *J Pediatr Surg* 1979;**14**:675.

12. Nezhat C, Nezhat F, Nezhat C, Seidman DS. Operative laparoscopy: redefining the limits. *J Soc Laparoendoscop Surg* 1997;**1**(3):213–216.

13. Seidman DS, Nezhat F, Nezhat C, Nezhat C. Gynecological operative laparoscopy: new training programs are needed. *Surg Technol Int* 1997;**6**:235–238.

14. Laufer MR. Identification of clear vesicular lesions of atypical endometriosis: a new technique. *Fertil Steril* 1997;**68**: 739.

15. Nezhat CR, Nezhat FR, Swan AE. Long term outcome of laparoscopic adhesiolysis in women with chronic pelvic pain after hysterectomy. *J Am Assoc Gynecol Laparosc* 1996;**3**:S33–34.

16. Sampson JA. The development of the implantation theory for the origin of peritoneal endometriosis. *Am J Obstet Gynecol* 1940;**40**:549.

17. Meyer R. Uber entzundliche neterope Epithelwucherungen im weiblichen Gentalgebiet und uber eine his in die Wurzel des Mesocolon ausgedehnte benigne Wucherung des Darmepithel. *Virchows Arch Pathol Anat* 1909;**195**:487.

18. Halban J. Hysteroadenosis metastica. *Wien Klin Wochenschr* 1924;**37**:1207.

19. Halme J, Becker S, Haskill S. Altered maturation and function of peritoneal macrophages: possible role in pathogenesis of endometriosis. *Am J Obstet Gynecol* 1987;**156**:783.

20. Marsh EE, Laufer MR. Endometriosis in premenarcheal girls who do not have an associated obstructive anomaly. *Fertil Steril* 2005;**83**(3):758–760.

21. Houston D. Evidence for the risk of pelvic endometriosis by age, race and socioeconomic status. *Epidemiol Rev* 1984;**6**:167–191.

22. Stavroulis AI, Saridogan E, Creighton SM, Cutner AS. Laparoscopic treatment of endometriosis in teenagers. *Eur J Obstet Gynecol* 2006;**125**:248–250.

23. Ranney B. Endometriosis. IV. Hereditary tendency. *Obstet Gynecol* 1971;**37**:734.

24. Simpson JL, Elias S, Malinak LR et al. Heritable aspects of endometriosis: I. Genetic studies. *Am J Obstet Gynecol* 1980; **137**:327.

25. Sanfilippo JS, Wakim NG, Schikler KN, Yussman MA. Endometriosis in association with uterine anomaly. *Am J Obstet Gynecol* 1986;**154**:39–43.

26. Laufer MR, Sanfilippo J, Rose G. Adolescent endometriosis: diagnosis and treatment approaches. *J Pediatr Adolesc Gynecol* 2003;**16**(suppl):S3–11.

27. Sanfilippo JS. Endometriosis in adolescents. In: Wilson EA (ed) *Endometriosis*. New York: Alan R Liss, 1987;161–172.

28. Yamamoto K, Mitsuhashi Y, Takaike T et al. Tubal endometriosis diagnosed within one month after menarche. A case report. *Tohoko J Exp Med* 1997;**181**:385–387.

29. Whitehouse H. Endometriosis invading the bladder removed from a patient who had never menstruated. *Proc R Soc Med* 1925–1926;**19**:15.

30. Koninckx PR, Meuleman C, Demeyere S, Lesaffre E, Comillie FJ. Suggestive evidence that pelvic endometriosis is a progressive disease, whereas deeply infiltrating endometriosis is associated with pelvic pain. *Fertil Steril* 1991;**55**:759–765.

31. D'Hooghe TM, Bambra CS, Raeymaekers BM, Koninckx PR. Serial laparoscopies over 30 months show that endometriosis in captive baboons (*Papio anubis, Papio cynocephalus*) is a progressive disease. *Fertil Steril* 1996;**65**:645–649.

32. Nezhat F, Allan CJ, Nezhat C. Non-visualized endometriosis at laparoscopy. *Int J Fertil* 1991;**36**(6):340–343.

33. Chatman K, Ward A. Endometriosis in adolescents. *J Reprod Med* 1982;**27**:156–160.

34. American College of Obstetricians and Gynecologists. *Endometriosis in Adolescents*. ACOG Committee Opinion No. 310. Washington, DC: ACOG, 2005.

35. Ling FW, for the Pelvic Pain Study Group. Randomized controlled trial of depot leuprolide in patients with chronic pelvic pain and clinically suspected endometriosis. *Obstet Gynecol* 1999;**93**:51.

36. Gambone JC, Mittman BS, Munro MG. Consensus statement for the management of chronic pain and endometriosis: proceeding of an expert-panel consensus process. *Fertil Steril* 2002;**78**:961.

37. Propst AM, Laufer MR. Endometriosis in adolescents: incidence, diagnosis, and treatment. *J Reprod Med* 1999;**44**: 751.

38. American Society for Reproductive Medicine. Revised American Society for Reproductive Medicine classification of endometriosis: 1996. *Fertil Steril* 1997;**67**:817.

39. Davis GD, Thillet E, Lindemann J. Clinical characteristics of adolescent endometriosis. *J Adolesc Health* 1993;**14**:362.

40. Redwine DB. Age-related evolution in color appearance of endometriosis. *Fertil Steril* 1987;**48**:1062.

41. Martin DC, Hubert GD, Vander Zwagg R et al. Laparoscopic appearances of peritoneal endometriosis. *Fertil Steril* 1989;**51**:63.

42. Demco L. Mapping the source and character of pain due to endometriosis by patient-assisted laparoscopy. *J Am Assoc Gynecol Laparosc* 1998;**5**:241.

43. Nisolle M, Berliere M, Paindaveine B et al. Histologic study of peritoneal endometriosis in infertile women. *Fertil Steril* 1990;**53**:984.

44. Emmert C, Romann D, Riedel HH. Endometriosis diagnosed by laparoscopy in adolescent girls. *Arch Gynecol Obstet* 1998;**261**:89–93.

45. Group Italiano per lo Studio dell'Endometriosi. Relationship between stage, site and morphological characteristics of pelvic endometriosis and pain. *Hum Reprod* 2001;**16**(1):2668–2671.

46. Ylikorkala O, Viinikka L. Prostaglandins and endometriosis. *Acta Obstet Gynaecol Scand* 1983;**113**(suppl):105.

47. Moore J, Kennedy S, Prentice A. Modern combined oral contraceptive for pain associated with endometriosis. *Cochrane Database of Systematic Reviews* 1997, Issue 4. Art. No.: CD001019.

48. Miller L, Hughes JP. Continuous combined oral contraceptive pills to eliminate withdrawal bleeding: a randomized trial. *Obstet Gynecol* 2003;**101**:653–661.

49. Lu P, Ory SJ. Endometriosis: current management. *Mayo Clin Proc* 1995;**70**:453–463.

50. Vercellini P, Cortesi I, Crosignani PG. Progestins for symptomatic endometriosis: a critical analysis of evidence. *Fertil Steril* 1997;**68**:393–401.

51. Prentice A, Deary AJ, Bland A. Progestagens and anti-progestagens for pain associated with endometriosis. *Cochrane Database of Systematic Reviews* 2000;(2): CD002122.

52. Gupta N, O'Brien R, Jacobsen LJ et al. Mood changes in adolescents using depot-medroxyprogesterone acetate for contraception: a prospective study. *J Pediatr Adolesc Gynecol* 2001;**14**:71–76.

53. Ballweg ML. Big picture of endometriosis helps provide guidance on approach to teens: comparative historical data show endo starting younger, is more severe. *J Pediatr Adolesc Gynecol* 2003;**16**(suppl):S21–26.

54. Cromer BA, Blair JM, Mahan JD et al. A prospective comparison of bone density in adolescent girls receiving depot medroxyprogesterone acetate (Depo-Provera), levonorgestrol (Norplant), or oral contraceptives. *J Pediatr* 1996;**129**(5):671–676.

55. Scholes D, Lacroix AZ, Ott SM et al. Bone mineral density in women using depot medroxyprogesterone acetate for contraception. *Obstet Gynecol* 1999;**93**:233–238.

56. US Food and Drug Administration. Black box warning added concerning long-term use of Depo-Provera contraceptive injection. Rockville, MD: US FDA, 2004. Available online at: www.fda.gov/bbs/topics/ANSWERS/2004/ANS01325.html.

57. Dmowski WP, Cohen MR. Antigonadotropin (danazol) in the treatment of endometriosis: evaluation of post-treatment fertility and three-year follow up data. *Am J Obstet Gynecol* 1978;**130**:41.

58. Barbieri RL. New therapy for endometriosis. *N Engl J Med* 1988;**318**:512–514.

59. Mahutte NG, Arici A. Medical management of endometriosis-associated pain. *Obstet Gynecol Clin North Am* 2003;**30**(1):133–150.

60. Dlugi AM, Miller JD, Knittle J. Lupron depot (leuprolide acetate of depot suspension) in the treatment of endometriosis: a randomized placebo-controlled double-blind study. *Fertil Steril* 1990;**54**:419–427.

61. Henzel HM, Corson SL, Moghissi K et al. Administration of nasal nafarelin as compared with oral danazol for endometriosis. *N Engl Med* 1988;**318**:485–489.

62. Dawood MY, Lewis V, Ramos J. Cortical and trabecular bone mineral content in women with endometriosis: effect of gonadotropin releasing hormone agonist and danazol. *Fertil Steril* 1989;**52**:21.

63. Agarwal SK. Impact of six months of GnRH agonist therapy for endometriosis. Is there an age-related effect on bone mineral density? *J Reprod Med* 2002;**47**:530.

64. Matkovic V. Nutrition, genetics and skeletal development. *J Am Coll Nutr* 1996;**15**(6):556–569.

65. Barbieri RL. Hormone treatment of endometriosis: the estrogen threshold hypothesis. *Am J Obstet Gynecol* 1992;**166**:740–745.

66. Surrey ES, Hornstein MD. Prolonged GnRH agonist and add-back therapy for symptomatic endometriosis: long-term follow up. *Obstet Gynecol* 2002;**99**:709–719.

67. Kiesel L, Schweppe KW, Sillem M, Siebzehnrubl E. Should add-back therapy for endometriosis be deferred for optimal results? *Br J Obstet Gynaecol* 1996;**103**(suppl 14):15–17.

68. Lubianca JN, Gordon CM, Laufler MR. Addback therapy for endometriosis in adolescents. *J Reprod Med* 1998;**43**:164.

69. Zeitoun KM, Bulun SE. Aromatase, a key molecule in the pathophysiology of endometriosis and a therapeutic target. *Fertil Steril* 1999;**72**:961–969.

70. Attar E, Bulun S. Aromatase inhibitors: the next generation of therapeutics for endometriosis? *Fertil Steril* 2006;**85**:1307–1318.

71. Ailawadi RK, Jobanputra S, Kataria M, Gurates B, Bulun SE. Treatment of endometriosis and chronic pelvic pain with letrozole and norethindrone acetate: a pilot study. *Fertil Steril* 2004;**81**:290–296.

72. Amsterdam LL, Gentry W, Jobanputra S, Wolf M, Rubin SD, Bulun SE. Anastrazole and oral contraceptives – a novel treatment for endometriosis. *Fertil Steril* 2005;**84**:300–304.

73. Nezhat C, Nezhat F, Metzger AD, Luciano AA. Adhesion reformation after tubal surgery by videolaparoscopy. *Fertil Steril* 1990;**53**:1008–1011.

74. Lundorf P, Hahlin M, Kallfelt B et al. Adhesion formation after laparoscopic surgery in ectopic pregnancy: a randomized trial versus laparotomy. *Fertil Steril* 1991;**55**:911–915.

75. Nezhat C, Nezhat F. Safe laser endoscopic excision or vaporization of peritoneal endometriosis. *Fertil Steril* 1989;**52**(1):149–151.

76. Soong YK, Chang FH, Chou HH et al. Life table analysis of pregnancy rates in women with moderate or severe endometriosis comparing danazol therapy after CO_2 laser laparoscopy plus electrocoagulation versus danazol therapy only. *J Am Assoc Gynecol Laparosc* 1997;**4**:225–230.

77. Vernon MW, Beard JS, Graves K et al. Classification of endometriotic implants by morphologic appearance and capacity to synthesize prostaglandin F. *Fertil Steril* 1986;**46**:801–806.

78. Nezhat C, Silfen SL, Nezhat F et al. Surgery for endometriosis. *Curr Opin Obstet Gynecol* 1991;**3**:385.

79. Nezhat C, Nezhat F. Postoperative adhesion formation after ovarian cystectomy with and without ovarian reconstruction. Paper presented at the 47th Annual Meeting of the American Fertility Association, Orlando, FL, October 21–24, 1991.

80. Beretta P, Franchi M, Ghezzi F et al. Randomized clinical trial of two laparoscopic treatments of endometriomas: cystectomy versus drainage and coagulation. *Fertil Steril* 1998;**70**:1176–1180.

81. Nezhat C, Nezhat FR. Safe laser endoscopic excision or vaporization of peritoneal endometriosis. *Fertil Steril* 1989;**52**(1):149–151.

82. Sesti F, Pietropolli A, Capozzolo T et al. Hormonal suppression treatment or dietary therapy versus placebo in the control of painful symptoms after conservative surgery for endometriosis stage III-IV. A randomized comparative trial. *Fertil Steril* 2007;**88**(6):1541–1547.

CHAPTER 21

Management of Chronic Pelvic Pain in the Adolescent

Kenneth A. Levey
New York University Medical Center, New York, NY, USA

Introduction

Chronic pelvic pain has many similarities to other chronic pain disorders and more specific pain syndromes such as migraine headaches, fibromyalgia, chronic fatigue syndrome, temporomandibular joint syndrome, generalized neuropathic pain, regional sympathetic dystrophy (RSD) and low back pain. Similarities include but are not limited to the multifactorial nature of the disorders, association with comorbid medical problems, and association with comorbid and premorbid psychiatric disorders. These similarities exist in the adolescent in a similar way to an adult.

However, there are special considerations with regard to management that must be made in the adolescent. In this regard, it is important to recognize differences in pain physiology, responsiveness, side effects and tolerance to various therapies, social factors, and issues in potential lifelong management. It is critical not to dwell on specific diseases with the purpose of developing a recipe for managing specific problems. This will almost always lead to a very myopic therapeutic regimen that will likely result in repeated and frustrating treatment failures. Rather, it is important to recognize that many disease processes implicated in the etiology of chronic pelvic pain have crossover symptoms, and similar therapeutic regimens may treat similar symptoms.

In this chapter, while specific diseases will be mentioned to illustrate a point, the focus is to create a general understanding of various modalities and how they work synergistically to create overall improvement in quality of life and potential cure.

The multidisciplinary model

The multidisciplinary model is well proven to confer efficacy in the management of all pain syndromes. Fordyce in 1973, as well as Painter [1] and Price [2] in 1980, demonstrated the efficacy of the multidisciplinary model in general pain syndromes. Other notable work in the multidisciplinary management of chronic pain syndromes was done by Newman [3] who evaluated the model for efficacy on low back pain, Skultety [4] who evaluated the model for efficacy in general intractable pain, and Lemstra who proved efficacy of multidisciplinary management in migraine headaches. Critical work in chronic pelvic pain was done by Kames [5] in 1990 and Peters in 1991 [6].

Peters performed a trial of 106 patients randomized to traditional therapy of laparoscopy and psychotherapy if laparoscopy failed to confer improvement versus multidisciplinary management including primary psychotherapy, medical therapy, nutrition, and physical therapy. The multidisciplinary group had significantly greater improvement in quality of life and sexual function scores versus the traditional management group.

There are no studies specifically evaluating the utility of multidisciplinary pelvic pain management in adolescents. However, it is reasonable to assume that this model would be equally, if not more, effective in adolescents as it is in

Pediatric, Adolescent, & Young Adult Gynecology. Edited by A. Altchek and L. Deligdisch. © 2009 Blackwell Publishing, ISBN: 978-1-4051-5347-8.

Box 21.1 Disciplines involved in the multidisciplinary team

Psychiatry
Psychology
Anesthesiology/pain management
Gynecology
Rheumatology
Gastroenterology
Physical therapy
Acupuncture
Social work
Neurology
Physical and rehabilitation medicine

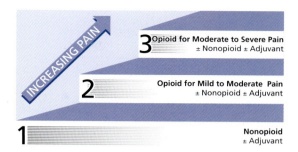

Figure 21.1 WHO pain ladder (source: World Health Organization).

adults. At NYU Medical Center, we use a multidisciplinary model that includes psychiatrists, psychologists, gastroenterologists, rheumatologists, anesthesiologists, gynecologists, physical therapists, nutritionists, social workers, and acupuncturists (Box 21.1). Involving this group has allowed us, over a 6–7 month period, to achieve a 50% rate of improvement in 70% of our patients. Factors associated with this rate of improvement include age (younger patients improve faster), body mass index (BMI), baseline depression, compliance with psychiatric care, and presence of a diagnosis (versus not having a diagnosis).

Specific therapeutic modalities

In general, a wide variety of therapeutic regimens exists for both the general management of chronic pelvic pain and the specific etiologies implicated in the pathogenesis of chronic pelvic pain. It is critical to ensure a clear understanding of the proposed management regimen between the physician and the adolescent as this age group may be more susceptible to rumor and Internet-related falsehoods. It may be preferable to offer a menu of options that in any combination will be acceptable and gradually phase in a full management plan over time.

Nonnarcotic analgesics

Analgesics are the mainstay of chronic pain management. The management of chronic pain using analgesics should always follow the widely accepted World Health Organization's pain management ladder (Figure 21.1). When taking the history it is important to understand the timing of the pain such that analgesic therapy can be tailored to

that. Additionally, it is important to educate the patient to take pain medication before the pain starts and continue taking medication throughout the pain episode. If she waits until pain symptoms peak this is likely to lead to lower efficacy and perceived treatment failure. When this happens, the patient will report that a variety of pain medications do not work when the reality is that they were administered incorrectly.

Acetaminophen is a useful first-line agent in doses of 325–650 mg up to a maximum of 4000 mg per day. Adverse side effects with acetaminophen are rare, so it is an excellent analgesic for mild pain in patients with asthma, peptic ulcer disease, gastrointestinal bleeding, and aspirin hypersensitivity [7].

Naproxen up to 500 mg bid, ibuprofen started at 400–600 mg up to qid, peroxicam 10–20 mg qd-bid or nabumetone 500–750 mg are common nonsteroidal anti-inflammatory drugs (NSAIDs) that may be prescribed as initial therapy. However, there are many other NSAIDs available and the practitioner must choose which is best. In patients chronically using NSAIDs, caution must be taken to protect against gastric ulcers. A once-daily dose of lansoprazole 30 mg is effective prophylaxis against gastric or duodenal ulcers.

The COX-2 inhibitors have been shown to have efficacy in a wide variety of chronic pain syndromes and for specific symptoms including dysmenorrhea. The only COX-2 inhibitor that remains on the market in the US is celecoxib. However, outside the US, other COX-2 inhibitors remain available and are very useful for a multitude of chronic pain conditions. With regard to pelvic pain, COX-2 inhibitors have been studied extensively in primary dysmenorrhea. Lumiracoxib 400 mg qd or bid and rofecoxib 25 or 50 mg daily are both effective therapy [8,9]. Valdecoxib 20 mg daily and celecoxib 200 mg daily may be used as well. They may also have efficacy in the long-term management of endometriosis [10].

Narcotic analgesics

After use of nonnarcotic analgesics has been maximized or as an adjunct to nonnarcotic analgesics, narcotic analgesics may be used. A major concern of both patients and parents is the possibility for addiction to narcotic analgesics when used over a long period. In a properly monitored setting (i.e. a pain management clinic), the rate of addiction among appropriately selected patients is low [11–15]. Additionally, it is advisable to have your patient sign a narcotics agreement with you so there is an understanding of the circumstances under which you will both continue to and no longer continue to prescribe narcotics. Examples of such an agreement can be found online from various sources. If the patient's need for combinations of narcotics, antidepressants, anxiolytics, and antiseizure medications, among others, arises then it is advisable to consult a anesthesiologist specializing in pain management and/or a psychopharmacologist.

Tramadol 50 mg is an effective mild narcotic that has inhibitory effects on both serotonin and norepinephrine reuptake as well as its primary effect on the μ-receptor. A typical starting dose is 50 mg bid-tid. If the patient is getting relief from round-the-clock dosing it is advisable to start her on an extended-release formulation of tramadol. If there is no effect from the tramadol then other narcotics should be tried. Hydrocodone/acetaminophen 5/500 and oxycodone/acetaminophen 5/325 (with increasing doses to 10/650) are appropriate next-step medications. With all narcotic combinations containing acetaminophen patients must be instructed not to use more than a total of 4000 mg per day as this leads to increased risk of hepatotoxicity. If pain relief is achieved with interval dosing, then a longer acting formulation should be considered such as extended-release morphine 15–30 mg qd-bid and/or intermediate-release morphine or oxycodone.

A simple approach to narcotic dosing in adolescents once narcotic tolerance, need, and efficacy have been established is to start a long-acting transdermal formulation of fentanyl. This will increase compliance and lead to more steady pain relief. Transdermal fentanyl is available in a 72-hour release formulation; however, clinical experience has shown that the effect may decrease at 48 hours. In this situation it is advisable to tell your patient to put on a

Table 21.1 Recommended fentanyl transdermal therapeutic system (TTS) dosage based on 24-hour oral morphine dose [16]

24-hour oral morphine (mg/24 hours)	Fentanyl TTS dosage (µg/hour)
45 to 134	25
135 to 224	50
225 to 314	75
315 to 404	100
405 to 494	125
495 to 584	150
585 to 674	175
675 to 764	200
765 to 854	225
855 to 944	250
945 to 1034	275
1035 to 1124	300

second patch and remove the first one at the full 72 hours. Table 21.1 is a guide for converting patients from oral morphine to transdermal fentanyl [16]. Patients and parents must be educated about narcotic side effects such as pruritus, nausea, constipation and warning signs such as oversedation and respiratory depression.

Hormonal management

In addition to their widely known effects on inflammation in and development of female reproductive tract disease, it is becoming clearer that both estrogen and progesterone play an important role in central pain modulation [17–19]. The first line of therapy for chronic pelvic pain that is cyclical in nature, regardless of the timing, is combined oral contraceptives with an NSAID. Traditionally, a 30 or 35 µg pill has been used with a 21-day active drug and seven-day placebo withdrawal period. This is an effective regimen, but for women who have other symptoms associated with the menses, such as those associated with premenstrual dysphoric disorder (PMDD), this may not be the best approach. A better approach may be to use an extended-dose regimen with an 84-day active pill cycle and a seven-day withdrawal period. This can be done with a pre-packaged 91-day pack or the patient may be instructed to combine four 28-day packs, skipping the placebos in the first three packs. There are both safety and efficacy data to support this regimen 20].

The IUD containing levonorgestrel (LNG-IUD) has proven efficacy in both endometriosis-related pelvic pain and for primary dysmenorrhea. It may also be beneficial for postoperative management of endometriosis-associated pain [21,22]. There is clear evidence that the LNG-IUD is better tolerated than gonadotropin-releasing hormone agonists (GnRHa). Additionally, the LNG-IUD can be used for five years while the GnRHa only have one-year safety data [23]. While LNG-IUDs are excellent therapy for endometriosis and other hormonally responsive conditions, it can be difficult to educate teens and their parents about the benefits of this therapy.

Depot medroxyprogesterone acetate (DMPA) 150 mg IM every three months has proven benefit as a second-line therapy in endometriosis but is also effective in general pelvic pain syndromes such as pelvic congestion syndrome. However, the side effects of this therapy, such as weight gain and abnormal bleeding, may be unacceptable to an adolescent. Additionally, there is evidence that bone mineral density development may be slowed by prolonged use of DMPA. Low-dose tamoxifen may also confer some relief in women with isolated dysmenorrhea that has been nonresponsive to traditional hormonal regimens [24]. This is largely experimental and should be considered third-line therapy.

GnRHa may be used in adolescents but should be considered second- or third-line therapy as considerations for bone mineral density must be taken into account. There are adequate one-year safety data in adults using depot leuprolide acetate 3.75 mg monthly when combined with calcium and a hormone replacement regimen such as conjugated equine estrogens 0.625 mg and norethindrone acetate 5 mg [23]. However, there are no such data in women who have not reached their peak bone mineral density and may not have even reached the point of full epiphyseal closure. Thus caution must be exercised when using GnRHa in adolescents. GnRHa should not be used as a diagnostic tool for any hormonally responsive pain etiology as isolated central pain disorders may respond well to this class of medications.

Aromatase inhibitors (AIs) are an emerging therapy in endometriosis and may be useful in the future for general treatment of other pelvic pain-associated disorder such as interstitial cystitis. Aromatase catalyzes the final step in producing estrogen locally and endometriosis is associated with an aromatase overexpression. AIs such as anastrazole 1 mg [25] or letrozole 2.5 mg have demonstrated efficacy in the medical management of endometriosis. Regardless of the regimen chosen, some form of ovulation

suppression must be included. This can be achieved with GnRHA, DMPA or combined oral contraceptives.

Surgical management

There are a select few chronic pelvic pain problems that may be prominent in the adolescent that may also be responsive to surgical management. While other pelvic pain disorders may be responsive to surgical management, they would not be expected to present in an adolescent. Diseases that may be responsive to surgical management which are found in adolescents include chronic hydrosalpinx, pelvic peritoneal fibrosis, pelvic floor hernias, endometriosis, and adenomyosis. The best evidence for improvement in pain with surgical management exists for endometriosis and adenomyosis. The surgical therapy for adenomyosis is hysterectomy and this is unacceptable in an adolescent. So, the best evidence-based reason to operate on an adolescent with chronic pelvic pain is a high index of suspicion for endometriosis. The diagnosis of endometriosis has been outlined in the previous chapter.

Depending on the volume and location of disease as well as the patient's symptoms, surgery may be considered as first-line therapy or a last resort. Unfortunately, the choice between medical and surgical management of endometriosis is not clearly defined. However, if an endometrioma is present the first line for management is surgical excision of the cyst wall. Simple laparoscopic fenestration, drainage, and destruction of the cyst wall are not adequate as there is a higher chance of losing ovarian reserve and worsening the effect of the endometriosis on future fertility [26]. Drainage of the cyst, with either surgical or guided aspiration, results in high rates of recurrence – up to 97% in the largest study [27]. For endometriosis not associated with an endometrioma, radical resection of endometriotic lesions is the surgical approach most likely to lead to a significant and long-term improvement in quality of life [28]. Adolescents must be counseled that endometriosis is a lifelong disease and that continuous monitoring and therapy may be needed.

Surgery for abdominopelvic adhesions has not been shown to provide any long-term benefit. Among patients with chronic abdominal pain and known adhesions, there is no difference between performing laparoscopic adhesiolysis and simple diagnostic laparoscopy [29]. In fact, the more surgical procedures a patient has for the purpose of removing adhesions, the more likely the pain will remain. Such diminishing returns do not justify repeated surgery on a patient with adhesions. Once adhesions have been diagnosed surgically, the mainstay must be multidisciplinary medical and other techniques of management that do not involve entering the peritoneal cavity. Once all medical options have been exhausted, it may be beneficial to place a spinal cord stimulator. While this option may not appeal to an adolescent, the long-term benefit in other pain syndromes is clear and this intervention is likely to decrease the chance of long-term depression, narcotics use, dependence, and social dysfunction.

Antidepressants

In general, antidepressants have proven benefit in chronic pain syndromes. The American Society of Anesthesiology states that "the literature supports the use of antidepressants for reducing chronic pain without notable adverse effects." Antidepressants have neuromodulatory effects that may improve both depression and pain. However, although there is no clear evidence supporting utility of empiric therapy with antidepressants for women with the chronic pelvic pain syndrome [30], there is certainly a role for antidepressants in a variety of conditions associated with chronic pelvic pain. Once a specific diagnosis has been made then it may be appropriate to start such therapy. Depression, for example, is common in chronic pain patients as both a premorbid and a comorbid condition. Depression that is clearly identified should be treated in accordance with current guidelines for treating depression outside chronic pain syndromes while taking into account the larger picture of the chronic pelvic pain.

The selective serotonin reuptake inhibitors (SSRIs) have utility in treating primary dysmenorrhea and premenstrual dysphoric disorder (PMDD). They have benefit for the pain symptoms, other physical symptoms such as bloating, and for the psychobehavioral symptoms of mood change, loss of sleep, dysthymia, and irritability. When used primarily for menstrual type symptoms, the SSRIs may have efficacy in days rather than weeks [31] as would be expected in treatment for isolated depression. Fluoxetine may be started at 20 mg daily but is also effective at 20 mg daily only during the luteal phase. Sertraline is also effective and well studied and can be started at 25 mg daily for seven days and increased to 50 mg daily. The most commonly reported side effects of SSRIs are insomnia, gastrointestinal disturbances, decreased libido, and fatigue. Recently, there has been some evidence that antidepressants, especially the SSRIs, may increase suicidal thinking in teenage patients. However, in a closely monitored setting where there is frequent contact between physicians and patients, this therapy may be safe.

When used as empiric therapy for chronic pain, the tricyclic antidepressants (TCAs) are started at lower doses than would otherwise be effective for depression. TCAs have benefit in some specific disorders associated with chronic pelvic pain such as generalized/provoked vulvodynia, interstitial cystitis, and fibromyalgia as well as sources of neuropathic pain such as nerve entrapments in the abdominal wall or pelvic floor.

Anticonvulsants

Anticonvulsants have demonstrated efficacy in disorders associated with neuropathic pain as well as in generalized chronic pain [32]. Carbamazepine, valproate, lamotrigine, oxcarbazepine, tiagabine, gabapentin, and pregabalin have been studied with varying levels of success in specific as well as general pain disorders. Some of the anticonvulsants may offer benefit beyond pain relief as they may act as mood stabilizers and anxiolytics. Gabapentin has been shown to have efficacy over amitriptyline in treating generalized chronic pelvic pain [33]. Doses may start at 300 mg per day and increase by 300 mg per day every two weeks until 300 mg tid is reached. This dose should then be titrated up to a maximum of 3600 mg per day in divided doses. The most common side effect reported is fatigue. All anticonvulsants should be tapered when it is planned to stop the drug.

Psychiatry, psychology, and behavioral approaches

The important role of psychologists, psychiatrists, and counselors in general chronic pain management is well documented in the literature. As the biopsychosocial model of understanding the pathogenesis of chronic pain has developed, so has the need for a variety of psychologically based treatment approaches. When treating the adolescent with chronic pelvic pain, the approach to measuring response to therapy is different from that in an adult. It is important to use a set of developmentally appropriate questions and explanations as well as providing several chances to answer similar questions. Some tools that are more appropriate for adolescents include word-graphic rating scales and multidimensional pain scales [34].

In addition to pain reduction, one critical outcome of chronic pelvic pain management in the adolescent is improvement in quality of life. Adolescents with chronic pain differ from healthy controls on several psychosocial factors [35]: they have significantly worse psychologic functioning, physical functioning, functional status, lower satisfaction with life, poorer perceived health status, and worse social functioning [36,37]. All of these may translate into poor long-term psychologic outcomes. It is important to prepare the adolescent regarding fluctuations in pain, medication outcomes, and their own behavioral changes. When referring an adolescent for psychotherapy, it is important to find a practitioner who is experienced in chronic pain management and the development of coping mechanisms in chronic pain patients [38].

Physical therapy

Physical therapy has demonstrated efficacy in chronic pelvic pain for a number of related disorders. Primarily physical therapists are utilized for the management of pelvic floor spasm and weakness. They can also be useful in the diagnosis and management of musculoskeletal disease associated with chronic pelvic pain such as chronic low back pain, piriformis syndrome, gait abnormalities, and other muscular problems that affect the pelvic musculoskeletal architecture.

Several modalities are primarily used by physical therapists. Biofeedback depends on the patient's ability to change her physiologic responses based on information given to her about disease processes (i.e. muscle spasm). Internal and external massage of tender and trigger points may have benefit in the short term but no long-term benefit has been demonstrated with this modality as monotherapy. Transcutaneous electrical nerve stimulation (TENS) has been shown to be effective for pain relief in a variety of conditions. Electrodes are placed on the skin and electric current applied at different pulse rates and intensities is used to stimulate these areas so as to provide pain relief. In dysmenorrhea, TENS is thought to work by alteration of the body's ability to receive or perceive pain signals rather than by having a direct effect on the uterine contractions. Education with home exercise programs may have the longest benefit of all these modalities as it allows a motivated patient to work at her own pace. There are no significant data on these modalities in adolescents but it is reasonable to presume the mechanics are the same.

Acupuncture

While there are few randomized trials demonstrating the utility of acupuncture in chronic pain management, it does not appear to confer any harm to the patient's general health or to the disease process. There is very little evidence to support its use outside pelvic girdle syndrome in pregnancy [39] and primary dysmenorrhea [40]. However, there is a growing body of evidence to support its use in general pain syndromes, migraine headaches, and temporomandibular joint (TMJ) syndrome. Thus, given its low likelihood of harm and known benefit in other pain syndromes, acupuncture may be recommended to most pelvic pain patients. A major consideration in making an acupuncture referral is the experience and training of the acupuncturist. There is likely a major difference between an acupuncturist who was licensed after a short course and a physician who completed training in traditional Chinese medicine and acupuncture with experience.

Common conditions and specific therapies

There are several common conditions that lend themselves to specific therapies not previously discussed. Endometriosis has been discussed above in the sections on hormonal management and surgical management. Clearly, there is a need, as there is with all chronic pelvic pain-related disorders, for both multidisciplinary and multimodal management in endometriosis patients.

Interstitial cystitis

Interstitial cystitis (IC) may also be called urgency-frequency-pain syndrome and is often seen in combination with endometriosis [41]. As many of the symptoms occur in both diseases it is not surprising that some of the therapeutic modalities, such as hormonal management, are the same.

Several therapeutic modalities are specific to IC. Pentosan polysulfate (PPS) is a mainstay of IC therapy. Compliance may be difficult in adolescents as the 100 mg dose is tid. There are no significant side effects associated with its use. Patients must be counseled that the drug needs to be used for six months or longer. TCAs are effective when combined with PPS. Desipramine starting at 25 mg, amitriptyline 10 mg or imipramine

25 mg can all be appropriate starting doses for TCAs in combination with PPS. Hydrodistension in the operating room has produced varying results and may not be more effective than education alone. Urethral dilation has absolutely no role in the management of interstitial cystitis.

Often there exists a secondary pelvic floor disorder that will benefit from physical therapy. When other modalities have failed, bladder instillations with varying combinations of dimethyl sulfoxide (DMSO), lidocaine, gentamicin, dissolved PPS, sodium bicarbonate, heparin, and triamcinolone may be used. A common mixture may include DMSO 50 cc, lidocaine 1% 20 cc, heparin 20,000 units, sodium bicarbonate 8.4% 50 cc, and triamcinolone 20 mg. The solution is placed via a urethral catheter and with each instillation the patient is instructed to hold it in longer and longer, with the goal being 2–3 hours. Instillations are done weekly for 4–6 weeks. Patients with interstitial cystitis may frequently present with acute exacerbations. It is important to be careful not to miss a urinary tract infection during these times as repeated unrecognized infections will only make the disease worse.

Vulvodynia

As with other specific diseases, the model of multidisciplinary and multimodal management applies to all categories of vulvodynia (localized/general, provoked/unprovoked). Adolescent patients must first be educated about the disease. They need to be advised to avoid any self-medicating, over-the-counter topical creams, ointments or lotions. These may lead to a contact dermatitis that will make it more difficult to control the symptoms. A careful discussion about hygiene and avoiding tight and/or synthetic clothing may be necessary.

As discussed above, antidepressants and anticonvulsants have value in treating general pain. This is also true in vulvodynia. Amitriptyline starting at 10 mg daily and increasing up to 100–150 mg daily as tolerated is useful first-line therapy. Topical therapy should include an initial trial of lidocaine 5% every night for six weeks as this is likely to alter the way the local nerve endings perceive pain [42]. Other topical therapies that may be attempted include topical ketoprofen 10% mixed with lidocaine 5%, gabapentin 6%, and triamcinolone 1% in a liposomal base daily for six weeks. Topical and injectable steroids may be effective, although caution should be exercised

due to the risk of atrophy. Interferon-α has demonstrated efficacy as a down-the-line therapy. Injections are done three times per week for 4–6 weeks but are poorly tolerated. As a treatment of last resort, surgery may be performed. Vulvar vestibulectomy is associated with a high rate of satisfaction at 26- [43] and 39-month [44] follow-up. Of all the management techniques described in the literature, the most successful in the long term has been vestibulectomy.

Very often there is a comorbid pelvic floor spasm that may be under-recognized and the reason for treatment failures. A careful evaluation of the pelvic floor is important. If such spasm is detected, physical therapy with biofeedback and muscle awareness and strengthening exercises should be started. If spasm is still present after a trial of physical therapy then botulinum toxin A may be used. This is an effective therapy when administered in properly selected patients [45].

Irritable bowel syndrome

Irritable bowel syndrome (IBS) is a functional bowel disorder characterized by intermittent episodes of diarrhea and constipation, cramping, bloating, and chronic abdominal and pelvic pain. Many of the therapies already described in this chapter have efficacy in treating IBS. These include depot leuprolide acetate [46]. There is a clear association between IBS and stress and anxiety so psychotherapy with behavioral modification may also help with IBS-associated pain. TCAs have benefit in relieving IBS-associated pain but not other gastrointestinal symptoms [47]. There is some promise in probiotics. The probiotic VSL#3 reduces flatulence and retards colonic transit without altering bowel function.

Individuals with IBS tend to have a large number of food intolerances. Unfortunately, there does not seem to be any known biologic correlation [48]. The patient should be her own guide when it comes to an appropriate diet. For constipation-predominant IBS, tegaserod 6 mg bid for up to six weeks is effective. However, caution must be exercised in patients with known intraperitoneal adhesions. As discussed above, a multimodal and multidisciplinary plan must be used. This may include psychotherapy, antidepressants, and behavioral modification. An intervention as simple as a onetime, multidisciplinary class for patients with IBS was associated with improvement in symptoms and health-promoting lifestyle behavior [49].

Managing expectations

In treating adults with chronic pelvic pain and other chronic pain syndromes, it may be difficult for the patient to understand the chronic nature of their disease. This problem is amplified in adolescents who are not only influenced by their parents' views but also have misconceptions of their own. They must understand the concept that when chronic pain exists there also may be neurologic change in the brain and spinal cord. It can be explained to the patient that the pain is not just in their pelvis but in their nerves as well and it takes a long time to change the way the brain perceives pain. It is appropriate to tell patients that it may take six months to one year before they see significant improvement. Taking the time to offer this type of explanation in my experience increases compliance and decreases therapies that have "failed" due to misconceptions about time course of therapy.

Role of the parents

In addition to being biologically complex, chronic pelvic pain has a complex set of environmental factors. An important factor may be the parental involvement, or lack thereof, and the quality of such involvement. It is known that parents are undereducated on the need for pain relief in their children [50,51]. It is important to explain therapy to the parents as well as the patients. In older adolescents, it may be important to balance the time spent with the patient alone and time spent with patient and parents, as parents may incite anxiety as well as relieve it when properly educated. Time alone with parents is not recommended.

Conclusion

There is no clear formula or algorithm for managing chronic pelvic pain in adolescents. While there may exist recipes for treating various diagnoses, most patients have symptoms that may suggest multiple possible diagnoses and therapy must be individualized and tailored to that patient's needs.

References

1. Painter JR, Seres JL, Newman RI. Assessing benefits of the pain center: why some patients regress. *Pain* 1980;**8**:101–113.

2. Price CL, Pawlicki RE. The pain clinic: a multidisciplinary approach to long term pain. *WeatherVane* 1980;**49**:2–3.

3. Newman RI, Seres JL, Yospe LP, Garlington B. Multidisciplinary treatment of chronic pain: long-term follow-up of low-back pain patients. *Pain* 1978;**4**:283–292.

4. Skultety FM, Meilman PW, Guck TP, Berman BM. Results of treatment of chronic pain at a multidisciplinary pain center. *Nebr Med J* 1986;**71**:93–97.

5. Kames LD, Rapkin AJ, Naliboff BD, Afifi S, Ferrer-Brechner T. Effectiveness of an interdisciplinary pain management program for the treatment of chronic pelvic pain. *Pain* 2007; **41**:41–43.

6. Peters AAW, Vandorst E, Jellis B, Vanzuuren E, Hermans J, Trimbos JB. A randomized clinical trial to compare 2 different approaches in women with chronic pelvic pain. *Obstet Gynecol* 1991;**77**:740–744.

7. Cooper SA. Comparative analgesic efficacies of aspirin and acetaminophen. *Arch Intern Med* 1981;**141**:282–285.

8. Bitner M, Kattenhorn J, Hatfield C, Gao J, Kellstein D. Efficacy and tolerability of lumiracoxib in the treatment of primary dysmenorrhoea. *Int J Clin Pract* 2004;**58**:340–345.

9. Morrison BW, Daniels SE, Kotey P, Cantu N, Seidenberg B. Rofecoxib, a specific cyclooxygenase-2 inhibitor, in primary dysmenorrhea: a randomized controlled trial. *Obstet Gynecol* 1999;**94**:504–508.

10. Cobellis L, Razzi S, De Simone S et al. The treatment with a COX-2 specific inhibitor is effective in the management of pain related to endometriosis. *Eur J Obstet Gynecol Reprod Biol* 2004;**116**:100–102.

11. Slagle MA. Pain management. Medication update. *South Med J* 2001;**94**:771–774.

12. Ward J, Hall W, Mattick RP. Role of maintenance treatment in opioid dependence. *Lancet* 1999;**353**:221–226.

13. Cherry DA, Gourlay GK. Pharmacological management of chronic pain: a clinician's perspective. *Agents Actions* 1994;**42**:173–174.

14. Hojsted J, Sjogren P. Addiction to opioids in chronic pain patients: a literature review. *Eur J Pain* 2007;**11**(5):490–518.

15. Jensen MK, Thomsen AB, Hojsted J. 10-year follow-up of chronic non-malignant pain patients: opioid use, health related quality of life and health care utilization. *Eur J Pain* 2006;**10**:423–433.

16. Jeal W, Benfield P. Transdermal fentanyl. A review of its pharmacological properties and therapeutic efficacy in pain control. *Drugs* 1997;**53**:109–138.

17. Hellstrom B, Anderberg UM. Pain perception across the menstrual cycle phases in women with chronic pain. *Percept Mot Skills* 2003;**96**:201–211.

18. Hucho TB, Dina OA, Kuhn J, Levine JD. Estrogen controls PKCepsilon-dependent mechanical hyperalgesia through

direct action on nociceptive neurons. *Eur J Neurosci* 2006;**24**:527–534.

19. Lacroix-Fralish ML, Tawfik VL, Nutile-McMenemy N, DeLeo JA. Progesterone mediates gonadal hormone differences in tactile and thermal hypersensitivity following L5 nerve root ligation in female rats. *Neuroscience* 2006;**138**:601–608.

20. Edelman A, Gallo MF, Nichols MD, Jensen JT, Schulz KF, Grimes DA. Continuous versus cyclic use of combined oral contraceptives for contraception: systematic Cochrane review of randomized controlled trials. *Hum Reprod* 2006;**21**:573–578.

21. Abou-Setta AM, Al Inany HG, Farquhar CM. Levonorgestrel-releasing intrauterine device (LNG-IUD) for symptomatic endometriosis following surgery. *Cochrane Database of Systematic Reviews* 2006;CD005072.

22. Vercellini P, Frontino G, De Giorgi O, Aimi G, Zaina B, Crosignani PG. Comparison of a levonorgestrel-releasing intrauterine device versus expectant management after conservative surgery for symptomatic endometriosis: a pilot study. *Fertil Steril* 2003;**80**:305–309.

23. Hornstein MD, Surrey ES, Weisberg GW, Casino LA. Leuprolide acetate depot and hormonal add-back in endometriosis: a 12-month study. Lupron Add-Back Study Group. *Obstet Gynecol* 1998;**91**:16–24.

24. Pierzynski P, Swiatecka J, Oczeretko E, Laudanski P, Batra S, Laudanski T. Effect of short-term, low-dose treatment with tamoxifen in patients with primary dysmenorrhea. *Gynecol Endocrinol* 2006;**22**:698–703.

25. Soysal S, Soysal ME, Ozer S, Gul N, Gezgin T. The effects of post-surgical administration of goserelin plus anastrozole compared to goserelin alone in patients with severe endometriosis: a prospective randomized trial. *Hum Reprod* 2004;**19**:160–167.

26. Hart R, Hickey M, Maouris P, Buckett W, Garry R. Excisional surgery versus ablative surgery for ovarian endometriomata: a Cochrane Review. *Hum Reprod* 2005;**20**:300–307.

27. Zanetta G, Lissoni A, Dalla VC, Trio D, Pittelli M, Rangoni G. Ultrasound-guided aspiration of endometriomas: possible applications and limitations. *Fertil Steril* 1995;**64**:709–713.

28. Angioni S, Peiretti M, Zirone M et al. Laparoscopic excision of posterior vaginal fornix in the treatment of patients with deep endometriosis without rectum involvement: surgical treatment and long-term follow-up. *Hum Reprod* 2006;**21**:1629–1634.

29. Swank DJ, Swank-Bordewijk SC, Hop WC et al. Laparoscopic adhesiolysis in patients with chronic abdominal pain: a blinded randomised controlled multi-centre trial. *Lancet* 2003;**361**:1247–1251.

30. Engel CC Jr, Walker EA, Engel AL, Bullis J, Armstrong A. A randomized, double-blind crossover trial of sertra-line in women with chronic pelvic pain. *J Psychosom Res* 1998;**44**:203–207.

31. Freeman EW, Rickels K, Sondheimer SJ, Polansky M. Differential response to antidepressants in women with premenstrual syndrome/premenstrual dysphoric disorder: a randomized controlled trial. *Arch Gen Psychiatr* 1999;**56**:932–939.

32. Wiffen PJ. Evidence-based pain management and palliative care in issue four for 2005 of The Cochrane Library. *J Pain Palliat Care Pharmacother* 2006;**20**:33–35.

33. Sator-Katzenschlager SM, Scharbert G, Kress HG et al. Chronic pelvic pain treated with gabapentin and amitriptyline: a randomized controlled pilot study. *Wien Klin Wochenschr* 2005;**117**:761–768.

34. Tesler MD, Savedra MC, Holzemer WL, Wilkie DJ, Ward JA, Paul SM. The word-graphic rating scale as a measure of children's and adolescents' pain intensity. *Res Nurs Health* 1991;**14**:361–371.

35. Merlijn VP, Hunfeld JA, van der Wouden JC, Hazebroek-Kampschreur AA, Koes BW, Passchier J. Psychosocial factors associated with chronic pain in adolescents. *Pain* 2003;**101**:33–43.

36. Hunfeld JA, Passchier J, Perquin CW, Hazebroek-Kampschreur AA, Suijlekom-Smit LW, van der Wouden JC. Quality of life in adolescents with chronic pain in the head or at other locations. *Cephalalgia* 2001;**21**:201–206.

37. Hunfeld JA, Perquin CW, Duivenvoorden HJ et al. Chronic pain and its impact on quality of life in adolescents and their families. *J Pediatr Psychol* 2001;**26**:145–153.

38. Rudy TE, Kerns RD, Turk DC. Chronic pain and depression: toward a cognitive-behavioral mediation model. *Pain* 1988;**35**:129–140.

39. Elden H, Ladfors L, Olsen MF, Ostgaard HC, Hagberg H. Effects of acupuncture and stabilising exercises as adjunct to standard treatment in pregnant women with pelvic girdle pain: randomised single blind controlled trial. *BMJ* 2005;**330**:761.

40. Tzafettas J. Painful menstruation. *Pediatr Endocrinol Rev* 2006;**3**(suppl 1):160–163.

41. Chung MK, Chung RP, Gordon D. Interstitial cystitis and endometriosis in patients with chronic pelvic pain: the "Evil Twins" syndrome. *J Soc Laparoendosc Surg* 2005;**9**:25–29.

42. Zolnoun DA, Hartmann KE, Steege JF. Overnight 5% lidocaine ointment for treatment of vulvar vestibulitis. *Obstet Gynecol* 2003;**102**:84–87.

43. Goldstein AT, Klingman D, Christopher K, Johnson C, Marinoff SC. Surgical treatment of vulvar vestibulitis syndrome: outcome assessment derived from a postoperative questionnaire. *J Sex Med* 2006;**3**:923–931.

44. Bergeron S, Bouchard C, Fortier M, Binik YM, Khalife S. The surgical treatment of vulvar vestibulitis syndrome: a follow-up study. *J Sex Marital Ther* 1997;**23**:317–325.

45. Ghazizadeh S, Nikzad M. Botulinum toxin in the treatment of refractory vaginismus. *Obstet Gynecol* 2004;**104**:922–925.

46. Mathias JR, Clench MH, Abell TL et al. Effect of leuprolide acetate in treatment of abdominal pain and nausea in premenopausal women with functional bowel disease: a double-blind, placebo-controlled, randomized study. *Dig Dis Sci* 1998;**43**:1347–1355.

47. Holten KB. Irritable bowel syndrome: minimize testing, let symptoms guide treatment. *J Fam Pract* 2003;**52**:942–950.

48. Monsbakken KW, Vandvik PO, Farup PG. Perceived food intolerance in subjects with irritable bowel syndrome – etiology, prevalence and consequences. *Eur J Clin Nutr* 2006;**60**:667–672.

49. Saito YA, Prather CM, Van Dyke CT, Fett S, Zinsmeister AR, Locke GR III. Effects of multidisciplinary education on outcomes in patients with irritable bowel syndrome. *Clin Gastroenterol Hepatol* 2004;**2**:576–584.

50. Finley GA, McGrath PJ, Forward SP, McNeill G, Fitzgerald P. Parents' management of children's pain following 'minor' surgery. *Pain* 1996;**64**:83–87.

51. McGrath PJ, Finley GA. Attitudes and beliefs about medication and pain management in children. *J Palliat Care* 1996;**12**:46–50.

CHAPTER 22

Adolescent Anovulatory Dysfunctional Uterine Bleeding and Menorrhagia

Albert Altchek

Mount Sinai School of Medicine and Hospital, New York, NY, USA

Introduction

Most cases of anovulatory dysfunctional uterine bleeding are mild and self-limiting. Mild irregular bleeding is not unusual at the start of menstrual life. Most pediatricians consider it to be a variation of normal due to intermittent ovulation. Management is empiric because of a lack of long-term controls.

However, anovulatory dysfunctional uterine bleeding (ADUB) may present as an emergency in the adolescent. It requires prompt clinical evaluation to decide if hospitalization is required and often oral contraceptive pills (OC) to control the bleeding. The bleeding may also be due to an inherited or acquired coagulation defect or pregnancy complication (Quick Take 22.1).

Pathophysiology

Anovulatory dysfunctional uterine bleeding is a leading cause of an emergency in the adolescent. Contrary to intuitive reasoning, at menarche only 50% of adolescents are ovulating. With ovulation there are regular menstrual periods at about 21–35 day intervals (from the first day of one period to the next period) usually lasting 4–7 days with a total menstrual blood loss of less than 40 mL, with uniform shedding of the compact endometrium at one time,

---

Pediatric, Adolescent, & Young Adult Gynecology. Edited by A. Altchek and L. Deligdisch. © 2009 Blackwell Publishing, ISBN: 978-1-4051-5347-8.

> **Quick Take 22.1**
>
> **Abnormal vaginal bleeding in the adolescent**
>
> - Anovulatory dysfunctional uterine bleeding
> - Complication of pregnancy
> - Coagulation defect causing menorrhagia (long, heavy periods)
> - Local causes of bleeding (trauma, tumor in vagina or cervix)
> - Hormone-producing ovarian neoplams

with premenstrual molimina (fluid retention, breast fullness and some discomfort, abdominal distension, mild bilateral lower abdominal cramps) and sometimes with dysmenorrhea (Quick Take 22.2). Anovulatory "menstrual" bleeding is less regular, without premenstrual molimina or dysmenorrhea, and may arrive without warning (Quick Take 22.3). In those who do not ovulate, it may be several months to two years before ovulation develops and even then at first it is often irregular. About 5% of adolescents never ovulate and are later found to have polycystic

> **Quick Take 22.2**
>
> **Ovulatory menses**
>
> - Regular monthly
> - Premenstrual molimina
> - Often with mild dysmenorrhea
> - Starts and stops abruptly with complete shedding of compact endometrium

ovarian syndrome (POS). About 10% of these may have underlying, atypical congenital adrenal hyperplasia.

There are two types of clinical presentation of anovulatory bleeding (Quick Take 22.4). The more frequent of the two is complete irregularity of bleeding. Less common but characteristic is episodes of about three months of amenorrhea followed by one month of irregular bleeding and then repetition of this cycle of events.

The pathophysiology of anovulatory dysfunctional uterine bleeding is lack of ovulation. There is irregular shedding of the surface of the tall but very loose and spongy endometrium which cannot be physically supported, resulting in irregular shedding. With continuous estrogen stimulation there are attempts by the body to repair the surface. This explains the first type of irregular bleeding. The second type occurs with a slow build-up of the tall but loose endometrium for up to three months following which it is too thick to be supported and there is slow irregular shallow shedding (because the continuous circulating estrogen repairs it). However, it takes about a month before it can adequately reach the basal layer (Chapter 46).

Anovulatory dysfunctional uterine bleeding also tends to occur again towards the end of menstrual life at about ages 49–52 when menses tend to occur at 21-day intervals. At that time, however, there is a different approach because of concern about possible atypical endometrial

adenomatous hyperplasia or endometrial cancer. At the end of menstrual life or in the postmenopause endometrial biopsy is done promptly for irregular bleeding. Other adult causes include endometrial polyp, submucous fibroid, adenomyosis (endometriosis of the myometrium), and pelvic inflammatory disease (Quick Take 22.5).

A common urgent situation occurs when the frightened mother and young patient come to the office or clinic believing that the patient is hemorrhaging! The physician should be prepared with a basic plan of diagnosis and management. The immediate problem is to decide whether the patient is acutely ill requiring immediate hospitalization or whether she can safely be followed at home (Quick Take 22.6).

Evaluation (Quick Take 22.7)

History

The history includes details of the onset of abnormal bleeding, and whether it was preceded by the usual early puberty breast development, pubic and axillary hair and linear growth. Is it pubertal or prepubertal? Is there dysmenorrhea, premenstrual molimina, and regularity? Were there any other illnesses or medications when the unusual bleeding began? Is there any bleeding tendency, mucocutaneous bleeding or does the patient bruise readily? Has she had surgical procedures or tooth extractions which caused unusual bleeding? Is there a family history of bleeders? Could there be a pregnancy complication (threatened abortion, ectopic, hydatidiform mole)?

Estimate the total blood lost by how many external pads or tampons were used daily, what was the size of the pad and was each one fully soaked? Although it is difficult to estimate the blood loss because patients often exaggerate and occasionally underestimate, nevertheless more than 15 blood-soaked pads per menstrual period is of concern. Were there clots? Is she still bleeding and how much? If the physician is not comfortable in managing an acutely ill patient then immediate consultation should be made or referral to a large hospital emergency department (see Quick Takes 22.6, 22.7).

Physical examination

This includes pulse, blood pressure, checking for conjunctival pallor, mucocutaneous bleeding, bruising, ecchymoses, lymph nodes, and hepatosplenomegaly. Very often the patient and mother are reluctant to have vaginoscopy or insertion of a narrow vaginal speculum to rule out a local vaginal cause of bleeding. The patient and mother might permit vaginal insertion of a wet cotton-tipped applicator stick which can measure the depth of the vagina, which might provoke bleeding suggesting a vaginal source, and for cytology and maturation index of vaginal mucosa.

Ideally the entire vagina should be inspected with an adult-length, narrow, virginal bivalve vaginal speculum to detect laceration, pregnancy complication, rare aborting cervical neoplasm, benign or malignant vaginal polyp or foreign body (forgotten tampon or rigid object). A test for gonorrhea, chlamydia, and streptococcus of the cervix may be done. Bimanual one-finger vaginal examination may reveal pelvic tenderness or mass (pelvic inflammatory disease, ovarian cyst, neoplasm, enlarged uterus). Rectal examination should be considered. It is not always necessary to do a pelvic examination (especially if the patient and mother are nervous about it at the moment). It is a matter of clinical judgment and patient cultural pattern. If feasible, do a basic evaluation including general history, family history, general examination and some basic laboratory tests such as complete blood count (CBC), platelet count, quantitative hCG, prothrombin time (PT), partial activated thromboplastin time (APTT), von Willebrand disease (vWd) panel tests (blood type O may have low vW factor) (Chapter 24), comprehensive metabolic screen, thyroid function (TSH, T4), prolactin, pelvic ultrasound (probe on lower abdomen, not in vagina) (to check for polycystic ovaries, ovarian neoplasm, and rare polyp of the endometrium, cervix or vagina).

Office management for mild cases

Most cases of ADUB are mild, with no significant blood loss, normal blood count, and no disturbance of lifestyle (Quick Take 22.8, 22.9). They can be managed at home with observation, especially if there are suggestions of occasional ovulations. The patient is instructed to keep a menstrual calendar record of dates of bleeding and amount (numbers of pads or tampons daily, and whether they were fully soaked). Advice is given regarding healthy diet and perhaps oral iron. She should understand that despite apparent lack of ovulation she still has a risk of pregnancy (as well as sexually transmitted disease). Close communication is required.

With the usual mild ADUB most cases do not need oral contraceptives with the expectation of later spontaneous ovulation and regular menses. The patient and mother are told that normal body hormonal co-ordination is anticipated within a year or two and therefore future

Quick Take 22.8

Management of mild cases of ADUB without OC

- Observation and monitoring
- Periodic office visits and blood tests
- Keep menstrual calendar with dates and severity of bleeding
- Report heavy bleeding promptly
- Record premenstrual molimina and dysmenorrhea
- Advise on healthy lifestyle, diet, vitamin and iron supplement
- If desired, basal body temperature, serum progesterone (increases after ovulation, usually tested one week after ovulation) or home urine tests for ovulation

Quick Take 22.10

Plan for mild to moderate managed cases

- If mild, observe, offer supportive therapy, consider oral iron with expectation of later spontaneous ovulation
- If moderate, use cyclic OC to regulate menses. If bleeding is not controlled by OC in about two days, re-evaluate
- Continue OC for about six months
- If the patient is sexually active, continue OC
- If she is not sexually active, stop OC after six months and observe. If there is 2–3 months of amenorrhea, check blood estradiol and give oral progestin for 7–10 days which should induce withdrawal bleeding to prevent recurrence of ADUB. If the blood estradiol is low and there is no withdrawal bleeding it implies pituitary failure so consider skull-pituitary MRI

spontaneous fertility is expected. Both are advised not to discuss the situation with nonprofessional persons (see Quick Takes 22.8, 22.9).

Fertility drugs are not used but might be considered later in life when pregnancy is desired but not achieved.

With moderate ADUB managed at home there may be mild to moderate anemia (from blood loss) down to 9–10 g hemoglobin, because of heavy or irregular bleeding, but usually there are no symptoms related to the anemia. Oral contraceptives (OC) should be used after blood is taken for special coagulation tests. The usual OC used is monophasic norgestrel (0.3 mg) or levonorgestrel (0.15 mg) with 30 μg of ethinyl estradiol (EE) in the routine fashion for contraception. Start cyclic OC as soon as possible rather than waiting for a Sunday start day. If it controls the abnormal bleeding, continue it for about six months otherwise ADUB may recur. If it does not stop the abnormal bleeding within two or three days, re-evaluate and consider using increased amounts of OC as described for emergency hospitalized cases (Quick Take 22.10).

Quick Take 22.9

Possible basic evaluation for mild cases

- Prompt initial blood tests – CBC with WBC, differential, platelet count, comprehensive metabolic screen (with hepatic and renal tests), quantitative hCG, PT, APTT (Chapter 23)
- Pelvic ultrasound (Chapter 41)

Ideally the OC pills are stopped after six months when the patient is at home (rather than away at summer camp or school) and when life is tranquil (no examinations, etc.). The patient is carefully observed thereafter. If she is sexually active the OC pills are continued. If there is amenorrhea for two months consider oral progestin pills for 7–10 days to induce withdrawal bleeding and prevent recurrence of ADUB, and repeat for further episodes of amenorrhea. If there is no withdrawal bleeding after progestin consider repeating blood estradiol and if low, consider an MRI of the skull to rule out a craniopharyngioma or microadenoma of the pituitary. Atypical mild congenital adrenal hyperplasia may be suggested by family and personal history of acne, hirsutism or androgenicity (Chapter 4). Moderate or severe ADUB tends to recur, especially if there has not been any preceding normal menses.

The standard method of treating ADUB is with OC to regulate bleeding. Historically prior to the OC some adolescents required repeated transfusions and dilation and curettage of the uterus. Continued anovulation has led to relatively early endometrial hyperplasia, polyps and cancer in later life.

Hospitalization

Hospitalization is appropriate for continuing heavy vaginal bleeding, probable significant anemia, unstable vital signs, suspicion of coagulation defect, vaginal laceration, pregnancy complication, vaginal tumor or foreign body, or if the patient cannot be followed at home (see Quick Take 22.7). Basic laboratory tests to consider include CBC, platelet count, hCG, comprehensive metabolic screen, prolactin, estradiol, and thyroid function. Coagulation tests (see Quick Take 22.9) include PT, APTT, vWD tests (antigen, ristocetin, multimere), factor VIII, hemophilia, and platelet function (Chapter 23). vWD may affect 1% of the population. It is difficult to diagnose and may require repeated tests.

Estrogen therapy (as with OC) may disguise the condition. Therefore blood should be drawn before OC are prescribed. Most cases are mild but may be more severe with blood type O. Hematology consultation is helpful.

Coagulation defects (congenital or acquired) characteristically cause heavy prolonged menses (menorrhagia) at regular intervals (implying ovulation).

In addition to the basic blood tests (Quick Takes 22.9, 22.11), consider a hematology consultation, especially if there is heavy, prolonged, regular ovulatory bleeding (menorrhagia) which suggests a coagulation defect (Chapter 23). Some coagulation tests require a special coagulation laboratory. Hormone tests to consider include prolactin, follicle-stimulating hormone (FSH), luteinizing hormone (LH), estradiol (E2), progesterone, androgens (testosterone, dehydroepiandrosterone sulfate – DHEAS), and 17-hydroxyprogesterone (17-OHP). A high LH:FSH ratio of 3:1 or more and elevated androgens suggest polycystic ovarian syndrome (Chapter 31).

Pelvic ultrasound and/or pelvic MRI should be considered to rule out a hormone-producing neoplasm of the ovary, a metallic vaginal foreign body or a rare tumor of the uterus or vagina.

Management of the hospitalized heavy bleeding patient (Quick Takes 22.12–22.14)

Call a hematologist consultant immediately and give intravenous fluids.

I usually prescribe monophasic OC with 0.5 mg norgestrel and 0.05 mg ethinyl estradiol one pill three times a day, and usually the bleeding will stop or greatly diminish within 48 hours. If not, the patient should be re-evaluated. The OC may cause nausea and vomiting.

Some have used empiric intravenous Premarin 25 mg which is thought to stop the bleeding within a few hours even though the defect is lack of progestin. The disadvantage is that this has been associated with deep venous thromboses. The mechanism of action is unknown. IV Premarin should be followed by OC otherwise there may be recurrent bleeding.

Since the defect is lack of progestin some use high oral doses of progestin. Theoretically if there has been heavy bleeding the endometrial surface may be raw with only the basalis remaining and progestin alone might not be too effective. Nevertheless high-dose progestin, testosterone or estrogen alone or in combination can stop bleeding.

Traditionally OC have been used to stop bleeding for a few days and then discontinued to provoke withdrawal bleeding, termed "medical curettage." This may occur with heavy flow, clots, and cramps. I avoid this because it is uncomfortable, frightening and results in additional blood loss. My usual protocol is to stop the bleeding using one OC pill three times daily for 1–2 days, then reduce the OC dose to one daily for three weeks, then stop for one week for withdrawal bleeding. Then restart cyclic monthly OC and continue for about six months (see

Quick Take 22.13

OC emergency treatment for serious heavy bleeding in hospital or at home

- After coagulation tests are drawn, start OC

- I usually prescribe OC with norgestrel 0.3 mg with 30 mg ethinyl estradiol (EE) or levonorgestrel 0.15 mg with 30 mg EE. One pill every 4–6 hours after food

- Prescribe several packets of OC with instructions to discard the last seven placebo pills

- The main problem with several OC pills daily is nausea. Take them after meals. Consider antiemetics or skin patches (some have estrogen, others have estrogen and progestin)

- Progestin without estrogen may not control bleeding if there has been heavy bleeding with a raw endometrium down to the basalis

- Infrequently IV Premarin 25 mg has been used if the patient has severe bleeding, cannot tolerate OC or if on nil by mouth. It may cause deep venous thrombosis

- Rapid cessation of bleeding by estrogen within hours may be due to endometrial hydration. Usually OC are effective and IV estrogen is rarely used

- If IV estrogen is used, start OC several hours afterwards or the next day

Quick Take 22.14). Discontinuing earlier usually results in recurrence of abnormal bleeding.

If the first withdrawal bleeding is heavy and long, restart cyclic OC after only 2–3 days of bleeding. After stopping the OC for six months, if there is no spontaneous menses after 2–3 months give progestin, such as medroxyhydroprogesterone, for 5–10 days or oral progesterone, to

Quick Take 22.14

Review use of OC

- One pill twice or three times a day which should stop the bleeding within 48 hours or re-evaluate diagnosis

- After bleeding stops, reduce OC to one pill daily for three weeks (avoid placebo pills) to stop bleeding for three weeks, thereby avoiding further blood loss

- Then OC monthly cycling for six months

- Then discontinue OC, observe for spontaneous menses; if none then progestin at eight-week intervals to induce withdrawal bleeding for about three cycles

- About 5% never ovulate and later present as polycystic ovarian syndrome

cause withdrawal bleeding and avoid recurrence of heavy ADUB. This may be done for about three months, with about six-week intervals to see if spontaneous menses occurs (see Quick Take 22.14).

If there is no spontaneous menses recheck the serum estradiol after a rest period without hormone therapy for about three weeks. If the estradiol is low or the prolactin elevated or if there are visual disturbances or headaches, consider a brain MRI to rule out pituitary microadenoma or craniopharyngioma.

It may take 1–2 years of menarche before spontaneous ovulation and regular menses occur.

About 5% of adolescents go into young adulthood and never ovulate. As adolescents they present heavy irregular bleeding while in young adulthood they present with oligo- or amenorrhea, infertility, and polycystic ovarian syndrome.

DUB with amenorrhea or excessive bleeding may be associated with anything which prevents ovulation such as:
- severe disturbance of the general health (renal, hepatic, anemia, excessive weight, partial starvation)
- emotional stress (out-of-town school, intense study, making decisions, etc.), physical stress from excessive sport (practicing for marathon race, intensive ballet, etc.)
- anorexia nervosa, body image distortion
- over-active and underactive thyroid, other hormonal disturbances
- X-O chromosome mosaic of partial ovarian dysgenesis with premature menopause and elevated FSH.

Empiric dilation and curettage for ADUB is not done because there may be damage to the cervix, because of emotional disturbance, and because malignant conditions of the uterus and uterine tumors are very rare.

Some hospital reports indicate that a 10% incidence of adolescents hospitalized for DUB have coagulation defects. This is exaggerated because of patient selection. The hospital incidence represents inherited and acquired coagulation defects. More than 90% of DUB cases are managed at home.

Although there is no large, long-term study of the management of ADUB, there is a relatively unanimous empiric approach based on practical experience.

These cases should be carefully followed to rule out predisposing long-term problems such as atypical congenital adrenal hyperplasia, polycystic ovarian syndrome, infertility, oligomenorrhea, chronic renal or hepatic diseases, and premature menopause.

CHAPTER 23

Bleeding Disorders in the Adolescent Female

Aaron R. Rausen
New York University Medical Center, New York, NY, USA

Introduction

With the onset of menstruation, the adolescent female may experience menorrhagia. This may be the first manifestation of an underlying bleeding disorder. The relationship is not straightforward, however. Although 10–15% of women experience menorrhagia during their lifetime, the prevalence of bleeding disorders among women with menorrhagia is up to 20% [1]. This equates to over 2 million American women. Thus, although menorrhagia should raise the suspicion of an underlying bleeding disorder, the majority of women with menorrhagia do not have such a disorder.

Menorrhagia, defined as heavy, regular menstrual bleeding, should be differentiated from metrorrhagia, which is defined as irregular menstrual bleeding. Although a subjective term, a quantitative definition of menorrhagia is more than 80 mL of blood a month associated with anemia [2]. A set of working predictors of abnormal menstrual flow includes clots greater than 1 inch in diameter, changing pads more frequently than hourly, and a low serum ferritin as an indicator of iron deficiency, with or without anemia [3].

The most common inherited bleeding disorder in women is von Willebrand disease (VWD), although it represents only about one-half of female bleeding disorders. The diagnosis of VWD is based on a personal bleeding history, a family history and a low level of von Willebrand

factor (VWF). Prevalence of VWD among females with menorrhagia is estimated as high as 20% [4–8]. Conversely, more than 90% of females with VWD have menorrhagia, typically presenting at menarche [9]. Based on the above classic criteria for diagnosis of VWD, the prevalence is 0.6–1.3% of the population [10,11]. Most will have mild symptoms. Thus, the presence of menorrhagia alone in the adolescent female should arouse suspicion that a bleeding disorder exists.

Other less common bleeding disorders are associated with menorrhagia; these include hemophilic carrier state, afibrinogenemia, combined factors V and VIII deficiencies, factors XI and XIII deficiencies, Glanzmann thrombasthenia and Bernard–Soulier syndrome. A more detailed differential diagnostic list of bleeding disorders to be considered in the adolescent female is given in Table 23.1 [12].

Anovulatory cycles are more likely to occur in adolescence. They are associated with heavier menstrual bleeding. Thus during the first few years after menarche young women with VWD or other bleeding disorders are more likely to experience severe menorrhagia [13].

When an adolescent female has menorrhagia, the primary physician should use history, physical examination, and screening laboratory tests to help determine whether patients should be referred to a hematologist to rule out an underlying bleeding disorder.

History

The history should include a personal bleeding history as well as questions regarding family bleeding history. Use of

Pediatric, Adolescent, & Young Adult Gynecology. Edited by A. Altchek and L. Deligdisch. © 2009 Blackwell Publishing, ISBN: 978-1-4051-5347-8.

Table 23.1 Bleeding disorders in the adolescent female [12]

Coagulation	Platelet	Vessel wall
Congenital		
Hemophilia A, B carrier	von Willebrand disease	Hereditary
Factor XI deficiency	Bernard–Soulier syndrome	Hemorrhagia, telangiectasia
Other factor deficiencies	Glanzmann thrombasthenia	Ehlers–Danlos syndrome
	Storage pool disease	
Acquired		
Anti-VIII inhibitor	ITP	Physical: Valsalva, weight lifting
Vitamin K deficiency	TTP	Infection
Liver disease	Drug: ASA, NSAID, antibiotics, chemo Rx	Drugs: necrosis 2° to coumadin, heparin
DIC	Collagen: SLE	Dysproteinemias
Drugs: coumadin, heparin, antibiotics	Renal disease	Cutaneous vasculitis
	Leukemia	
	Myeloproliferative disorders	

medications, particularly aspirin and nonsteroidal anti-inflammatory drugs, which alter platelet function, should be ascertained. The site of bleeding as well as its severity, frequency, and spontaneity should be determined. As an example, epistaxis lasting more than 10 minutes, apparent spontaneous bruising, prolonged or heavy bleeding after dental work or operative procedures suggest an underlying bleeding disorder [14,15]. Inquiry should be made regarding the presence of associated medical conditions affecting the thyroid, kidney or bone marrow. Additionally, the presence of a bleeding tendency in male and/or female family members, particularly if of known etiology, should be determined.

Physical examination

Evidence of skin or mucosal membrane bleeding suggests impaired platelet plug formation (a defect in primary hemostasis) whereas hematomas or hemarthroses suggest impaired coagulation and subsequent fibrin clot formation (a defect in secondary hemostasis). Additionally, skin, oral or nasal mucosal telangiectases suggest a vascular wall abnormality. Lymphadenopathy or hepatosplenomegaly would raise the suspicion of systemic disorders with a secondary acquired hemostatic abnormality (such as thrombocytopenia secondary to leukemic marrow replacement or coagulation protein deficiencies secondary to hepatitis or sepsis-associated intravascular coagulation).

Laboratory evaluation

If a careful history and/or physical examination are suggestive of a bleeding disorder, it is appropriate for the primary physician to obtain some preliminary laboratory evaluation prior to deciding on the need for referral in the nonurgent clinical setting. Such tests would include a complete blood count, prothrombin time, activated partial thromboplastin time, and fibrinogen. The blood count would determine a quantitative decrease in platelets as well as anemia associated with blood loss. An isolated prolongation of the prothrombin time suggests the rare presence of factor VII deficiency; when combined with a prolonged activated partial thromboplastin time, on the other hand, it indicates an intrinsic pathway deficiency such as that of factor VIII, IX, XI, XII, prekallikrein, high molecular weight kininogen or, more commonly, VWD. It should be stressed, however, that in up to 50% of patients with VWD, the activated partial thromboplastin time is normal. Thus, referral for more definitive testing for VWD is not precluded by having a normal activated partial thromboplastin time, in the presence of a suspicion of an underlying bleeding disorder as suggested by menorrhagia.

In overly simplistic terms, referral to a hematologist with access to reliable laboratory resources for detailed hemostasis testing and, ideally, expertise in coagulation disorders is appropriate if platelet or coagulation test abnormalities were detected or no platelet number or coagulation test abnormalities were found but the clinical history and/or physical examination are significantly suspicious of a bleeding disorder. When available, my preference would be referral to a knowledgeable pediatric hematologist with the aforementioned ready access to a laboratory capable of performing and interpreting special tests of coagulation protein quantity and function, as well as assays of platelet functional defects.

There are a number of factors that may confound a precise association of a low level of VWF with a bleeding tendency. Since type I VWD is autosomal dominant with variable penetrance, its contribution to a bleeding tendency may vary widely even within families, and may seem to be unrelated to a given level of VWF. Additionally, ABO blood type affects the level of VWF. Blood group O individuals have a 25–35% lower level than blood group A, B or AB individuals [16].

A prolonged activated partial thromboplastin time should be studied by a mixing test, to differentiate factor deficiencies from factor inhibition, as well as a thrombin time, when appropriate, to evaluate possible heparin contamination. When necessary, uncommon platelet functional disorders of adhesion and aggregation should be evaluated. Platelet adhesion disorders suggest the congenital Bernard–Soulier syndrome or acquired defects as in immune thrombocytopenia or a myeloproliferative disorder. Platelet aggregation defects suggest congenital Glanzmann thrombasthenia or acquired disorders such as renal disease.

Recognizing the frequent problem of overlap of laboratory findings and symptoms between normals and patients with VWD and the absence of a definitive single diagnostic test, the diagnosis of VWD can be problematic. The recent development of a "bleeding score" appears, when positive, to correlate directly with surgical and/or procedural bleeding and indirectly with VWF:Ristocetin cofactor, VWF:antigen, and factor VIII levels, making the score a useful predictor of the risk of bleeding in patients suspected of having type 1 VWD [17].

General management

In the at-risk patient, liaison between the hematology consultant and the primary physician regarding a current and projected treatment plan, as well as family testing, is expected. Response to DDAVP (desmopressin) testing to determine its potential use with future surgery should

Table 23.2 Bleeding score for von Willebrand disease

Symptoms	Assigned score	Events
Epistaxis	0	no or trivial
	1	present
	2	packing/cauterization
	3	transfusion/replacement
Cutaneous	0	no or trivial
	1	petechiae/bruises
	2	hematomas
	3	medical consultation
Minor wounds	0	no or trivial
	1	present (1–5/year)
	2	medical attention
	3	surgical/transfusion
Oral bleeding	0	no or trivial
	1	present
	2	medical attention
	3	surgical/transfusion
GI bleeding	0	no or trivial
	1	present
	2	medical attention
	3	surgical/transfusion
Postpartum bleeding	0	no or trivial
	1	present/medical attention/Fe Rx
	2	transfusion/D&C/suture
	3	hysterectomy
Muscle/joint bleed	0	no or trivial
	1	present
	2	medical attention
	3	transfusion/intervention
Tooth extraction (most severe episode)	0	no or trivial replacement Rx
	1	present
	2	suture/packing
	3	transfusion
Surgery (most severe episode)	0	no or trivial
	1	present
	2	suture/resurgery
	3	transfusion
Menorrhagia	0	no or trivial
	1	present
	2	consult/pill use/Fe Rx
	3	transfusion/hysterectomy/D&C/ replacement Rx

be determined; however, testing should be done more than three weeks before projected surgery to avoid suboptimal preoperative response by depleting VWF stores. All patients with bleeding disorders should be vaccinated against hepatitis A and B, and be advised against the use of aspirin and nonsteroidal anti-inflammatory drugs. Since VWF levels increase during pregnancy and are often normal in the third trimester in affected women, retesting in the eighth month of pregnancy is recommended to determine the need for prophylaxis at the time of delivery.

Treatment

The treatment of menorrhagia in the adolescent with a bleeding disorder usually begins with the use of oral contraceptives. Even though reported to reduce blood loss and resultant iron deficiency anemia, oral contraceptive agents alone may be ineffective in 76% of women with bleeding disorders [12]. When menorrhagia is not controlled with a low-dose estrogen pill the pediatrician/primary physician in collaboration with a gynecologist may try moderate-dose estrogen or, if need be, continuous combined hormonal contraception to induce temporary amenorrhea. Limitations of estrogen use may include migraine headaches and cardiovascular disease.

The major hemostatic agent of use in type 1 VWD is DDAVP, a synthetic vasopressin analog (1-desamino-8-d-arginine vasopressin) which releases VWF from stores in endothelial Weibel–Palade bodies via cyclic AMP [18]. When given as a 30-minute intravenous infusion of 0.3 μg per kilogram, DDAVP is effective for mucosal bleeding [12]. Another formulation of DDAVP for intranasal administration, Stimate®, when used along with hormonal therapy, may work to reduce menorrhagia. The recommended dose is 150 μg (0.1 mL of a 1.5 mg/mL solution) as one puff in one nostril if less than 50 kg body weight or one puff in each nostril if equal to or greater than 50 kg body weight. Although menstrual flow becomes less heavy, this therapy may not reduce menorrhagia significantly [19]. These methods are limited by tachyphylaxis after depletion of endothelial stores as well as side effects of headache, flushing and, rarely, antidiuretic effects of hyponatremia or fluid overload if excess fluid intake occurs.

On occasion, when hormonal therapy or DDAVP is insufficient to reduce menorrhagia, antifibrinolytic amino acid therapy such as epsilon amino caproic acid (Amicar) at 50 mg/kg IV given every 6 hours for the 5–7 days of the menstrual cycle is suggested by some, although others feel there is insufficient evidence to strongly support its use [20]. Hemostatic control of menorrhagia in pa-

tients with type 1 VWD can also be accomplished with plasma-derived VWF-containing concentrate given intravenously. These products, however, are extremely costly and prone to the risk of transmissible infection. In dire circumstances, surgical intervention by dilation and curettage is usually of short-term, if any, benefit and needs DDAVP or VWF concentrate support.

The cytokine interleukin 11 (Neumega), which increases VWF levels in VWF-deficient animal models [21,22], is currently undergoing clinical trials.

A recent commentary emphasizes the need for a public health approach to lessen the significant compromises in lifestyle in adolescent and other premenopausal women due to menorrhagia secondary to a bleeding disorder [23]. These areas include a need:
• to improve the patient's self-awareness of the potential existence of a bleeding disorder (i.e. that it is not necessarily "normal")
• for the primary caregiver (the pediatrician or family physician) to think of the possibility of a bleeding disorder in any adolescent patient with menorrhagia
• for the hematology community to insure an adequate supply of well-trained and highly visible subspecialists to see such patients
• to develop improved screening methods to identify pathologic bleeding for the adolescent woman (particularly for VWD)
• to improve the available treatments for VWD and other bleeding disorders in affected adolescent women.

References

1. Shaw RW. Treating the patient with menorrhagia. *Br J Obstet Gynaecol* 1994;**101**:8–14.
2. Ragni M, Bontempo F, Cortese-Hassett AL. Von Willebrand disease and bleeding in women. *Haemophilia* 1999;**5**:313–317.
3. Warner P, Critchley H, Lumsden M et al. Menorrhagia 1: measured blood loss, clinical features, and outcome in women with heavy periods: a survey with follow-up data. *Am J Obstet Gynecol* 2004;**190**:1216–1223.
4. Edlund M, Blomback B, von Schoultz B, Andersson O. On the value of menorrhagia as a predictor for coagulation disorders. *Am J Hematol* 1996;**53**:234–238.
5. Kadir R, Economides D, Sabin C, Owens D, Lee CA. Frequency of inherited bleeding disorders in women with menorrhagia. *Lancet* 1998;**351**: 485–489.

6. Dilley A, Drews C, Miller C et al. Von Willebrand disease and other inherited bleeding disorders in women with diagnosed menorrhagia. *Obstet Gynecol* 2001;**97**:630–636.

7. Goodman-Gruen D, Hollenbach K. The prevalence of von Willebrand disease in women with abnormal uterine bleeding. *J Women's Health Gend Based Med* 2001;**10**:677–680.

8. Woo YL, White B, Corbally R et al. Von Willebrand's disease: an important cause of dysfunctional uterine bleeding. *Blood Coagul Fibrinol* 2002;**13**:89–93.

9. Fraser IS. Menorrhagia – a pragmatic approach to the understanding of causes and the need for investigations. *Br J Obstet Gynaecol* 1994;**101**(suppl 11):3–7.

10. Werner EJ, Broxon EH, Tucker EL, Giroux DS, Shults J, Abshire TC. Prevalence of von Willebrand disease in children: a multiethnic study. *J Pediatr* 1993;**123**:893–898.

11. Biron CB, Mahieu A, Rochette X et al. Preoperative screening for von Willebrand disease type 1: low yield and limited ability to predict bleeding. *J Lab Clin Med* 1999;**134**:605–609.

12. James AH, Ragni MV, Picozzi VJ. Bleeding disorders in premenopausal women: (another) public health crisis for hematology. *Hematology Am Soc Hematol Educ Program* 2006:474–485.

13. Silwer J. Von Willebrand's disease in Sweden. *Acta Paediatr Scand* 1973;**238**(suppl):1–159.

14. Drews CD, Dilley AB, Lally C, Beckman MG, Evatt B. Screening questions to identify women with von Willebrand disease. *J Am Med Women's Assoc* 2002;**57**:217–218.

15. Laffan, M, Brown SA, Collins PW et al. The diagnosis of von Willebrand disease: a guideline from the UK Haemophilia Centre Doctors' Organization. *Haemophilia* 2004;**10**:199–217.

16. Gill JC, Endres-Brooks J, Bauer PJ, Marks WJ, Montgomery RR. The effect of ABO group on the diagnosis of von Willebrand disease. *Blood* 1987;**69**:1691–1695.

17. Tosetto A, Rodeghiero F, Castaman G et al. A quantitative analysis of bleeding symptoms in type 1 von Willebrand disease: results from a multicenter European study (MCMDM – 1VWD). *J Thromb Haemost* 2006;**4**:766–773.

18. Kaufmann JE, Oksche A, Wollheim CB, Gunther G, Rosenthal W, Vischer VM. Vasopressin induced von Willebrand factor secretion from endothelial cells involves V2 receptors and cAMP. *J Clin Invest* 2000;**106**:107–116.

19. Leissinger C, Becton D, Cornell C Jr, Gill JC. High dose DDAVP spray (Stimate®) for the prevention and treatment of bleeding in patients with mild haemophilia A, mild or moderate type 1 von Willebrand disease and symptomatic carriers of haemophilia A. *Haemophilia* 2001;**7**:258–266.

20. Mannucci M. Treatment of von Willebrand's disease. *N Engl J Med* 2004;**351**:683–694.

21. Denis CV, Kwack K, Saffaripour S et al. Interleukin 11 significantly increases plasma von Willebrand factor and factor VIII in mild type and von Willebrand disease mouse models. *Blood* 2001;**97**:465–472.

22. Olsen EHN, McCain AS, Merricks EP et al. Comparative response of VWF in dogs to up-regulation of VWF mRNA by interleukin-11 versus Weibel–Palade body release by desmopressin (DDAVP). *Blood* 2003;**102**:436–441.

23. Picozzi VJ. Bleeding disorders in premenopausal women. *Hematology Am Soc Hematol Educ Program* 2006: 483.

CHAPTER 24

Congenital Gynecologic Anomalies I – Rokitansky Syndrome (MRKH Syndrome)

Albert Altchek
Mount Sinai School of Medicine and Hospital, New York, NY, USA

Introduction

Congenital absence of the uterus and vagina is known as Rokitansky syndrome, von Rokitansky syndrome, Mayer–Rokitansky–Küster–Hauser syndrome (MRKH) and Müllerian agenesis or aplasia. The ovaries are present and have normal function regarding hormones and ovulation. Therefore the patient has normal growth and development and is completely female, psychologically and physically. The chromosomes are the normal 46 XX. The disorder is not considered familial. The current theory is that it is usually due to many unknown factors (etiologic, heterogeneity or polygenic/multifactorial).

The incidence is though to be approximately 1/5000 female births. The only way to be precise would be to examine all newborns with inspection of the vulva and the passage of a urethral catheter into the vagina to make sure the vagina is patent and of the normal 4 cm depth. If there is any question then a pelvic ultrasound and/or MRI could be done. With the usual case there is no vagina but a shallow dimple where the vagina should be. Biopsy of the dimple shows normal vaginal mucosal cells even though there is no vagina. The dimple is the wall of the embryonic urogenital sinus whose mucosa could not grow inward to line a vaginal cavity. The condition develops at about eight weeks of fetal life when there is a failure of fusion of the

Müllerian ducts to form a single uterus. The upper part normally does not fuse and forms two separate fallopian tubes. Usually these uterine vestiges are nonfunctional, do not menstruate, and do not cause any symptoms.

Diagnosis

In the usual gynecologic practice such a patient is seen at about 5-year intervals. However, if adolescents are evaluated for primary amenorrhea an amazing 15% may have MRKH! Usually there is a delay in diagnosis because nature fools us. There is normal growth and development. Unfortunately time and resources are often wasted with x-rays for bone age, serum hormones, thyroid function and chromosomes, all of which are normal, while anxiety mounts. Once there is concern the patient should be referred for examination before extensive testing. In most cases the diagnosis is delayed until the ages of 13–17 (Quick Take 24.1).

The body contours are perfectly normal feminine (Fig. 24.1). The breasts are normal and there is sexual hair. The vulva looks perfectly normal including the labium majus and minus, clitoris and urethra (Fig. 24.2). Where the vagina should be there is a characteristic dimple of ruffled mucosa approximately 1.5–2 cm in diameter. No vaginal opening can be seen. There may be a vestigial hymen around the edges (Fig. 24.3). More often, the dimple has a variable appearance, often with blind 1–2 mm openings (Fig. 24.4). The physician is tempted to use a narrow metal lacrimal probe in the openings but this will cause a

Pediatric, Adolescent, & Young Adult Gynecology. Edited by A. Altchek and L. Deligdisch. © 2009 Blackwell Publishing, ISBN: 978-1-4051-5347-8.

Quick Take 24.1

Puberty without menstruation

- Before extensive, expensive testing the patient should be referred for examination.
- Examination takes only a few minutes and with adequate experience is relatively reliable.
- Early diagnosis avoids a prolonged build-up of severe anxiety.
- The physician must understand the marked psychodrama of the mother and patient when the diagnosis is revealed.

perforation into the bladder or rectum and may result in bleeding and scarring. If there is any probing it should be done gently with a soft urethral catheter or cotton-tipped applicator stick.

The condition may be confused with imperforate hymen (Chapters 2, 25). I have had patients operated upon with that misdiagnosis. On rectal examination no cervix is felt, but one may feel prominent taut sacrouterine ligaments bilaterally which meet in the midline. Pelvic and renal ultrasound is the standard diagnostic procedure, but ultrasound is not always reliable. In a personal series of about 100 cases, in four there was an optimistic misdiagnosis by competent radiologists of a small normal uterus being present. This gives the misleading hope that hormone therapy might make the uterus grow. The fact is the patient already has normal amounts of estrogen hormone and whatever uterine analog might be there will not grow further. In questionable cases laparoscopy may have to be performed (Fig. 24.5). In former years laparoscopy

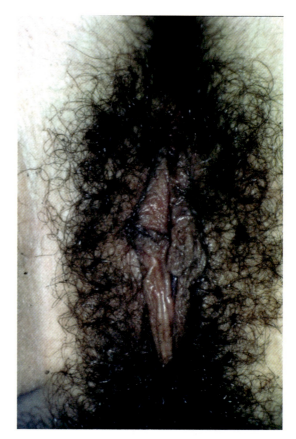

Figure 24.2 Normal vulva, normal pubic hair.

was routinely done before vaginal construction. In recent years, with more certain diagnosis, it is often omitted. I have done laparoscopic biopsies of the uterine analog section of the Müllerian duct. Most do not have an endometrial cavity. A few nonmenstruating Müllerian ducts have a nonfunctioning endometrium.

I had one case of a menstruating left Müllerian duct vestigial uterus with a cervix with menstrual blood collecting in the distended vagina cap around the cervix and causing pain. I made a distal surgical vagina to exit the menstrual blood using the distended cap of vagina and avoiding a skin graft because the patient was too young and emotionally immature.

In the usual case of Rokitansky syndrome the adnexa are high on the pelvic brim and not in the usual location deep in the pelvis. Unless the laparoscope is tilted to

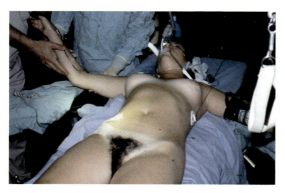

Figure 24.1 Normal female body contours, breasts and sexual hair in Rokitansy syndrome (patient in operating room, whole-body view)

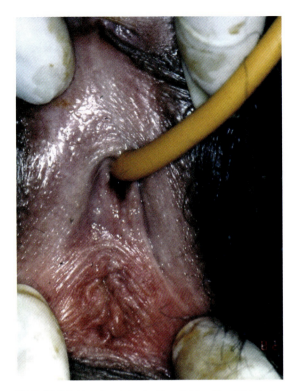

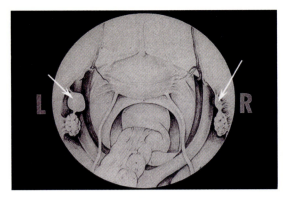

Figure 24.5 Laparoscopic view of pelvis. Left Müllerian duct (*arrow*) primitive hemiuterus is intraperitoneal with a small mesentery. Right Müllerian duct is retroperitoneal (*arrow*). Both sides have a round ligament of the ovary going to the primitive hemiuterus.

Figure 24.3 Rokitansky syndrome characteristic picture. "Vaginal dimple" of ruffled mucosa/ where the vagina should be. Normal labia and urethra.

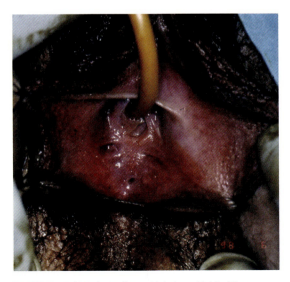

Figure 24.4 Rokitansky syndrome. Variation with blind 2 mm openings.

the side, the surgeon might erroneously believe that there were no ovaries. There are bilateral unfused Müllerian ducts. On each side there is a spindle-shaped swelling in the Müllerian ducts about 3 or 4 cm in length and 1.5–2.0 cm in width representing the primitive unfused uterine analog. The primitive uterus (Müllerian duct) may be bulging in the retroperitoneal space with no mesentery or it may be intraperitoneal with a short mesentery. A fallopian tube may or may not be present. The normal ovaries are always present together with the round ligament of the ovary (uteroovarian ligament) attached to the vestigial adjacent uterine analog (see Fig. 24.5).

Clinical differential diagnoses include androgen insensitivity which has a normal (high) male serum testosterone, karyotype XY, scanty sex hair, a short or absent vagina, no uterus, and often inguinal hernias containing a gonad (Chapter 5). Other diagnoses include agglutination of the labia minora, microperforate hymen, imperforate hymen (Chapters 2, 25) and distal complete transverse vaginal septum (Quick Take 24.2).

Management of absent vagina with a menstruating uterus requires differentiation from imperforate hymen and distal transverse vaginal septum (Chapter 25). With simple imperforate hymen the hymen appears thin and bulging, and has a dark blue-black tint above it due to old retained menstrual blood. With distal transverse vaginal septum and with absent vagina the hymen site does not bulge, does not have a dark tint and has a solid appearance. Rectal examination may be of help. If there is

---

Quick Take 24.2

Differential diagnosis of no vaginal opening

- Rokitansky syndrome
- Imperforate hymen
- Microperforate hymen
- Agglutination of the labia minora (not found in the newborn because of maternal estrogen)
- Complete distal transverse vaginal septum
- Large periurethral cyst of newborn (Chapter 2) conceals vaginal opening
- Androgen insensitivity, no vagina or short vagina (Chapter 5)

Quick Take 24.3

Rokitansky syndrome – practical approach to emotional support

- No one in the world is perfect
- You are fortunate not to have a life or death anomaly
- You are fortunate to have a loving, supportive family
- You are intelligent, attractive and have "the whole world in front of you"
- About 15–25% of married couples with a uterus do not get pregnant
- You can achieve satisfaction and recognition by excelling in studies, sports, leadership roles, community help, music, arts, etc.
- There are several methods of making a vagina
- Many of my patients have had successful, happy marriages, careers, have adopted children and some arranged for a surrogate mother
- There is every reason to feel that one day you will find someone whom you wish to marry and who wishes to marry you because of you
- There is no emergency to do anything surgically in the usual case without a menstruating uterus

---

an incorrect diagnosis of imperforate hymen the surgeon may encounter dense fibrous tissue of unknown depth and risk injury to rectum or bladder.

There may be other associated congenital anomalies in structures which form at the same period of early embryologic life. About 25% have an absent or pelvic kidney, about 15% have vertebral anomalies, and a smaller percentage have limb anomalies. Although rare, fused cervical vertebrae may present with a short neck (Klippel–Feil syndrome) resembling the webbed neck of gonadal dysgenesis (Turner syndrome) which has XO karyotype mosaic, short stature and small single uterus (Chapter 5). Perhaps because of increased investigation, mitral valve prolapse seems more common. Some cases have associated hearing defects.

Management plan and emotional support of patient

The patient and mother are anxious to learn the diagnosis because of concern about the lack of onset of menstrual periods. When the diagnosis is revealed there is a psychodrama that always unfolds. They are told that the patient will never menstruate, never be pregnant and, unless something is done, never have the usual sex activity. The patient and her mother go into a state of acute depression. I suggest a psychiatric consultation which the patient usually refuses, saying "I'm not crazy." I try to explain that this is a very stressful situation and she needs professional help. I urge her not to discuss it with friends to avoid gossip.

I have the patient and mother return in about six weeks at which time they are more calm. Even if the patient sees a therapist the therapist needs to understand the medical aspects so I have devised a practical superficial psychotherapeutic support [1,2] (Quick Take 24.3; Chapter 13). At subsequent visits I point out that no one in the world is normal. The patient is fortunate to have a loving, supportive family and not to have an anomaly which might be a life or death matter. She is also informed that anywhere from 15% to 25% of all married couples with the uterus do not get pregnant. The physician has to encourage self-esteem and confidence and emphasize the positive. If with time there are serious discussions of marriage and having children, it would be ethical to indicate that they are blessed to have found each other and would probably have to adopt children. All physicians caring for these patients agree that emotional support is equal in importance to the procedures to make a vagina and is important in the final result.

I review the current various options for the patient, pointing out that there is no emergency about any of these in the usual case because there is no functioning uterus,

---

Quick Take 24.4

Vaginal dilators (Frank method)

- The first thing to do if the patient is emotionally prepared
- Although old-fashioned, it should be attempted by almost all patients
- Candidate should be motivated
- Vaginal dimple nontender, soft, pliable
- Advantages – nonsurgical, might create an adequate vagina; if later surgery required, it is easier; the patient learns how to use a vaginal stent postoperatively to avoid contracture
- Requires frequent visits to the office to be certain patient is doing it properly and not dilating the urethra, checking progress, encouragement, and using progressively larger dilators

Quick Take 24.5

Possible options for creating a vagina surgically

- No method is ideal, which is why there continue to be various approaches
- Consider the advantages and disadvantages of each
- The patient should understand the options and which would be easiest for her to manage physically and emotionally
- Psychologic aspects and motivation are important in the final result of any procedure
- For the usual patient with Rokitansky syndrome, there is no emergency
- In general vaginal dilation is the best initial procedure

---

there is no pain, there is no obstruction of menstrual flow, and there is no retrograde menstruation which would predispose to pelvic endometriosis. The patient should be evaluated for other organ anomalies which also form at eight weeks, such as renal and skeletal.

Vaginal dilation

When the patient is emotionally adjusted and wishes to proceed, I always start with the possibility of dilators to develop a vagina [3]. If the area of the vaginal dimple is nontender, soft and pliable and if the patient is motivated, she is a perfect candidate for dilators. The advantage of vaginal dilators is that it makes subsequent surgery easier because it may develop a small vagina and also the patient becomes aware that whatever procedure is used to make the vagina, she would have to use vaginal stents for a number of months afterwards to maintain patency and to avoid secondary stricture. Ideally the dilators are used once or twice daily, about 15 minutes each time. Privacy is essential. If she lives at school she should have a private room. She has to learn by palpation how to avoid the urethra, and push the dilators in slightly posteriorly using a lubricating jelly. She should be seen frequently at 2–4 week intervals for encouragement, to check progress, to be certain that the urethra is not being dilated and to receive advice on using progressively larger dilators (Quick Take 24.4).

When vaginal dilation does not work

If the patient is unsuccessful with dilators and wishes to have a surgical procedure, explain the various options with the pros and cons (Quick Takes 24.5, 24.6) [4–8]. In former years surgery was postponed until several months before marriage. This concept is no longer valid because the patient may never develop an outgoing self-esteem, which will reduce her ability to socialize, and premarital sex has become acceptable.

Every few years a new surgical procedure is reported to create a neovagina. The modified McIndoe vaginoplasty "is recommended as the procedure of choice for women unable or unwilling to obtain a neovagina with dilatation methods. Women with a flat perineum with no dimple or pouch have no alternative other than the McIndoe vaginoplasty to obtain a neovagina for comfortable sexual relations" [4]. The vast majority of my cases have used the modified McIndoe procedure with good results.

The experience, preference and skill of the individual surgeon are important in deciding the surgery. All agree that the first operation gives the best chance of success, that excellent postoperative care is critical and that the patient should be emotionally adjusted and motivated. In the USA the most common procedure is the McIndoe operation [6] which is usually done by the gynecologist and avoids a laparotomy or laparoscopy. In the original McIndoe procedure a space was dissected between bladder and rectum and lined with one large piece of split-thickness skin graft. McIndoe used a hard, oval-shaped plastic mold to sew in the neovaginal space for six months and then

Quick Take 24.6

After initial trial of vaginal dilatation, consider possible options

- McIndoe technique (most common procedure in the USA)
- Dissecting a space and keeping it open with stents until the mucosal cells of the dimple grow inward (Wharton method) abandoned by Wharton because of postoperative stricture
- Dissecting a space for the neovagina and lining it with:
  - an inert material
  - peritoneum
  - transplanted rectum, colon or small bowel from the same patient
  - fresh human amnion
  - cultured human skin from a newborn foreskin to stimulate inward growth of vaginal mucosal cells of the introitus; experimental, one case report with long-term follow-up [12]
  - skin and muscle flaps
  - tissue expanders to develop extra skin for split-thickness or full thickness skin graft
- Williams external pouch
- Vecchietti operation

removed it surgically. He could not reduce the 2% incidence of rectovaginal fistula which was caused by the constant pressure of the hard plastic stent. There were also urethral and vesicovaginal fistulas from compression against the pubic symphysis bone. At present a soft mold is used to avoid fistula formation.

Several months after the McIndoe report, in 1938, Virgil Counseller, Chief of Surgery of the Mayo Clinic, USA, reported a similar procedure [7]. It is not generally known that McIndoe had been a fellow under Dr Counseller and therefore it is not certain who developed the concept. Counseller used a soft mold for surgery and later used a hard, plastic torpedo-shaped stent to prevent contracture with a knob protruding from the introitus. The patient could remove the stent, wash it and reinsert. Thus fistulas were avoided. Although the Counseller stent had been extensively used for prevention of late strictures, I found that it was too small. The original stent is no longer available.

Some have used a lining of inert material to prevent adhesions by keeping the raw dissected walls apart. The purpose is to allow the vaginal mucosal cells of the introitus to grow inward and cover the raw surface of the neovagina. Only a few cases have been done and the procedure is not used very often today. In the past peritoneum

was transplanted to cover the raw area of the new vagina but this too has not been popular.

Transplanted rectum, colon and small bowel have been used to line the neovagina. All these have the tendency for profuse secretion. They also require either laparotomy or laparoscopy to prepare the bowel segment.

Vecchietti devised a technique which is the reverse of the Frank test tube method [8]. Instead of pushing in the vaginal dimple, the Vecchietti operation pulls it in. Originally a laparotomy was done, but this is now being replaced by laparoscopy, passing a thin wire through the pelvis and the area between the bladder and rectum to emerge at the vaginal dimple. After attaching an olive-shaped plastic ball to the thin wire, it is kept under constant tension by a device on the abdomen which slowly pulls it up. This may cause the vagina to form in about 7–10 days by pulling in the dimple. A vaginal stent has to be kept in temporarily to prevent postoperative contracture. The advantage is that the neovagina is constructed with the patient's own vaginal mucosa. It is not FDA approved in the USA. A new modification is being done in the University of Tübingen, Germany.

Fresh human amnion from the delivery room has been used to line the new vagina. However, this has been discontinued for fear of spreading HIV or other illness.

Williams devised a completely different approach [9]. Rather than dissect a space between bladder and rectum, he created an external pouch by a U-shaped incision on the vulva. The advantage is that it is relatively safe, and simple, with minimum bleeding. The disadvantage is a bizarre appearance, different angulation and the external pouch results in distortion of the urinary stream. It is useful after previous unsuccessful McIndoe procedures with dense scarring (and sometimes fistula repair) and after radical oncologic surgery. In select cases I have used the Williams technique but I do not make the outer wall high enough to distort the urinary stream. The loss of depth may be made up with dilators for the scarred original dimple.

Skin and muscle flaps have been developed from the lower abdomen and inner thighs to line the new vagina. These have never been popular because of resulting scarring of the donor sites. The flaps with reattached circulation are very tedious and time-consuming procedures because the many small vessels can readily obstruct. In recent years tissue expanders (balloons placed subcutaneously in the groin and the labia majora) have been used to stretch the skin, excise it and use it as a skin graft for the neovagina. Hair grows in the new vagina if it came from the labia majora.

Menstruating uterus without a vagina

The only situation in which it is urgent to act occurs in about 9% with an absent vagina combined with a functioning uterus which may result in retrograde menstrual flow, episodes of acute pelvic pain, and possible pelvic endometriosis. Usually in these cases there is a single fused uterus with a cervix and a cap of normal vaginal mucosa around the cervix. I have noticed that whenever there is a cervix there is also a surrounding cap of vaginal mucosa which has endocervical histology without stratified squamous cells. This cap of mucosa can distend but eventually there is retrograde menstrual flow through the fallopian tubes. It can be detected on rectal exam when the lower pole of the distended vagina may be felt (Fig. 24.6). Imaging may also reveal this condition. If the condition is discovered relatively early before there is a large sac of old blood then surgery should be done promptly to avoid retrograde menstruation and pelvic endometriosis.

At Johns Hopkins (Baltimore), Jones recommended dissecting the space but without a split-thickness skin graft because the emotionally immature patient will not use stents postoperatively and is not emotionally prepared to have the skin graft from the buttocks. Accordingly he recommended dissecting the space and implanting a rigid plastic tube in the neovagina, keeping it in place for about nine months at which time it is removed and the vagina is found to be epithelialized by ingrowth of the cells of the vaginal dimple [4]. I found that at a later date the vagina would have to be made larger (wider) by the split-thickness skin graft technique. The other possibility is medication to stop menstrual flow until the child matures emotionally which might take perhaps six months or a year or two. This latter approach usually has not succeeded despite the theory.

If the distended upper vagina is not discovered until after it has enlarged and by downward pressure moved closer to the perineum, then the vaginal dimple is opened and dissected upward, reaching and mobilizing the distended sac, opening it to drain, suturing the sac edges to the introitus, and using a postoperative relatively soft mold to avoid contracture. If the distal dissected vaginal

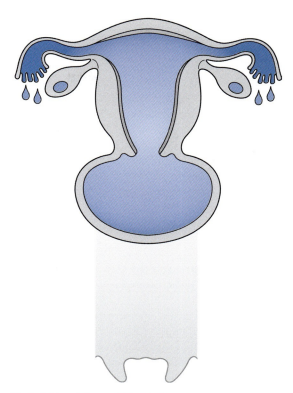

Figure 24.6 Rectal examination palpation – menstruating uterus, distended vaginal cap, retrograde menstrual flow, absent vagina.

width is very narrow, consideration should be given to widening it using meticulous hemostasis. Although some have recommended it, it is not wise to wait for the upper vaginal cap to distend significantly to make it feasible to reach by dissection upward from the dimple. If surgery is delayed for months the patient may experience progressive pelvic pain and recurrent retrograde intraperitoneal menstruation with an increased chance of causing pelvic endometriosis which may give a menstrual life of pain and reduced fertility. The retrograde menstruation is often discovered by emergency surgery for presumed acute appendicitis.

In about 1% of cases of absent vagina, there is a menstruating uterus without a cervix or vaginal cap. Attempts to create a surgical vagina and cervix have generally not been successful because the cervix fistula closes. The traditional consensus is that the uterus should be removed because there have been fatal infections with attempts at surgical correction. I have had two cases without a cervix.

The first was an emotionally immature 15-year-old who had previous unsuccessful surgery to create a vagina. I made a surgical vagina and cervix using amnion membrane. She did not use the postoperative mold to avoid stricture and despite repeated attempts to keep the vagina and cervix open, she finally had a subtotal hysterectomy. There was pelvic endometriosis. The second patient was emotionally mature, older, had not had prior surgery and was motivated. I used the McIndoe technique and created a "cervix" fistula lined with the split-thickness skin graft. It was successful but the patient was alerted to the absent cervix, possible later stenosis and difficulty in possible future pregnancy.

Personal approach to the McIndoe procedure (Quick Take 24.7)

This is a practical clinical approach based on approximately 100 personal surgical procedures over many years. The patient should be significantly emotionally mature regarding making an important decision, understanding the lengthy course of treatment, having the desire and motivation, and understanding that she has to be responsible for her own care and use the vaginal stent to prevent postoperative stricture which may take many months because of individual variation and the onset of coitus. She should understand the risks of any surgery and what results may be expected. Because of a normal vulva, labia, clitoris, and levator muscle pelvic floor, orgasm should occur. Of course initial coitus even in the normal female usually does not result in orgasm. It may take months or sometimes years and may never occur. With surgery to create a vagina, there is even more anxiety.

Unless there is an unusual menstruating uterus surgery is delayed at least a year to allow emotional acclimatization. Ideally the surgery should be done without school disturbance, such as during the summer vacation. This also avoids the need to fabricate reasons why the patient missed school. Try to do the surgery about six weeks before school. It is wise to avoid surgery on girls age 17 or younger. I do most cases after high school and before or during college vacations or even later. There is no rush. The patient should be in a private room to avoid the adjacent patient asking questions. The unadjusted patient will be miserable, will not use the stent, risking postoperative

---

Quick Take 24.7

Checklist for use prior to the McIndoe procedure

1. Patient emotionally prepared, understands and is motivated.
2. Prolonged postoperative care has been planned.
3. Enema or cathartic one day prior to surgery.
4. Written consent of parent and patient.
5. Preoperative evaluation, consider coagulation or thrombogenic defect because of postoperative bedrest.
6. Usually general anesthesia with endotracheal intubation.
7. If a plastic surgeon is to participate in taking the split-thickness skin graft there should be preoperative consultation with the patient trying on a swimsuit and graft marking outlined
8. Take the skin graft before the dissection of the neovaginal space if the gynecologic surgeon does not anticipate an unusual problem which might cause cancellation, such as bladder or rectal injury or prolonged surgery such as single pelvic kidney. The buttock graft is taken first with the patient positioned on one side. If necessary, a second graft may be needed from the opposite buttock. The donor site is dressed and then the patient is repositioned for lithotomy. Thus there is a minimum of patient manipulation under anesthesia. While the neovaginal space is dissected, the plastic surgeon can be suturing the graft over the stent with the raw surface exposed. This saves time and there is minimal repositioning.
9. Although often not necessary for diagnosis, if a laparoscopy is to be performed it should be done first for precise diagnosis of unusual anomalies which might affect the surgical plan. If the diagnosis seems reasonable and laparoscopy is desired, the laparoscopy is done after taking the graft and before the dissection of the neovaginal space.
10. Surgeons, anesthesologists and nurses must all participate in a checklist and co-ordination of patient placement while under anesthesia.
11. Good headlight, retractors, good assistants, long narrow instruments, comfortable seat for the surgeon for vaginal dissection, consider ultrasound harmonic hemostasis clamp, meticulous hemostasis, and avoid rushing.

---

stricture, and distress the physician. The surgery in the usual case is not necessary for health.

The oldest patient that I operated upon was age 40. Twenty years previously she had been erroneously told nothing could be done. She had a 20-year psychologic nightmare through having to reject close relationships.

Nevertheless she was now engaged to marry. She had a good result. Despite concern about bedrest for the first week postoperatively there were no complications.

General surgical management

The surgery should be done by someone with adequate experience regarding correct diagnosis and the actual surgery. The procedure is done infrequently in most hospitals because there are relatively few cases and most gynecologic residents never have the opportunity to do an adequate number. Adverse events include injury to the rectum and bladder, causing a fistula, hemorrhage preventing the take of the graft, failure of the patient to use the stent postoperatively because of inadequate psychologic preparation, and scarring resulting in contracture of the neovagina. Repeat procedures are more difficult because of scar tissue.

I usually operate on patients during summer vacations so the patient can be healed by the time the new academic year begins in August or September. I advise the patient and the parents not to discuss the details with visitors, and caution the medical staff not to discuss it with the relatives to avoid gossip. The patient is given moral support and encouragement privately without the parent because the patient has to use the stent by herself.

An enema or cathartic is given the day before the procedure to be certain that the rectum is empty. Stool in the rectum makes the surgery hazardous as well as increasing contamination due to the repeated rectal examinations. The hospital staff nurses and house doctors require special orientation. Whereas the usual gynecologic patient gets out of bed the day after surgery, these patients remain in bed for about 5–8 days postoperatively. For the first two days the patient remains flat in bed with pneumatic leg compression. If she coughs or vomits, the nurse checks the vaginal mold to be certain that it has not torn the retaining heavy braided silk labial stitches and been expelled. This becomes an emergency because if the graft comes out with the mold, it will die and must be immediately reinserted. It takes about two to three days for delicate capillaries to start to grow from the raw dissected space and nourish the graft. Movement of the graft will shear and tear the capillaries. On the third postoperative day the patient is allowed a larger pillow and is "log rolled" by the nurse to one side or the other. This aerates the back and takes pressure off the buttock donor site. The suprapubic bladder urine drain is left open continuously. If the physician

suspects it is not reliable, an additional soft indwelling urethral catheter should be placed at surgery. If the suprapubic drain fails it is extremely difficult to pass a urethral catheter postoperatively because of pressure of the inflatable stent (mold). On the fifth day the patient is allowed to turn side to side by herself. A low-residue diet is used to reduce the need for a bowel movement. Prophylactic antibiotic (usually a cephalosporin) is given prior to surgery. Urine analysis and culture is done. Since some have only one or a pelvic kidney, it is critical to watch for urinary tract infections. Some continue antibiotics as a daily routine until the second trip to the operating room. This does reduce the foul odor when the original mold is removed.

The patient is returned to the operating room about postoperative day 7 for a second short procedure best done under a light general anesthesia. Doing the procedure in the hospital bed is difficult because of inadequate light, exposure, painful removal of the large labial sutures, removal of the foul-smelling mold and estimating the graft take. The suprapubic urine drainage tube and urethral catheter if present are removed. The neovagina is gently irrigated. The original mold is discarded and replaced by another soft mold, either inflatable (valve opened when sterilized) or sponge rubber covered with a condom (gas sterilized). The patient is shown the mold prior to surgery. When the patient is awake and back in her room or on the next day the surgeon and the nurse show the patient how to remove, wash and reinsert the mold. This is done daily, especially before bowel movements. The nurse should be empathetic, encourage the patient and be prepared to help the patient reinsert the mold. The patient is allowed out of bed after the second visit to the operating room and is usually discharged two days later to be "on her own" at home. There may be temporary orthostatic hypotension.

About 2–3 weeks later a hard mold (usually called a "stent") is used to prevent postoperative contraction. It is easier to handle and clean in contrast to the soft mold. There are a variety of stents. Ideally it should have a bottle-shaped configuration with the wide side inserted obliquely and then rotated to lie flat, manipulated by a neck handle which is also used to remove it. It can be made to order using dental acrylic plastic or silastic. The flat shape is the same as the normal vaginal space (unlike the round shape of the Counseller and usual type stent) and it has less chance of falling out. The patient should be seen by the surgeon or educated nurse at two-week intervals to be certain that she keeps using the stent. After several months the use of the stent may be gradually reduced by leaving it out for increasing periods of time during the day, moving to only at night and then every other night. Eventually if there is adequate coitus, the stent may be discontinued. There is great individual variation in tendency to stricture. I have had patients who had been married several years and then divorced, stopped coitus for two years and at that time there was a severe stricture.

Even with regular coitus or use of the stent, all patients should have an annual examination of the entire neovagina because of a very small chance of benign or malignant neoplasms [10].

Schedule of surgical events

I have found that the most efficient surgical plan (assuming experienced staff with a typical patient), using minimum movement of the anesthetized patient and for time efficiency, is to follow this sequence.

1 Have adequate staff to reposition the patient under anesthesia. She is given general anesthesia with endotracheal anesthesia, lying on her back.

2 Then turn the patient to the right side to expose the buttock, if the gynecologic surgeon does not anticipate an unusual problem which might prolong or cancel the surgery such as bladder or rectal injury (especially due to previous scarring and adhesions) or complex pelvic kidney. The split-thickness graft is taken from the exposed buttock in one piece or two pieces. If necessary, do the dressing and move the patient to expose the opposite buttock to take an extra split-thickness skin graft.

3 Then have one surgeon sew the graft with the raw surface outermost over the mold, keeping the graft moist. If the graft falls on the floor, retrieve it, wash thoroughly and use it for the procedure with the expectation of normal healing. Use prophylactic antibiotics.

4 While the graft is being sewn, carefully reposition the patient to the lithotomy position. If a laparoscopy is necessary, it is done before placing the patient in lithotomy.

5 The gynecologic surgeon then dissects the space for the vagina with meticulous hemostasis.

6 The graft-draped mold is inserted into the raw vaginal space, sewn in place and a suprapubic urine drainage tube is made indwelling using sutures.

Preparation of skin graft and stent

For clarity, I refer to the initial operative soft form which is used to support the graft as a "mold." After a few weeks of healing, a hard plastic form is used to maintain patency (but not to dilate or stretch) for many months; I refer to this as a "stent." These are two different devices with different purposes.

The split-thickness skin graft is 17/1000 to 18/1000 inch thickness and is usually taken from the buttocks in an area covered by the swimsuit. The graft skin is thick enough to be transplanted to the dissected space while the residual skin is sufficient to re-epithelialize the donor site. In former years the skin graft was taken from the anterior thigh. Although it is easier, it is a psychologic disaster. Whenever the patient undresses or goes to the beach she will be reminded of her condition and people will ask questions.

A sheet of skin should be a full 4 inches width and 8 inches in length. Very often the graft is not that size and additional skin is taken from the same buttock or the opposite one to avoid a tight fit of the graft over the stents, which may impede healing, and to allow for possible later contracture. Despite some initial donor site bleeding, it stops spontaneously in a short while. A nonadherent Telfa® or Xeroform® impregnated gauze is used to dress the donor site, thus avoiding tearing the healing skin when the dressing is changed at the second procedure. When changing the dressing later, do not pull off an adherent gauze because it will cause trauma and bleeding. Simply cut the loose edges until the central area heals and the overlying gauze falls away by itself like an autumn leaf.

A dermatome drum (using skin glue) or an electric dermatome (resembling a hair clipper) (using skin lubricant) may be used while the skin is held taut with a flat instrument. The graft is draped over the mold with the raw surface outermost to be in apposition to the raw surface of the dissected vaginal space. The edges of the rectangular graft bilaterally are sutured with a fine absorbable suture to each other on either side, similar to a glove draping. Some surgeons place a shredder over the graft before placing it over the mold to expand the surface of the graft and create spaces which can permit discharge of any trapped blood or serum between the dissected space and the graft. Most surgeons do not shred, relying on excellent hemostasis.

The inflatable mold has a straight sausage shape, with a central midline drainage tube throughout the length of the mold extending beyond the mold to the exit 2 cm outside the vaginal introitus. There is a second longer tube for inflation. It is gas sterilized. Before using it, test the balloon

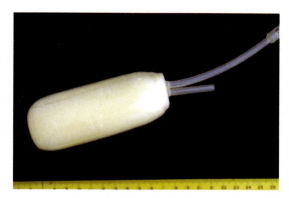

Figure 24.7 Inflatable vaginal mold. Short tube is for drainage from apex of vagina, long tube is for infections.

integrity and then empty it. The stent never completely collapses because it has a soft rubber core around the central drainage tube (Fig. 24.7). The graft covering the stent is kept moist with Ringer's lactate solution with the distal end of the graft near the introitus unsutured. I usually use a 12 or 14 cm length inflatable mold initially. I have a special model made of the 12 cm length mold which has a slightly wider circumference which works better to produce an ample vagina. The advantage of the inflatable stent is that it is ready to use. The disadvantage is that it is expensive, disposable, might be punctured as the graft is sewn over it, and, despite careful use of a ball lock and additional thumb screw clamp on the inflation tube, the mold is usually found partially deflated at the second procedure.

The other type of stent (made by the surgeon) is a sterilized, carved upholsterer's sponge rubber stuffing covered by a large, wide condom. The usual condom is not wide enough. This requires carving the stent in the operating room or preparing several sizes in advance. The alternative is to sew the graft over a wide sponge rubber form without the condom. Another technique involves placing a wide condom over a wide metal tube and inserting the sponge rubber or using the metal tube to direct the sponge rubber directly into the gloved graft as it is inserted into the dissected space. The Counseller vaginal stent is too small for the first operation and often gives an unsatisfactory result because of the resulting small neovagina.

Dissection of the vaginal space

The labia minora or majora are sutured laterally for exposure. An indwelling Foley catheter is placed and left

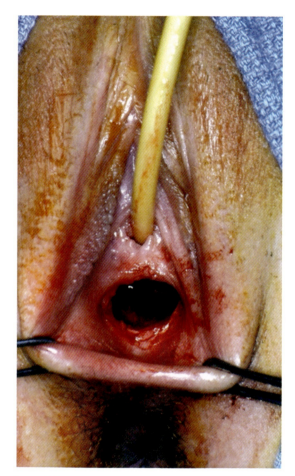

Figure 24.8 Transverse incision in vaginal dimple.

open. Rectal examination is done with double gloves. A transverse incision is made in the vaginal dimple, being slightly closer to the perineum than the urethra. This may cause some bleeding. After about 2 cm depth of incision, a relatively bloodless plane is reached (Fig. 24.8). Using a finger or a test tube, very gently dissect on each lateral edge of the incision cephalad. There may or may not be a midline sagittal septum from bladder to rectum which may require a very cautious incision (Fig. 24.9). Gentle one-finger blunt dissection is continued cephalad and lateral. Create a space for the neovagina larger than its final size to allow for some postsurgical stricture. A three-finger vaginal width above the introitus is desirable. If necessary, lateral incisions are made about 2–3 cm on either side into

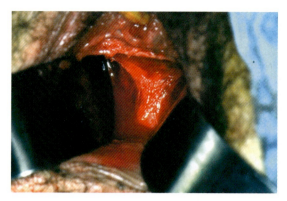

Figure 24.9 Midline septum connecting bladder to rectum, two curved retractors, one on each side.

the levator pelvic floor. It is easy to injure large vessels. Perfect hemostasis is critical because a hematoma under the graft will cause local necrosis. Suture ligatures may be needed deep in the lateral vagina. Care is taken to avoid injury to bowel or bladder and this is checked periodically. Avoid monopolar electric coagulation for midline bleeding because an underlying necrosis may occur. The introitus itself should be a little less than three fingers' width in order to contain a hard, self-retaining stent at a later time. The blunt dissection is carried up to the peritoneum until an exposure of 4 cm is made (Fig. 24.10). Further dissection may result in later enterocele. There may be congenital vascular anomalies with an extensive vascular plexus of collateral vessels from the inferior mesenteric-superior rectal, and from the internal iliac-internal pu-

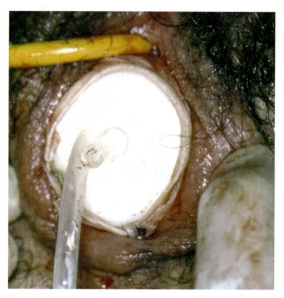

Figure 24.11 Inflatable mold covered with graft, raw surface outermost, in apposition to vaginal raw surface being inserted into the dissected vaginal space.

dendal arteries. This has occurred in two of my cases. It may be associated with a pelvic kidney and fusion of the bulbocavernosus muscle and unusual rectosigmoid vascular plexus. In the vast majority of cases there is no or minimal blood loss.

Placement of the graft-covered stent

The dissected space must be dry. Repeat rectal examination is done to check integrity. Remove any sutures found in the rectum. Repair any rectal tear meticulously and bring in lateral adjacent loose tissue for coverage. Check bladder integrity. Is the urine clear? Consider filling the bladder with diluted methylene blue or sterile skim milk, then empty the bladder. Any bladder tear is repaired without tension. Insert the deflated mold covered with graft, raw surface outermost, into the dissected vaginal space (Fig. 24.11). Sew the distal edges of the graft with interrupted sutures to the vestibule epithelium. Distend the bladder and place an indwelling large suprapubic urine drainage tube, which is kept open, and sew it in place. Gently fill the inflatable stent with about 50–100 mL of water or saline. Close the valve of the inflation tube and use an additional thumb screw or small hemostat clamp. Place two or three retaining heavy braided silk retention

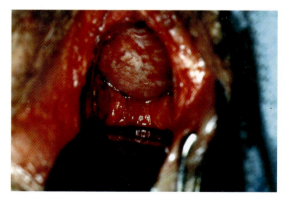

Figure 24.10 The liberally dissected, adequately exposed vaginal space – bladder anterior, rectum posterior. Good hemostasis.

sutures with an attached large sharp needle, using a deep bite through the labia majora above and below the stent tubes. Use bolster tubing to protect the labia. If it is certain that the suprapubic tube drains adequately, the urethral catheter may be removed. If the condom-covered foam rubber stent is used, it is inserted untied to allow trapped air to escape. The labia majora are sutured together to retain the mold.

The patient is taken to the recovery room where a sample mold is shown to the nurse with instructions to call if the mold comes out or if the suprapubic bladder tube is obstructed. The orders are reviewed again with the reminder that the patient remains almost flat in bed for 48 hours. This is unusual in gynecologic surgery. Postoperative pain occurs from the buttock donor site, the pelvic dissection and the retention labial sutures. After two days the latter causes almost all the pain. A small amount of vaginal bleeding may occur. Check the urine analysis and culture, blood count, and vital signs. Start clear fluids on postoperative day 1 and advance the low-residue diet cautiously. Some surgeons prescribe medication to prevent bowel movements but this may cause later hard stool rectal impaction.

Second stage of surgery

The patient is returned to the operating room 5–7 days later with a light general anesthesia for a short procedure. The retaining braided silk sutures are removed. The original stent is removed and discarded. The neovagina is gently irrigated and visualized. Usually there is an excellent take of the graft except at the introitus where the retention sutures have compressed the tissue. This does not cause a problem since later examination shows vaginal mucosa has grown inward rapidly for 2 cm from the vaginal dimple remnant. The patient is fitted with a new soft mold, often slightly smaller. The 14 cm length stent is replaced by a 12 cm. The 12 cm stent is usually retained even if it is slightly tight. The stent is held in by a binder.

The patient is allowed to dangle her legs on the day of surgery and is assisted out of bed the next day with elastic stockings to avoid orthostatic hypotension. She is also taught how to remove the stent, wash it and reinsert it immediately. Different binder devices are tried. The patient is usually discharged on the second postoperative day with instructions to return in 1–2 weeks, and call immediately if she cannot reinsert the stent. The buttock donor site is inspected and redressed but any adherent dressing is not pulled off to avoid bleeding and slow healing. Over the years there is further gradual healing and occasionally the scar is almost impossible to see.

After about 3–6 weeks the soft mold is replaced with a hard stent. The ideal is a hard plastic, acrylic or silastic stent with a flat bottle shape. The wider end is inserted first so that the narrow neck appears at the introitus. This stent is self-retaining because of the levator muscle, pelvic floor muscle and fascia. Nevertheless, an external pad may be helpful.

After several months the stent may be left out for gradually increasing periods of time until it is left out during the whole day. Progressively, it may be used for two or three nights a week and finally stopped when there is sexual activity. If coitus discontinues even after several years, the vagina may start to contract. Orgasm develops as with other normal girls. Urinary tract infections are of concern especially if there is absent or pelvic kidney.

There should be an annual complete visualization of the neovagina because there have been very rare benign and malignant neoplasms.

Types of stent and reasons for failure

There is no simple, readily available vaginal stent to prevent contracture. Although most authors refer to it as "dilation," in reality this procedure is prevention of a fibrous contractile stricture which is an inherent disadvantage of the procedure and the reason for the initial liberal overdissection of the space. Once there is fibrous stricture, dilation is often ineffective and it may require secondary surgical opening. The hard stent is started about 3–6 weeks after the initial operation when the graft is sufficiently healed and can withstand the pressure. The hard stent is easier to manipulate and cleaner than the soft mold.

The hard Counseller vaginal stent used to be the standard and was readily available but is no longer manufactured. Another manufacturer has produced the Counseller stent in silastic but I found it relatively too long, too slender, too heavy and it caused pressure on the vault apex. Dental laboratories can make acrylic vaginal stents to order.

The silastic stents of Jones are made in different sizes by Johns Hopkins technicians. They have a round cross-section and a slight bottle shape with a knob handle. The bottle shape helps to prevent expulsion. It is easy for the patient to handle (Fig. 24.12).

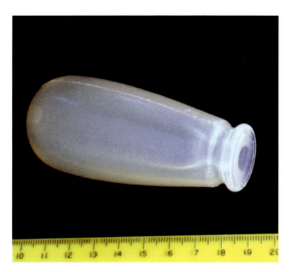

Figure 24.12 Silastic stent designed by Dr Howard Jones II when at Johns Hopkins.

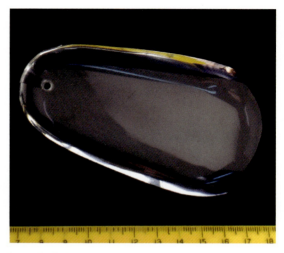

Figure 24.13 British stent, flat tear drop. Hole made at distal end to attach string for removal.

The ideal shape for a hard vaginal stent should derive from the shape of the vagina which is only a potential space and which is always flat. The traditional round stent has a round cross-section and presses on the bladder and may cause discomfort. Like vaginal tampons, it might predispose to lower urinary tract infection. The normal vaginal entrance is vertical. In order to be self-retaining and be flat, the stent has to be the shape of a flat bottle. The stent shoulders are held up by the levator pelvic floor (or puborectalis muscle fascia). The neck is narrow and the handle is a vertical knob which can be readily grasped between the thumb and index fingers. The knob avoids the urethra and is directed posteriorly. A British company manufactures a flat teardrop-shaped stent using a clear hard plastic. There is no handle. It is easy to insert and is self-retaining but impossible to remove. I had a hole drilled into the neck to attach a string to remove it (Fig. 24.13).

Live casts of the normal vagina have a flat bottle shape but in addition, on lateral view they have a slight convexity at the deep proximal end where the vagina lies on the pelvic floor and accommodates the posterior fornix and cervix. The ideal stent should have such a curve and a handle and should be inserted almost like an arched vaginal contraceptive diaphragm.

Thus the ideal stent should have an appropriate size, have a flat bottle-shaped body, with the proximal up-

per end slightly convex, narrow neck and knob handle, smooth surface easily inserted and removed, easy to clean, of relatively light weight but not fragile, and if possible slightly soft.

Graft sites may not take because of underlying hematoma, compression or infection, and granulation tissue forms. This may be treated by curettage or silver nitrate cauterization. If the area is small (less than 4 cm) the surrounding transplanted skin may grow over it. If the raw area is larger or in the upper vagina, it tends to persist and may require a patch graft. If the area is near the introitus vaginal dimple, the introitus mucosa will usually cover it.

Personal reflections on the McIndoe procedure

It was previously thought that the transplanted split-thickness skin graft in the neovagina became vaginal mucosa. However, this is not the case. If vaginal mucosa appears, it simply grew from the introitus dimple to cover over raw spaces where the original transplanted skin did not take. In cases where there is a complete take of the graft one finds postoperatively that the new vagina has a complete skin coverage and in addition, there are dark patches because of the original skin color compared to the pink of the normal vagina. Also, biopsies show skin sweat glands. There is no hair growth on the skin transplant from the buttocks.

Human epidermis (keratinocytes) taken from the intact skin of burn victims can be cultured *in vitro* and within three weeks develop enough skin surface to cover the entire body. This has been used to cover raw surface skin if there is no pressure placed on it. It is very thin and delicate. It was used once elsewhere for the McIndoe procedure to line the neovagina. The thin layer of epidermis was destroyed by pressure necrosis from the vaginal stent.

In vitro culture of human skin and vaginal mucosa has been done in a relatively thick spongy layer of bovine collagen to protect it from pressure and provide a framework for multilayers [11]. It should not be rejected, should not be destroyed by pressure, would avoid the need for a large graft and should result in a mucosa-lined vagina.

I have performed one case in an emotionally mature, motivated patient who insisted on a McIndoe procedure without a skin graft and who would use a postoperative stent. I used living, human, bilayered skin cultured from a newborn foreskin with a good long-term result. This is still experimental. Although the cultured skin had lost its early rejection response, later rejection occurred two weeks afterward. Nevertheless, the numerous growth stimulants caused rapid ingrowth of the vaginal mucosal cells of the dimple and there was a good result [12]. This is also experimental.

No method is ideal. Despite overall patient satisfaction, the McIndoe procedure gives a flat vaginal wall, in contrast to the folds of the normal vagina, may be dry and require lubrication, and gives a Pap cytology report of "anucleated squamous cells." If done carefully, the transplanted skin persists. It retains the color of the original donor site rather than the normal pink vaginal mucosa color. Biopsy proves it to be skin with keratin and occasionally skin sweat glands. Occasionally there may be a slight malodor. Areas where the skin transplant did not survive are covered by mucosa growing up from the introitus. Some textbooks erroneously suggest that the skin transmutes into mucosa but it is just a replacement process. When viewed externally, it appears to be a perfectly normal vagina, although occasionally persistent skin may be visible with a wide introitus. There may be a susceptibility to postoperative stricture if there is no coitus or use of a stent.

The Vecchietti operation to create a vagina by pulling the vaginal dimple in has been popular in Europe. In the USA the original abdominal line tension apparatus did not have FDA approval but laparoscopy and laparotomy techniques give similar results [13]. The neovagina is the patient's own vaginal mucosa and the vagina can be created in about 10 days. New instruments made by Karl Storz, Tuttlingen, Germany, have been compared with the original apparatus designed by Vecchietti in the laparoscopic Vecchietti operation and were found to be a "small but significant improvement" [14]. At the University of Tübingen in Germany, a new version of the Vecchietti operation is being done using improved laparoscopy instruments made by Storz for this operation [15]. Holding an ultrasound transducer against the vaginal dimple, "endovaginal sonography" can guide the penetrating wire from the abdomen between the bladder and rectum [16].

The Williams operation for the MRKH syndrome was improved in 2001 by the Creatsas modification [17].

I now have a number of patients who, after extensive counseling, have started to use surrogacy motherhood in which the patient's eggs are fertilized with her husband's sperm *in vitro* and then implanted in the uterus of another woman. The new child is a biologic child of the patient with the Rokitansky syndrome.

There is speculation about the future possibility of human uterus transplantation in select cases (International Conference on Transplantation of the Uterus, Sahlgrenska Academy at Göteborg University, Sweden, April 1, 2007, at which I was a participant).

References

1. Altchek A. Congenital absence of the uterus and vagina. In: Altchek A, Deligdisch L (eds) *The Uterus: Pathology, Diagnosis and Management.* New York: Springer Verlag, 1991:272–293.
2. Altchek A. Psychologic aspects of adolescent obstetric and gynecologic conditions. In: Heacock DR (ed) *A Psychodynamic Approach to Adolescent Psychiatry. The Mount Sinai Experience.* New York: Marcel Dekker, 1980:239–278.
3. Frank RT. The formation of an artificial vagina without operation. *Am J Obstet Gynecol* 1938;**35**:1053–1055.
4. Rock JA, Beech LL. Surgery for anomalies of the Müllerian duct. In: Rock JA, Jones HW III (eds) *Te Linde's Operative Gynecology*, 9th edn. Philadelphia, PA: Lippincott, Williams and Wilkins, 2003.
5. ACOG. *Vaginal Agenesis: Diagnosis, Management and Routine Care.* Committee Opinion No. 355. Washington, DC: ACOG, 2006:1605–1609.

6. McIndoe AH, Bannister JB. An operation for the cure of congenital absence of the vagina. *J Obstet Gynaecol Br Emp* 1938;**5**:490–494.

7. Counseller VA. Congenital absence of the vagina and traumatic obliteration of vagina and its treatment with inlaying Thiersch grafts. *Am J Obstet Gynecol* 1938;**36**:632–638.

8. Vecchietti G. The neovagina in the Rokitansky–Kuster–Hauser syndrome. *Rev Med Suisse Romande* 1979;**99**(9):593–601.

9. Williams EA. Congenital absence of the vagina – a simple operation for its relief. *J Obstet Gynaecol Br Commonw* 1964;**71**:511.

10. Altchek A, Deligdisch L, Idrees MT. Squamous papilloma with hyperpigmentation developing in the skin graft of the neovagina in Rokitansky syndrome. *J Pediatr Adolesc Gynecol* 2006;**19**(2):154.

11. Doillon CJ, Altchek A, Silver FH. Method of growing vaginal mucosal cells on a collagen sponge matrix. Results of preliminary studies. *J Reprod Med* 1990;**35**(3):203–207.

12. Altchek A, Brem H. Case report: the first reported successful use of human skin equivalent (APLIGRAF®) to line new vagina in Rokitansky syndrome. *J Pediatr Adolesc Gynecol* 2005;**18**:215–218.

13. Borruto F, Camoglio FS, Zampieri N, Fedele L. The laparoscopic Vecchietti technique for vaginal agenesis. *Int J Gynecol Obstet* 2007;**98**(1):15–19.

14. Fedele L, Bianchi S, Berlanda N, Fontana E, Bulfoni A, Borruto F. Laparoscopic creation of a neovagina with the laparoscopic Vecchietti operation: comparison of two instrument sets. *Fertil Steril* 2006;86(2):694–699.

15. Brucker S, Gegusch W, Zubke K et al. Neovagina creation in vaginal agenesis: development of a new laparoscopic Vecchietti-based procedure and optimized instruments in a prospective comparative interventional study in 101 patients. *Fertil Steril* 2008. Epub ahead of print.

16. Csermely T, Halvax L, Vizer M et al. The application of 'endovaginal' sonography during a laparoscopy-assisted Vecchietti operation. *Acta Obstet Gynaecol Scand* 2007;86(10):1231–1235.

17. Creatsas G, Deligeoroglou E, Makrakis E, Kontoravdis A, Papadimitriou L. Creation of a neovagina following Williams vaginoplasty and the Creatsas modification in 111 patients with Mayer–Rokitansky–Küster–Hauser syndrome. *Fertil Steril* 2001;**76**(5):1036–1040.

CHAPTER 25

Congenital Anomalies II – "No Eponym Syndrome," and Diagnostic Problems

Albert Altchek

Mount Sinai School of Medicine and Hospital, New York, NY, USA

The "no eponym" syndrome

I have used this name to designate a syndrome of uterus didelphys, double vagina with unilateral distal vagina aplasia resulting in outflow obstruction and ipsilateral renal agenesis. It is considered to be extremely rare. The incidence is less than that of Rokitansky syndrome but still considerable. It is under-reported because of difficulty in diagnosis, lack of a name, making it difficult to find it in an index or a review of the literature, and the relatively few case reports each of which uses different descriptions.

It is infrequently discovered in the newborn when an obstructed vaginal mucosal wall bulges through the hymen. This is due to a low unilateral vaginal agenesis which distends due to maternal estrogen-induced endocervical secretion and it bulges at the hymen. The diagnosis is suggested by an absent kidney on the obstructed side. The bulge may gradually retract as the distending mucus is absorbed. The patient should be observed if she is asymptomatic but should have surgical correction at puberty.

Depending on the capacity of the obstructed vagina, the dysmenorrhea may start with the first menses or after many months. Diagnosis and management require special expertise and the patient should be referred.

Before there is extensive dilation of the upper obstructed vagina, vaginoscopy might be able to reach the

Pediatric, Adolescent, & Young Adult Gynecology. Edited by A. Altchek and L. Deligdisch. © 2009 Blackwell Publishing, ISBN: 978-1-4051-5347-8.

> **Quick Take 25.1**
>
> **When to suspect the "no eponym" syndrome**
>
> - Progressively severe unilateral dysmenorrhea despite apparently unobstructed menstrual flow and despite oral contraceptives
> - Later, continuous unilateral pain
> - Palpation may indicate a tender tense cystic unilateral lower abdominal mass
> - Rectal examination reveals a tender tense cystic mass on one side of the vagina and posteriorly
> - With one-finger vaginal examination, there is medial vaginal wall bulging into the vagina

unobstructed cervix which may show the external os with a wide abnormal opening and displaced medially and either anteriorly or posteriorly.

The typical case presents in late puberty with regular menstrual periods accompanied by severe pelvic pain, usually unilateral. The obstructed vagina and uterus become distended with old menstrual blood and there is unilateral retrograde menstruation causing peritoneal endometriosis. If the patient and parent permit, a one-finger vaginal examination reveals a paravaginal, slightly posterior, tense cystic mass. It can also be appreciated by rectal examination. The height of the mass indicates the level of the obstruction. Pelvic and renal ultrasound reveal a cystic mass and an ipsilateral absent kidney (Quick Take 25.1). The cystic mass may be misdiagnosed as an ovarian cyst, leading to an incorrect abdominal surgical

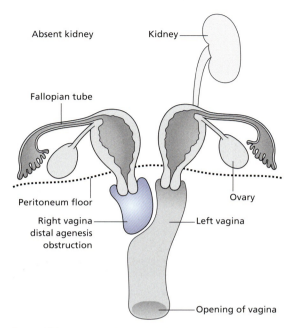

Figure 25.1 "No eponym" syndrome. Before the onset of menses there are no symptoms. Uterus didelphys, aplasia distal right vagina, absent right kidney.

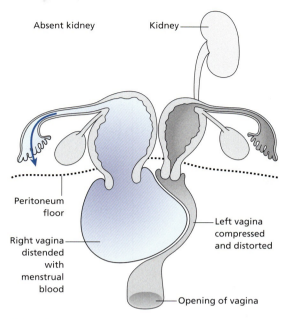

Figure 25.2 After the onset of menses the right vagina distends with retained menstrual blood and cyclic right lower quadrant pain begins months later.

approach (Figs 25.1–25.3). The pelvic ultrasound may report possible bicornuate or septate uterus with uncertainty regarding the cervix. MRI will give a better picture of the cervix. Renal ultrasound is recommended for close relatives.

The introitus of the vagina appears normal. Rarely, with a low vaginal obstruction the bulging vagina presents itself (Fig. 25.4). A higher or smaller obstructed vagina may have to be pulled down for exposure (Fig. 25.5).

The therapy is a vaginal surgical approach. The typical patient varies in age from 12 to 15 years with a long, narrow vagina. The ideal procedure is complete marsupialization of the bulging upper vagina to form a single vagina. It should be done only by an experienced surgeon. It requires a good headlight, expert assistance, good retractors, and long narrow instruments. An operating hysteroscope has been used. Before cutting into the presumed obstructed upper vagina, aspirate old menstrual blood to verify location (Fig. 25.6).

The goal is to remove a large part of the median wall of the distended vagina by marsupialization at one time. The problems are adequate visualization and avoiding

injury to the bladder or rectum. In addition, the wall varies in thickness and vascularity. Hemostatic running locked sutures and interrupted figure-of-eight sutures tend to result in a "pursestring effect" with narrowing of the opening, which also tends to narrow with healing. Nonelectric (to avoid burn injury), crushing, coagulation,

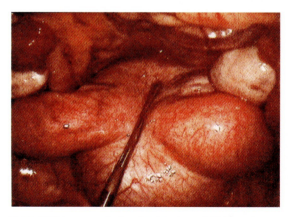

Figure 25.3 Laparoscopic view showing uterus didelphys and marked distension of the upper obstructed vagina.

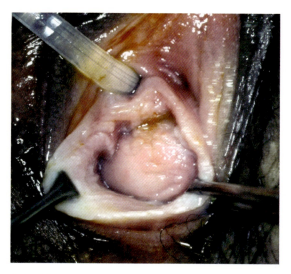

Figure 25.4 Distended upper left vagina protruding from introitus.

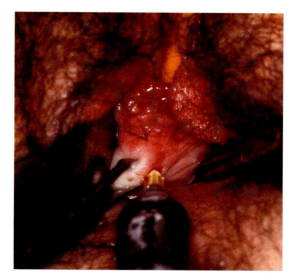

Figure 25.6 Aspiration of old blood to verify location of obstructed upper vagina.

ultrasound-type forceps are helpful (Ethicon harmonic scalpel Ace® and Sure-Seal, Valley Lab, Tycos®) to reduce the "purse string" tendency (Quick Take 25.2).

If it is not possible to do a complete marsupialization, perform a partial procedure to relieve the obstruction and consider a second vaginal operation several months later to complete the opening. There is danger of closure and infection. If a second procedure fails, consider an abdom-

inal approach to remove the obstructed uterus (Quick Take 25.3).

Occasionally, the obstructed vagina has minute openings which permit infection which may require urgent surgery for vaginal drainage. With recurrent closure, the obstructed vagina may become a sac of pus. There is the danger of ascending infection and the obstructed uterus may have to be removed from above.

If one uterus requires removal it might be done by laparoscopic morcellation. Its fallopian tube may require removal because of damage by pyosalpinx or hematosalpinx.

At observational laparoscopy in an otherwise uncomplicated case with hematosalpinx, there is no unanimity on whether to evacuate it through the open fimbria or

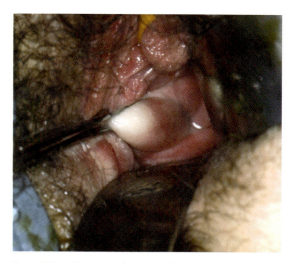

Figure 25.5 Pulling down obstructed left upper distended vagina.

Quick Take 25.2

Surgery for "no eponym" syndrome

- Requires experience and expert assistance
- The approach is vaginal, not abdominal
- It is difficult because the vagina is narrow in the young patient, the bladder or rectum may be injured, and it may be difficult to do an adequate marsupialization of the obstructed vagina

Quick Take 25.3

Considerations at the first surgery for "no eponym" syndrome

- If the marsupialization is inadequate, do a second vaginal operation to enlarge it
- If the marsupialization has closed, either do a second vaginal marsupialization (which has a risk for infection) or via laparoscopy or laparotomy remove the obstructed uterus
- With the latter, consider removal of the obstructed hematosalpinx to avoid infection and possible later ectopic pregnancy. The ovary is preserved on the obstructed side

leave it alone, assuming that relief of the vaginal obstruction would allow spontaneous evacuation.

Follow-up of fertility is not adequate. Intuitively one assumes later pregnancy should be in the unobstructed uterus. A patient on whom I had done a right vaginal marsupialization later had a successful pregnancy and vaginal delivery at 36.5 weeks in the previously obstructed right uterus. The postpartum examination showed a small normal right cervix and a patulous, less formed left cervix. This is counterintuitive. Others have noticed this also. Aside from the fact that it is standard practice to simply do a marsupialization and leave both of the uteri, try not to remove the obstructed uterus. Despite suggestions that there is an unfavorable prognosis for a later successful pregnancy, my experience suggests a relatively good prognosis. There may be a tendency for labor to start three or four weeks early because of the small size of the uterus. The cervix may dilate slowly in labor because of an increased amount of fibrous tissue and there is a possibility of cesarean section.

There is a rare variant in which one uterus lacks a patent cervix. I had such a case with an ipsilateral absent kidney and only one vagina. The cervix site had a dimple which was bluntly opened and a stent was left indwelling. The stent was expelled in two weeks. Postoperative MRI showed cervix closure and hematometra of the affected uterus and hematosalpinx. It took several months before the cyclic pain recurred. Rather than risk infection, this patient was reoperated and had a laparoscopic morcellation of the left obstructed uterus and removal of the hematosalpinx. The normal ovary was left in place. There was early peritoneal endometriosis. Because of an absent kidney on the obstructed side, there is no ureter to avoid

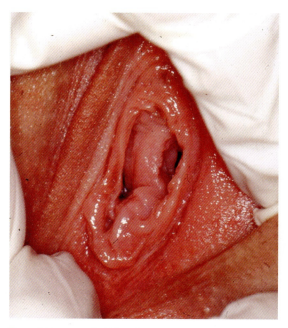

Figure 25.7 Unusually thick midline longitudinal vaginal septum visible from the introitus.

during surgery. There was no sign of the cervix. Postoperative examination showed an indurated left pelvis.

As with Rokitansky syndrome, failure of fusion of the embryonic Müllerian ducts at eight weeks results in an extraordinary variety of uterine anomalies ranging from the least affected arcuate uterus, to septate uterus, bicornuate uterus, didelphic uterus, unicollis uterus and finally to the most affected Rokitansky syndrome. The latter retains the unfused ducts. With these fusion failures there are other embryonic developmental failures also occurring at eight weeks, especially renal and skeletal.

Longitudinal vaginal septum

The midline longitudinal vaginal septum is asymptomatic. It may be discovered by routine examination and can be visualized by holding the labia apart (Fig. 25.7). Sometimes the patient discovers it by palpation while inserting a vaginal tampon and when two tampons are required.

The septum may extend to the vaginal vault with a uterus didelphys or may end before reaching the vault. If it disturbs the patient emotionally, surgery is appropriate.

It is also done for dyspareunia and prior to pregnancy if desired (Quick Take 25.4).

Although the surgery seems simple, complications do arise. The preparation is similar to that of the "no eponym" syndrome (see Quick Take 25.2).

There is a normal tendency to start by cutting the anterior edge because the septum holds it down. It is better to start with the posterior edge otherwise if the entire anterior edge was cut, it would be awkward to hold up the septum to cut posteriorly. Excessive pulling on the septum may result in excising too wide an area. If this occurs on both walls, anterior–posterior adhesions may occur. In addition, excessive pulling may result in injury to the bladder or rectum. If this occurs, identify it at once and repair it in layers. Leave an indwelling bladder catheter if injured. Healing should be uneventful. Being overly cautious may leave a residual septum base. This is usually not a problem unless the patient places her finger in the vagina when inserting the tampon.

If the septum is thin, if visualization is not ideal, and if speed is essential, simply cut the septum in the midline leaving residue on the anterior and posterior walls (Quick Take 25.5).

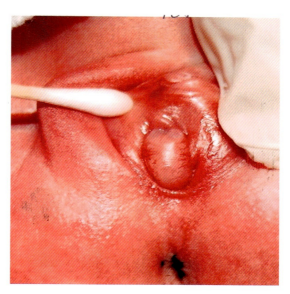

Figure 25.8 Imperforate hymen in a newborn; bulging vagina due to endocervical mucus stimulated by maternal estrogen (gloves should be worn).

Imperforate hymen

Imperforate hymen may be discovered at birth on routine examination or because of a pelvic mass. Maternal estrogen can stimulate endocervical mucus which accumulates in the vagina and the hymen will bulge. It may be imaged by ultrasound and palpated by rectal examination. Previously management was simply to have the patient return in early puberty for surgery. The proper management is periodic observation and surgery if the vagina distends significantly before puberty.

Infrequently the newborn (Fig. 25.8) has a distended abdomen causing cardiorespiratory distress due to excessive endocervical mucus distending the obstructed vagina by imperforate hymen or complete transverse vaginal septum. Figure 25.9 shows an imperforate hymen in an infant. Figure 25.10 shows an unusual case of imperforate hymen in an infant which bulged when crying.

Dependent on case selection and routine practice, many cases are not discovered until menarche. Cyclic pain does not occur until after several months of concealed menstruation because the vagina can distend. There is a palpable suprapubic mass, a distended imperforate hymen and a cystic mass on rectal examination. The pelvic

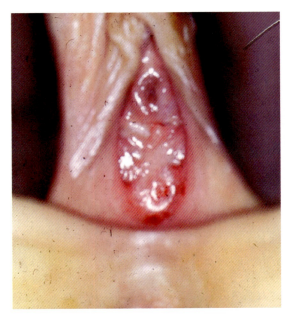

Figure 25.9 Imperforate hymen in an infant. Although the usual presentation is a smooth wall, occasionally the surface is irregular.

mass is the distended vagina and a distended bladder from pressure on the bladder neck. The hymen is thin, distended and has a dark blue tint (Figs 25.11, 25.12). A

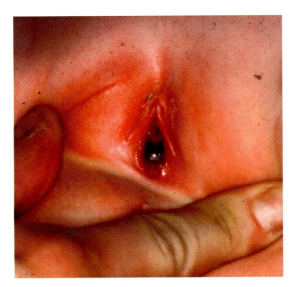

Figure 25.10 Shiny imperforate hymen that bulges when crying, dark blue color due to small hematocolpos for another reason. (Gloves should be worn.)

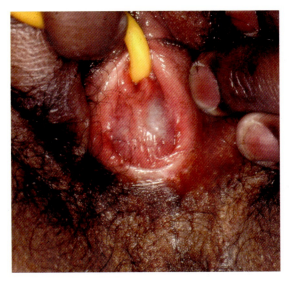

Figure 25.11 Distended thin dark blue imperforate hymen in an adolescent, after several months of concealed menses accumulated in the distended vagina without pain.

simple incision results in a gush of old dark menstrual blood. It is dangerous to do only an incision and drainage as the cut edges may close over in a few days, resulting in the vagina becoming a sac of pus. The old blood and the distended vaginal wall with its impaired small vessel blood supply make it extremely susceptible to infection, especially with the nearby anus. Therefore, in addition to the simple incision, the central part of the hymen should be excised to permit spontaneous slow drainage of old blood. The alternative is a cruciate incision. A drain is

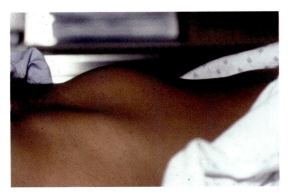

Figure 25.12 Adolescent with a distended lower abdomen due to hematocolpos and bladder neck compression.

not reliable. Correspondingly, avoid contamination during surgery. There must be a follow-up examination to be certain the hymen remains patent.

In early puberty surgery should be done prophylactically. The correct diagnosis is important. General anesthesia should be employed to avoid patient movement. Delicate small instruments are used. Consider using adjacent injection of a small amount of diluted vasopressin to reduce bleeding with a tuberculin syringe. Good lighting, exposure and an optical loop are helpful in avoiding injury to the urethra. The tissue is friable and bleeds readily, so needle electrode unipolar coagulation may be helpful. Another concern is incorrect diagnosis such as congenital absence of the vagina or distal vaginal agenesis. If that happens the surgery should be immediately discontinued to avoid injury to bladder or rectum and to avoid scarring which will make later surgery more difficult.

Microperforate hymen

This is often overlooked and under-reported. It mimics imperforate hymen and also may be a cause of recurrent urinary tract infections.

The original report of microperforate hymen showed an incorrect artist's conception. With the classic form only the urethral meatus is visible. With gentle downward retraction a second orifice is observed (microperforate hymen). When the traction is released the opening disappears under the urethra (Figs 25.13, 25.14). It tends to cause urinary tract infections because it acts like a urogenital sinus. Most of the urine passes on voiding but some dribbles into the vagina through the closed hymen. The stagnant urine breeds bacteria which gets back into the urethra and bladder. There is often postvoid dribbling (Quick Takes 25.6, 25.7).

Microperforate hymen is discovered by routine examination and suggests an imperforate hymen or absent vagina. Examination should be done if there is recurrent urinary tract infection. Surgical enlargement of the hymen posteriorly is considered for urinary tract infection, prior to the onset of menstruation or before coitus. Sometimes the orifice of the microperforate hymen is discovered after a fused labia minora is opened (Fig. 25.15).

There is a variation with a hymen opening high on the anterior hymen with a visible opening just below the

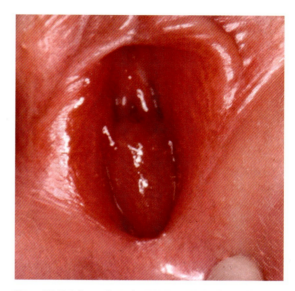

Figure 25.13 Microperforate hymen concealed under urethra (gloves should be worn).

urethra. This may also cause recurrent UTI and postvoid dribbling and may require surgical enlargements as well (Fig. 25.16).

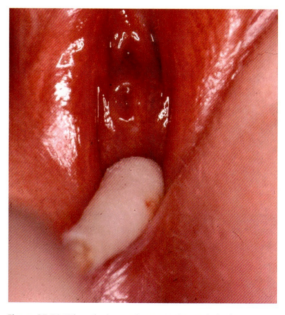

Figure 25.14 When the hymen is retracted posteriorly the microperforate opening is visualized; when released, it springs back under the urethra. (Gloves should be worn.)

Complete transverse vaginal septum

Complete transverse vaginal septum is rare and may oc-cur in the mid or upper vagina with a patent lower vagina and open hymen. It may have a confusing presentation in the newborn with a distended upper vagina (from endo-cervical mucus) which, if large, may elevate the abdomen and diaphragm, resulting in cardiorespiratory distress. It may also present in childhood, especially in inbred groups. It may be misdiagnosed as an ovarian or abdom-inal cyst. Before doing a laparotomy with resection of the "ovarian cyst" (and then discovering that the small uterus was removed with the upper distended vagina), do a vaginoscopy. If there is a complete transverse septum it should be opened, resected and drained and then the patient improves.

With a complete transverse septum there is vagina above and below the septum. Below the vagina is mucosa, above it is columnar epithelium. An experienced surgeon is required to resect the septum, reducing the chance of postoperative stricture by avoiding raw surfaces, using "Z" type plastic techniques (difficult to do), and using a vaginal stent with a central drain (or a simple wide ring pipe stent).

There is a related anomaly of absent distal vagina with a normal uterus. The distended upper vagina gradually ex-

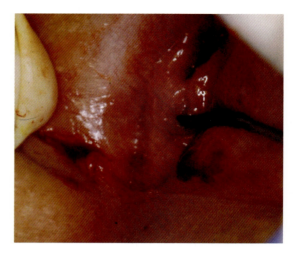

Figure 25.15 Microperforated hymen with probe discovered when labial fusion was done.

erts pressure caudad towards where the hymen should be. Unless routine examination has discovered it, it may not present until there is cyclic pain without external men-struation and a pelvic mass (Fig. 25.17). With surgical dissection upward, the lower pole of the distended upper

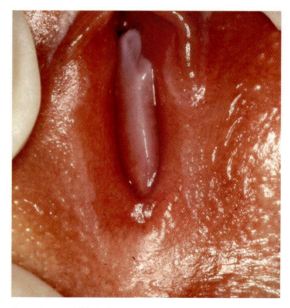

Figure 25.16 Visible high opening anterior hymen, just under urethra which is not visible.

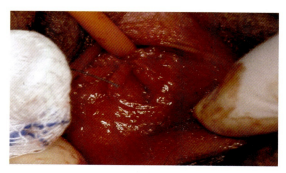

Figure 25.17 Puberty. Absent distal vagina, menstruating uterus, open hymen, above is bulge of upper vagina dissecting downward as it enlarges. It resembles Rokitansky syndrome, imperforate hymen and androgen insensitivity.

vagina is reached. Its lining looks unusual because it is thin, stretched, inflamed from old blood and is made of single cell columnar epithelium similar to the endocervical canal rather than the normal vaginal stratified thick mucosa. This lack of mucosa occurs in all cases of lack of access to ingrowth of vaginal mucosal cells from the wall of the embryonic urogenital sinus. There may be confusion if a biopsy if done (Chapter 24).

Paraurethral cyst

This is present at birth but often overlooked if the vulva is not carefully examined, and is under-reported because usually after a few days or a week the cyst spontaneously ruptures. It completely disappears within one minute because it is thin and tense, leaving only its contents of a milky-white viscous fluid which also disappears in about three minutes. In an obstetric unit with 3000 deliveries a year, there will be at least one case.

When first seen it presents as a terrifying, tense, milk-white, smooth cyst with a surface covering of bright fine "capillary" vessels embedded in a thin transparent covering membrane. This cyst may fill the entire introitus. The urethra is not visible and usually the vagina is not seen. With gentle traction the cyst is pulled downward to reveal the urethra. The cyst usually has its base at the distal posterior urethra but occasionally it is on either side of the urethra and rarely anterior to the urethra. With upward traction, the cyst will reveal the posterior hymen and vagina. Patency and depth of the vagina (normal

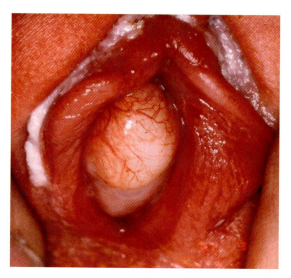

Figure 25.18 Large paraurethral cyst. The urethra and vagina are concealed. Thin stretched posterior hymen covers the posterior cyst.

3.5–4.0 cm) can be determined with a catheter or applicator stick. If there is concern about the diagnosis, a free part of the cyst may be excised for biopsy which shows stratified squamous epithelium. On opening the cyst, it will immediately rupture and collapse. Do not attempt to excise the edges to avoid injury to the adjacent urethra. It is not known whether these children will have a suburethral cyst or diverticulum in later life (Fig. 25.18).

If the clinical diagnosis is confirmed by an experienced observer then it may simply be punctured. The lesion has also been referred to as cyst of the introitus (Chapter 2).

Polyps of the hymen

Polyps of the hymen are usually benign. It is not unusual to have a prominent protruding posterior lip of the hymen suggesting a small polyp with a yellow tint (Chapter 2). With a loss of maternal estrogen this hymen tag may dessicate and fall away in a few days. The hymen may have a true, larger, often cystic or solid polyp, usually from the posterior half of the hymen. These usually persist. The important thing is to identify the base of the polyp. If it originates in the vagina above the hymen, especially the anterior vagina, the entire polyp should be removed as it

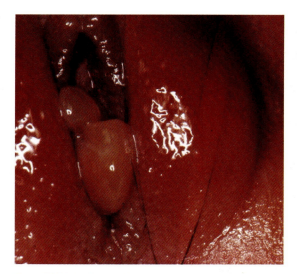

Figure 25.19 Newborn with polyps of the hymen.

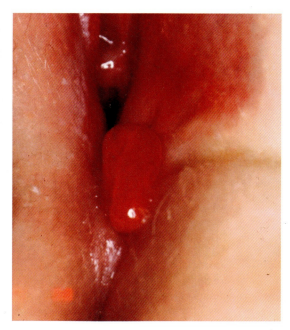

Figure 25.21 Perineal granuloma following repair to deep perineal trauma.

might be a rare rhabdomyosarcoma (Chapters 2, 8, 49). Prominent or large hymen polyps, even though benign, may bleed if torn (Figs 25.19, 25.20).

Polyps of the hymen may contain benign mucous cell nests.

Differential diagnosis

Perineal granuloma

Repair of deep perineal injury may result in a polypoid granuloma with a narrow base close to the posterior fourchette protruding from the skin closure site. It may bleed with slight trauma but it is benign. It should be removed flush with the skin, sent to pathology and the pinpoint opening cauterized with a silver nitrate stick (Fig. 25.21).

Occasionally the prepubertal vagina and hymen over-react to topical estrogen to become very hyperplastic and may simulate vaginal rhabdomyosarcoma (Fig. 25.22).

Agglutination of the labia minora

This is common, especially with atopic dermatitis which causes it to be recurrent. Many cases have one-third posterior agglutination which is asymptomatic. More extensive agglutination may extend anteriorly to leave only a small area to allow passage of urine. The opening is sometimes only a pinpoint. This causes distortion of the voided urinary stream, postvoid dribbling (seen in the child without diapers), and a tendency to recurrent urinary tract

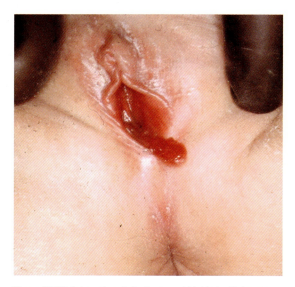

Figure 25.20 Polyps of posterior hymen which bled with trauma, age 3.

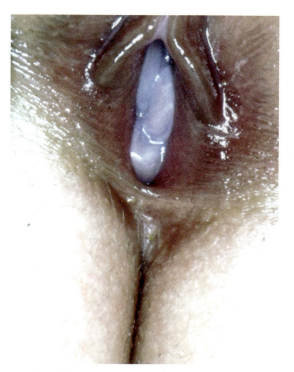

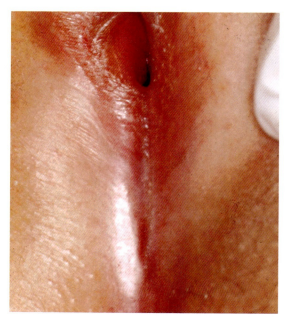

Figure 25.23 Classic agglutination of labia minora with closure of posterior labia and small opening anteriorly which required treatment.

Figure 25.22 Prepubertal over-reaction to topical estrogen simulating vagina rhabdomyosarcoma.

infection despite repeated courses of antibiotics. The reason is the functional urogenital sinus made of the vestibule lining of the inner surface of the labium majus. Since these cases are not hospitalized the pediatric house staff may not see them until they do office or clinic practice. The condition simulates congenital adrenal hyperplasia with a single perineal opening.

Occasionally the agglutination is posterior and anterior with the opening in the middle (Figs 25.23–25.25).

In former years the labia were torn apart in the office. This results in the child having pain, bleeding, fear of future examinations and rough raw surfaces which promptly glue together.

Children who require treatment are normally prescribed topical estrogen which usually causes spontaneous opening within two weeks. Prolonged use may cause tender enlarging breasts (which reduce in size after the medication is discontinued). Rarely there is labial pigmentation and hair growth which usually persists. Topical estrogen is not FDA approved for this purpose ("off label") and

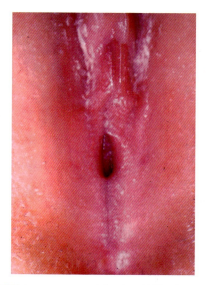

Figure 25.24 Less common agglutination of labia minora with central opening.

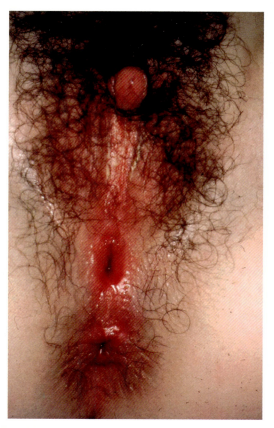

Figure 25.25 For differentiation from labial agglutination, an unusual complex congenital anomaly with large clitoris anteriorly, android pelvis which caused posterior location of single perineal opening leading to large urogenital sinus and urinary hydrocolpos, high imperforate hymen, early puberty; menstruation had not started, requiring extensive surgical reconstruction. Different from congenital adrenal hyperplasia.

the brochure reads that estrogen may cause endometrial cancer and estrogen is contraindicated in pregnancy. Nevertheless, it is generally agreed that it is appropriate therapy and preferable to surgery. The warning is based on estrogen pills for adults and postmenopausal women.

If there is a severe urinary tract infection not responding to antibiotics, consider urgent surgical opening.

If the agglutination of the labia minora has been chronic it may become fibrotic and not respond to topical estrogen.

For the child who no longer uses diapers, one topical application of estrogen at night is sufficient. For the child with diapers requiring frequent changing and cleaning, topical estrogen may have to be used three times daily.

After opening the agglutination by topical estrogen or surgery, consider atopic dermatitis-like care to avoid recurrent irritation of the skin which might cause a recurrence.

Distal longitudinal vaginal mucosal folds

I was the first to observe distal vaginal longitudinal mucosal folds and report it at a North American Society for Pediatric and Adolescent Gynecology (NASPAG) poster session about ten years ago and a second one in 2007 [1]. They are usually in the distal posterior vagina at about 6 and 8 o'clock (Fig. 25.26). They occur in about 20% of prepubertal children and can be visualized by vaginoscopy. With a relaxed child, a relatively wide hymen opening and a bright light, they may be visualized from the outside with an oblique view. If the folds reach as far as the hymen they fuse with it to form a "bump" which is readily seen from the outside and may be confused with old trauma from molestation (Fig. 25.27). The distal vaginal longitudinal mucosal fold does not have a fibrous core. An external direct view gives the incorrect impression of molestation and hymen injury (Fig. 25.28). The vaginal folds seen in the vagina may be confused with rhabdomyosarcoma. These folds usually disappear within a few months at puberty, presumably because of estrogen causing enlargement of the vagina.

This anomaly has been overlooked because prepubertal vaginoscopy, which reveals the condition, is rarely done. In my referral practice children are sent for vaginoscopy to investigate bleeding, recurrent vaginitis, suspicion of foreign body or anomaly and diethylstilbestrol (DES) exposure. The folds disappear after puberty when patients have vaginal examinations. Autopsies on prepubertal children never examine the vagina. After fetal exposure to maternal DES there are often benign, gross, anatomic distortions of the vagina and/or cervix. When followed over the years, these distortions may resolve very slowly because of the fibrous tissue base [2].

Prepubertal unilateral fibrous hyperplasia of the labium majus

With four cases operated upon by me and four others surgeons, we reported and named the prepubertal

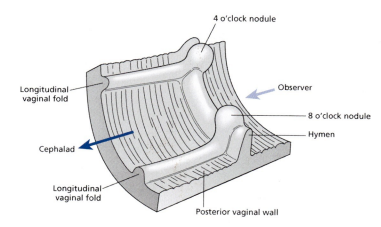

4 o'clock nodule

Longitudinal vaginal fold

Observer

8 o'clock nodule

Hymen

Cephalad

Longitudinal vaginal fold

Posterior vaginal wall

Figure 25.26 Sketch of prepubertal distal longitudinal vaginal folds usually at 6 and 8 o'clock; if they reach the hymen, a "bump" is formed.

unilateral fibrous hyperplasia of the labium majus [3] (Fig. 25.29). Apparently we were the first to identify it in an abstract of 2000 [4]. We also were the first to report ethnicity, religion, and geographical location, thereby raising questions of genetic or environmental predisposition or perhaps case selection. Seven of the eight cases were Ashkenazi Jewish girls from a closed community in one part of New York City, the other was Chinese who

lived nearby (this might be due to case selection). We were the first to find that the growth could not be completely removed because it extended into the contiguous levator pelvic floor as proven by MRI. We also established that despite prepubertal rapid growth in a few months to about 6 cm in size without palpable borders and apparent infiltration, it was not malignant. In two cases the lesion was present for three and three and a half years prior to

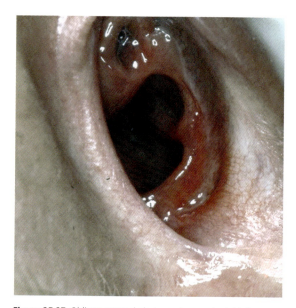

Figure 25.27 Oblique external photograph, prepubertal left longitudinal vaginal mucosal fold which reaches the hymen to form a "bump" (reproduced with permission from reference 1).

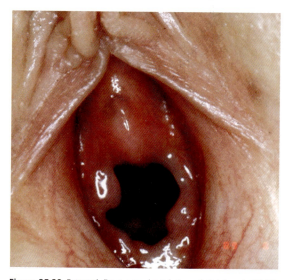

Figure 25.28 External direct prepubertal view of distal vaginal folds forming hymen "bumps." There is a "bump" at 10–11 o'clock. At 9 o'clock the relatively narrow hymen incorrectly suggests a "cleft" from an old tear (reproduced with permission from reference 1).

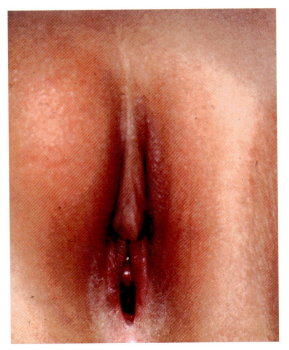

Figure 25.29 Prepubertal unilateral fibrous hyperplasia of the right labium majus. Early surface changes of indurated tan and peau d'orange overlying skin of anterior labium majus.

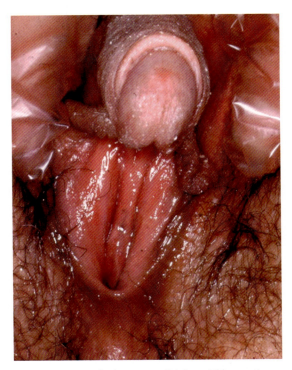

Figure 25.30 Large clitoris, no urogenital sinus, visible separate urethra and vagina indicate androgenic stimulus after birth.

surgery without further growth after puberty. This was also true of the operative cases. We found evidence that the physiologic increase in adrenal secretion leading to puberty stimulated growth. We were the first to describe the overlying indurated tan peau d'orange skin, and two cases with fine small hairs seen by colposcopy. This may help clinical diagnosis.

Ectopic ureter

Most cases are not discovered until young adulthood. The symptoms are a gush of purulent watery fluid from the vagina when getting out of bed in the morning. The distal ectopic ureter is often widened and tortuous and usually exits into the anterolateral vagina where the fluid also tends to collect. For the rest of the day there may be a slow watery dribble. It does not look or smell like urine because the origin of the ectopic ureter is the cephalad part of the kidney where the urine is not concentrated.

Rarely the ectopic ureter exits close to the urethra and is visible (Chapter 7).

Large clitoris

Figure 25.30 shows a large clitoris without a urogenital sinus. This indicates that the androgenic stimulus occurred after birth. If it was present at birth there would also be a single perineal orifice which leads to a urogenital sinus which drains the urine from the urethra and the vaginal introitus. The typical congenital adrenal hyperplasia presents with a large clitoris and a single perineal orifice. Clitoris enlargement after birth may be due to atypical late-onset adrenal hyperplasia, testosterone from an ovarian neoplasm or progestin therapy in pregnancy.

Inverted nipples (Fig. 25.31)

Although inverted nipples in the adult is a sign of breast cancer, in the young infant it is normal to have inverted

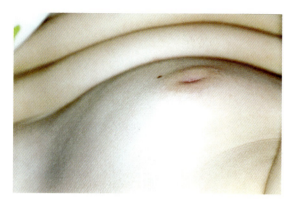

Figure 25.31 It is normal to have inverted nipples in the young child before further growth and development of the areola.

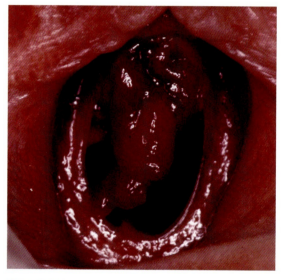

Figure 25.32 Partial hymen septum, attached anteriorly, rough surface. Some have a smooth surface, midline just below urethra. It may protrude and bleed.

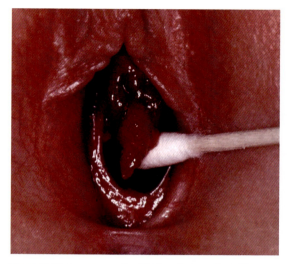

Figure 25.33 Same case as Fig. 25.32, posterior aspect is free.

Partial hymen septum

Partial hymen septum (Figs 25.32, 25.33) may be misdiagnosed as vaginal rhabdomyosarcoma because it is a protrusion of a mass from the anterior vaginal wall and may bleed. Rhabdomyosarcoma usually orginates high in the anterior vaginal wall near the anterior fornix and presents in separate masses.

The partial hymen septum is attached to the anterior distal vagina just below the urethra.

References

1. Altchek A, Deligdisch L. Update on prepubertal distal longitudinal vaginal mucosal folds. *J Pediatr Adoles Gynecol* 2007;**20**(2):127–128.
2. Altchek A, Wasserman B, Deligdisch L. Original studies, prepubertal distal longitudinal vaginal folds. *J Pediatr Adolesc Gynecol* 2008;**21**: 351–354.
3. Altchek A, Deligdisch L, Norton K, Gordon RE, Greco MA, Magid MS. Prepubertal unilateral fibrous hyperplasia of the labium majus. *Obstet Gynecol* 2007;**111**(1):103–108.
4. Magid MS, Walsh MM, Greco RE et al. Novel fibrous proliferation of the vulva. *Mod Pathol* 2000; **13**:205A

nipples when the mammary tissue is growing rapidly. The latter may have a round cystic feel and may be tender. This tends to occur with premature thelarche in girls from age one to four.

CHAPTER 26

Laparoscopy in the Pediatric and Adolescent Female

Robert K. Zurawin

Baylor College of Medicine, Houston, Texas, TX, USA

Introduction

Gynecologic laparoscopy as we know it today began with laparoscopic tubal sterilization in 1962 [1] by Palmer with major advances developed by Semm [2] and others. Laparoscopy was well established among gynecologists by the 1970s, but it did not gain popularity among general surgeons until the late 1980s when it was first applied to cholecystectomy [3]. Within ten years, laparoscopy became the technique of choice for many general surgery procedures. However, its wide adoption by pediatric surgeons took another decade for several reasons. The instrumentation devised for adult laparoscopy was not compatible with infants, and many surgeons felt that the shorter recovery time and analgesic requirements of children made the need to develop minimally invasive procedures less urgent [4]. Pediatric hospitals were reluctant to purchase the capital equipment to support the procedures [5].

Few gynecologists are thoroughly trained in the surgical management of pediatric and adolescent pathology, and even fewer are familiar with the minimally invasive treatment of these conditions, especially congenital abnormalities. There have been very few controlled studies evaluating pain, length of hospital stay, and cost of laparoscopy in pediatric patients [6]. In the last decade, these obstacles have been largely overcome and minimally invasive surgery (MIS) has replaced open approaches for many general surgical procedures [7,8].

Pediatric, Adolescent, & Young Adult Gynecology. Edited by A. Altchek and L. Deligdisch. © 2009 Blackwell Publishing, ISBN: 978-1-4051-5347-8.

Instrumentation

A full treatise on laparoscopic surgery is beyond the scope of this chapter, and many excellent sources are available. There are several important considerations when performing MIS in pediatric and adolescent patients. Optimal visualization is the key to all endoscopic surgery, and is critical in surgery on children. Ideally, the endoscope and all operative instruments should be able to fit through the smallest ports possible to minimize trauma. Improvements in fiberoptic technology and high-resolution video imaging allow the use of smaller endoscopes. It is not necessary to use anything larger than a 5 mm endoscope, which allows excellent imaging, especially when both 0° and 30° scopes are employed. Smaller rod-lens scopes are available but they are easily damaged. Fogging of the lens can be reduced by preheating the laparoscope with warm water [9] and using an insufflator system containing warm, humidified air. When operating on very small children, the use of unhumidified and unwarmed air can contribute to hypothermia in prolonged cases [10].

Most minimally invasive gynecologic procedures in children may be performed without laparoscopic suturing thanks to the development of tissue coagulation, fusion, and cutting devices that fit through a 5 mm port. The energy sources vary from monopolar and bipolar electrosurgery to harmonic energy. Tissue effect is monitored using continuous impedance-based feedback allowing delicate dissection in confined spaces, minimizing collateral thermal injury to bowel and vascular structures. The removal of specimens may be accomplished without large incisions, except in cases of malignancy, by placing the tissue in a bag through a 10 mm port, or by morcellating the specimen.

Technique of peritoneal access

Safe peritoneal access is imperative in all laparoscopic surgery. Injury to vascular structures on initial port placement is the greatest cause of complications in laparoscopic surgery [11–13]. Trocar injuries may be minimized by careful attention to anatomy and surgical technique. The umbilicus is still the most common point of access because it is an avascular locus where all layers of the abdominal wall fuse, and whose thickness is independent of the patient's obesity. Safe laparoscopic entry into the peritoneal cavity via the umbilicus may be accomplished even in patients with previous abdominal surgery. The establishment of a pneumoperitoneum using carbon dioxide gas is the widely accepted method of preparation for optical trocar placement. Direct trocar placement has been described in both adult and pediatric surgery [14] but there is increased hazard of inadvertent injury to bowel and vascular structures [11]. Some surgeons prefer open trocar placement using the Hassan cannula, especially in patients with previous abdominal surgery and scarring, but studies have not borne out improved safety over careful closed insufflation [15]. Palmer's point (Fig. 26.1) may be selected in obese patients and those with prior lower

abdominal surgery or large pelvic masses rising to the umbilicus [16].

In the young patient, the distance between the umbilicus and the aortic bifurcation is only a few centimeters. Elevation of the abdominal wall is essential to reduce vascular injury, and the use of towel clips at the umbilicus has been shown to significantly decrease the incidence of trauma compared with elevation using the hand [17]. The hanging drop technique confirms proper intraperitoneal placement of the Veress needle prior to insertion and helps avoid preperitoneal insufflation as well as perforation of a viscus. The Veress needle should be inserted vertically to take advantage of the fusion of the abdominal layers and to minimize preperitoneal tracking. Once the pneumoperitoneum has been established, the use of optical trocars allows the surgeon to safely enter the peritoneal cavity. Optical trocars may be used in the accessory ports to avoid injury to the epigastric vessels. An accessory port should always be placed, because it is impossible to adequately perform a diagnostic laparoscopy with only one port, even those 10 mm scopes with an in-line operative channel. A separate site for probes and graspers is imperative.

Anesthesia and pain management

The assessment of postoperative pain in children is difficult, and recently the concept that children feel less pain and recover more quickly than adults has been challenged. Consequently, surgeons are paying more attention to preemptive pain management, intraoperative techniques to reduce pain, and postoperative analgesia. The majority of postoperative pain associated with laparoscopy is located at the trocar sites and subdiaphragmatically. There are no large randomized prospective studies of preoperative and postoperative use of infiltrative anesthesia at trocar sites. Several studies involving small numbers of patients suggest that local injection may reduce the use of postoperative narcotics and antiemetics [18,19]. The variability in outcome may be related to the failure of the surgeon to wait long enough for the anesthetic to take effect – usually ten minutes – before making the incisions and inserting the trocars.

General anesthesia must be modified for the very young patient. Systemic accumulation of CO_2 may necessitate an increase in ventilation by as much as 68% to maintain

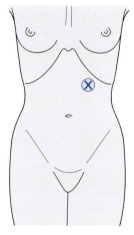

Figure 26.1 Palmer's point.

normal levels. Combining the effects of anesthesia, reverse Trendelenburg and CO_2 insufflation of the peritoneal space can lead to a 50% reduction in cardiac index. Children also have an exaggerated vagal response to peritoneal insufflation [20]. In smaller children, pressure limits on the insufflator should be 6–8 mmHg and in older children, the pressure should range between 12 and 15 mmHg [9]. Hypothermia in smaller children must be monitored carefully and controlled using external warming and the use of warmed humidified CO_2 [21,22].

Inspection of the peritoneal cavity

Once the umbilical trocar has been placed, the endoscope should be inserted vertically under direct visual guidance so that the areas immediately below the umbilicus may be inspected for any injury related to insufflation and trocar placement. Particular attention should be paid to the omentum, the bowel mesentery and the lower aorta, vena cava, and iliac vessels. The upper abdomen, diaphragm, liver, gallbladder and stomach should be inspected and all adhesions should be noted. The endoscope should then be placed through the accessory port to inspect the umbilical site to check for bleeding and injury to any adherent structures.

A careful and systematic anatomic evaluation of the pelvis is a precursor for any operative intervention. The appendix should be inspected, especially in cases of pelvic pain. In addition to appendicitis and adhesions, the appendix is a site for endometriosis implants. The ureters should be identified at the pelvic brim and traced throughout their course in the pelvis, noting their relationship to the ovarian vessels, the pelvic side walls, ovaries, and uterosacral ligaments. Beginning at the left infundibulopelvic ligament and moving clockwise, all pelvic structures should be evaluated, noting adhesions, cysts, endometriosis, congenital abnormalities, color, and amount of peritoneal fluid. The fimbriae are examined for patency and adhesions, tracing the fallopian tube to the cornu. The ovary should be grasped at the utero-ovarian ligament and gently rotated out of the cul-de-sac and inspected on all sides, along with the entire lateral pelvic side wall. The left uterosacral ligament and pouch of Douglas are examined for endometriosis and peritoneal window defects. The insertion of the left round ligament into the canal of Nuck should be evaluated for herniation. Note that the inferior

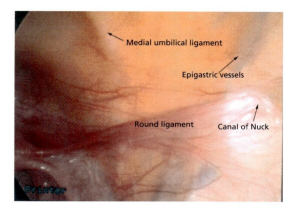

Figure 26.2 The peritoneal cavity.

epigastric vessels exit the pelvis in the fossa bordered medially by the obliterated umbilical ligament and laterally by the round ligament (Fig. 26.2). The anterior broad ligament over the bladder is then traced to the right side of the pelvis where the identical algorithm is followed.

Laparoscopic procedures in the pediatric and adolescent patient

The surgical management of many gynecologic conditions is similar for adult and adolescent patients, but there are some procedures unique to the young female that require special consideration. Ovarian pathology in a child or adolescent carries a special burden to preserve the affected ovary when simple removal would be indicated in an older woman. Obstructive congenital anomalies appear shortly after menarche and their correction using minimally invasive techniques necessitates individualization of approach. The diagnosis and management of pelvic pain in the adolescent are challenging and depend on the surgeon's ability to recognize the many presentations of endometriosis, along with the surgical ability to treat it effectively. Finally, the preservation of fertility in a child with cancer is an additional challenge to the gynecologic surgeon.

Adnexal masses

The incidence of ovarian, paraovarian, and paratubal cysts (Figs 26.3, 26.4) in the pediatric and adolescent population is not known. The widespread availability of

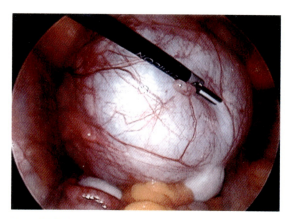

Figure 26.3 Paratubal cyst.

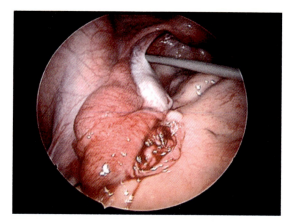

Figure 26.4 Laparoscopic excision of paratubal cyst.

ultrasound over the past 20 years has caused an explosion in the diagnosis of ovarian cysts, the vast majority of which are asymptomatic, discovered incidentally during the work-up of other conditions. Once these cysts are diagnosed, the combination of anxiety on the part of the parent and the uncertainty of management on the part of the physician frequently leads to more aggressive treatment than necessary.

The frequent use of prenatal ultrasound has led to an increased diagnosis of neonatal ovarian cysts, which are almost universally asymptomatic. These cysts may be managed expectantly and will normally resolve within six months. Simple unilocular cysts over 4 cm have an increased risk of torsion and may be aspirated under ultrasound guidance or surgically removed [23,24]. Torsion

of a neonatal cyst is not uncommon, especially in larger cysts. Autoamputation is the most frequent complication and yet laparoscopy is the favored method of treatment – in the most recent series the average age of the patient was 3.7 months [25].

Templeman reviewed a series of 140 patients under the age of 21 with adnexal masses who underwent surgery over a period of 18 years [26]. The most common finding (62%) was a functional ovarian cyst. The majority of these lesions may be treated laparoscopically, even when the cysts are large. In the adult population, Sagiv reviewed 21 patients with very large ovarian cysts managed laparoscopically without complications. The mean cyst volume in this series was 2844 cc [27]. Goh described the management of large ovarian cysts treated with a combination of laparoscopic drainage and extracorporeal cystectomy through the trocar site [28].

The distribution of pathology of ovarian tumors in the pediatric and adolescent population is different from that in adults, with a larger proportion of germ cell tumors. Epithelial malignancies are in children compared to women of reproductive age, and are largely borderline tumors found in older adolescents.

Before attempting laparoscopic management of the pediatric and adolescent ovarian tumor, it is advisable to obtain tumor markers AFP, LDH, inhibin, β-HCG and CA-125 [29]. In contrast to the surgical management of gynecologic malignancy in adults, pediatric surgeons and oncologists have not widely adopted staging laparotomy with lymph node sampling. In a recent series of 131 girls with stage I and II pediatric ovarian germ cell tumors, only 1% had bilateral node sampling [30]. Nezhat reviewed 1101 patients younger than 55 years of age with adnexal masses and found that 80% of the lesions were benign, hormone-dependent cysts or endometriomas, 8% were benign neoplasms and only 0.4% were malignant [31]. However, ovarian enlargement detected by ultrasound in females 21 years or less represented a borderline or malignant ovarian neoplasm in 5.7% of cases [32,33]. Germ cell tumors represent 67–85% of the malignancies in this age group. These tumors may be managed with unilateral salpingo-oophorectomy and staged laparoscopically. With this approach, fertility-preserving treatment for malignant germ cell tumors, even in advanced stages, allowed for a 76% pregnancy success rate [34].

The management of mature cystic teratomas (Fig. 26.5) has evolved significantly. Historically, concerns about

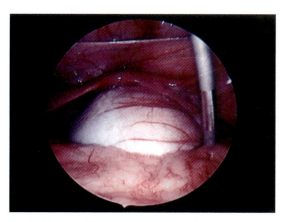

Figure 26.5 Mature teratoma in a prepubertal girl.

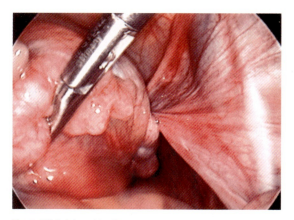

Figure 26.6 Adnexal torsion.

laparoscopic resection centered on spillage and the possibility of malignancy [35]. Several large retrospective studies have demonstrated that the laparoscopic approach is associated with less postoperative pain, blood loss, hospital stay, and total cost. There is a higher incidence of intra-abdominal spillage compared to laparotomy but this was not associated with any increase in morbidity or fertility. There was a significantly higher risk of recurrence – 7.6% versus 0% after two years [36]. The size of the lesion is associated with increased risk of malignancy and it is recommended that frozen section be obtained in lesions greater than 5 cm to assess the neural elements of the tumor so that prompt staging may be achieved [37].

One of the most common presentations of the adnexal mass is in association with torsion (Fig. 26.6). Adnexal tor-

sion may account for up to 2.7% of acute abdominal pain in children and is much higher in adolescents. Although most commonly associated with adnexal pathology such as teratomas, ovarian and paratubal cysts and other neoplasms (Table 26.1), up to 25% of young patients with torsion have normal ovaries [38], suggesting that children and adolescents may have excessively mobile mesovaria. In prepubertal children, the ovary is an abdominal and not a pelvic organ, and the protective effect of the ovary residing in the cul-de-sac is diminished.

The prompt and accurate diagnosis of adnexal torsion is often challenging. The classic symptoms are intermittent colicky pain in association with an adnexal mass. However, pain may be constant or even absent in cases where torsion is chronic. Torsion may occur in the absence of

Table 26.1 Torsion in relation to pathology

Pathology	Evidence of torsion in OR n = 50(%)	No evidence of torsion in OR n = 10(%)
Paratubal cyst	14 (33%)	0
Hemorrhagic cyst	7 (16%)	1 (14%)
Ovarian teratoma	5 (14%)	3 (43%)
Ovary c/w torsion	6 (14%)	0
Ovarian biopsy c/w hemorrhage	4 (9%)	0
Follicular cyst	0	2 (29%)
Serous cystadenofibroma	2 (5%)	0
Serous cystadenoma	1 (2%)	0
Papillary serous cystadenofibroma	1 (2%)	0
Appendix	0	1 (14%)
Other*	2 (5%)	

* Fibrovascular tissue w/edema; hemorrhagic fallopian tube wall with partial oophorectomy.

enlarged adnexa. Additionally, the sensitivity of Doppler imaging of the adnexa is unfortunately disappointing. Up to 50% of torsed adnexa show blood flow on Doppler studies, and an equal number of ovaries with absent Doppler flow are normal at the time of surgery. In the most recent large series, there was no statistically significant association between the ultrasound characteristics studied and the presence or absence of adnexal torsion as determined at the time of surgery except for adnexal size greater than 5 cm [39]. Surprisingly, symptomatic corpus luteum cysts comprise only a small portion of cases of adnexal torsion in the adolescent compared to torsion of a paratubal cyst (16% versus 33% of all cases of torsion).

Consequently, it is reasonable to proceed with diagnostic laparoscopy in cases of adnexal mass and absence of blood flow on ultrasound. It is equally important to avoid delay in patients with pelvic pain and adnexal mass even in the presence of Doppler flow. In one series of 102 children with torsion treated with immediate cystectomy, 71.4% were diagnosed with ovarian dysfunction at a later date, reinforcing the importance of prompt diagnosis and management [40]. Other studies have shown normal folliculogenesis on follow-up ultrasound [41,42]. When torsion has been present for some time, the ovary will undergo enlargement and edema (Fig. 26.7). In these cases, there is no cyst to remove after detorsion has been accomplished. Similarly, torsion associated with hemorrhagic corpus luteum cyst does not lend itself to resection because of bleeding and unnecessary loss of normal ovarian cortex. In these cases, the question arises of how to

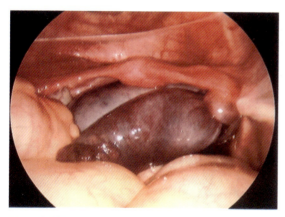

Figure 26.7 Torsion with ischemia and edema of right fallopian tube and ovary.

manage the ovary following detorsion. Until the ovary can recover its blood supply and return to normal size, oophoropexy may be performed to reduce the chance of recurrent torsion. However, there are no long-term data on the effect of oophoropexy in the management of torsion, or on its effect on fertility [43].

Less than 20 years ago, laparotomy with salpingo-oophorectomy was the standard approach to adnexal torsion due to lack of laparoscopic instrumentation and skill as well as the concern about embolism from ovarian vein thrombosis caused by prolonged venous stasis. Detorsion with or without cystectomy is now the preferred management of adnexal torsion. The same criteria to determine laparoscopic versus open cystectomy should be followed in cases of torsion.

Pelvic pain and endometriosis

The management of chronic pelvic pain in adolescents is often frustrating to the physician and exasperating to the parent. Clearly, many cases are functional and due to poor diet, anxiety or manipulative behavior. The patient frequently sees many specialists and undergoes multiple radiologic and other diagnostic tests without a definitive diagnosis.

Almost half of adolescents who underwent diagnostic laparoscopy following a thorough but otherwise negative work-up for abdominal and pelvic pain were found to have endometriosis when surgery was performed by a clinician experienced in the recognition of the disease [44,45]. Early diagnosis, prompted by a high index of suspicion, is key to the optimal treatment of endometriosis. The appearance of endometriosis in adolescents is protean and the classic powder burn lesions seen in adults are not the most common presentation in younger women. Lesions in the adolescent are frequently clear and vesicular, or petechial. An area of injected hyperemic erythematous peritoneum will frequently yield endometriosis on biopsy (Fig. 26.8). It is imperative to follow the systematic evaluation of the abdomen and pelvis described above when performing laparoscopy for pelvic pain.

The standard surgical treatment of endometriosis has been ablation of the lesions using a variety of energy sources, ranging from monopolar and bipolar electrosurgery to endocoagulation, laser vaporization, and harmonic energy. However, endometriosis is rarely confined to the peritoneal surface and is frequently deeply invasive, especially in the rectovaginal space. Optimal therapy

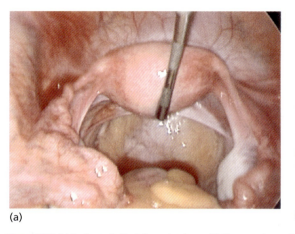
(a)

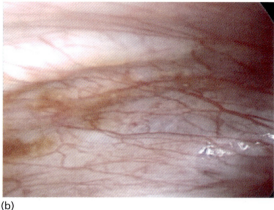
(b)

Figure 26.8 (a) Erythema in the left ovarian fossa. (b) Close-up shows clear vesicles.

requires excision of the visible lesions in order to obtain a definitive surgical diagnosis as well as to achieve optimal excision of the endometriosis. It is preferred to excise the lesions sharply or with an energy source with minimal lateral thermal spread [46]. When lesions overlie the ureter, rectum or uterine vessels (Fig. 26.9), hydrodissection or cavitation using harmonic energy may be used to elevate the affected peritoneum away from the vital structures. Endometriosis involving the appendix is common in advanced cases. However, even in mild to moderate cases of endometriosis involving significant pelvic pain, appendectomy is advised [47]. In advanced cases, it is advisable to prescribe a 3–6 month course of leupro-

lide therapy followed by chronic suppression using oral contraceptives.

When endometriosis is diagnosed in a young adolescent, the primary objective of therapy is to treat the pain and then prevent recurrence and preserve fertility for as long as possible, since it may be many years before she is ready to become pregnant. There are no long-term randomized prospective studies evaluating the optimal combination of medical and surgical therapies for endometriosis stratified according to disease stage in adolescents. They key to treatment is early diagnosis and adequate resection followed by suppressive therapy.

Congenital anomalies

Developmental abnormalities of the female genital tract are related to the interaction between the Müllerian and Wolffian duct systems and their ultimate joining with the vaginal plate. They may be divided into disorders of lateral and vertical fusion. Vertical defects range from the simple imperforate hymen to transverse septa causing outflow obstruction at various levels of the vagina. These lesions are managed transvaginally. Lateral fusion defects encompass a range of conditions from septate to bicornuate to didelphic uteri (Fig. 26.10) and may present with varying degrees of communication of the respective horns. Surgery is necessary when there is an obstructive anomaly. Frequently the patient presents with primary amenorrhea and cyclic pain and the diagnosis is straightforward. However, in uterine duplications where one side is patent and the other is obstructed, the diagnosis is frequently

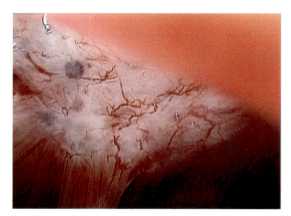

Figure 26.9 Classic nodule of endometriosis on uterosacral ligament.

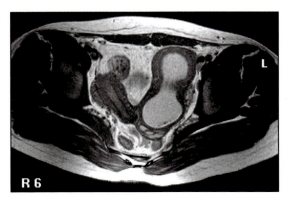

Figure 26.10 MRI image of didelphic uterus with noncommunicating horn. Note thin avascular band separating the horns.

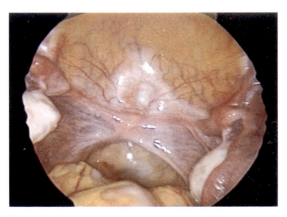

Figure 26.11 MRKH with bilateral rudimentary horns and midline raphe.

delayed until the girl presents with a large abdominal mass.

Magnetic resonance imaging is the best diagnostic modality for congenital anomalies of the pelvis. It is not without flaws, however, and complete diagnosis requires a combined radiologic and laparoscopic evaluation [48]. Uterine duplications with obstructed horns may be managed by laparoscopic excision of the affected horn. The plane between the two horns is usually avascular. Careful dissection of the retroperitoneal space is important because of the frequent occurrence of anomalous insertions of the uterine vessels combined with urologic abnormalities, including absence of the ipsilateral kidney and ureter and ureteral duplications [49,50].

Mayer–Rokitansky–Küster–Hauser (MRKH) syndrome is a rare anomaly, estimated at 1 in 5000 females (Fig. 26.11). Creation of a neovagina using progressive vaginal dilators is the mainstay of therapy. Dilation is never indicated in children and should be utilized only in women who are sexually active. Some patients are unwilling or unable to tolerate dilator therapy. The traditional surgical repair is the McIndoe and Bannister procedure, utilizing split-thickness skin grafts (Chapter 24). The procedure requires long hospitalization and immobilization, with significant graft rejection, donor site complications, and postoperative stenosis. Several alternative laparoscopic approaches are now available. The laparoscopic modification of the Vecchietti procedure utilizes an "olive" that is placed on the vaginal dimple. Wires running from the olive on the perineum

to a device on the patient's abdomen are connected by threading them laparoscopically into the pelvis and exiting the lower lateral abdominal wall (Fig. 26.12) [51]. Incremental traction using the spring-loaded device rapidly advances the olive over the course of approximately two weeks and creates a very satisfactory vagina without the need for any graft. The neovagina is maintained with intercourse and vaginal dilators.

An alternative procedure is the Davydov operation [52] in which a space is dissected between the rectum and the bladder in the manner of a McIndoe repair. Laparoscopy is performed concomitantly and the peritoneum in the pouch of Douglas is directed toward the vaginal incision where it is grasped from below and opened. The edges of

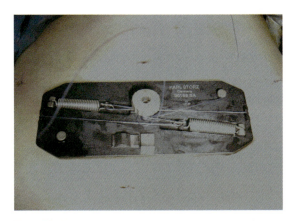

Figure 26.12 Vecchietti device.

the peritoneum are then sewn to the perineum and the upper aspect of the neovagina is created by placing two pursestring sutures using anterior and lateral peritoneum and large bowel serosa. A vaginal dilator is sewn in place for one week after which mold insertion and dilation is performed for six weeks [53].

These advanced reconstructive laparoscopic procedures should be performed by surgeons with extensive experience in vaginal reconstruction and laparoscopic surgery. A multidisciplinary team consisting of clinical nurse specialists and psychologists is important in obtaining optimal postoperative outcome.

Conclusion

The twin goals of surgery on the pediatric and adolescent female genital tract are organ preservation and maintenance of future fertility. Advances in technique and improvement in instrumentation have enabled surgeons to tackle increasingly complex operations using a laparoscopic approach instead of open laparotomy. The pathologic states of the pediatric and adolescent female are particularly suited to minimally invasive surgery and yet specialized training is required in order to properly address these conditions. It is reasonable to anticipate that most laparotomies for gynecologic pathology in this age group will be performed using a minimally invasive approach in the near future.

References

1. Palmer MR. Essais de stérilisation tubaire coelioscopique par électrocoagulation isthmique. *Bull Fed Soc Gynecol Obstet Lang Fr* 1962;**14**:298–305.
2. Semm K. New methods of pelviscopy (gynecologic laparoscopy) for myomectomy, ovariectomy, tubectomy and adnectomy. *Endoscopy* 1979;**11**:85–93.
3. Mühe E. Long-term follow-up after laparoscopic cholecystectomy. *Endoscopy* 1992;**24**:754–758.
4. Schechter NL. The undertreatment of pain in children: an overview. *Peditar Clin North Am* 1989;**36**:781–794.
5. Waldhausen JH, Tapper D. Is pediatric laparoscopic splenectomy safe and cost-effective? *Arch Surg* 1997;**132**:822–824.
6. Rangel SJ et al. Small evidence for small incisions: pediatric laparoscopy and the need for more rigorous evaluation of novel surgical therapies. *J Pediatr Surg* 2003;**38**(10):1429–1433.
7. Zitsman JL. Current concepts in minimal access surgery for children. *Pediatrics* 2003;**111**(6 Pt 1):1239–1252.
8. Zitsman JL. Pediatric minimal-access surgery: update 2006. *Pediatrics* 2006;**118**(1): 304–308.
9. Mansuria SM, Sanfilippo JS. Laparoscopy in the pediatric and adolescent population. *Obstet Gynecol Clin North Am* 2004;**31**(3):469–483, vii.
10. Ott DE, Reich H, Love B et al. Reduction of laparoscopic-induced hypothermia, postoperative pain and recovery room length of stay by pre-conditioning gas with the Insuflow device: a prospective randomized controlled multi-center study. *J Soc Laparosc Surg* 1998;**2**(4):321–329.
11. US Food and Drug Administration (FDA). *Laparoscopic Trocar Injuries.*: Center for Devices and Radiological Health (CDRH) Systematic Technology Assessment of Medical Products (STAMP) Committee. www.fda.gov/cdrh/medical-devicesafety/stamp/trocar.html
12. Chen MK, Schropp KP, Lobe TE. Complications of minimal-access surgery in children. *J Pediatr Surg* 1996;**31**(8):1161–1165.
13. Esposito C et al. Complications of pediatric laparoscopic surgery. *Surg Endosc* 1997;**11**(6):655–657.
14. Yokomori K et al. A new technique applicable to pediatric laparoscopic surgery: abdominal wall 'area lifting' with subcutaneous wiring. *J Pediatr Surg* 1998;**33**(11): 1589–1592.
15. Vilos GA, Ternamian A, Dempster J, Laberge PY. Laparoscopic entry: a review of techniques, technologies, and complications. *J Obstet Gynecol Can* 2007;**29**(5):433–447.
16. Jansen FW, Kolkman W, Bakkum EA et al. Complications of laparoscopy: an inquiry about closed- versus open-entry technique. *Am J Obstet Gynecol* 2004;**190**(3):634–638.
17. Cakir T, Tuney D, Esmaeilzadem S, Aktan AO. Safe Veress needle insertion. *J Hepatobiliary Pancreat Surg* 2006;**13**(3): 225–227.
18. Hasaniya NW et al. Preinsertion local anesthesia at the trocar site improves perioperative pain and decreases costs of laparoscopic cholecystectomy. *Surg Endosc* 2001;**15**(9):962–964.
19. Stringer NH et al. On-Q system for managing trocar site pain after operative laparoscopy. *J Am Assoc Gynecol Laparosc* 2000;**7**(4):552–555.
20. Means LJ, Green MC, Bilal R. Anesthesia for minimally invasive surgery. *Semin Pediatr Surg* 2004;**13**(3):181–187.
21. Kalfa N et al. Tolerance of laparoscopy and thoracoscopy in neonates. *Pediatrics* 2005;**116**(6):e785–791.
22. Hazebroek EJ, Haitsma, JJ, Lachmann B et al. Impact of carbon dioxide and helium insufflation on cardiorespiratory function during prolonged pneumoperitoneum in an experimental rat model. *Surg Endosc* 202;**16**:1073–1078.
23. Bryant AE, Laufer MR. Fetal ovarian cysts: incidence, diagnosis and management. *J Reprod Med* 2004;**49**(5):329–337.

24. Esposito C et al. Laparoscopic management of ovarian cysts in newborns. *Surg Endosc* 1998;**12**(9):1152–1154.

25. Tseng D, Curran TJ, Silen ML. Minimally invasive management of the prenatally torsed ovarian cyst. *J Pediatr Surg* 2002;**37**(10):1467–1469.

26. Templeman C et al. Noninflammatory ovarian masses in girls and young women. *Obstet Gynecol* 2000;**96**(2):229–233.

27. Sagiv R, Golan A, Glezerman M. Laparoscopic management of extremely large ovarian cysts. *Obstet Gynecol* 2005;**105**(6):1319–1322.

28. Goh SM et al. Minimal access approach to the management of large ovarian cysts. *Surg Endosc* 2006.

29. Gadducci A et al. Serum tumor markers in the management of ovarian, endometrial and cervical cancer. *Biomed Pharmacother* 2004;**58**(1):24–38.

30. Billmire D et al. Outcome and staging evaluation in malignant germ cell tumors of the ovary in children and adolescents: an intergroup study. *J Pediatr Surg* 2004;**39**(3):424–429.

31. Nezhat F et al. Four ovarian cancers diagnosed during laparoscopic management of 1011 women with adnexal masses. *Am J Obstet Gynecol* 1992;**167**(3):790–796.

32. Diamond M et al. Occurrence of ovarian malignancy in childhood and adolescence: a community-wide evaluation. *Obstet Gynecol* 1988;**71**(6):858–860.

33. Gershenson DM. Fertility-sparing surgery for malignancies in women. *J Natl Cancer Inst Monogr* 2005;**34**:43–47.

34. Tangir J et al. Reproductive function after conservative surgery and chemotherapy for malignant germ cell tumors of the ovary. *Obstet Gynecol* 2003;**101**(2):251–257.

35. Hilger WS, Magrina JF, Magtibay PM. Laparoscopic management of the adnexal mass. *Clin Obstet Gynecol* 2006;**49**(3):535–548.

36. Laberge PY, Levesque S. Short-term morbidity and long-term recurrence rate of ovarian dermoid cysts treated by laparoscopy versus laparotomy. *J Obstet Gynaecol Can* 2006;**28**(9):789–793.

37. Einarsson JI, Edwards CL, Zurawin RK. Immature ovarian teratoma in an adolescent: a case report and review of the literature. *J Pediatr Adolesc Gynecol* 2004;**17**(3):187–189.

38. Breech L, Hillard P. Adnexal torsion in pediatric and adolescent girls. *Curr Opin Obstet Gynecol* 2005;**17**(5):483–489.

39. Adigun YE, Boswell HB, Wesson DE, Braverman R, Zurawin RK. Predictive value of ultrasound in the diagnosis of adnexal torsion in the pediatric and adolescent population. Submitted for publication to *J Pediatr Adolesc Gynecol.*

40. Cohen S et al. Laparoscopy versus laparotomy for detorsion and sparing of twisted ischemic adnexa. *J Soc Laparosc Surg* 2003;**7**:295–299.

41. Celik A et al. Long-term results of conservative management of adnexal torsion in children. *J Pediatr Surg* 2005;**40**(4):704–708.

42. Oelsner G et al. Minimal surgery for the twisted ischaemic adnexa can preserve ovarian function. *Hum Reprod* 2003;**18**(12):2599–2602.

43. Crouch NS et al. Ovarian torsion: to pex or not to pex? Case report and review of the literature. *J Pediatr Adolesc Gynecol* 2003;**16**(6):381–384.

44. Laufer MR et al. Prevalence of endometriosis in adolescent girls with chronic pelvic pain not responding to conventional therapy. *J Pediatr Adolesc Gynecol* 1997;**10**(4):199–202.

45. Laufer MR, Sanfilippo J, Rose G. Adolescent endometriosis: diagnosis and treatment approaches. *J Pediatr Adolesc Gynecol* 2003;**16**(3 suppl):S3–11.

46. Stavroulis AI et al. Laparoscopic treatment of endometriosis in teenagers. *Eur J Obstet Gynecol Reprod Biol* 2006;**125**(2):248–250.

47. Lyons TL, Winer WK, Woo A. Appendectomy in patients undergoing laparoscopic surgery for pelvic pain. *J Am Assoc Gynecol Laparosc* 2001;**8**(4):542–544.

48. Economy KE, Barnewolt C, Laufer MR. A comparison of MRI and laparoscopy in detecting pelvic structures in cases of vaginal agenesis. *J Pediatr Adolesc Gynecol* 2002;**15**(2):101–104.

49. Silva PD, Welch HD. Laparoscopic removal of a symptomatic rudimentary uterine horn in a perimenarchal adolescent. *J Soc Laparosc Surg* 2002;**6**:377–379.

50. Fedele L, Bianchi S, Zanconato G, Berlanda N, Bergamini V. Laparoscopic removal of the cavitated noncommunicating rudimentary uterine horn: surgical aspects in 10 cases. *Fertil Steril* 2005;**83**(2):432–436.

51. Fedele L, Busacca M, Candiani M, Vignali M. Laparoscopic creation of a neovagina in Mayer-Rokitansky-Küster-Hauser syndrome by modification of Vecchietti's operation. *Am J Obstet Gynecol* 1994;**171**:268–269.

52. Davydov SN. Colpopoeisis from the peritoneum of the uterorectal space. *Akusherstvo i ginekologiia* 1969;**45**(12):55–57.

53. Ismail IS, Cutner AS, Creighton SM. Laparoscopic vaginoplasty: alternative techniques in vaginal reconstruction. *Br J Obstet Gynecol* 2006;**113**(3):340.

CHAPTER 27

Disorders of the Young Breast

Yasmin Jayasinghe[1] *& Patricia Simmons*[2]

[1]Department of Gynaecology, Royal Children's Hospital, Melbourne, Australia
[2]Mayo Clinic, Rochester, MN, USA

Introduction

Clinical problems of the breast occur throughout life, even in the very young. These conditions may be congenital, developmental, inflammatory, endocrine or neoplastic in nature. Neonates and young children may have persistent breast nodules (buds) that need to be distinguished from premature thelarche or precocious puberty. Common congenital anomalies include polythelia and nipple inversion. Breast asymmetry is common in adolescents and may be due to asynchronous development, hyperplastic conditions such as juvenile hypertrophy, hypoplastic conditions, breast masses or trauma. The overwhelming majority of breast masses in the young are benign, representing fibroadenomas or inflammatory processes. Recognition of these conditions and expeditious clinical management, including counseling, may significantly reduce the psychologic distress and concern associated with breast disorders. This chapter will address the common breast disorders of female children and adolescents, including an approach to evaluation and management. An evidence-based approach to breast care in the young will also be discussed.

Early breast development

Development of the mammary ridge, between the axilla and inguinal region, begins during the fifth gestational week. The areola develops after the fifth month of prenatal life and the nipple soon after birth. The developed

Pediatric, Adolescent, & Young Adult Gynecology. Edited by
A. Altchek and L. Deligdisch. © 2009 Blackwell Publishing,
ISBN: 978-1-4051-5347-8.

breast is composed of 15–20 lobules containing ductal and glandular tissue within fibrofatty stroma.

Persistent breast nodules in the neonate

Breast nodules are present in nearly all term newborns, and in the first two weeks are largely due to breast engorgement related to the circulating maternal hormones of pregnancy. However, nodules may enlarge even up to 10 months of age under the influence of the infant's own endocrine activity [1,2]. Breast tissue may be quantitatively assessed in a standardized manner by measuring the vertical and horizontal diameters of the nodule and multiplying the two to yield the "breast unit" [3] or by comparing the diameters with standardized disks. Most commonly, a horizontal or horizontal and vertical diameters are measured. Average breast diameter at term birth is 8 mm, and size appears to be associated with increasing gestational age at birth and with birth weight [1]. Palpable breast nodules are rare under 32 weeks gestation, but may develop in premature newborns over the ensuing postnatal months. Female infants develop larger nodules which persist longer after delivery than male infants. Eventually the breast bud undergoes regression and remains barely palpable until puberty. This breast tissue is composed of rudimentary epithelium-lined ducts lying within fibro-connective tissue.

Galactorrhea in newborns

Galactorrhea may be expressed in the majority of term infants, most commonly from five to seven days after birth, and may persist in a significant number of infants at one month of age, and rarely after two months. This phenomenon is partly due to maternal progesterone withdrawal, but pituitary prolactin production by the infant takes on a more important role after two weeks of life. The fluid secretion resolves spontaneously. Attempting to express the fluid is discouraged due to the risk of inflammation and abscess. Rare causes of galactorrhea in the infant include congenital hypothyroidism and side effects of certain medications.

Bloody nipple discharge in neonates and infants

Bloody nipple discharge in neonates is rare, and may result from bacterial infection or mammary duct ectasia (dilation of the mammary duct, periductal fibrosis, and inflammation), sometimes causing a palpable subareolar nodule. Discharge in neonates may last for weeks to months and is often self-limiting, requiring observation only.

Bloody nipple discharge raises concern about malignancy or premalignancy, particularly if the discharge is persistent, uniductal, spontaneous and associated with a mass, although breast carcinoma has not been reported in neonates or young infants. One series reported the presence of secretory carcinoma in 17 children, the youngest of whom was three years of age. None of the children had nipple discharge [4]. Such reports of carcinoma in children are exceptional and because of the risk of iatrogenic amastia from surgery involving the breast bud, a conservative approach to the evaluation of breast masses in this age group is generally recommended. Ultrasound to evaluate the mass and continued observation as long as the patient is asymptomatic are preferred. Where surgical biopsy is considered necessary, acknowledgment and discussion of the high risk of long-term breast deformity secondary to removal or disruption of the breast bud should be held with the family [5].

Thelarche

Thelarche is the onset of breast development and normally occurs between eight and 13 years of age. During early puberty, fat deposition, stromal growth, and ductal proliferation occur under the influence of estrogen. Development of the alveolar units of the breast lobules occurs under the influence of progesterone, mainly after menarche, and is complete after pregnancy. Growth hormone, glucocorticoids, insulin, thyroxine, and prolactin influence the development of breast stroma and local growth factors also contribute to breast growth and development.

Box 27.1 Tanner stages of human breast development [9]

Stage B1	Elevation of the papilla only (preadolescent)
Stage B2	Elevation of breast and papilla and areola diameter (small breast bud)
Stage B3	Further enlargement of breast and areola (small breast)
Stage B4	Projection of the papilla and areola above the level of the breast (secondary mound)
Stage B5	Projection of papilla only above the mature breast

Thelarche is usually the first sign of pubertal development, although it may be preceded by adrenarche, particularly in African-American girls [6,7]. Normal breast development is characterized by five Tanner stages or sexual maturity ratings (Box 27.1), and takes 2–4 years for completion [8].

Premature thelarche

Premature thelarche is defined as isolated breast development occurring before the age of eight years, in the absence of other signs of puberty. Classic premature thelarche usually presents before the age of two years. In the majority, breast development occurs after documented regression of the neonatal breast nodule. However, in about 30%, the breast nodule is present from birth and in the past has traditionally been accepted as a form of premature thelarche when it persists beyond 10 months. Unfortunately, there is little normative evidence regarding breast nodule size and duration in normal infants, and studies are under way to determine normal parameters which may facilitate assessment of infants with breast enlargement. Those with classic premature thelarche typically have breast buds that are bilateral and around 2–4 cm in diameter. The condition is often cyclic and ultimately remits after a few years [10]. The mechanism is thought to be transient activation of the hypothalamic-pituitary axis and/or end-organ sensitivity to sex steroids. Serum follicle-stimulating hormone (FSH) may be normal or slightly elevated and gonadotropin-releasing hormone (GnRH)-stimulated FSH may be elevated but all other investigations, including growth parameters and bone age, are normal and there is no impact on puberty and final height. "Nonclassic" or "atypical premature thelarche" occurs in slighter older girls, usually 6–8 years of age, and may be associated with progression to central precocious puberty. Therefore, management includes observation over time for other signs of early pubertal development.

Precocious puberty

Precocious puberty is defined by the Lawson Wilkins Pediatric Endocrine Society as secondary sexual characteristics occurring before the age of seven years in caucasian or six years in African-American girls [11], although advanced pubertal development occurring after these ages is not always benign. Central precocious puberty is the result of early activation of the hypothalamic-pituitary axis and is idiopathic in 90% of females, but may result from a central nervous system (CNS) disorder. Peripheral or "incomplete" precocious puberty is caused by a steroid-producing tumor, exogenous steroid exposure or hypothyroidism. Girls with precocious puberty are at risk of advanced growth and skeletal maturation and, therefore, ultimately short stature. While in 90% of girls with isosexual precocious puberty the etiology is idiopathic, one must be concerned about the possibility of an underlying cause, including intracranial, ovarian or adrenal etiology as well as hypothyroidism. Investigation for precocious puberty is addressed in Chapter 18.

Congenital anomalies

Inverted nipples are seen at birth and usually normalize within the first month of life. If persistent, blockage of lactiferous ducts may occur, which can lead to mastitis. In the long term, lactation dysfunction may occur, which is not resolved by surgical correction. Other nipple anomalies include bifid and depressed nipples.

Polythelia (supernumerary nipples) occurs in up to 6% of girls and is more common than *polymastia* (supernumerary breasts, which more often present during pregnancy). They may be found anywhere along the mammary ridge but are most commonly located in the axilla or on the chest wall. They appear as small macules, nipple-areola complexes or glandular tissue, which may cause cyclic discomfort or swelling after puberty and particularly during pregnancy. Conservative management is usually all that is required for simple polythelia. Those with a glandular component require long-term follow-up, as there are occasional reports of malignancy developing in this tissue, but usually not before the fifth decade of life. Indications

for surgical excision in adolescence are cosmesis, pain, irritation or change in size or character of the tissue.

Athelia (absence of the nipple), *amazia* (absence of breast glandular tissue), and *amastia* (absence of both the nipple and glandular tissue of the breast) are uncommon and usually associated with other congenital or familial anomalies. Surgical augmentation is the only form of therapy to create breasts for these patients. Unilateral athelia or amastia with pectoralis muscle defect occurs in Poland sequence along with upper limb, spine, and/or other associated anomalies. Treatment of Poland sequence, which occurs in 1 in 20,000, involves chest wall reconstruction as well as breast augmentation. Young women with amazia due to congenital causes need to be distinguished from those with delayed thelarche. The distinction lies in the fact that those with congenital amazia have normal bone age, ovarian function, pubertal levels of sex steroids, and development of other secondary sexual characteristics.

Tuberous breast deformity is a hypoplastic breast disorder arising from constriction of breast base diameter with herniation of breast tissue into the nipple-areola complex, giving a characteristic appearance considered similar to a tuberous plant. Awareness of the condition facilitates counseling, since this condition does not resolve with maturity. Breast feeding may be compromised. The only treatment option is plastic surgery.

Developmental anomalies

Hypomastia (small breasts) may result from delayed thelarche (absent breast development by 13 or 14 years), may represent only recent onset of puberty or may be found in someone who has completed secondary sexual development but has constitutionally small breasts. Those with constitutionally small breasts have normal growth and secondary sexual development, and hormonal therapy is unlikely to be of benefit. Those with delayed puberty require endocrinologic investigation and management for induction of puberty with hormone replacement therapy under experienced medical supervision.

Breast atrophy occurs with weight loss and hypoestrogenism and therefore should respond to treatment of the underlying cause.

Juvenile or virginal hypertrophy describes rapid pubertal or postpubertal overgrowth of one or both breasts, and has been attributed to end-organ increased sensitivity to sex steroids, but the underlying cause is not known. This condition may have significant physical and psychologic sequelae. Breast pain and distension are common but tissue necrosis and skin rupture, postural problems, avoidance of physical and social activities, and school disruption may also occur. These patients are otherwise healthy and have normal serum hormones. While the breast growth may cease spontaneously, when it is severe the only therapeutic option is reduction mammoplasty. Timing of surgery should be individualized based on maturity, severity, and course. It is difficult to determine how much tissue to remove in the growing breast, so early surgery may be inadequate and result in the need for further resection. Future breast feeding in patients who have undergone surgery is often possible when adequate subareolar tissue preservation and pedicle transposition of the nipple-areolar complex occur. Adequate breast support and education play an important role in the care of young patients with breast hypertrophy. When obesity or weight gain is a contributing factor in breast enlargement, weight loss is advised.

Breast asymmetry is common and usually physiologic. When secondary to asynchronous development, improvement generally occurs by late adolescence. However, many patients have two normal breasts of different size, in which case asymmetry will persist. Less commonly, asymmetry results from unilateral hypoplasia which may occur due to congenital anomalies or as a result of damage to the breast bud, including from breast biopsy or thoracostomy tube placement, trauma or burns. Juvenile hypertrophy and breast masses due to inflammatory or neoplastic processes may also result in asymmetry. Musculoskeletal conditions such as scoliosis or chest wall lesions may cause pseudoasymmetry. Management should be individualized depending on the cause, severity of asymmetry, and degree of psychosocial distress. Contractures from previous trauma should be released in early adolescence to allow growth of breast tissue. Measures such as the temporary use of a brassiere insert or external prosthesis for the smaller breast may be all that is required. Plastic surgery may be indicated in more severe cases, with a view to revision after completion of growth. Timing is a challenge but with injectable saline implants, gradual growth of a much smaller breast may be achieved. Some patients benefit from reduction of the larger breast or from a combination of augmentation of the smaller

and reduction of the larger breast to achieve the desired result. Complications of breast surgery include scarring, infection, hematoma, lactation dysfunction, possible loss of nipple sensation, and fat necrosis.

Mastitis

The incidence of mastitis shows a bimodal distribution with peaks in the first few weeks of life and in the peripubescent years. Risk factors for mastitis are lactation, hormonal factors (such as withdrawal of maternal hormones after birth, puberty, and pregnancy), ductal metaplasia and ectasia, nipple inversion, presence of an underlying breast mass or cyst, and nipple trauma (including nipple hair plucking, shaving, stimulation, and piercing) [12]. Investigations should include culture of any purulent discharge, and breast ultrasound in the presence of a suspected abscess or mass. A mass may be detected more easily after infection resolves and should be actively sought in relapsing mastitis. Treatment with oral or parenteral antibiotics which include staphylococcus cover is recommended. If the initial antibiotic therapy fails, then additional anaerobic antibiotic coverage is recommended. Gram-negative bacteria may also cause mastitis. First-line treatments are cephalexin or amoxicillin-clavulinic acid. Clindamycin may be used if there is a history of penicillin or cephalosporin allergy [12,13]. Abscesses require surgical drainage or sometimes repeated percutaneous aspiration under ultrasound guidance.

Breast masses

Breast masses in children

Breast masses in children are nearly always benign and rarely require biopsy. Asynchronous thelarche has been reported to account for up to 35% of clinical presentations for breast mass in a series of children 18 years and younger [14]. Other considerations in the differential diagnosis are abscess, cyst, soft tissue mass (such as lipoma, hemangioma, and neuroma) and masses due to trauma such as hematoma and fat necrosis. Observation and reassurance are appropriate in most cases when infection has been excluded. Masses in patients with a known history of cancer or chest radiation therapy or that are growing, associated with skin changes or worrisome signs or symptoms (constitutional symptoms, lymphadenopathy, organomegaly) should undergo biopsy with great care to reduce the risk of damage to the breast bud.

Breast masses in adolescents

The overwhelming majority of breast masses in adolescents are benign.

Fibrocystic change is a common clinical diagnosis in adolescence, and focal change may be clinically indistinguishable from a breast neoplasm. Patients with fibrocystic changes often have bilateral breast nodularity associated with cyclic mastalgia. Cysts often resolve over a couple of cycles, but occasionally larger persistent cysts may require percutaneous drainage for symptom relief. *Mastalgia* may be independent of fibrocystic change. Empiric measures (such as reducing intake of caffeine, fat or dairy, wearing a well-fitting brassiere, the use of simple analgesia, evening primrose oil, and menstrual suppression with a continuous oral contraceptive pill or oral progesterone) have improved mastalgia in anecdotal reports rather than systematic studies. Noncyclic and/or localized mastalgia may be suggestive of a focal lesion in the breast or chest wall and merits further investigation.

Fibroadenomas are benign fibroepithelial tumors and, as the most common tumor of the adolescent breast, account for 44–94% of histologic diagnoses and up to 63% of breast masses in clinical series [14–29]. Fibroadenomas usually present after puberty, as a mobile rubbery mass in the upper outer quadrant, and are more common in the older adolescent. They may be bilateral in up to 15% of patients. Giant fibroadenomas are those weighing over 500 g or greater than 5–10 cm in diameter, or replacing over four-fifths of the breast. Cellular fibroadenomas have a dense cellular appearance and are more likely to become giant types. Juvenile fibroadenomas refer to rapidly growing tumors in adolescence. Complex fibroadenomas demonstrate cystic change, sclerosing adenosis or apocrine metaplasia and are not common in adolescence. Malignant change of the epithelial component of a fibroadenoma is extremely rare, particularly in women under 30 years. Most small fibroadenomas may be managed conservatively and observed for regression. Adult series have demonstrated that approximately 50% of fibroadenomas regress by five years [30]. A longitudinal study of adolescent females with solitary breast masses demonstrated resolution rates of 39% over 1–12 months, but persistence in 61% after 3–40 months. No

solid masses seen on ultrasound resolved (although one-third decreased in size), suggesting that the majority of the lesions that resolved completely were focal cystic changes rather than fibroadenomas [29].

Phyllodes tumor is a fibroepithelial tumor closely related to fibroadenoma but displaying increased stromal cellularity. These tumors are classified as benign, borderline or malignant. The term "cystosarcoma phyllodes" is no longer used, as these tumors are distinct from breast sarcomas. Eight percent of phyllodes tumors occur in young women mainly in their late teens, and the vast majority of these are benign. Recurrences may occur in histologically benign or malignant phyllodes tumors. Phyllodes may be clinically indistinguishable from fibroadenomas. These may become large, distorting breast architecture and causing overlying skin stretching or necrosis. Ultrasound scan may sometimes give a clue to diagnosis due to the presence of fluid-filled spaces, but often they are indistinguishable from fibroadenoma. The tumors can be locally infiltrative and in young women treatment of choice is wide local excision to achieve clear margins of 1–2 cm. Sometimes mastectomy is required for multiple recurrences or aggressive tumors with chest wall invasion. Tumor spread is hematogenous and nodal clearance is not required. Five-year survival approaches 100% in adolescents, although fatalities have been reported. Clinical behavior does not correlate well with tumor histopathology, so all phyllodes tumors should be excised and follow-up for recurrence or spread is recommended.

Epithelial masses, that is tubular adenomas and juvenile papillomatosis, are benign tumors which may present as solitary discrete masses similar to fibroadenoma, but are far less common. Juvenile papillomatosis may occur in young women with a family history of breast cancer although the malignant potential is unknown. "Proliferative disease" is a collective term to describe intraductal papilloma or sclerosing papillomatosis. These conditions are rare in adolescence and may present with a uniductal bloody discharge, with or without a subareolar mass. Natural history in adolescents is unknown but they are known to be premalignant in adults. Breast carcinoma is rare in adolescents.

Malignancy of the adolescent breast is rare and more often due to metastases or stromal malignancy (such as malignant phyllodes tumor) than to breast carcinoma. A breast mass may be the first sign of a malignancy elsewhere and rhabdomyosarcoma, non-Hodgkin lymphoma, and leukemia are the most common breast metastases in adolescence, though other malignancies have been reported, including neuroblastoma. The presence of constitutional symptoms (fatigue, anemia, fever, weight loss) [16], overlying skin changes, masses elsewhere or the presence of multiple superficial lumps in the subcutaneous tissue overlying the breast rather than within the breast itself raise increased concern for metastastic disease to the breast. *Breast carcinoma* is rare and has an age-specific incidence rate in girls between 15 and 19 years of less than 0.5 per 100,000 [31]. When this rare condition does occur in adolescents, diagnosis is often delayed due to delayed presentation, low index of suspicion by the care provider, low sensitivity of clinical examination (due to nodular breast tissue and carcinomas that appear clinically similar to fibroadenomas), and/or low sensitivity of imaging.

Evaluation of a breast mass in an adolescent

A detailed history is important and should include the duration of the mass and a history of enlargement, trauma, associated skin changes, and nipple discharge. Fibroadenomas and phyllodes tumor tend to present after puberty and are more commonly diagnosed in older teens. Fibroadenomas may have been present for months or years. Phyllodes tumor tends to have a long period of slow growth followed by a sudden rapid increase in size, but this course may not be apparent. A tender cyclic mass may indicate nodular fibrocystic change. A history of trauma and hematoma, areolar hair plucking or nipple piercing may suggest abscess, and a more distant history of trauma may indicate fat necrosis.

A detailed medical history, systems review, and family history are important. Concerning features for malignancy include a history of constitutional symptoms (such as fever, weight loss, sweats, anorexia, and malaise), a history of prior chest radiation or previous malignancy. Though rare, an epithelial malignancy may need consideration when there is a family history of breast or ovarian carcinoma in first-degree relatives and young age of diagnosis, or known BRCA 1/2 mutation. A family or personal history of mesenchymal tumors or familial p53 mutation increases the risk of a sarcomatous or fibroepithelial breast tumor. A history of previous breast disease may be significant. Menstrual history for chronic anovula-

---

Box 27.2 Concerning clinical features in adolescents who present with a breast mass

Medical history
Constitutional symptoms
Prior radiation
Previous malignancy
Rapidly growing mass

Family history
Significant family history of breast or ovarian carcinoma:
  in first-degree relatives
  with young age of diagnosis
Personal or family history of mesenchymal tumors
History of germline mutation (BRCA1/2, p53)

Clinical examination
Skin changes
Hard masses with an irregular edge
Skin tethering
Axillary lymphadenopathy
Bloody nipple discharge
Multiple masses not characteristic of fibrocystic changes

---

tion, oral contraceptive use, alcohol and smoking history should be obtained as they are risk factors for breast disease, though for manifestations later in life. Sexual history with attention to possible pregnancy or lactation is also relevant.

Explanation of the rationale and nature of the examination helps instill confidence, comfort, and co-operation in the patient, and a chaperone may be prudent. A general physical examination to exclude systemic disease and particularly lymphadenopathy and hepatosplenomegaly should be performed. The breast examination consists of first visual inspection for Tanner staging, evidence of trauma, congenital anomaly, asymmetry, visible masses, and skin changes. The four quadrants of each breast should be palpated with the patient sitting up and lying down. The majority of masses occur in the outer upper quadrant. Concerning features for worrisome breast pathology include hard masses with an irregular edge, skin tethering and/or axillary lymphadenopathy. Multiple masses may also raise concern, unless they have the character of fibrocystic changes. A mass that remains fixed in position after rotation of the patient when lying down may indicate a chest wall tumor.

A suspected fibroadenoma which is less than 5 cm in diameter, where there are no other concerning features on history or examination (Box 27.2), may be

Box 27.3 Indications for surgical excisional biopsy of an adolescent breast mass

1. Patients with concerning features on medical history, family history or examination
2. Masses ≥5 cm
3. Any mass that causes distortion of breast architecture
4. Rapidly growing masses
5. Persistent masses that have not shown signs of regression after 3–4 months
6. Multiple and bilateral breast masses if suspicious for malignancy where core biopsy is negative
7. Bloody uniductal nipple discharge associated with a mass
8. Concerning features on breast imaging

Box 27.4 Medications causing hyperprolactinemia

Amphetamines
Butyrophenones
Calcium channel blockers
Chemotherapeutic drugs (cisplatinum, adriamycin)
Estrogens (hormone therapy, oral contraceptive pill)
Histamine receptor antagonists
Methyldopa, metoclopramide, monoamine oxidase inhibitors
Opiates
Phenothiazines
Tricyclic antidepressants

managed with continued surveillance, with initial review after 1–2 months to observe for regression and then three monthly until regression is assured. At presentation, adolescents with breast carcinoma may not have any of these features, so all teenagers with a breast mass need follow-up.

Breast ultrasound scan helps differentiate the category of adolescent breast mass most of the time. Sensitivity for breast carcinoma is low, and ultrasound does not always make the distinction between a phyllodes tumor and fibroadenoma. As malignancy is rare, ultrasound is the imaging modality of choice, and recommended in patients with masses that are persistent or associated with any concerning features on history or examination, and for suspected breast abscess. Mammograms have poor sensitivity due to the increased breast density in young women and are not recommended in the evaluation of an adolescent. When malignancy is suspected from the clinical presentation or ultrasound, breast MRI should be considered. Fine needle aspiration cytology is insensitive. Core needle biopsy has a proven place in the investigation for adult breast cancer. Its role in adolescence has not been clearly established. The majority of breast masses in adolescents are fibroepithelial. Unfortunately, the distinction between a phyllodes tumor and fibroadenoma is not always clear after core biopsy, as phyllodes are heterogeneous tumors. Furthermore, masses that are large and show evidence of architectural distortion of the breast and overlying skin require surgical excision irrespective of a core biopsy result (Box 27.3). Core needle biopsy does play a role in suspected metastatic disease, as systemic rather than operative therapy may be the treatment of choice in these patients.

Evaluation of nipple discharge in an adolescent

Nipple discharge may be physiologic (due to temporary secretion from areola glands and Montgomery tubercles) or may be due to endocrine or ductal disorders. Careful history and physical examination are key to the diagnosis. One should determine the color of the discharge, whether it is unilateral or bilateral, and whether it is emanating from one location on the areola (uniductal) or multiple sites. Galactorrhea is usually milky, yellow or green, bilateral, multiductal and spontaneous, consistent with an end-organ response to hyperprolactinemia [32]. Galactorrhea can be differentiated from nonmilk discharge with a Sudan stain for fat. Prolactin levels may be raised due to physiologic conditions (pregnancy, lactation, stress, breast stimulation), hypothyroidism, prolactinoma, chronic medical conditions, and medications (Box 27.4).

Nipple discharge due to ductal lesions may be serous, mucinous, green-black or bloody. Duct ectasia is most commonly associated with bilateral green-black discharge which tests negative for occult blood but may be associated with serous, bloody or purulent discharge. If the discharge is multiductal, nonbloody and without an underlying mass, reassurance is all that is required. Fibrocystic change is associated with bilateral multiductal serous or light green discharge which is often provoked. If found in association with fine bilateral breast nodularity on examination, reassurance is appropriate. Bloody uniductal spontaneous discharge raises concern for intraductal papilloma or, more rarely, ductal carcinoma in situ (DCIS) or malignancy. Studies in adults have demonstrated that the diagnosis of malignancy is very unlikely in the absence of a breast mass or imaging abnormality. Evaluation of nipple discharge should include general examination for signs of endocrinopathy, lymphadenopathy and masses elsewhere.

Assessment for the presence of nipple discharge should be part of the routine breast examination. Discharge may be reproduced by palpating the breasts in a radial fashion from the periphery towards the centre of the breast. The nature of the discharge, its origin (from a single duct, multiductal or bilateral), and the presence of an associated subareolar mass should be noted. Most papillomas are within 1–2 cm from the areola edge. If history and examination suggest galactorrhea, investigations should include assessment for pregnancy, serum prolactin, thyroid function, a review of medication history, and head MRI if fasting morning prolactin levels are persistently elevated. Investigation of uniductal bloody nipple discharge with an underlying mass may include ultrasound, exfoliative duct cytology (although this lacks sensitivity and requires expert cytopathologic interpretation) or excisional duct biopsy. Galactography and ductal endoscopy are showing some early success in increasing preoperative diagnostic accuracy in adults [33] but the role of these technologies in adolescents has not been established.

Breast health

Breast screening

There are currently no data to justify routine breast self-examination (BSE), breast screening or BRCA testing in adolescents because of the very low incidence of malignancy and risk of false-positive results. In select groups, however, they may play a role. BSE is recommended for all young women who have had a previous malignancy or previous chest radiation therapy. Young women who have a family history of BRCA mutations or known carriers may benefit from BSE, although surveillance is not recommended before 18 years of age.

Risks for breast cancer

Risk factors for breast cancer, that is adenocarcinoma, later in life include chronic anovulation, tobacco smoking, alcohol consumption, and unopposed estrogen as well as genetic predisposition. Therefore, as part of health maintenance, patients should be counseled on these risks. Additional risk factors for malignancy involving the breast

are prior history of cancer and chest radiation therapy, and these can manifest during adolescence.

Oral contraceptive pill (OCP) and the risk of breast cancer

Breast epithelium appears to be vulnerable to carcinogens during the time between puberty and the final differentiation that occurs with first full-term pregnancy. Some studies have demonstrated that use of the oral contraceptive pill before age 20 years confers a modest increase in risk for premenopausal breast cancer (relative risk of ever-users being 1.19 times that of never-users) [34]. Risk decreases with time since last use and after 10 years since last use, there is no increased risk associated with age at first use [35]. The absolute risk of developing breast cancers due to oral contraceptive exposure is extremely small (estimated to be 0.5 excess cases and 1.5 excess cases per 10,000 women aged 16–19 and 20–24 respectively up to ten years after discontinuation of the OCP) [35]. A careful risk–benefit assessment before use in young patients is part of routine care.

Nipple piercing

Nipple piercing has gained popularity in the young and for some adolescents it may be a marker for high-risk behaviors. Preliminary reports have suggested that the practice can be associated with mastitis rates of up to 20%, delayed healing, foreign body granuloma, nipple hypertrophy, sensory loss, blood-borne infection, bacterial endocarditis in those at risk, potential lactation dysfunction, and neurogenic hyperprolactinemia. Until further studies are available, the practice of nipple piercing should be discouraged, particularly in those who are expected to be at highest risk of complications, such as those with breast implants, subacute bacterial endocarditis risk, immunosuppression, coagulation disorders, and skin diseases.

References

1. McKiernan J, Hull D. Breast development in the newborn. *Arch Dis Child* 1981;**56**:525–529.
2. Schmidt I, Chellakooty M, Haavisto A et al. Gender difference in breast tissue size in infancy: correlation with serum estradiol. *Pediatr Res* 2002;**52**(5):682–686.
3. Capraro VJ, Dewhurst CJ. Breast disorders in childhood and adolescence. *Clin Obstet Gynecol* 1975;**18**(2):25–50.

4. Karl SR, Ballantine TV, Zaino R. Juvenile secretory carcinoma of the breast. *J Pediatr Surg* 1985;**20**(4):368–371.

5. George A, Donnelly P. Bloody nipple discharge in infants. *Breast* 2006;**15**:253–254.

6. Wu T, Mendola P, Buck GM. Ethnic differences in the presence of secondary sex characteristics and menarche among US girls: the Third National Health and Nutrition Examination Survey, 1988–1994. *Pediatrics* 2002;**110**:752.

7. Biro FM, Huang B, Crawford PB et al. Pubertal correlates in black and white girls. *J Pediatr* 2006;**148**(2):234–240.

8. Marshall WA, Tanner JM. Variations in pattern of pubertal changes in girls. *Arch Dis Child* 1969;**44**:291.

9. Tanner JM. *Growth in Adolescence*, 2nd edn. Oxford: Blackwell Scientific Publications, 1962.

10. Traggiai C, Stanhope R. Disorders of pubertal development. *Best Pract Res Clin Obstet Gynaecol* 2003;**17**(1):41–56.

11. Kaplowitz PB, Oberfield SE and the Drug and Therapeutics and Executive Committees of the Lawson Wilkins Pediatric Endocrine Society. Reexamination of the age limit for defining when puberty is precocious in girls in the United States: implications for evaluation and treatment. *Pediatrics* 1999;**104**:936–941.

12. Faden H. Mastitis in children from birth to 17 years. *Pediatr Infec Dis J* 2005;**24**(12):1113.

13. Stricker T, Navratl F, Forster I, Hurumann R, Sennhauser F. Non-puerperal mastitis in adolescents. *J Pediatr* 2006;**148**:278–281.

14. West KW, Reseorla FJ, Schere LR, Grosfeld JL. Diagnosis and treatment of symptomatic breast masses in the pediatric population. *J Pediatr* 1995;**30**:182–187.

15. Bock K, Duda VF, Hadji P et al. Pathologic breast conditions in childhood and adolescence. Evaluation by sonographic diagnosis. *J Ultrasound Med* 2005;**24**:1347–1354.

16. Simmons P, Wold L. Surgically treated breast disease in adolescent females: a retrospective review of 185 cases. *Adolesc Pediatr Gynecol* 1989;**2**:95–98.

17. Dehner L, Hill A, Deschryver K. Pathology of the breast in children, adolescents, and young adults. *Semin Diagn Pathol* 1999;**16**(3):235–247.

18. Cifti AO, Tanyel FC, Buyukpamukcu N, Hicsonmez A. Female breast masses during childhood: a 25 year review. *Eur J Pediatr Surg* 1998;**8**:67–70.

19. Daniel W, Mathews M. Tumors of the breast in adolescent females. *Pediatrics* 1968;**41**:743.

20. Turbey W, Buntain W, Dudgeon D. The surgical management of pediatric breast masses. *Pediatrics* 1975;**56**:736.

21. Bower R, Bell M, Ternberg J. Management of breast lesions in children and adolescents. *J Pediatr Surg* 1976;**11**:337.

22. Stone A, Shenker I, McCarthy K. Adolescent breast masses. *Am J Surg* 1977;**134**:275.

23. Gogas J, Sechas M, Skaleas G. Surgical management of diseases of the adolescent female breast. *Am J Surg* 1979;**137**:634.

24. Ligon R, Stevenson D, Diner W et al. Breast masses in young women. *Am J Surg* 1980;**140**:779.

25. Goldstein D, Miler V. Breast masses in adolescent females. *Clin Pediatr* 1982;**21**:17.

26. Elsheikh A, Keramopoulos A, Lazaris D, Ambelia C, Louvrou N, Michalas S. Breast tumors during adolescence. *Eur J Gynaec Oncol* 2000;**XXI**(4):408–409.

27. Vargas HI, Vargas P, Eldrageely K et al. Outcomes of surgical and sonographic detection of breast masses in women younger than 30. *Am Surg* 2005;**71**:716–719.

28. Sadove AM, van Aalt JA. Congenital and acquired pediatric breast anomalies: a review of 20 years' experience. *Plast Reconstr Surg* 2005;**115**:1039–1050.

29. Neinstein LS, Atkinson J, Diament M. Prevalence and longitudinal study of breast masses in adolescents. *J Adolesc Health* 1993;**13**:277–281.

30. Cant PJ, Madden MV, Coleman MG et al. Non-operative management of breast masses diagnosed as fibroadenoma. *Br J Surg* 1995;**82**:297.

31. Surveillance, Epidemiology, and End Results (SEER) Program. Available online at: www.seer.cancer.gov.

32. Falkenberry SS. Nipple discharge. *Obstet Gynecol Clin North Am* 2002;**29**(1):21–29.

33. Vargas HI, Romero L, Chlebowski RT. Management of bloody nipple discharge. *Curr Treat Options Oncol* 2002;**3**(2):157–161.

34. Kahlenborn C, Modugno F, Potter DM, Severs WB. Oral contraceptive use as a risk factor for pre-menopausal breast cancer: a meta-analysis. *Mayo Clin Proc* 2006;**81**:1290–1302.

35. Collaborative Group on Hormonal Factors in Breast Cancer (CGHFBC). Breast cancer and hormonal contraceptives: collaborative reanalysis of individual data on 53 297 women with breast cancer and 100, 239 women without breast cancer from 54 epidemiological studies. *Lancet* 1996;**347**:1713–1727.

CHAPTER 28

Contraceptive Choices in Pediatric, Adolescent, and Young Adult Gynecology

Albert George Thomas Jr

Mount Sinai School of Medicine, New York, NY, USA

Introduction

Unplanned pregnancy and childbirth among teenagers living in the United States is the lowest ever recorded. This remarkable feat is a result of improved knowledge about and access to strategies aimed at preventing unplanned teen pregnancy and childbirth. Many teens, especially those aged 17–19, are choosing to delay their sexual debut. In addition, sexually active teens use condoms in addition to more effective hormonal contraceptive choices more often than ever before. Dual use of complementary methods such as condoms and oral contraceptive pills to prevent infection and pregnancy is increasing. Progestin-only emergency contraceptive pills are finally available as an over-the-counter option for couples aged 18 and above. Access to this modality has the estimated potential to prevent nearly 1 million abortions per year among US women experiencing unprotected coitus.

Despite these positive findings, teens in the US still experience the highest rates of pregnancy, childbearing, and abortion compared to teens in other developed countries. In addition, the teen birth rate in the US rose in 2006 for the first time since 1991. US teens also experience the highest rates of sexually transmitted infection compared to teens in other developed countries. Healthcare disparities in the United States continue to persist along racial and economic groups. If you are poor, African-American or Spanish speaking, you are at higher risk of experiencing an unplanned pregnancy or acquiring a sexually transmitted disease as compared to affluent white teens. This discrepancy persists despite the disproportionate improvements in unplanned pregnancy and infections occurring among blacks, whites, and Hispanics over the last decade.

The goal of this chapter is to define adolescent pregnancy trends in the United States, to describe the effects of contraceptive use on these trends, and to discuss the advantages and disadvantages of each method.

United States adolescent birth rates

Teenage childbearing has declined significantly over the last six decades in the United States. This teen birth rate, defined as the number of births per 1000 women aged 15–19, has steadily decreased since the late 1950s, except for a sharp increase from the late 1980s through 1991 [1]. The high US teen birth rate was attributed to high rates of unprotected sexual intercourse and decreased availability of effective, long-term contraceptive options. The US birth rate in the year 2000 for teens aged 15–19 years (48.7 per 1000) is half the rate recorded in 1957 (96.3 per 1000) and 11% lower than the rate in 1940. It has been estimated that the decrease in teen birth rates over the last decade has led to approximately 546,000 fewer births (Fig. 28.1).

The Centers for Disease Control and Prevention (CDC) recently reported another exception to the overall decline in the teen birth rate. The US rate rose in 2006 for the first time since 1991, according to preliminary birth

Pediatric, Adolescent, & Young Adult Gynecology. Edited by A. Altchek and L. Deligdisch. © 2009 Blackwell Publishing, ISBN: 978-1-4051-5347-8.

Quick Take 28.1

United States contraceptive timeline

1929 Pomeroy bilateral tubal ligation

1957 Enovid-10®, G.D. Searle and Co. (9.850 mg norethynodrel and 150 µg mestranol). First combined hormonal pill approved for treatment of "menstrual disorders"

1960 Enovid-10® approved for cyclic control of ovulation (the "Pincus pill" for birth control)

1960–1987 Intrauterine uterine devices (IUDs; Margulies Spiral™)

1976–2002 Progestasert® IUD

1973 Progestin-only pills (POPs) 0.350 mg norethindrone (NE)

1973 Low-dose oral contraceptive pills (OCPs) approved

1974 POP containing 0.075 mg norgestrel (NG)

1974 Ultra low-dose OCP available (<20 µg EE)

1982 Biphasic combination OCP

1984 Triphasic combination OCP

1986 Cu-7 IUD withdrawn by G.D. Searle

1989 Gonane progestin norgestimate (Ortho-Cyclen®) approval

1990 Female condom

1990 Cu T380A IUD (Paragard™)

1990–2002 Subdermal levonorgestrel implant (Norplant®)

1992 Gonane progestin desogestrel (Desogen®, Orthocept®)

1992 Depot medroxyprogesterone acetate (Depo-Provera®)

1997 Ortho Tri-Cyclen approved for treatment of acne vulgaris

1998–2004 Emergency contraceptive pill (ECP) (Preven®)

1999 Emergency contraceptive pill (Plan B®)

2000 Levonorgestrel IUD (Mirena®)

2000–2002 Monthly injectable combination contraceptive (Lunelle®)

2001 Transdermal contraceptive patch (Evra®)

2001 New 17 α-spironolactone progestin drospirenone (DRSP) (Yasmin®)

2001 Vaginal ring (NuvaRing®)

2002 Essure®. Microinsert nonincisional hysteroscopic sterilization

2003 First extended 91-day (84/7) cycle OCP (Seasonale®)

2006 Shortened pill-free interval OCP DRSP Regime (24 + 4 Yaz®)

2006 Subdermal etonorgestrel implant (Implanon®)

2006 Plan B ® ECP "over the counter" (OTC) status for adults >18 years

2006 Shorter hormone-free interval OCP (Loestrin 24 FE®)

2006 Short hormone-free interval OCP containing DRSP (Yaz®)

2006 Extended 91-day OCP with short hormone-free interval (Seasonique®)

2007 Yaz® approved for triple indication: birth control, premenstrual dysphoric disorder, and acne

2007 365-day extended-cycle OCP without pill-free intervals or placebo (Lybrel®)

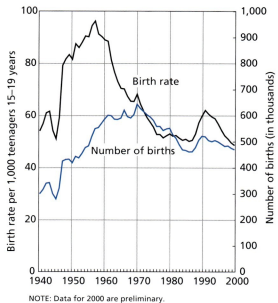

NOTE: Data for 2000 are preliminary.

Figure 28.1 Number of births and birth rates for teenagers 15–19 years: United States, 1940–2000.

statistics released by the CDC in *Births: Preliminary Data for 2006* at the website: www.cdc.gov/nchs/pressroom/07newsreleases/teenbirth.htm. The report shows that between 2005 and 2006, the birth rates for teenagers 15–19 rose 3%, from 40.5 live births per 1000 females in 2005 to 41.9 births per 1000 in 2006. This follows the 14-year downward trend in which the teen birth rate fell by 34% from its recent peak of 61.8 births per 1000 in 1991.

International birth rates are lower

Although the 2002 US teenage birth rate was the lowest ever recorded (43 per 1000 women aged 15–19) it is double the rate in Canada (20 per 1000) and quadruple the rates in Germany (10 per 1000) and France (8 per 1000) [2] (Table 28.1). Twenty-two percent of US teens reported having a child before age 20. This figure was lower in Great Britain (15%), Canada (11%), France (6%), and Sweden (4%). In addition to higher birth rates, US teens also have higher pregnancy, abortion and sexually transmitted disease rates than teens from Great Britain, Canada, Sweden and France.

Darroch et al conducted an international study that utilized survey information and government data to analyze the roles of sexual activity and contraceptive use

Table 28.1 Number of births per 1000 women 15–19 years of age: United States, 2002, and selected countries, most recent year available

Country	Number of births per thousand
United States	43
United Kingdom	31
Portugal	21
Canada	20
Australia	17
Belgium	12
Germany	10
France	8
Sweden	7
Spain	8
Italy	7
Netherlands	6
Japan	5

Source: United Nations Demographic Yearbook, 2001 New York: United Nations, 2003

in teenage pregnancy rate differences in these four countries and the US [3]. Two key points were revealed by this analysis. The first was that US teens were not more sexually active than European teens. The proportion of women aged 20–24 who had first intercourse before 20 was similar for all five countries: Sweden (86%), Great Britain (85%), France (83%), United States (81%), and Canada (75%). The second point was that higher US teen pregnancies could be partially attributed to lower overall use of contraception as well as a tendency to use less effective hormonal methods. Potential reasons for discrepant cross-country variations in contraceptive use include:

• societal attitudes about adolescent sexual activity that may influence the provision of reproductive services to teenagers

• adolescent attitudes about use of contraception including accuracy of knowledge of how to use the methods and fear of side effects

• the level of confidentiality, and the extent of parental support or opposition.

Decrease in sexual activity and increase in contraceptive use among US teens leads to decline of birth rate

Teenage birth rates and sexually transmitted infection (STI) rates are higher in the US than in Europe. These US rates are similarly in sync with European rates that are declining. This decline resulted from the availability of integrated, comprehensive sex education programs in several centers throughout the United States. Ventura et al, using birth certificates filed for babies born in the US, reported that the teen birth declines from 1991 to 2000 were associated with decreased sexual activity reflecting changing attitudes toward premarital sex, increases in condom use, and acceptance of cutting-edge, effective hormonal contraception, such as implants and injectables [1]. Abma et al, utilizing data analyzed from the National Survey of Family Growth (NSFG), noted significant declines in teen sexual activity [2]. Between 1998 and 2002, sexual activity declined from 51% to 46% and 60% to 46% for female and male teenagers, respectively [2]. Teenagers also reported postponing sex until older ages. In 2002, 13% of never-married female teens had had sex before age 15 compared with 19% in 1995; 15% of males initiated sex before age 15 compared to 21% in 1995 [2]. Santelli et al analyzed the determinants of the 30% decline in rates of pregnancy among women aged 15–17 between 1991 through 2001 using national data from the Youth Risk Behavior Survey (YRBS), contraceptive failure rates from the 1988 and 1995 NSFG, and pregnancy rates from the National Vital Statistics System. The authors concluded that 53% of decreased US teen pregnancy was attributed to decreased sexual experience and 47% to improved contraceptive use [4]. An updated study by the same authors based on 1995 and 2002 NSFG data for women aged 15–19 concluded that the overall pregnancy risk index declined 38%, with 86% of the decline attributable to improved contraceptive use. Among adolescents aged 15–17 years, 77% of the decline in pregnancy risk was attributable to improved contraceptive use [4a]. These findings suggest that as in other developed countries, improved contraceptive use is the primary determinant of declining US adolescent pregnancy rates.

Increased contraceptive use among sexually active US teens

Two studies examined trends in adolescent contraceptive use between 1991 and 2003 [5,6]. Anderson et al, using YRBS data and multivariate methods, analyzed the 30% of high-school students who reported that they had been sexually active in the previous three months. Condom use increased significantly from 46.2% to 63%. The percentage reporting use of either no method or withdrawal declined from 32.6% to 18.8%. In 2003, withdrawal or no method was greater among females, Hispanics, those who had been pregnant or had caused a pregnancy, and those who reported feeling sad or hopeless or had considered suicide. This high-risk group who engaged in poorly protected sex accounted for 6.4% of high-school students.

Santelli et al concluded that although overall teen hormonal use changed little between 1991 and 2003, teens tended to use more effective hormonal contraceptive. For example, the decrease in teen use of oral contraceptive pills (OCPs) from 25% to 20% was offset by a 5% increase use of more effective injectable contraceptives. Injectable hormones are well known to have lower typical failure rates over one year of use (2–3%) than oral contraceptives (8%), which in part helps to explain falling teenage pregnancy rates [7].

Dual-method use

Concomitant use of a hormonal contraceptive with condoms (dual use) prevents STI and is associated with lower contraceptive failure rates. Dual-use rates among teens increased from 3% in 1991 to 8% in 2003. This finding suggested that teens were increasingly considering the prevention of pregnancy along with protection from disease [6].

The next section will describe how increased utilization of more effective contraception by teenagers affects pregnancy rate.

Contraceptive failure rates

Typical use and perfect use

"Contraceptive efficacy" refers to how well a contraceptive method works in clinical trials. The term "effectiveness" refers to how well it works in actual practice [8]. According to Trussell et al, contraceptive failure rates during typical use (user effectiveness) show how effectively a method prevents pregnancy during actual use, that includes inconsistent or incorrect use. Contraceptive methods requiring user intervention before penile–vaginal contact have higher typical failure rates compared with published perfect-use failure rates (method effectiveness). Method effectiveness describes how effective methods can be when always used as directed and implies correct and consistent use.

Perfect-use failure rates are usually published following clinical trials that are conducted under strict conditions that prompt participants to continue to use the method with every coital event. Typical failure rates are usually generated by large surveys that estimate contraceptive failures as the proportion of method users who experience failure within a certain time period [7].

A review by Trussell illustrates the idea of some contraceptive methods being more forgiving than others when used imperfectly. In addition, imperfect use often depends on how difficult a contraceptive is to use [8]. This review included more than 165 articles and estimated the probability of pregnancy during the first year of typical use of each available method in the United States in 2004. This rate is compared to the best-guess estimates of perfect-use pregnancy probabilities and includes one-year continuation rates [9]. According to the analysis of the 1995 NSFG and the 1994–1995 Abortion Patient Survey (APS) by Fu, when contraceptive methods are ranked by effectiveness over the first 12 months of use, the implant and injectables, both user-independent choices, have the lowest failure rates (2–3%), followed by the pill (8%), the diaphragm and cervical cap (12%), the male condom (14%), periodic abstinence (21%), withdrawal (24%), and spermicides (26%). Failure rates were higher in the certain socio-economic subgroups that mirror healthcare disparities of the US in general [10]. These groups included cohabiting and otherwise unmarried women, among those with an annual income below 200% of the federal poverty level, among black and Hispanic women, among adolescents and among women in their 20s [7]. For example, adolescent women who are not married but are cohabiting experience a failure rate of 31% in the first year of contraceptive use while the 12-month failure rate among married women aged 30 or older is only 7%. Black women have a contraceptive failure rate of about 19% that did not vary by rate of family income. Overall 12-month rates were lower for Hispanic women (15%) and white women (10%) but vary by income, with poorer women having substantially greater failure rates than more affluent women.

An analysis of the 1988 and 1995 NSFG illustrates that contraceptive failure rates declined in the second year of use, possibly due to increased learner experience with the method [11]. The average failure rate for all reversible methods declined from 13% to 8% from the first year of method use to the second year. First-year rates were highest for women using spermicides, withdrawal, and periodic abstinence (on average 23–28% in the first year), and lowest for women relying on long-acting methods and oral contraceptives (4–8%).

In an analysis of contraceptive practices in women seeking abortions, 46% of women used no contraceptive method in the month they conceived [12]; 33% of this group perceived that they were at low risk of conception (6% thought that they or their partner was sterile) and 32% had concerns about the contraceptive methods themselves. Such concerns included problems with the methods in the past (20.2%), fear of side effects (13.3%), beliefs that methods would make sex less fun (3.1%), that methods would be too difficult to use (1.1%), and that methods would be too messy (0.6%). The male condom was the most commonly reported method among these women (28%) followed by the pill (14%). Inconsistent method use was the main cause of pregnancy for 49% of condom users and 76% of pill users; 42% of condom users cited condom slippage or breakage as a reason for pregnancy. Substantial proportions of pill and condom users indicated perfect method use (13–14%). It has been estimated that 51,000 abortions were averted by the use of emergency contraceptive pills in 2000 [12].

Contraceptive choices

Adolescent contraceptive use is increasing. According to the 2002 NSFG, of at least 9.5 million females and 10.1 million males between the ages of 15 and 19 who were unmarried and reported ever having intercourse, approximately one-third reported having sexual intercourse in the previous three months [2]. This illustrates the substantial numbers of sexually active teenagers requiring effective contraception. Several available reversible contraceptives choices are appropriate for use by adolescents [13]. These choices include abstinence, oral contraceptive pills, emergency contraception, barrier methods, injectables and implants, intrauterine devices, and periodic abstinence. Permanent contraceptive methods such as those that ligate the fallopian tubes by laparoscopy (bilateral tubal ligation) or hysteroscopy (transtubal ligation; Essure) are usually inappropriate for young people less than 21 years of age (Table 28.3).

Most young people who report being sexually active have used some form of contraception [2]. In 2002 the percentage of females aged 15–19 who ever used condoms was 93.7%. The percent of ever use of the oral contraceptive pill was 61.4%, making this the most frequently used hormonal method. Doubled reported utilization of contraceptive injectables occurred between 1995 and 2002 (9.7% and 20.7% respectively). This is a significant finding in that such contraceptives have considerably lower failure rates compared to other hormonal methods that are user dependent; 8.1% also reported using the transdermal patch, another method associated with lower failure rates.

Abstinence

Sexual abstinence is an essential component of successful comprehensive adolescent education that aims to reduce STI and unintended pregnancies [14]. One study suggests that approximately 53% of the decrease in the adolescent pregnancy rate is attributed to teen abstinence and 47% is due to improved use of contraception [4]. Although abstinence is considered an ideal goal, many teens practicing this method alone will ultimately engage in high-risk sexual behavior. According to the YRBS 2005, 33.9% of students had had sexual intercourse with one person or more during the three months preceding the survey [15]. This means that abstinence-only programs can put at risk teens who cannot or will not utilize the method by discouraging condom use.

Larger numbers of adolescents are delaying initiation of sexual intercourse [2]. Between 1988 and 2002 the percentage of sexually experienced female teens aged 15–19 decreased from 51.1% to 45.5%. In males aged 15–19 the same trend of decreasing sexual experience occurred, from 60.4% to 45.7%. It was notable that the largest percentage decrease in sexual experience occurred among younger teens aged 15–17, versus older teens aged 18–19. The sexual experience of females aged 18–19 from 1988 to 2002 dropped from 73% to 69% while males decreased from 77% to 64%.

Abstinence intervention usually stresses delayed sexual intercourse or reducing its frequency [16]. Adolescent perceptions about abstinence may differ from the public health definitions that emphasize refraining from sexual contact, i.e. no vaginal, anal or oral intercourse [14]. Abstinence as a stand-alone strategy has gained in popularity

Table 28.2 Percentage of women experiencing an unintended pregnancy during the first year of typical use and the first year of perfect use of contraception and the percentage continuing use at the end of the first year. United States

Method (1)	% of women experiencing an unintended pregnancy within the first year of use		% of women continuing use at one year[3] (4)
	Typical Use[1] (2)	Perfect Use[2] (3)	
No method[4]	85	85	
Spermicides[5]	29	18	42
Withdrawal	27	4	43
Fertility awareness-based methods	25		51
Standard days method[6]		5	
Two-day method[6]		4	
Ovulation method[6]		3	
Sponge			
Parous women	32	20	46
Nulliparous women	16	9	57
Diaphragm[7]	16	6	57
Condom[8]			
Female (Reality)	21	5	49
Male	15	2	53
Combined pill and progestin-only pill	8	0.3	68
Evra patch	8	0.3	68
NuvaRing	8	0.3	68
Depo-Provera	3	0.3	56
IUD			
ParaGard (copper T)	0.8	0.6	78
Mirena (LNG-IUS)	0.2	0.2	80
Implanon	0.05	0.05	84
Female sterilization	0.5	0.5	100
Male sterilization	0.15	0.10	100

Emergency contraceptive pills: treatment initiated within 72 hours after unprotected intercourse reduces the risk of pregnancy by at least 75%.[9]

Lactational amenorrhea method: LAM is a highly effective, *temporary* method of contraception.[10]

Source: Trussell J. Contraceptive efficacy. In: Hatcher RA, Trussell J, Nelson AL, Cates W, Stewart FH, Kowal D. (eds) *Contraceptive Technology*, 19th rev. edn. New York: Ardent Media, 2007.

[1] Among *typical* couples who initiate use of a method (not necessarily for the first time), the percentage who experience an accidental pregnancy during the first year if they do not stop use for any other reason. Estimates of the probability of pregnancy during the first year of typical use for spermicides, withdrawal, fertility awareness-based methods, the diaphragm, the male condom, the pill, and Depo-Provera are taken from the 1995 National Survey of Family Growth corrected for under-reporting of abortion; see the text for the derivation of estimates for the other methods.

[2] Among couples who initiate use of a method (not necessarily for the first time) and who use it *perfectly* (both consistently and correctly), the percentage who experience an accidental pregnancy during the first year if they do not stop use for any other reason. See the text for the derivation of the estimate for each method.

[3] Among couples attempting to avoid pregnancy, the percentage who continue to use a method for one year.

[4] The percentages becoming pregnant in columns (2) and (3) are based on data from populations where contraception is not used and from women who cease using contraception in order to become pregnant. Among such populations, about 89% become pregnant within one year. This estimate was lowered slightly (to 85%) to represent the percentage who would become pregnant within one year among women now relying on reversible methods of contraception if they abandoned contraception altogether.

[5] Foams, creams, gels, vaginal suppositories, and vaginal film.

[6] The ovulation and two-day methods are based on evaluation of cervical mucus. The standard days method avoids intercourse on cycle days 8 through 19.

[7] With spermicidal cream or jelly.

[8] Without spermicides.

[9] The treatment schedule is one dose within 120 hours after unprotected intercourse, and a second dose 12 hours after the first dose. Both doses of Plan B can be taken at the same time. Plan B (one dose is one white pill) is the only dedicated product specifically marketed for emergency contraception. The Food and Drug Administration has in addition declared the following 22 brands of oral contraceptives to be safe and effective for emergency contraception: Ogestrel or Ovral (one dose is two white pills), Levlen or Nordette (one dose is four light-orange pills), Cryselle, Levora, Low-Ogestrel, Lo/Ovral or Quasence (one dose is four white pills), Tri-Levlen or Triphasil (one dose is four yellow pills), Jolessa, Portia, Seasonale or Trivora (one dose is four pink pills), Seasonique (one dose is four light-blue-green pills), Empresse (one dose is four orange pills), Alesse, Lessina or Levlite (one dose is pink pills), Aviane (one dose is five orange pills), and Lutera (one dose is five white pills).

[10] However, to maintain effective protection against pregnancy, another method of contraception must be used as soon as menstruation resumes, the frequency or duration of breastfeeds is reduced, bottle feeds are introduced, or the baby reaches six months of age.

Table 28.3 Major methods of contraception and some related safety concerns, side effects, and noncontraceptive benefits

Method	Dangers	Side effects	Noncontraceptive benefits
Combined hormonal contraception (pill, and presumably Evra patch, and NuvaRing)	Cardiovascular complications (stroke, heart attack, blood clots, high blood pressure), depression, hepatic adenomas, increased risk of cervical and possibly liver cancers, earlier development of breast cancer in young women	Nausea, headaches, dizziness, spotting, weight gain, breast tenderness, chloasma	Decreases dysmenorrhea, menorrhagia, anemia and cyclic mood problems (PMS); protects against ectopic pregnancy, symptomatic PID, and ovarian, endometrial, and possibly colorectal cancer; reduces acne
Progestin-only pill	May avoid some dangers of combined hormonal contraceptives	Less nausea than with combined pills	Lactation not disturbed
IUD	Infection post insertion, uterine perforation, anemia	Menstrual cramping, spotting, increased bleeding with non-progestin-releasing IUDs	Mirena decreases menstrual blood loss and menorrhagia and can provide progestin for hormone replacement therapy
Male condom	Anaphylactic reaction to latex	Decreased sensation, allergy to latex	Protects against STIs, including HIV; delays premature ejaculation
Female condom	None known	Esthetically unappealing and awkward to use for some	Protects against STIs
Implanon	Infection at implant site; may avoid some dangers of combined hormonal contraceptives	Headache, acne, menstrual changes, weight gain, depression, emotional lability	Lactation not disturbed; decreases dysmenorrhea
Depo-Provera	Depression, allergic reactions, pathologic weight gain, bone loss; may avoid some dangers of combined hormonal contraceptives	Menstrual changes, weight gain, headache, adverse effects on lipids	Lactation not disturbed; reduces risk of seizures; may protect against ovarian and endometrial cancers
Sterilization	Infection; possible anesthetic or surgical complications; if pregnancy occurs after tubal sterilization, high risk that it will be ectopic	Pain at surgical site, psychologic reactions, subsequent regret that the procedure was performed	Tubal sterilization reduces risk of ovarian cancer and may protect against PID
Abstinence	None known		Prevents STIs, including HIV, if anal and oral intercourse are avoided as well
Diaphragm, sponge	Vaginal and urinary tract infections, toxic shock syndrome; possible increase in susceptibility to HIV/AIDS acquisition if exposed to positive partner	Pelvic discomfort, vaginal irritation, vaginal discharge if left in too long, allergy	
Spermicides	Vaginal and urinary tract infections; possible increase in susceptibility to HIV/AIDS acquisition if exposed to positive partner	Vaginal irritation, allergy	
Lactational amenorrhea method (LAM)			Provides excellent nutrition for infants under six months old

since the late 1980s due to the political context surrounding sex education [17]. This has led to the expenditure of millions of dollars on abstinence-only educational initiatives. A national survey was conducted in 1999 to attempt to characterize what teacher attitudes and priorities were regarding sexuality education in the United States. The authors concluded that sex education in secondary public schools was increasingly focused on abstinence and less likely to present students with comprehensive teaching that included necessary information on topics such as birth control, abortion and sexual orientation [17].

One randomized controlled trial of 659 African-American adolescents at risk for acquisition of infection with the human immunodeficiency virus (HIV) compared abstinence intervention, safer sex intervention that stressed condom use, and a control intervention concerning health issues unrelated to sexual behavior [16]. Jemmott et al concluded that both abstinence and safer sex interventions can reduce HIV risk behaviors, but safer sex interventions may be especially effective with sexually experienced adolescents and may have longer effects [16]. Ott et al emphasized that adolescents are likely to be best served by placing abstinence education back within the framework of broader sexuality education. This would provide adolescents with the information and decision-making skills to evaluate relationships, develop communication within relationships, and accurately assess their own level of readiness [14]. The effective clinician may approach the celibacy issue by recognizing the adolescent's need for intimacy in relationships that can be addressed by skills building related to noncoital ways to achieve closeness and connection [18].

It is possible that the recent higher percentage expenditure on abstinence-only programs may be responsible for the recent CDC report of the first teen birth rate rise for 15 years, in 2006.

Combination oral contraceptive pills

Oral contraceptive pills (OCPs) containing estrogen and progestin are the most popular method of hormonal contraception used in the US. Innovative chemists, including Russell Marker, Carl Djerassi, and Percy Lavon Julian, were first credited with the discovery of pathways that led to mass production of precursor steroids essential to progesterone and cortisone production [19,20].

According to the 2002 NSFG, 82% of women aged 15–44 had used or were using the pill; 19% of women aged 15–

44 named OCPs as their current contraceptive [21]. Ever-use of OCPs among teens aged 15–19 increased between 1995 and 2002 from 51.6% to 61.4% and current use at last intercourse among teens 15–19 was 34% [2].

Mechanism of action

The combination pill prevents ovulation by inhibiting gonadotropin secretion via an effect on both pituitary and hypothalamic centers of the brain [19]. The progestin agent suppresses luteinizing hormone (LH) secretion, thus suppressing ovulation. The estrogenic agent suppresses follicle-stimulating hormone (FSH), thus inhibiting the selection and emergence of the dominant ovarian follicle. Therefore, the estrogenic component also contributes to the contraceptive efficacy. However, if follicular growth and development were not sufficiently inhibited, the progestin component would prevent the LH surge, a requirement for ovarian egg release [19]. The estrogen also stabilizes the endometrium, preventing breakthrough bleeding and providing cycle control. This is important to adolescents who often interpret breakthrough staining and spotting as a sign of ineffectual contraception which in turn often leads to method termination and/or method dissatisfaction, with consequent increase in pregnancy risk [22–24].

Estrogen also potentiates the action of the progesterone agent, allowing reduction in the progesterone doses in the pill. Progesterone is also known to block sperm entry into the uterus, inhibit sperm capacitation, slow fallopian tube motility, disrupt transport of the fertilized ovum, and induce endometrial atrophy [9].

Adverse events and contraindications

The original high-dose OCP formulations used during the 1960s were extremely effective at preventing pregnancy [25]. The benefits of this revolutionary compound, pioneered by biologist Gregory Goodwin Pincus and gynecologists John Rock and Celso Ramon Garcia, undoubtedly saved many women's lives by preventing unintentional pregnancies that often ended in illegal septic abortion [26,27]. It is likely that faulty study design of early pill formulations led to the false conclusion that combination pills with lower hormonal content were associated with higher failure rates [27]. During the 1960s, the high estrogen dose contents of these pills were associated with increased risk of arterial and venous thrombosis resulting in stroke, myocardial infarction (MI) (especially in

Table 28.4 Available combination oral contraceptives

	Name	Progestin (mg)	Type of estrogen (μg)
50 μg estrogen	Ogestrel/Ovral	Norgestrel (0.5)	EE (50)
	Necon/Nelova/Norethin/Norinyl/ Ortho-Novum 1/50	Norethindrone (1.0)	Mestranol (50)
	Ovcon 50	Norethindrone (1.0)	EE (50)
	Norlestrin 1/50	Norethindrone acetate (1.0)	EE (50)
	Demulen 50/Zovia 1/50	Ethynodiol diacetate (1.0)	EE (50)
<50 μg estrogen plus monophasic	Lo-Ovral/Low-Ogestrel	Norgestrel (0.3)	EE (30)
	Ovcon 35	Norethindrone (0.4)	EE (35)
	Desogen/Orthocept	Desogestrel (0.15)	EE (30)
	Levlen/Levora/Nordette	Levonorgestrel (0.15)	EE (30)
	Ortho-Cyclen	Norgestimate (0.25)	EE (35)
	Necon/Nelova/Norinyl/Norethrin/ Ortho-Novum 1/35	Norethindrone (1.0)	EE (35)
	Lo/Ovral	Norgestrel (0.3)	EE (30)
	Brevicon/Modicon/Necon/Nelova 0.5/35	Norethindrone (0.5)	EE (35)
	Loestrin 1.5/30	Norethindrone acetate (1.5)	EE (30)
	Alesse/Levlite 0.1/20	Levonorgestrel (0.1)	EE (20)
	Seasonale .15/30	Levonorgestrel (0.15)	EE (30)
	Lybrel	Levonorgestrel (0.09)	EE (20)
	Loestrin 1/20	Norethindrone acetate (1.0)	EE (20)
	Demulen/Zovia 1/35	Ethynodiol diacetate (1.0)	EE (35)
<50 μg estrogen plus multiphasic	Ortho-Novum 7/7/7	Norethindrone (0.5, 0.75, 1.0)	EE (35, 35, 35)
	Tri-Levlen/Triphasil/Trivora	Levonorgestrel (0.05, 0.075, 0.125)	EE (30, 40, 30)
	Jenest	Norethindrone (0.5, 1.0)	EE (35, 35)
	Necon/Nelova/Ortho-Novum 10/11	Norethindrone (0.5, 1.0)	EE (35, 35)
	Ortho Tri-Cyclen	Norgestimate (0.18, 0.215, 0.250)	EE (35, 35, 35)
	Tri-Norinyl	Norethindrone (0.5, 1.0, 0.5)	EE (35, 35)
	Estrostep	Norethindrone acetate (1.0, 1.0, 1.0)	EE (20, 30, 35)
	Mircette	Desogestrel (0.15)	EE (0.02, 0.01)
Other	Yasmin	Drospirenone (3)	EE (30)
	Yaz	Drospirenone (3)	EE (20)

EE, ethinyl estradiol.
Adapted from Rebar R. (ed) *Contraception*. Available at: endotext.org.

smokers), deep vein thrombosis (DVT), and pulmonary embolism (PE) [28]. The first combination pill available in the US was named Enovid-10 and was manufactured by G.D. Searle and Co. The formulation of Enovid was 150 μg of the estrogen mestranol and 9.850 mg of the progestin norethynodrel. This was approximately four times the dose of estrogen and 10 times the dose of progestin in today's pills [29]. A dose-related effect between estrogen dose and DVT led to a four-decade trend of decreasing

hormonal content to improve the safety and side-effect profile of the combination OCP.

Progestin and estrogen components in OCPs

Most progestins contained in the OCPs approved for US distribution are derived from 19-nortestosterone. They belong to the estrane (norethindrone, norethindrone acetate, ethynodiol diacetate) or gonane (norgestrel, levonorgestrel, desogestrel, norgestimate) category. Drospirenone is a non-19-nortestosterone progestin derived from 17α-spironolactone.

Norgestimate and desogestrel became available in 1989 and 1992 respectively and both were notably less androgenic progestins *in vitro*. This property was developed to minimize the adverse lipid profiles that were associated with use of the earlier generation progestins. The beneficial lipid profiles resulting from use of these OCPs never translated into lower rates of clinical disease.

OCP formulations were considered first generation if they contained greater than 50 μg of ethinyl estradiol (EE), second generation if they contained levonorgestrel, norgestimate or other members of the levonorgestrel (LNG) family and contained 30 or 35 μg of EE. Third-generation OCPs were defined as those containing desogestrel or gestodene with 20 or 30 μg of EE [19]. Gestodene is not approved for use in the US.

Desogestrel (DSG) and gestodene (GSD) became controversial in 1995 when three reports found an approximately twofold increased risk of venous thromboembolism (VTE) for oral contraceptives containing DSG versus older formulations. The risk of nonfatal VTE with the use of hormonal contraceptives containing DSG and GSD is relatively benign as compared to pregnancy and activities of daily living (Table 28.5). It is estimated that 20–30 cases of nonfatal VTE per 100,000 users of third-generation OCPs containing these progestins can be expected compared to 10–15 cases per 100,000 users of OCPs containing LNG. Pregnancy, on the other hand, confers an increased risk of about 60 cases of nonfatal VTE per 100,000 women [30]. Thus discontinuation of OCPs in patients at risk of pregnancy could have serious public health consequences. A recent report regarding norgestimate (NGM) suggests that this gonane does not share the same DVT risk with DSG and GSD [31].

The World Health Organization (WHO) does not recommend special hematologic testing to find the 1–2% of women with inheritable risk factors for thrombophilic disorders [28]. Such disorders include activated protein C resistance or changes on the factor V chain (factor V Leiden). Although routine coagulation tests are not justified, taking a family and personal history is recommended prior to use of OCPs [32].

Drospirenone (DRSP), a novel progestin analog of spironolactone, is presently available in two low-dose OCP formulations. This unique progestin exhibits anti-

Table 28.5 Voluntary risks in perspective

Activity	Risk of death
Risk per year	
While skydiving	1 in 1000
From an accident	1 in 2900
From an automobile accident	1 in 5000
From a fall	1 in 20,000
From a fire	1 in 50,000
From riding your bicycle	1 in 130,000
In an airplane crash	1 in 250,000
From being struck by lightning	1 in 2,000,000
Risk per year for women preventing pregnancy	
Using combined oral contraceptives (and presumably the patch and ring as well)	
Nonsmoker	
Aged 15–34	1 in 1,667,000
Aged 35–44	1 in 33,300
Smoker	
Aged 15–34	1 in 57,800
Aged 35–44	1 in 5200
Undergoing tubal sterilization	1 in 66,700
Risk per year from using tampons	1 in 5,734,000
Risk from pregnancy	1 in 8700
Risk from spontaneous abortion	1 in 142,900
Risk from legal induced abortion	
Mifepristone/misoprostol	1 in 162,500
Surgical	1 in 142,900
≤8 weeks	1 in 1,000,000
9–10 weeks	1 in 500,000
11–12 weeks	1 in 250,000
13–15 weeks	1 in 58,800
16–20 weeks	1 in 29,400
≥21 weeks	1 in 11,200

mineralocorticoid, antiandrogenic activity and no androgenic effect. This is in distinction to the 19-nortestosterone progestins that exhibit a minimal androgenic effect. The product labeling for DRSP includes additional precautions about its use in conditions predisposing to hyperkalemia, such as renal insufficiency, hepatic dysfunction, and adrenal insufficiency or if taking potassium-sparing drugs, supplements, heparin or chronic nonsteroidal anti-inflammatory drugs (NSAIDs) [31]. A 1998 review article was reassuring about the use of DRSP even in high hyperkalemia-risk populations [32]. A ultra-low dose DRSP formulation (Yaz™) 24/4-day regime containing 3 mg DRSP (equal to 25 mg of the diuretic spironolactone) and 20 μg EE has been approved for treatment of emotional and physical symptoms associated with premenstrual dysphoric disorder (PMDD). The diuretic effect, which many women find beneficial, is believed to be a mild one that tapers off after the first few months.

Despite the development of new progestin compounds within OCP formulations, over the last 20 years, the estrogen components have remained relatively stable. The two available estrogens in the US are EE and mestranol. The original OCPs contained considerably higher doses of estrogen (150 μg), that were approximately six times more potent than formulations existing today. Low-dose OCPs are defined as those containing less than 50 μg of estrogen and ultra-low dose OCPs contain 25 or 20 μg. Most formulations contain 30–35 μg.

OCP formulations may be monophasic or multiphasic. Monophasic formulations are those where each active pill contains the same doses of estrogen and progestin. Multiphasic regimes contain varying amounts of estrogen and progestin in the pills. Multiphasics can be considered either biphasic or triphasic. Biphasic formulations have two different combinations of estrogen and progestin in the pills. Triphasic formulations have three different combinations of estrogen and progestin [9]. The triphasic formulations were developed to minimize hormonal dosing by closely mimicking the hormonal milieu of a natural menstrual cycle.

Substantial reductions in estrogen and progestin doses in OCPs evolved both to reduce nuisance side effects experienced by patients and improve the safety profile for users [33,34]. Decreased estrogen would mean less nausea and breast tenderness, as well as lower thrombosis risk, for example. However, too low a dose of estrogen is associated with more episodes of breakthrough bleeding and more user dissatisfaction.

The combination OCPs traditionally were formulated as 28-day pill packs that consisted of 21 days of hormonally active pills ending with seven placebo pills (21/7) to allow hormonal withdrawal bleeding prior to beginning the next pill pack. The use of many low-dose 21/7 OCP regimes has been associated with hormone withdrawal symptoms including pelvic pain, breast tenderness, bloating, swelling, and increased usage of pain medications during the conventional seven-day hormone-free interval (HFI) [35]. Many hormone withdrawal symptoms resulted from maintaining the seven-day HFI in the new low-dose OCPs. The decreased hormonal content resulted in lower ovarian suppression, increased production of endogenous hormones, and more ovarian activity that translated into menstrual-associated symptoms [36].

One strategy to avoid HFI adverse effects is to administer active pills continuously with a 91-day extended-cycle pack that extends the time between menses to once every three months (84/7 active pill/placebo pill regime). This approach of four menses per year was extremely useful, for example, in the group of women suffering from hormone withdrawal headaches.

The first extended regime introduced in 2003 consisted of a "triple decker" pill pack of containing 84 active pills (0.15 mg LNG/30 μg EE) followed by seven placebo pills (Seasonale™). Breakthrough bleeding and spotting are common with extended regimes. Decreasing the HFI to 3–4 days when bothersome breakthrough bleeding and/or spotting occurs has been recommended as one successful strategy [37]. Decreasing the HFI to 3–4 days was found useful during management of breakthrough bleeding when comparing a 21/7 OCP with a 168-day extended regime of an OCP containing 3 mg of drospirenone and 30 μg of EE [36]. Another 91-day extended regime was developed containing 84 active pills (0.15 mg LNG/30 μg EE) ending with seven low-dose (10 μg) EE tablets substituted for the placebo to address this breakthrough bleeding (Seasonique™) [38]. Bleeding was reported as similar to other oral contraceptive regimes.

A systematic review of six randomized controlled trials comparing extended regimes with conventional formulations of OCPs generally showed similar compliance rates, safety profiles, and contraceptive efficacy. Discontinuation rates for breakthrough bleeding were also similar. Bleeding patterns were similar or better for extended regimes. Favorable outcomes for extended regimes were notable as compared to standard 28-day regimes including improvement in terms of headaches, genital irritation, bloating, tiredness, and menstrual pain [39].

Contraindications

In order to properly anticipate concerns that teens have about hormonal contraception, providers must balance the numerous benefits with the known adverse events associated with their use.

The main adverse metabolic effect of the estrogenic component is increased hepatic synthesis of proteins, especially those that enhance venous and arterial thrombosis [25]. Progestins may adversely affect the lipid profile while estrogen may cause an increase in serum levels of triglycerides. Although there are cardiovascular effects associated with OCPs, these events are rare, especially in young people who avoid smoking [28]. The introduction of low-dose OCPs has markedly improved the safety profile. The decrease in the estrogen component has decreased the incidence of VTE. The risk of myocardial infarction and stroke in users is rare with formulations containing less than 50 μg of estrogen. Thus the safety-related concerns associated with use of OCPs and cardiovascular health have lessened over time [28].

Neoplastic concerns associated with the OCPs include an increased risk for development of adenocarcinoma of the cervix, and a slightly increased risk of breast cancer among current but not past users. OCPs have been associated with a decreased risk of endometrial and ovarian cancer, a benefit that persists for many years after discontinuation. They have also been associated with a decreased risk of colorectal carcinoma. The results of one analysis suggest that the effect of OCPs in US women is to slightly reduce the risk of invasive cancer by age 60, a result that held for black and white women between the ages of 20 and 59 [28]. The authors state that the public health impact varies by site of invasive cancer. Overall, there was a decreased risk for ovarian and endometrial cancer and a slight increased risk for breast and cervical cancer detection. The putative increase for liver cancer and reduced risk for colorectal cancer remain uncertain.

Noncontraceptive benefits

Noncontraceptive benefits of the OCP are well known, and include prevention of abnormal uterine bleeding, decreased number of functional ovarian cysts, reduced acne vulgaris, reduced dysmenorrhea, and maintenance of bone density [25]. The OCP has also been associated with decreased pelvic inflammatory disease and ectopic pregnancy. OCPs are also useful mainstream medications that decrease pain associated with endometriosis, need for hysterectomy, and risk for benign breast disease like fibroadenoma and fibrocystic changes, and serve as a treatment for menorrhagia and polycystic ovarian syndrome.

OCPs containing DRSP have been approved for the treatment of PMDD. A new formulation of DRSP is available as a 24/4 regime containing 20 μg EE/3 mg DRSP

Box 28.1 Classification of categories

1. A condition for which there is no restriction for the use of the contraceptive method.
2. A condition where the advantages of using the method generally outweigh the theoretical or proven risks.
3. A condition where the theoretic or proven risks usually outweigh the advantages of using the method.
4. A condition which represents an unacceptable health risk if the contraceptive method is used.

---

that shortens the HFI to four days. The bleeding profile was similar to other OCP regimes [40]. A study evaluated the use of an extended monophasic drospirenone contraceptive continuously for six months. A high continuation rate of 92% was reported for the six-month period. Breakthrough bleeding was effectively managed by decreasing the HFI rather than continuing active pills [36].

WHO medical eligibility criteria for contraceptive use

Prior to dispensing hormonal or nonhormonal contraception, the provider must consider if conditions (medical or individual) are present that might contraindicate its use. This information must also be balanced with an understanding of the effect that pregnancy will have on the pre-existing condition or individual. Evidence-based guidelines, *Medical Eligibility Criteria for Contraceptive Use* (third edition), were published by the WHO in 2004 to determine who could use contraceptive methods safely [41]. Conditions affecting eligibility to receive the contraceptive method (see Box 28.1) have been classified under one of four categories. The four eligibility categories are applied in practice according to clinical judgment as shown in Table 28.6 [41]. For example, a category 3 medical condition might warrant the specialist to consider use of a particular method with careful clinical judgment and access to clinical services. If unavailable, then this condition would be then considered category 4 and the woman is not eligible for the method.

Flexibility in applying these guidelines is based on the clinical judgment of the provider. The WHO states that adolescents are eligible to use any method of contraception and must have access to a variety of contraceptive choices [41]. Proper education and counseling both before and at the time of the method selection can help adolescents address their specific problems and make informed

Table 28.6 Using the categories in practice

Category	With clinical judgment	With limited clinical judgment
1	Use method in any circumstances	Yes (Use the method)
2	Generally use the method	
3	Use of method not usually recommended unless other more appropriate methods are not available or not acceptable	No (Do not use the method)
4	Method not to be used	

and voluntary decisions. Every effort should be made to prevent service and method costs from limiting the options available.

WHO medical eligibility criteria for combined oral contraceptives

Examples of category 1 diseases that are absolutely allowed with combined OCPs are fibroids, PID, STIs, AIDS, and depression. Cateogory 4 diseases that are not allowed include known thrombogenic mutations such as factor V Leiden, prothrombin mutations, protein S, protein C and antithrombin deficiencies, less than six weeks postpartum, age 35 or greater while smoking 15 cigarettes daily or more, presence of multiple risks for arterial cardiovascular disease like older age, smoking, diabetes, and hypertension, history of DVT, history of ischemic heart disease, stroke, pulmonary hypertension or atrial fibrillation, or history of subacute bacterial endocarditis, active viral hepatitis, cirrhosis of the liver or liver tumors.

WHO selected practice recommendations for contraceptive use and immediate initiation of hormonal contraception – Quick Start

A complementary publication entitled *Selected Practice Recommendations for Contraceptive Use* (second edition) was developed by the WHO to provide guidance on how to use contraceptive methods safely and effectively, once they are deemed to be medically appropriate [42].

One of the questions posed by this document was "when can a woman start combined oral contraceptives (COCs)?". Based on these evidence-based guidelines, one may start the pill by traditional or complementary means. Traditional means include taking the first contraceptive

Box 28.2 When can a woman start combined oral contraceptives (COCs)?

Note: The woman may be provided with COCs in advance with appropriate instructions on pill initiation, provided she is medically eligible.

Having menstrual cycles

- She can start COCs within five days after the start of her menstrual bleeding. No additional contraceptive protection is needed.

- She also can start COCs at any other time, if it is reasonably certain that she is not pregnant. If it has been more than five days since menstrual bleeding started, she will need to abstain from sex or use additional contraceptive protection for the next seven days.

Amenorrheic

- She can start COCs at any time, if it is reasonably certain that she is not pregnant. She will need to abstain from sex or use additional contraceptive protection for the next seven days.

pill within the first five days of menstruation. The guidelines state that the woman is also allowed to start at any other time, if it is reasonably certain that she is not pregnant. Reasonable certainty of nonpregnancy is defined as:

- has not had intercourse since the last menses
- has been correctly and consistently using a reliable method of contraception
- is within the first seven days after a normal period
- is within four weeks postpartum for nonlactating women
- is within the first seven days postabortion or miscarriage
- is fully or nearly fully breastfeeding, amenorrheic, and less than six months postpartum.

If a sensitive urine pregnancy test is available, this may also be used to confirm nonpregnancy. If it has been more than seven days since menstrual bleeding started, the patient will need to abstain from sex or use additional back-up contraceptive protection until she has taken seven consecutive pills. If she has had unprotected intercourse in the 120 hours prior to OCP initiation, she should be instructed to take two tablets of LNG emergency contraception (EC), Plan B™, immediately. She should take the first pill in her regular pill pack the following day and remember to use a back-up method for eight days (including the EC day) [43]. This Quick Start method of oral contraceptive pill initiation has been shown to be acceptable for adolescent and adult clients alike [44,45].

One prospective study concluded that patients who elected to initiate the OCP on the day seen in clinic were more likely to continue using a second pill pack than those who did not (adjusted odds ratio 2.8, 95% confidence interval 1.1–7.3) [45]. All patients making this choice had a negative sensitive urine pregnancy test and were given emergency contraception when deemed appropriate. Quick Start was also found to be an appropriate method when applied for immediate initiation of other combined hormonal choices such as the vaginal contraceptive ring (NuvaRing™), depot medroxyprogesterone acetate (Depot Provera™), and the transdermal patch (Ortho Evra™) [46–51]. Patients given the opportunity to use Quick Start with their method of choice had higher continuation rates with the ring and injection but not the patch.

Dual-method use of condoms and hormonal contraception

It is imperative that teens are encouraged to practice dual-method use of condoms and hormonal contraceptives since adolescents bear the highest risk of acquiring and transmitting STIs. Teens may think that dual-method use is redundant or unnecessary. Thus, it is necessary to tailor counseling to account for the adolescent's perceived risk of pregnancy and acquisition of STIs [52].

Combined hormonal systems

New delivery systems of combination hormonal contraception are suitable for all sexually active women. However, in our experience, teens are often skeptical about new methods. Cutting-edge choices seem to be more ac-

ceptable to the client already versed in the benefits of oral contraceptives, who is looking for convenience.

Transdermal contraceptive patch

The transdermal combination hormonal contraceptive system has been available since 2001 (Ortho Evra™) and had been used by approximately 8.1% of teens aged 15–19 in 2002 [2].

Mechanism of action

This contraceptive patch contains EE and norelgestromin (NGMN), a primary active metabolite of norgestimate. This is a matrix system consisting of three layers: an outer protective layer of polyester, a medicated, adhesive middle layer, and a clear polyester release liner that is removed with each patch application. This novel delivery system circumvents the gastrointestinal tract and allows once-weekly application with the potential to increase compliance and decrease typical failure rates as compared to daily oral contraceptives. This 20 cm^2 matrix delivery system is placed onto the skin once weekly for three weeks with a one-week patch-free interval to induce menstruation. Each patch delivers 20 μg of EE and 150 μg of NGMN daily. These constant blood levels inhibit ovulation up to nine days, which allows for a two-day margin of error. The patch may be applied on the day of the office visit if pregnancy can be adequately ruled out (see Quick Start section above) or during the first 24 hours of a normal menstrual cycle or on a Sunday after the menses with a one-week back-up method such as the condom.

The patch may be applied to dry, healthy skin on the abdomen, buttock, upper outer arm or upper torso, excluding the breast. It must be rotated to prevent skin irritation. The preferred application sites for adolescents in one study were the buttock (40%) and the lower abdomen (32%) [53]. Creams, ointments, and moisturizers must be avoided in the area of patch placement to allow proper adhesion. An extra patch is usually dispensed as a back-up in case of detachment. There is an approximate 1.1% detachment rate during activities such as exercise, swimming or using a sauna. Complete and partial detachment rates were higher in adolescents, ranging from 35.5% to 53% [53,54]. The patch had high acceptability and good rates of short-term compliance, but consistent dual usage with the condom was only 15% in one study [53]. High continuation rates were noticed among teenagers. A comparative study of extended use (84 days) and standard 28-day use found that those in the extended group experienced fewer mean headache days during the HFI [55].

Efficacy

Typical failure rates are 8% for one year of use, which is similar to the OCP [8]. Two-thirds of patients using the patch were previous OCP users [56].

Adverse events and contraindications

One comparative study of the patch and the OCP reported a higher incidence of breast tenderness and dysmenorrhea in patch users. All other side effects were similar [57]. Transient breast tenderness or nausea, both estrogen effects, usually vanish after the first three months. Teens must be told about this before they start. The patch has the same contraindications as combination OCPs and the vaginal ring. Caution is advised in patients with valvular heart disease, severe hypertension, diabetes with vascular involvement, headaches with focal neurologic symptoms, acute or chronic hepatocellular disease with abnormal liver function, and hypersensitivity to any component within the patch.

Drug interactions

Drug effectiveness may be reduced when hormonal contraceptives are co-administered with some antibiotics, antifungals, anticonvulsants, and other drugs known to increase metabolism of contraceptive steroids. Some possible potential drug interactions with barbiturates, griseofulvin, rifampin, phenylbutazone, phenytoin, carbamazepine, felbamate, oxcarbazepine, topiramate, and possibly with ampicillin may decrease serum levels of the hormones. Oral administration of tetracycline did not seem to affect the pharmacokinetics of NGMN or EE. There have been reports in a pooled analysis of clinical trial data that the contraceptive patch may be less effective in women weighing greater than 198 lbs (90 kg). However, pregnancies reported in this cohort of women only represented 3% of the study population. Subsequent studies suggest that this decreased efficacy in heavier women may be an effect that is not unique to patch use and may also be demonstrated with low-dose OCPs [58,59].

In November 2005, the FDA noted higher serum concentrations of EE in patch users, approximately 60% higher than those found in OCPs. This led to a package insert labeling change for patch users that advised patients of the potential of increased adverse events associated with elevated estrogen doses. A recent nested case–control study comparing the patch and a norgestimate OCP found similar rates of VTE in each group [60]. Controversy exists since another unpublished study purports a twice-greater rate of VTE in patch versus OPC users [61,62].

In summary, the combination hormonal patch is a highly acceptable form of contraception with high continuation rates within the teenage population. To date, there is conflicting evidence about whether increased serum estrogen levels in patch users will translate into clinically significant cases of VTE. As with all hormonal contraception, condom use must be strongly encouraged if the patch is chosen.

Combined contraceptive vaginal ring

The combined contraceptive vaginal ring (CCVR; NuvaRing™), approved in 2002 for US use, is a combination hormonal method. It is a flexible, transparent, and colorless ring made of soft plastic ethylene vinyl acetate with an outer diameter of 54 mm and a cross-sectional diameter of 4 mm.

Mechanism of action

The ring contains both EE and the potent progestin etonogestrel (ETN), the precursor progestin of desogestrel, a third-generation progestin. ETN is also the active ingredient used in the subdermal implant Implanon™. Once placed vaginally, the CCVR releases steady serum concentrations of 120 μg of ETN and 15 μg of EE daily through the vaginal mucosa. The amount of estrogen released is lower than the amounts of estrogen released by either the OCP or the transdermal patch [63]. Conventional initiation begins on the first day of the menses or days 2–5 with a back-up. Although usage has not been reported in the 2002 NSFG statistics, increased use of this method by teens can be anticipated as more providers begin offering this method to their patients. High rates of user and partner acceptability, convenience, reliability and safety have been reported in large trials in Europe and the US [64,65].

One open-label randomized trial of self-selected women aged 18–40 from an urban US family planning clinic who were willing to try the vaginal ring were allotted to receive either the ring or a low-dose (25 μg EE) triphasic birth control pill. The study was designed to analyze acceptability and satisfaction with the Quick

Start method of immediate initiation of the contraceptive method on the day the patient is seen in the provider's office [47]. The authors concluded that the women allocated to initiate the vaginal ring on the day of the clinic visit were likely to be more satisfied with the method and to continue its use than the pill users. This finding was unrelated to patients' comfort with touching their genitals, greater frequency of masturbation, more comfort with intercourse, and past use of vaginal contraceptives and products [47].

CCVR and OCPs had acceptable bleeding patterns regardless of conventional or immediate start [46,65]. Westhoff et al concluded that CCVR users experienced fewer days or episodes of bleeding or spotting and shorter intervals of bleeding than those using the low-dose OCP [46]. Weight gain was not significantly different between OCP and ring users [66].

Efficacy

The typical failure rate for one year of use is 8%, which is similar to the OCP [8]. The contraceptive efficacy is unchanged if a misplaced ring is replaced within three hours.

Adverse events and contraindications

The most common adverse events experienced during CCVR use included vaginal discharge (1%), lower abdominal pain or dysmenorrhea (1%), headache (1%), and migraine (1%) [62]. Many experienced favorable bleeding patterns, decreased dysmenorrhea, and decreased premenstrual syndrome (PMS). Removal of the ring during intercourse is not necessary.

Contraindications to the use of combined rings containing estrogen are the same as those for OCPs and the patch, including but not limited to history of thrombosis, hypertension, gallbladder disease, and hepatic adenomas or benign liver tumors.

Lunelle

Lunelle® (Cyclofem) was marketed from 2000 to 2002. It is a monthly combined injectable contraceptive (CIC) containing 25 mg of medroxyprogesterone acetate (MPA) and 5 mg of estradiol cypionate (E_2C). The major advantage of this contraception was its minimal disruption of menstrual cycles when taken monthly. Lunelle was given within five days of the onset of a regular menses, within 10 days of a first trimester abortion, or between four and six weeks postpartum. This medication was voluntarily recalled from the US market when assurance of full potency of each prefilled syringe was questioned, possibly risking contraceptive failure. Cyclofem® is still available in several nations. It had the same contraindications as OCPs and the combined hormonal patch and vaginal ring.

Contraceptives containing progestins alone

Progestin-only contraceptives are available in a variety of formulations and delivery systems. In the US progestin-only pills (POPs) were approved in 1973. The subdermal levonorgestrel implant (Norplant®) and the injectable contraceptive depo-medroxyprogesterone acetate (DMPA; Depo-Provera®) became available in 1990 and 1992, respectively. The availability of both methods rapidly expanded method choices for US women and were credited with helping to decrease the US adolescent pregnancy rates over the last decade due to their lower typical failure rates when used over one year [8].

The distribution of Norplant ended in 2002 due to litigation concerns of the manufacturer, and it is no longer available in the US. Implanon™, a new one-rod implant containing 3-keto-desogestrel or ETN, has been approved for US distribution in 2006. ETN is the same progestin component of the combined contraceptive vaginal ring, NuvaRing®, discussed previously.

The safety profile of progestin-only contraceptives is a major advantage, especially for adolescents with medical contraindications to estrogen use [41]. According to the WHO *Medical Eligibility Criteria for Contraceptive Use*, third edition, candidates with medical conditions that contraindicate estrogen use are able to use progestin-only contraceptives. Such conditions include DVT, genetic mutations predisposing to thrombosis, history of ischemic heart disease, stroke, valvular heart disease, migraines, diabetes, gallbladder disease, and mild compensated cirrhosis. In such cases pregnancy avoidance with progestin compounds is generally safe.

Reviews of POPs concluded that this contraceptive method appeared to have no effect on coagulation factors and would be most appropriate for women who are at increased risk for cardiovascular disease (CVD) [67,68]. Thus, patients with a history of thrombosis or those who suffer from medical conditions contraindicating use of estrogen would still be candidates for these types of progestin-only methods. This fact must be reconciled with the reality that these formulations are often associated with breakthrough bleeding and patient dissatisfaction. Therefore, combined contraceptive methods containing estrogen are often considered as first-line contraceptive choices due to their superior cycle control and the relative rarity of CVD in the adolescent population. Progestin-only methods with novel delivery systems are especially suitable for adolescents at high risk for pregnancy.

It is perceived by many teenagers that breakthrough bleeding equates to lower efficacy and is unhealthy. This idea must be discussed with the teen during the counseling session to avoid discontinuation of the method [22,69].

Progestin-only contraceptive pills

In 1973, progestin-only pills (POPs or minipills) became available for distribution in the US [68]. POPs for use in the US contain either norgestrel or norethindrone. Examples include Ovrette® (0.075 mg norgestrel) and Micronor®, Nor-QD®, Camila®, and Errin® (0.35 mg of norethindrone). The prevalence of POP use varies widely among countries, in part due to varying levels of awareness about their advantages and disadvantages. According to OC sales figures from the early 1990s, approximately 1% of US women used POPs versus 15% in Sweden, 8% in Great Britain, 6% in Finland, and 3% in France [68]. POPs contain about a third of the progestin dose of combination OCPs. These formulations are useful choices for women seeking to minimize hormone intake for contraception.

Mechanism of action

The contraceptive effect of the POP is attributed to thickening of the cervical mucus, decreased tubal motility, and endometrial atrophy [67]. Approximately 40% of patients will ovulate normally during POP use, making this a secondary mechanism of action [70].

Efficacy

POP packs contain 28 active pills and no placebo pills. There are no hormone-free days as with traditional combination OCPs. Initiation of POPs is recommended on the first day of the menses, in nonpregnant women. A back-up method is recommended for seven days. In postpartum patients, POPs may be begun immediately postpartum in nonbreastfeeding or at six weeks in breastfeeding women. Breastfeeding on demand suppresses ovulation which is complementary to the contraceptive action of the POP.

This contraceptive effect of the POP is dependent on endometrial and cervical mucus effects since ovulation is not consistently suppressed [19]. This dual effect of hypothalamic suppression by lactation and progestin effects on the endometrium and cervical mucus enhances efficacy.

In order to insure efficacy, POPs must be taken at the same time daily, consecutively, to achieve adequate serum concentration. If the pill is taken greater than three hours off schedule, then the client is told to use a back-up for 48 hours. The circulating serum progestin levels are approximately 25% of those found in combination OCPs. This is sufficient to thicken cervical mucus for 22 hours. After that time, this action begins to diminish [19]. The typical failure rate for POPs is remarkably similar to the combined OCP, at 8% per year of usage [8]. This similar one-year failure rate may convince more providers to consider using POPs as a mainstream choice outside the context of breastfeeding women [67].

Adverse events and contraindications

As with all progestin-only contraceptives, anticipatory counseling about the high prevalence of irregular bleeding patterns with POPs is advised. Irregular bleeding while on progestin contraceptives may be managed by doubling up POP doses, using high-dose NSAIDs or adding low-dose estrogen [13].

Bleeding patterns of 358 nonlactating women attending a British family planning clinic were prospectively recorded for up to 150 months [71]. Ethynodiol (EDD 500 µg), LNG 30 µg and norethindrone (NET 350 µg) were the three progestins dispensed at this facility. Bleeding patterns were as follows: 39.8% reported mostly regular periods, 23.1% were mostly irregular, 7.7% experienced mostly amenorrhea and the balance a mixture of these categories. As expected, the major cause of premature discontinuation of this method was menstrual disturbances (47.5%) [71]. These authors concluded that POPs provided very acceptable contraception that should be actively promoted as a mainstream choice. Interestingly, the majority of women using POPs at this center were young, less than 35 years old (59.8%), and 10.6% were less than 25 years old. In addition, the majority of POP users (87.8%) were not lactating.

The serum levels of progestin in breastfed neonates with mothers using the POP are 1–6% of the levels found in maternal serum [68]. This was equivalent to the fully breastfed neonate receiving one minipill every 2–3 years [67].

Medical indications

Since minipills contain no estrogen, they pose few of the risks commonly associated with the combination pill. Despite these benefits, the irregular bleeding resulting from the absence of estrogen and experienced by the majority of users could lead to noncompliance and dissatisfaction if anticipatory counseling addressing these side effects is omitted. POPs are particularly suited to women who have contraindications to estrogen in combined OCPs (VTE, strokes, MI, etc.), for breastfeeding mothers, and for older women [68].

There are few medical contraindications for use of the POP according to the WHO *Medical Eligibility Criteria for Contraceptive Use* [41]. Conditions in which the advantages of POP use outweigh the theoretical or proven risks include previous ectopic pregnancy, multiple risk factors for arterial cardiovascular disease, severe hypertension (HTN), history of DVT, known thrombogenic mutations, ischemic heart disease, stroke, hyperlipidemia, migraine headache with aura, benign breast disease, AIDS on antiretroviral therapy, griseofulvin use, diabetes, gallbladder disease, and stable hepatitis carrier states. POPs should be avoided in patients with current DVT, breast cancer, active viral hepatitis, and cirrhosis of the liver [41].

A 2004 review found the safety profile of POPs was acceptable for patients with HTN even after 2–3 years of follow-up [72]. This contraceptive may also be used in teens with various medical conditions like sickle cell disease, heart disease, diabetes mellitus, hyperlipidemia, and systemic lupus erythematosus [13].

POPs have a higher absolute rate of ectopic pregnancy compared with other progestin-only contraceptives (POCs), but still less than using no method since they decrease the overall pregnancy rate.

Drug interactions

Patients using all POCs, including POPs, should be cautious while using medications known to increase metabolism of hormones such as the antitubercular drug rifampicin and anticonvulsants like phenytoin, carbamazepine, barbiturates, primodone, topiramate, and oxcarbazepine [41].

Depo-Provera

During the 1980s, few long-term contraceptives were available for US women. They included the intrauterine device (IUD) and permanent sterilization that were both unsuitable for sexually active teens. In addition, the developmental challenges of adolescence often interfered with consistent use of condoms or daily self-administration of oral contraceptives [73]. Even fewer choices were available for women with medical conditions contraindicating estrogen and combination OCPs. This lack of long-term contraceptive choices became a critical issue for sexually active patients with medical conditions that were often worsened by pregnancy. This led to a real need to consider safe contraceptive alternatives.

In 1960 the 400 mg/mL dose of the injectable pregnane progestin depo-medroxyprogesterone acetate (DMPA) was approved by the Food and Drug Administration (FDA) for treatment of endometriosis and habitual abortion [74]. This formulation was later approved for treatment of metastatic endometrial or renal carcinoma in the US. By 1980, the efficacy and safety of DMPA as a three-month injectable contraceptive led to its use in 80 countries worldwide for contraception [74]. This extensive worldwide clinical experience as a safe, effective contraceptive led to DMPA being offered at the Mount Sinai Medical Center Family Planning Clinic in 1984 as a primary form of hormonal contraception. This "off-label use" of this drug for contraception was justified by the extensive evidence of literature attesting to its safe use for this indication. Such DMPA use required intensive anticipatory counseling by trained nursing personnel and physicians and required informed consent. DMPA was especially useful as a contraceptive for women with medical conditions in which pregnancy or estrogen use was contraindicated [75]. Many women above the age of 35 found DMPA useful since use of the OCP was considered a contraindication in this age group. Patients signed a special, informed consent form outlining known benefits and risks of its use; 0.34 mL of the 400 mg/mL formulation totaling 150 mg was administered intramuscularly every 12 weeks.

Groups opposed to the approval of DMPA for contraception in the US were concerned about the potential for coercive use in vulnerable groups of women. In addition, there were concerns about the association of breast tumors in beagle dogs that were administered 20–25 times the normal human dose of DMPA. These results, however, cannot be extrapolated directly to women, since the beagle is prone to breast lumps and is known to be especially sensitive to progestins [67]. On balance, ample evidence was presented to the FDA describing DMPA as a safe, reliable contraceptive for women. This led to the FDA expanding the indications of DMPA for contraceptive use in 1992 after the WHO published results showing that users were not at increased risk of breast and gynecologic malignancies [74]. A 1 mL single-dose vial containing 150 mg was approved for injection once every 12 weeks in 1992. Depo-subQ Provera 104®, a new subcutaneous formulation containing 104 mg/0.65 mL, was approved for use in the US in 2004. It is indicated for contraception and for management of endometriosis-associated pain. It is also given once every three months.

The historically low US teenage pregnancy rates are continuing to decrease. Much of this decrease has been attributed to at-risk youth having access to effective long-acting hormonal contraceptives like DMPA and subcutaneous progestin implants [76]. The percentage of teens aged 15–19 who have ever used DMPA doubled between 1995 and 2002, from approximately 10% to 21% [2]. DMPA has been shown to have failure rates of 3% over one year [8]. This low rate makes DMPA a particularly good choice of contraception for teens.

Mechanism of action

High circulating blood levels of DMPA give it unique contraceptive properties in comparison with other low-dose progestins [19]. In addition to thickening of cervical mucus and alteration of the endometrium, the LH surge is blocked by the high circulating blood levels of the progestin. Suppression by DMPA of FSH levels is less intense compared with combination OCPs, allowing endogenous estrogen levels to be maintained at early follicular phase of the menstrual cycle [19]. Product labeling states that 150 mg of DMPA be given by deep IM injection in the gluteal or deltoid muscle during the first five days of a normal menstrual period. In the postpartum, nonbreast-feeding woman it may be given within the first five days as well. In the breastfeeding woman it may be initiated at six weeks if the woman is not at risk of pregnancy. WHO Selected Practice Recommendations state that it is reasonable to give progestin-only injectables like DMPA within seven days after the start of menstrual bleeding with no additional contraceptive protection required. One may also initiate the first injection at any time if it is reasonably

certain that the woman is not pregnant. If it has been more than seven days since menstrual bleeding started, then she will need to abstain from sex or use additional contraceptive protection for the next seven days [42]. Immediate initiation of DMPA is feasible, but early luteal-phase pregnancies can occur even when sensitive urine pregnancy tests and emergency contraception are administered [48,49].

Adverse events and contraindications

As with other POCs, menstrual irregularity is common. Initial unpredictable breakthrough bleeding followed by increasing amenorrhea rates are the hallmarks of DMPA use. Approximately 46% and 59% of DMPA users experience amenorrhea after three and nine months of use, respectively. Continued use leads to an approximate 70% amenorrhea experience at 12 months [74].

One small, randomized controlled trial attempted to anlayze if the IM route of administration of DMPA was a significant disincentive to DMPA use in teens. The study was conducted in an urban adolescent health center and compared injection site pain scores of two available concentrations of DMPA with continuation rates over one year. The hypothesis was that higher pain scores associated with the higher concentrated formulation would lead to lower adherence, but this was not observed. Continuation rates at one year were low in both groups and did not differ significantly (multidose and single-dose users were 36% and 23%, respectively). As with other larger studies, the predominant reason for discontinuation in both groups was menstrual disturbances [75]. DMPA continuation rates in one prospective, international study for three, six, nine, and 12 months were 68%, 67%, 55%, and 51% respectively [75]. Factors associated with increased continuation rates included the provision of information about returning to the clinic for side effects, and advising the patient as to the possibility of amenorrhea. These authors concluded that effective counseling by the provider led to higher continuation rates, especially in patients motivated to use the method due to large family size and spousal input [77].

The suppression of endogenous estrogens is associated with decreased bone mineral density in current users of DMPA. This led to a FDA regulatory action in 2004 that included a black box label warning about long-term use of DMPA. The warning states that bone mineral density may be lost over time and that it may not be completely

reversible. It also states that use over two years should occur only if other methods of birth control are inadequate.
This was deemed controversial since such a designation
could lead to hesitancy of many practitioners in the US to
continue using this effective contraceptive method [78]. It
is notable that women using DMPA experience reversible
bone loss less than the approximate 4% observed in lactating mothers [78]. In addition, adolescent pregnancy
also may be associated with bone loss [79,80].

Based on present usage of DMPA by over one million
adolescent girls in the US and the uncertain predictability
of using bone density as a surrogate marker for fracture,
many experts have released guidelines for practitioners
for continued use of this option [81]. The authors suggest
that patients be advised of the black box warning as a
routine part of anticipatory guidance. Routine bone density testing can be avoided, if calcium supplementation
is considered with exercise to promote bone health. The
WHO medical eligibility guidelines state that the benefits
of DMPA use in adolescents outweigh the theoretic risks
and that, in general, use of the method is appropriate [41].

Weight gain while using DMPA is a major complaint.
One short-term, placebo-controlled, randomized trial
evaluated DMPA users' energy intake and resting energy expenditure. It was concluded that preinjection, both
DMPA and placebo study participants consumed more
energy and expended more energy at rest in the luteal
phase than in the follicular phase. Comparison of pre- and
postinjection means showed that treatment with DMPA
had no significant effects on energy intake or expenditure
or caused weight gain in women aged 20–35 [82].

The WHO *Medical Eligibility Criteria for Contraceptive Use*, third edition, states that DMPA shares similar
advantages as detailed for POCs earlier in this chapter
[41]. Since progestins are not considered thrombogenic,
the benefits of use generally outweigh the risks in patients
with a history of DVT but use must be discontinued if an
active DVT develops.

Noncontraceptive benefits

Noncontraceptive benefits of DMPA include prevention
of endometrial cancer, anemia, PID, ectopic pregnancy,
and uterine myomas. It may be suitable for conditions
such as menorrhagia, dysmenorrheal pain due to en-
dometrioisis, seizure disorders, hemoglobinopathies, endometrial hyperplasia, vasomotor symptoms in postmenopausal women, pelvic pain of ovarian origin post

hysterectomy, metastatic breast cancer, and metastatic endometrial cancer [74]. Lastly, since DMPA does not protect against STI, concomitant condom use (the belt and
suspenders approach) should be encouraged.

Norplant®

In 1991, the Norplant® subdermal contraceptive implant
was the first new contraceptive system approved for use
in the US in 30 years [83]. It was the most extensively
tested contraceptive implant, with nearly 60,000 women
participating in clinical trials [84]. In 1995, approximately
1 million US women and 2.5 women worldwide were
using this contraceptive method.

Although the distribution of Norplant was discontinued in the US in 2002, a review will illustrate how this
innovative, five-year contraceptive choice was associated
with decreased unintended pregnancies in at-risk teen
populations. Although the increased use of condoms,
OCPs, Norplant, DMPA, and emergency contraception
(ECP) by teens is credited for the decreased teen pregnancy rates experienced from 1995 through 2002 [2],
long-term contraceptives are especially suitable for populations prone to experience repeat pregnancy. Adolescent
mothers have high repeat pregnancy rates that vary from
14% at one year to 35% at two year [76]. One study illustrated how teen access to the Norplant five-year subdermal contraceptive resulted in lower repeat pregnancies,
thus contributing to lower overall adolescent pregnancies
in the US. The pregnancy outcomes of 100 postpartum
adolescent mothers at an urban hospital seeking either
Norplant or oral contraceptive were compared [85]. The
Norplant group had higher continuation rates (95% versus 33%) and lower repeat pregnancy rates (one became
pregnant in the Norplant group versus 22 in the oral contraceptive group).

A case–control study comparing 94 teens 18 years of age
and younger who received Norplant with matched teens
using OCPs concluded that Norplant provoked more side
effects in the early months, but provided superior protection against pregnancy [86]; 43% of OCP users discontinued within six months versus none in the Norplant group.
Six patients became pregnant in the OCP group.

Mechanism of action

Norplant consists of six subdermal silastic capsules filled
with 216 mg of the crystalline progestin levonorgestrel
released at an average of 30 μg daily to achieve serum

elevations of 175–250 pg/mL. The capsules were placed in the inner aspect of the nondominant arm in a minor surgical procedure, requiring local anesthetic in an out-patient setting. Removal of the Norplant system, which could take place any time up to five years after insertion, also required local anesthesia but a slightly larger incision [87].

The high efficacy of Norplant can be attributed to the long-term release of low blood levels of the progestin levonorgestrel. These concentrations are sufficient to create an inhospitable environment for fertilization to occur. Cervical mucus is scant, thick, and hostile to sperm penetration with an endometrium not supportive of sperm capacitation or implantation. When Norplant is first inserted higher blood levels inhibit ovulation, but follicles still enlarge and produce near-normal amounts of estradiol [88]. In the first five years of use about half of cycles are ovulatory; however, most ovulatory cycles occur toward the later years of use when serum levonorgestrel levels begin to decline. Because ovulation occurs more often in the later years, bleeding is more likely to be regular after the implants have been in for two or more years and luteal progesterone production has become cyclical.

Efficacy

The five-year efficacy of Norplant surpassed that of surgical sterilization, yet it was completely reversible (typical failure rate 0.05% vs 0.5% failure rate within one year of use) [8].

Adverse events and contraindications

As with all POCs, irregular and untimely bleeding are the most common adverse events leading to premature discontinuation. The addition of estrogen, prostaglandin inhibitors, and progestin antagonists can reduce incidence of bleeding.

One of the first US studies, by Darney et al in 1990, characterized the five-year experience of 205 Norplant users in an urban center in San Francisco, many of whom were using Norplant II, a two-rod levonorgestrel system [89]. As can be predicted by Norplant's progestin-only properties, of the women participating in the trial, 95% experienced at least one side effect. Over 80% experienced menstrual changes, 32% weight changes, 24% headaches, 16% mood changes, and 15% acne. Nevertheless, because of dissatisfaction with other methods, the majority of women were willing to tolerate these side effects, as evidenced by a

53% five-year continuation rate. Interestingly, 61% of women who discontinued Norplant said they would use the method again. The authors concluded that Norplant appeared to be a highly acceptable method of contraception, despite the frequent occurrence of bothersome side effects in a group of fairly diversified women in an urban center. Despite frequent side effects, experiences of high acceptability are similar among many different groups of women, including adolescents [85,86,90].

According to the WHO eligibility criteria, Norplant is appropriate for those various medical conditions that contraindicate pregnancy or estrogen use [41].

Summary

In July 2002, Norplant distribution stopped in the US. The decision resulted from expensive litigation based on predictable adverse events and removal difficulties among less experienced providers. In some cases, poorly placed devices were inappropriately removed through larger incisions. Many such procedures lasted greater than one hour to remove all six implants. The withdrawal of Norplant from the US market led to greater use of DMPA as an effective alternative hormonal contraceptive for sexually active adolescents.

Implanon®

In 2006, Implanon became the second subdermal contraceptive system approved for use in the US. This single-rod, nonbiodegradable implantable contraceptive contains 68 mg of etonogestrel (ETN), a potent, precursor progestin of desogestrel.

Implanon is one of several one- and two-implant systems developed to address the side effects and removal problems that characterized earlier versions of subdermal implants such as Norplant. Clinical trials documented the high efficacy, benign adverse event profile, and ease of removal of one- and two-implant systems compared with the six-capsule Norplant [88]. Implanon is the subject of at least 17 clinical trials and has been marketed in over 30 countries. Since 1998, 2.5 million prescriptions have been dispensed widely in Europe, Australia, and Indonesia.

Implanon is 4 cm long and 2 mm wide and is composed of an ethylene vinylacetate (EVA) copolymer core, containing 68 mg of ETN, surrounded by a rate-limiting EVA copolymer membrane. Another difference between Implanon and Norplant is the supplied, preloaded sterile single-use applicator that facilitates insertion. This matchstick-sized implant is inserted subdermally on the inner aspect of the nondominant arm in the groove between the biceps and the triceps. named the sulcus biceptalis medialis. This insertion site is the same for Norplant. The serum release rate is 60–70 µg daily initially, decreasing to 25 µg daily by the end of the third year.

Mechanism of action

Ovulation inhibition is the main mechanism of action. No ovulation was observed for 30 months whereas two of 31 (6.5%) of subjects ovulated in year 3 with no resulting pregnancies. Contraceptive efficacy is augmented through thickening of the cervical mucus. While Implanon effectively suppresses ovulation, it does not completely suppress ovarian function to the point that the subject becomes hypoestrogenic. One study compared Implanon with a nonhormone IUD and found baseline bone mineral density was unchanged for both groups. In addition, the 17β-estradiol levels were similar for both groups. The investigators concluded that Implanon could be safely used in young women who have not achieved their peak bone mass [91].

Efficacy

Implanon is effective for three years, with postmarketing typical failure rates, estimated from nearly 205,000 implants used in Australia, to be 1/1000 or 0.1% over one year of use [92]. The 2006 cumulative pearl index, another measure of efficacy, is 0.38 pregnancies per 100 women-years of use based on six pregnancies reported in 20,648 cycles.

Adverse events and contraindications

An open-label, randomized, multicenter trial was carried out in China, comparing the efficacy and bleeding patterns of Implanon with the six-rod Norplant. This study concluded that Implanon was associated with less frequent bleeding than Norplant, and the incidence of infrequent bleeding and amenorrhea was higher with Implanon. Implanon was significantly quicker to insert (0.61 minutes versus 3.9 minutes) and remove (2.18 vs 11.25 minutes) than was Norplant [93].

A multicenter, open-label clinical trial done in the US summates the experience among 330 women, 13% aged between 18–20 [94]. Implanon® insertion was completed in 0.5 minutes and removed in 3.5 minutes. The continuation rate for this two-year study was 51% with the majority of discontinuations due to bleeding pattern changes and other adverse events. No pregnancies resulted during Implanon use. Eleven of 46 subjects discontinuing Implanon who failed to use alternative contraception became pregnant between one and 18.5 weeks later. The authors concluded that Implanon was safe and efficacious. There were no pregnancies during the trial. There was rapid return to normal menstrual cycles and fertility following removal. Uterine bleeding pattern abnormalities were common, leading to premature discontinuation in 13% of subjects. No significant changes of hemoglobin levels resulted in spite of these bleeding patterns. No clinically meaningful effects on laboratory parameters were noted. Similarly, most studies report no clinically meaningful changes in hemoglobin levels for other progestin-only options such as POPs [68]. One randomized comparative study between Implanon and Norplant undertaken to compare serum lipid levels demonstrated no significant differences between the two [95]. Weight gain in the US trial averaged 2.8 lbs and 3.7 lbs in the first and second year, respectively. Whether higher weight subjects experience lower efficacy remains unknown since participants weighing greater than 130% of ideal body weight were excluded.

Summary

It is recommended that Implanon insertion should be timed to coincide with days 1–5 of the menstrual cycle if no preceding contraception was used in the past month. Switching from combination methods is allowed any time within seven days of the last active combined dose. If a progestin-only method is used then one may switch as follows: on any day of the POP use, on the same day as implant or IUD removal, or on the day when the next contraceptive injection is due. Insertion may also be done within five days following a first trimester abortion, 3–4 weeks following childbirth or a second trimester abortion, or after the fourth postpartum week if exclusively breast-feeding. If deviating from the recommended timing of insertion, rule out pregnancy, use emergency contraception if appropriate, and use a nonhormonal back-up method of contraception for seven days after Implanon insertion.

According to the WHO eligibility criteria, POCs like Implanon and Norplant can be appropriate choices for those individuals with various medical conditions that contraindicate estrogen usage. This includes history of VTE.

Implanon usage worldwide has been associated with high compliance and acceptability rates, with typical failure rates that are lower than oral contraceptive pills. Success in the US is likely if clients receive appropriate anticipatory counseling by trained providers comfortable with device insertion and removal. It is likely that the integration of effective methods with high continuation rates, such as Implanon, will lead to continuing progress towards elimination of the US as the developed nation with the highest teen pregnancy rates. This may be achieved by combining the knowledge gained from the Norplant experience with the improved subdermal implant design of Implanon.

Emergency contraception

Emergency contraception (EC) is the postcoital use of a drug or device to prevent pregnancy after unprotected intercourse. In 2002, 4.2 % of sexually experienced women in the US aged 15–44 had used emergency contraception (EC). The corresponding percentage for teens aged 15–19 was higher at 8.1% [2,21]. Despite this fact, up to 30% of patients have never heard of EC and only 10% know how to access it [96,97].

In 1997, it was estimated that widespread use of EC could prevent 1 million abortions and 2 million unintended pregnancies that end in childbirth in the US [98]. More recent estimates have estimated that some 51,000 abortions in the year 2000 were averted by use of emergency contraceptive pills (ECPs) in the US [97].

EC options available in the US include oral contraceptive tablets, levonorgestrel-only contraceptive tablets, and the copper-T IUD.

Combined emergency contraceptive pills

Combined OCPs containing estrogen and progestin may be used as ECPs to prevent pregnancy when initiated within 72 hours of unprotected intercourse. Ethinyl estradiol (EE) with either LNG or norgestrel (NG) (NG contains both levo and dextro isomers of the progestin LNG) are the hormones most extensively studied in clinical trials as ECPs [97].

The Yuzpe method of EC was named for Albert Yuzpe, the Canadian physician who first described its use. This regime consisted of two doses of tablets taken 12 hours apart after unprotected sex. Each dose consisted of two tablets, each containing 50 μg of EE and 0.25 mg of LNG (100 μg EE and 0.5 mg LNG per dose). Thus the to-

tal amount taken is 200 μg of EE and 1.0 mg of LNG. Alternative regimes using NE and EE (two doses of two tablets of Ovcon 50® each containing 50 μg EE and 1 mg NE) rather than the Yuzpe-like method using NG and EE (two doses of two tablets Ovral® each containing 50 μg EE and 0.5 mg NG) suggest slightly higher efficacy for the Yuzpe (NG) method [97,99]. Preven®, the first dedicated combination ECP available in the US, became available in 1998. It consisted of two pills containing EE (100 μg each) and LNG (0.5 mg each), to be taken 12 hours apart. Preven was withdrawn from the US market in 2004.

Mechanism of action

ECs' main mechanism of action is inhibition and delay of ovulation [100]. Additional possible mechanisms include endometrial alterations, interference with corpus luteal function, thickening of cervical mucus, and alterations of tubal transport.

Efficacy

The use of the combined Yuzpe method reduces the pregnancy rate by about 75% when initiated within 72 hours [97,101]. This means that if 100 women had unprotected intercourse once during the second or third week of their cycle, about eight would become pregnant whereas after treatment with ECPs, only two would be pregnant, a 75% decrease. The present treatment schedule is one dose within 72 hours of unprotected intercourse and a second dose 12 hours after the first.

Adverse events and contraindications

Due to the high dose of estrogen present in this regime, 50% experience nausea and 20% vomit [97]. Fifty milligrams of meclizine (Bonine®), an over-the-counter motion sickness medication, reduces this side effect. Almost all women can safely use combined ECPs, though theoretically caution might be considered in those with a history of VTE or migraine with neurologic sequelae. Although clotting factors do not increase in patients using combined ECP, nonestrogen options are available, making this decision unnecessary [97,102].

There are 18 generic or branded combined oral contraceptive pills available in the US containing EE plus NG or LNG and one specially packaged combined ECP product (Preven®) that may be used for EC [97]. Recent recommendations have been made to extend the time limit for starting the Yuzpe method to 120 hours (five days) from 72 hours [103].

Lastly, according to the WHO guidelines, when taken as directed, the benefits of combined ECPs outweigh any potential risks in patients with pre-existing cardiovascular diseases [41].

Progestin-only ECPs

In 2006, Plan-B®, the progestin-only emergency contraceptive pill, was FDA approved for over-the-counter (OTC) use for women 18 and older. A prescription is still required for those 17 or younger, requiring that the medicine be held behind the pharmacy counter for age proofing or prescription [104].

The LNG ECP regime consists of one 0.75 mg LNG dose within 72 hours of unprotected intercourse followed by a second dose of 0.75 mg 12 hours later (total 1.5 mg LNG). If the dedicated product is unavailable, then another option is to substitute 20 Ovrette® minipills (each contains 0.075 mg norgestrel) for each of two doses 12 hours apart for a total of 40 pills. Twice as much norgestrel is required since each 1 mg of norgestrel contains 0.5 mg of LNG. Plan B® is a dedicated progestin-only ECP that has been available in the US since 1999. It consists of two tablets each containing 0.75 mg of LNG. The first dose of Plan B is to be taken within 72 hours of unprotected coitus followed by the second dose 12 hours later. Efficacy has been shown to be equivalent if both pills are taken at once.

Mechanism of action

Early treatment with progestin-only ECPs may inhibit or delay ovulation or interfere with sperm migration and function at all levels of the genital tract [97].

Efficacy, adverse events, and contraindications

One WHO double-blind, randomized trial recruited nearly 2000 women in 1988 to compare the LNG and Yuzpe regimes of ECPs. The progestin-only LNG regime was better tolerated and highly effective [97,105]. The LNG regime reduced the proportion of pregnancy by 85%. In addition, 50% less nausea and 70% less vomiting occurred with the LNG regime compared with the combined Yuzpe method (23.1% and 50.5% nausea, 5.6% and 18.8% vomiting, respectively) [105]. Subsequent trials showed that progestin ECPs are most effective when

used within 120 hours (five days) of unprotected coitus and that a single dose of 1.5 mg LNG is as effective as two 0.75 mg doses given 12 hours apart [97,106,107].

The effect of single-dose LNG ECPs on the timing and duration of the next menstrual period is dependent on the day that the pills were taken [108]. When taken in the first three weeks of the menstrual cycle, this regime significantly shortened that cycle as compared to a control group of women who did not use ECP. This same regime if taken later in the cycle had no effect on cycle length, but did cause prolongation of the next cycle. Intermenstrual bleeding was 8% in the ECP group and 4% in the controls.

Lastly, according to the WHO guidelines, when taken as directed, the benefits associated with progestin-only ECPs outweigh any potential risks in patients with pre-existing cardiovascular diseases [41].

Emergency contraception with copper IUDS

The copper T380A (Paragard™) can be inserted up to the time of implantation (5–7 days after ovulation) to prevent pregnancy. This option is limited in the teen population, however, since teens are at high risk of contracting STIs, a contraindication to IUD insertion. Emergency insertion of a copper IUD is significantly more effective than use of ECPs, reducing the risk of pregnancy by 99% [97].

Access to emergency contraception

Since EC's efficacy is time sensitive, it is prudent to prioritize pregnancy prevention for women by removing any barriers that impede immediate access to the medication. This can be accomplished by policy changes that allow:
- OTC purchase of ECPs at the neighborhood pharmacy
- purchase from the pharmacy directly without a provider subscription
- facilitation of purchase by phone via a website with a provider who calls in a prescription to that person's pharmacy without a physical exam [97].

Women, teens and teen mothers, given advanced access to EC used the method more frequently when needed, but did not compromise their use of routine contraception nor increase their sexual risk behavior [97,109–111]. This evidence concerning ECP OTC use contradicts the concerns of opponents of EC who feel that those utilizing ECPs would do so irresponsibly.

The recent US OTC approval of EC could decrease a large portion of the 3 million unplanned pregnancies that occur in the US. Many think that the FDA bar against teen use of EC missed an unparalleled opportunity to address the 800,000 teen pregnancies that occur yearly in the United States [112].

Emergency contraceptive resources include websites (http://not-2-late.com, http://ec.princeton.edu/), the telephone (1-888-NOT-2-LATE), and planned parenthood organizations.

Cost-effectiveness of emergency contraception

Emergency contraception is cost effective because it prevents the costly results of unplanned pregnancy. An analysis was done to evaluate the cost savings of combined ECPs, progestin-only ECPs and the IUD. All three methods were found to reduce expenditure on medical care [113]. Advance provision of ECPs to women using barrier contraceptives, spermicides, withdrawal or periodic abstinence saves from $263 to $498 annually in a managed care setting and from $99 to $205 annually in a public payer setting. The authors concluded that expanded use of EC could reduce the considerable medical and social costs of unintended pregnancy.

Nonhormonal methods

Condoms

Barrier methods of family planning are described in the writings of ancient civilizations of Egypt and Greece [114,115]. These methods prevent pregnancy by providing a physical or chemical barrier to keep sperm from entering the cervix. Contraceptive barriers included mixtures of honey, acacia, and crocodile dung that were placed in the vagina prior to intercourse. The ancient Egyptians also wore decorative sheaths over their penises as early as 1350 BC though it is less clear if these were ever used during the act of intercourse [9,113].

The earliest published description of linen penile sheaths appears in Gabriel Fallopio's *De morbo gallico* (Padua, 1563), Chapter 89. The method was named for Dr Condom, a physician at the court of Charles II (who ruled 1660–1685), and extensively used by Casanova (1725–1788), who called it an English riding coat, to prevent acquisition of infection. Condoms made from animal intestines were used for contraception in the 1700s. The condom as a birth control device gained wide usage after vulcanization of rubber occurred in 1844 [115].

Mechanism of action

The condom consists of a thin sheath placed over the glans and shaft of the penis primarily to act as a physical barrier to prevent the deposition of semen into the vagina during intercourse. This prevents pregnancy and transmission of STIs that are found in semen such as gonorrhea, chlamydia, trichomoniasis, human immunodeficiency virus (HIV), and hepatitis B. A recent longitudinal study also suggested the utility of consistent condom use to reduce the risk of cervical and vulvovaginal human papillomavirus (HPV) infection [116]. Other longitudinal studies also conclude that consistent use of condoms among discordant couples is highly effective in preventing the transmission of HIV [117]. This includes a 2002 Cochrane review of 14 longitudinal studies that calculated a proportionate reduction in HIV seroconversion with condom use of 80% [118].

Condom use by sexually active teens is particularly critical since teens have very high risks of STI acquisition, and heterosexual transmission of HIV is the most common route of infection. Of the 19,000,000 cases of STIs occurring in the US, approximately 9,000,000 (50%) are among persons 15–24 years of age [2,119]. Adolescents aged 10–19 are particularly vulnerable to acquisition of STIs because of the likelihood of having multiple and high-risk sexual partners [2,120]. The contraceptive method most frequently used by teens aged 15–19 in 2002 was the condom. Ninety-three percent of teens reported its use. In addition, the "belt and suspenders approach" of simultaneous use of the condom, to prevent STIs, with a more effective contraceptive method is increasing. The percentage of sexually active teens practicing dual use in 1988, 1995, and 2002 was 3.3%, 8.4%, and 19.5%, respectively [2]. One longitudinal study comparing 123 teens' use of condoms with OCPs found that consistent dual usage continues to be an elusive challenge. Only 45% of reported coital events were associated with this modality, with 20% of coital events still unprotected by either method [121].

There is a wide variety of condoms with various shapes, textures, colors, and flavors. Although the majority of condoms are composed of latex, new alternative nonlatex male barrier methods made from polyurethane (Avanti, Trojan Supra, eZ-on™) or synthetic elastomers like Tactylon (styrene ethylene butylenes styrene, SEBS, a material used to make nonlatex gloves) were designed for those individuals who could not or would not use latex due to allergies or to preferences. The eZ-on™ condom is marketed as the first bidirectional condom that unrolls in both directions onto the penis. The design prevents incorrect unrolling of the condom onto the penis, which is felt to be a major cause of condom breakage during coitus. Lambskin condoms are permeable to viral particles. Thus use of lambskin condoms should be restricted to contraception rather than prevention of infection [114,122,123].

Efficacy

Typical failure rates for condoms are typically higher for teens and less experienced users. Typical failure rates for condom use over one year is 15% [8]. Motivation and experience with all coitally dependent methods will lead to lower failure rates that approach the perfect failure rate of 2%. One prospective randomized clinical trial comparing the Tactylon nonlatex condom with a commercial latex condom concluded that the nonlatex condom had a higher frequency of breakage or slippage during intercourse or withdrawal (4.0%) versus latex condoms (1.3%). The six-cycle typical pregnancy rates did not differ significantly (10.8% versus 6.4%). The six-cycle perfect-use pregnancy rate was higher for the nonlatex condom (4.9% versus 1.0%). The recommendation was to promote latex condoms first, with recommendation of the nonlatex condom for those who could not or were unwilling to use latex condoms [124].

Approximately 3% of couples are latex allergic. The idea of having various condom choices to encourage wider use in sexually active couples seems reasonable based on acceptability studies comparing natural latex condoms with the nonlatex polyurethane and SEBS condoms [125]. Couples using condoms for pregnancy prevention were enrolled in a three-way crossover study. Although none of the condom types was statistically preferred overall, approximately two-thirds of male and female participants preferred one of the two condoms made of synthetic material, suggesting that consumers appreciate the availability of these products [125].

One recent review of randomized controlled trials compared nonlatex male condoms with latex condoms in terms of contraceptive efficacy, breakage and slippage, safety, and user preference. The eZ-on™ condom did not protect against pregnancy as well as its latex comparison. No differences were found in typical-use efficacy between the Avanti and the standard Tactylon condoms and their latex counterparts. The nonlatex condoms had significantly higher rates of clinical breakage than their latex counterparts (Peto odds ratio for clinical breakage ranged from 2.6 (95% CI 1.6–4.3) to 5.0 (95% CI 3.6–6.8)). However, substantial proportions of participants preferred the nonlatex condom or reported that they would recommend its use to others. The authors concluded that although the nonlatex condoms were associated with higher rates of clinical breakage than those made from latex, these new condoms still provided an acceptable alternative for those with allergies, sensitivities or preferences that might prevent the consistent use of latex condoms. More studies to evaluate the contraceptive efficacy of nonlatex condoms were recommended [124,126].

Adverse events and contraindications

The WHO does not recommend the use of condoms impregnated with the spermicidal agent nonoxynol-9 since these condoms have not been shown to have higher efficacy in preventing pregnancy. Additionally, there are also concerns about nonoxynol-9 use and increased HIV transmission in women at high risk for HIV infection or in those who have multiple daily acts of intercourse [41,114].

Female condom

The female condom (Reality®) is a polyurethane sheath available in the US since the early 1990s. This method was developed to allow women to participate in safe sexual practices with a new barrier method [127]. Shervington conducted a premarketing study among African-American women living in New Orleans. This focus group discussion revealed that this group of women did not perceive themselves to be at risk nor perceive the need to engage in safe sex practices. Additionally, the deep-rooted cultural norm of female submission and passivity was identified as a major barrier to preventing unprotected sex in this group. Importantly, once offered the female condom as an option, the women wholly endorsed its use since it allowed them control over safe sex practices without having to challenge the power of the male partner.

This illustrates the importance of the practitioner eliciting a social and sexual history that allows tailored care that is acceptable to the patient's needs. This information is crucial for risk assessment for acquisition of STIs and is readily obtained when asked in a culturally sensitive and professional manner.

One survey of a convenience sample of homeless, high-risk adolescents recorded attitudes towards female condoms and male condoms. The authors found that adolescent respondents agreed with their adult counterparts about the usefulness of having the female condom as a choice [128]. Sixty-three percent used the male condom as their primary contraceptive, with 48% stating that they always used the male condom consistently and 44% reported having sex without a condom in the previous two weeks. Although 73% of this group stated that they would prefer to use the male condom, male respondents mentioned that the female condom might be more comfortable than male condoms. The authors recommended that the female condom be made available in addition to male condoms since young respondents and males might be willing to try the female condom in the future.

Efficacy

The female condom has a typical failure rate of 16% over one year's use. This is higher than the male condom and lower than the diaphragm [8].

Other barrier methods

Other less frequently used barrier methods have higher failure rates than condoms. Teen providers will usually avoid these modalities due to their higher typical failure rates. Examples include the cervical cap and Lea's shield, which both require provider intervention, and the contraceptive sponge that is available OTC. One reanalysis of data from two clinical studies compared the contraceptive efficacy of the diaphragm, the sponge, and the cervical cap [129]. The typical probabilities of failure during the first year were 17% for the sponge, 18% for the cervical cap, and 13–17% for the diaphragm.

The contraceptive sponge is a nonoxynol-9 impregnated disk that is wet with tap water before coitus. This method was not available for many years due to production problems. A major advantage of the sponge was that it empowered women and was readily available. The diaphragm, cervical cap, and Lea's shield require fitting by providers in their offices, a major disadvantage. They also require use of contraceptive spermicidal jellies composed of nonoxynol-9 to immobilize sperm that circumvent the barriers if they become dislodged during coitus.

Intrauterine devices

Eligible adult women in the United States seeking effective, long-term contraception underutilize the intrauterine device (IUD). In 2002, 5.8% of women aged 15–44 had experienced using the IUD, but only 1.3% were current users [2]. By comparison, prevalence of IUD use is higher for women living abroad. Rates of use in Canada, the UK, Switzerland, Germany, Austria, Finland, and France are 3%, 5%, 6%, 6%, 9%, 18%, and 21%, respectively [130]. As expected, low US teenage use of this modality is also found; 0.2% of teens aged 15–19 use the IUD with half (0.1%) admitting current use [2].

Intrauterine device underutilization stems from the unique history experienced by many US women [130]. The Dalkon shield was used by approximately 4.5 million women between 1971 and 1974, and accounted for two-thirds of the US IUD market. This device had higher method failure rates than initially reported and was also associated with septic spontaneous abortion. The unique multifilament tail that was designed to remove the device without breakage had a serious flaw: it acted as a conduit for ascending infection from the cervix to the uterus. This flaw was especially disastrous when coupled with poor patient selection that in many cases included younger patients with higher exposures to STIs. This IUD was recalled from the market in 1974.

The poor patient and practitioner experience with the Dalkon shield has led to reluctance to use new improved devices. This legacy will be hard to overcome without concerted simultaneous education of patients and providers.

Two IUD types are approved in the US. The first contains copper (copper T380A, Paragard®). It was introduced in 1988 [131] and consists of a T-shaped polyethylene frame that holds 380 mm² of exposed wire: 320 mm² wound on the vertical shaft and 60 mm² on the horizontal shaft of the T. A polyethylene monofilament is tied to the base of the T to assist in removing the device once the 10 years of approved use have occurred.

The second device is a LNG-releasing intrauterine system (IUS). The Mirena™ was first marketed in Finland in 1990 and became available in the US in 2001. This device consists of a T-shaped polyethylene frame (T-body) with a steroid reservoir (hormone elastomer core) around the vertical stem. The reservoir consists of a cylinder, made of a mixture of levonorgestrel and silicone (polydimethylsiloxane), containing a total of 52 mg levonorgestrel. The reservoir is covered by a silicone (polydimethylsiloxane) membrane. The IUS is 32 mm wide and 32 mm high and is designed to release 20 μg of LNG daily for at least five years. A monofilament brown polyethylene removal thread is attached to a loop at the base of the vertical stem of the T-body for assistance in confirming the presence of the IUS and also to assist the provider with its eventual removal.

Mechanism of action

The mechanism of action of the Paragard IUD is inhibition of sperm capacitation by released copper ions and salts, in addition to leukocyte stimulation of the endometrium, with enhanced prostaglandin production and inhibition of various endometrial enzymes.

The mechanism of action of the Mirena IUS is to thicken cervical mucus, inhibit sperm motility, cause endometrial atrophy, and inhibit ovulation. Ultimately both IUDs are thought to also play a role in inducing a foreign body reaction that is spermicidal and prevents fertilization. Plasma concentrations of LNG in IUS users are substantially lower than levels in combination OCP users or peak levels in users of POP and Norplant®.

These IUDs are not abortifacients since neither device has been associated with disruption of an implanted pregnancy.

Efficacy

Paragard and Mirena are both highly effective methods of contraception with pregnancy rates of less than 1% [129]. Paragard is approved in the US for 10 years, has efficacy for 12 years, and has a one-year failure rate of 0.6–0.8%. Mirena is approved for five years, has efficacy for seven years, and has a one-year failure rate of 0.1–0.2%. Interestingly, this surpasses the efficacy of permanent sterilization that is 0.5% after one year [8].

Adverse events and contraindications

Paragard is associated with heavier bleeding and cramping than Mirena. Conversely, Mirena significantly decreases both menorrhagia and dysmenorrhea when compared with Paragard but leads to infrequent bleeding, regular spotting or amenorrhea [131]. Twenty percent of those using Mirena may experience amenorrhea after one year. Minor side effects usually abate after the first three months. The incidence of lower abdominal pain, acne, back pain, mastalgia, headache, vaginal discharge,

mood changes and nausea are all less than 2% at five years in Mirena users.

Since IUDs prevent pregnancy effectively, they will also protect women from ectopic pregnancies. However, patients with previous ectopic pregnancy should not use the Mirena. The progestin released from the IUS could inhibit tubal motility, leading to repeat ectopic pregnancies.

Noncontraceptive benefits

Copper IUDs like Paragard have been associated with reduced risk of endometrial cancer.

Mirena is useful for the treatment of menorrhagia, especially in patients with adenomycosis [131]. Mirena may also be considered as an alternative to medical therapy for patients with bleeding due to submucous fibroids, benign endometrial hyperplasia, or in perimenopausal or postmenopausal patients receiving estrogen replacement therapy. Patients with severe medical conditions and vaginal bleeding benefit by avoiding general anesthesia and surgery. Once endometrial sampling excludes carcinoma, Mirena can be presented as an alternative to endometrial ablation, resectoscopic removal of fibroids and hysterectomy [131].

Summary

Many authors believe IUD use should be considered in women of various reproductive ages [131]. The ideal IUD candidate is a parous, monogamous woman in a stable sexual relationship. She should be at low risk of STI, without history of PID. Use by a mature, multiparous 19-year-old seeking effective child spacing is one such example. An IUD candidate must be extensively counseled to contact their provider when she or her partner has new sexual liaisons that risk exposure to STIs. Both chlamydia and gonorrhea have been associated with PID and pelvic abscess in the IUD user. Patients must also be monitored for PID during the first 30 days after IUD insertion.

Patients with contraindications to estrogen contraceptives or who are interested in avoiding use of hormones can benefit from the long-term efficacy of the IUD.

Conclusion

The economic consequences of teenage pregnancy are staggering. According to the National Campaign to Prevent Teen Pregnancy, taxpayers spent $9 billion on teenage childbearing in 2004 [132] (www.teenpregnancy.org/

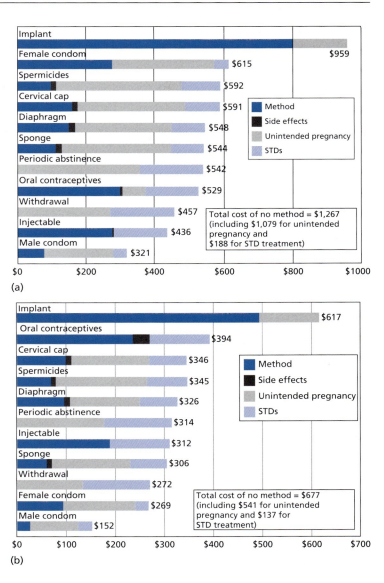

Figure 28.2 One-year cost of contraceptive use among adolescents under scenario 3, by method. (a) Private-sector setting. (b) Public-sector setting. Scenario 3 – acquiring and using a contraceptive method, treating side effects associated with contraceptive use or avoiding reproductive diseases, caring for an unintended pregnancy (birth, spontaneous abortion, induced abortion or ectopic pregnancy), assuming unwanted births will never occur but mistimed births will be postponed for two years, treating STDs.

default.asp). An analysis of of the economic consequences of adolescent contraceptive use by Trussell et al has concluded that use of any method is more cost effective than use of no method [133] (Fig. 28.2). Thus, use of effective contraception in the teen population not only decreases the negative consequences associated with teen pregnancy, but also makes sense from an economic point of view.

Lastly, recent US policy has been to expend billions of dollars on abstinence-only teen education. Undoubtedly, any analysis seeking to elucidate possible causes for the increased teen birth rates that occurred in 2006 will question the role of such policy. This analysis will also illustrate the effects that this policy change has had on teenage morbidity and mortality rates.

References

1. Ventura SJ, Mathews TJ, Hamilton BE. Births to teenagers in the United States, 1940–2000. *Nat Vital Stat Rep* 2001;**49**(10):1–23.

2. Abma JC, Martinez GM, Mosher WD, Dawson BS. Teenagers in the United States: sexual activity, contraceptive use, and childbearing, 2002. *Vital Health Stat* 2004;**24**:1–48.

3. Darroch JE, Singh S, Frost JJ. Differences in teenage pregnancy rates among five developed countries: the roles of sexual activity and contraceptive use. *Fam Plan Perspect* 2001;**33**(6):244–250, 281.

4. Santelli JS, Abma J, Ventura S et al Can changes in sexual behaviors among high school students explain the decline in teen pregnancy rates in the 1990s? *J Adolesc Health* 2004;**35**(2):80–90.

4a. Santelli JS, Lindberg LD, Finer LB, Singh S. Explaining recent declines in adolescent pregnancy in the United States: the contribution of abstinence and improved contraceptive use. *Am J Public Health* 2007;**97**(1):150–156.

5. Anderson JE, Santelli JS, Morrow B. Trends in adolescent contraceptive use, unprotected and poorly protected sex, 1991–2003. *J Adolesc Health* 2006;**38**(6):734–739.

6. Santelli JS, Morrow B, Anderson JE, Lindberg LD. Contraceptive use and pregnancy risk among US high school students, 1991–2003. *Perspect Sex Reprod Health* 2006;**38**(2):106–111.

7. Fu H, Darroch JE, Haas T, Ranjit N. Contraceptive failure rates: new estimates from the 1995 National Survey of Family Growth. *Fam Plan Perspect* 1999;**31**(2):56–63.

8. Trussell J. Contraceptive failure in the United States. *Contraception* 2004;**70**(2):89–96.

9. Hatcher RA, Trussell J, Stewart F et al (eds). *Contraceptive Technology*, 19th edn. 2007.

10. Smedley BD, Stith AY, Nelson AR (eds). *Unequal Treatment: Confronting Racial and Ethnic Disparities in Healthcare.* 2003.

11. Ranjit N, Bankole A, Darroch JE, Singh S. Contraceptive failure in the first two years of use: differences across socioeconomic subgroups. *Fam Plan Perspect* 2001;**33**(1):19–27.

12. Jones RK, Darroch JE, Henshaw SK. Contraceptive use among US women having abortions in 2000–2001. *Perspect Sex Reprod Health* 2002;**34**(6):294–303.

13. Greydanus DE, Patel DR, Rimsza ME. Contraception in the adolescent: an update. *Pediatrics* 2001;**107**(3):562–573.

14. Ott MA, Pfeiffer EJ, Fortenberry JD. Perceptions of sexual abstinence among high-risk early and middle adolescents. *J Adolesc Health* 2006;**39**(2):192–198.

15. Eaton DK, Kann L, Kinchen S et al. Youth risk behavior surveillance – United States, 2005. *MMWR Surveill Summ* 2006 9;**55**(5):1–108.

16. Jemmott JB 3rd, Jemmott LS, Fong GT. Abstinence and safer sex: HIV risk-reduction interventions for African American adolescents: a randomized controlled trial. *JAMA* 1998;**279**(19):1529–1536.

17. Darroch JE, Landry DJ, Singh S. Changing emphases in sexuality education in US public secondary schools, 1988–1999. *Fam Plan Perspect* 2000;**32**(5):204–211, 265.

18. Ott MA, Millstein SG, Ofner S, Halpern-Felsher BL. Greater expectations: adolescents' positive motivations for sex. *Perspect Sex Reprod Health* 2006;**38**(2):84–89.

19. Speroff L, Glass RH, Kase N (eds). *Clinical Gynecologic Endocrinology and Infertility*, 6th edn. 1999.

20. www.pbs.org/wgbh/nova/julian/ accessed on 02/19/07.

21. Chandra A, Martinez GM, Mosher WD, Abma JC, Jones J. Fertility, family planning, and reproductive health of US women: data from the 2002 National Survey of Family Growth. *Vital Health Stat* 2005;**25**:1–160.

22. Clark LR, Barnes-Harper KT, Ginsburg KR, Holmes WC, Schwarz DF. Menstrual irregularity from hormonal contraception: a cause of reproductive health concerns in minority adolescent young women. *Contraception* 2006;**74**(3):214–219.

23. Rosenberg MJ, Waugh MS, Meehan TE. Use and misuse of oral contraceptives: risk indicators for poor pill taking and discontinuation. *Contraception* 1995;**51**(5):283–288.

24. Rosenberg MJ, Burnhill MS, Waugh MS, Grimes DA, Hillard PJ. Compliance and oral contraceptives: a review. *Contraception* 1995;**52**(3):137–141.

25. Mishell J, Daniel R. State of the art in hormonal contraception: an overview. *Am J Obstet Gynecol* 2004;**190**(4, suppl 1):S1–S4.

26. Segal SJ. Gregory Pincus, father of the pill. *Popul Today* 2000;**28**(5):3.

27. Hannaford PC, Webb AMC (eds). *Evidence-Guided Prescribing of the Pill.* 1996.

28. Burkman R, Schlesselman JJ, Zieman M. Safety concerns and health benefits associated with oral contraception. *Am J Obstet Gynecol* 2004/;**190**(4, suppl 1):S5–S22.

29. Blackburn RD, Cunkelman A, Zlidar VM. Oral contraceptives – an update. *Popul Rep A* 2000;**28**(1):1–16, 25–32.

30. Westhoff CL. A perspective on the concept of "risk". *Dialogues Contracept* 1996;**5**(1):8–9.

31. Jick SS, Kaye JA, Russmann S, Jick H. Risk of nonfatal venous thromboembolism with oral contraceptives containing norgestimate or desogestrel compared with oral contraceptives containing levonorgestrel. *Contraception* 2006;**73**(6):566–570.

32. Winkler UH. Blood coagulation and oral contraceptives. A critical review. *Contraception* 1998;**57**(3):203–209.

33. Kaunitz AM. Enhancing oral contraceptive success: the potential of new formulations. *Am J Obstet Gynecol* 2004/;**190**(4, suppl 1):S23–S29.

34. Heinemann LA, Dinger J. Safety of a new oral contraceptive containing drospirenone. *Drug Saf* 2004;**27**(13):1001–1018.

35. Sulak PJ, Scow RD, Preece C, Riggs MW, Kuehl TJ. Hormone withdrawal symptoms in oral contraceptive users. *Obstet Gynecol* 2000;**95**(2):261–266.

36. Sulak PJ, Kuehl TJ, Coffee A, Willis S. Prospective analysis of occurrence and management of breakthrough bleeding during an extended oral contraceptive regimen. *Am J Obstet Gynecol* 2006;**195**(4):935–941.

37. Sulak PJ, Carl J, Gopalakrishnan I, Coffee A, Kuehl TJ. Outcomes of extended oral contraceptive regimens with a shortened hormone-free interval to manage breakthrough bleeding. *Contraception* 2004;**70**(4):281–287.

38. Anderson FD, Gibbons W, Portman D. Safety and efficacy of an extended-regimen oral contraceptive utilizing continuous low-dose ethinyl estradiol. *Contraception* 2006;**73**(3):229–234.

39. Edelman AB, Gallo MF, Jensen JT, Nichols MD, Schulz KF, Grimes DA. Continuous or extended cycle vs. cyclic use of combined oral contraceptives for contraception. *Cochrane Database of Systematic Reviews*, 2005, 3, CD004695.

40. Yonkers KA, Brown C, Pearlstein TB, Foegh M, Sampson-Landers C, Rapkin A. Efficacy of a new low-dose oral contraceptive with drospirenone in premenstrual dysphoric disorder. *Obstet Gynecol* 2005;**106**(3):492–501.

41. World Health Organization. *Medical Eligibility Criteria for Contraceptive Use*, 3rd edn. Geneva: World Health Organization, 2004.

42. World Health Organization. *Selected Practice Recommendations for Contraceptive Use*, 2nd edn. Geneva: World Health Organization, 2004:170.

43. Nelson AL, Sulak PJ. New Approaches in oral contraceptive regimes: breaking out of old models. *Forum* 2006;**45**(2):2.

44. Lara-Torre E, Schroeder B. Adolescent compliance and side effects with Quick Start initiation of oral contraceptive pills. *Contraception* 2002;**66**(2):81–85.

45. Westhoff C, Kerns J, Morroni C, Cushman LF, Tiezzi L, Murphy PA. Quick start: novel oral contraceptive initiation method. *Contraception* 2002;**66**(3):141–145.

46. Westhoff C, Osborne LM, Schafer JE, Morroni C. Bleeding patterns after immediate initiation of an oral compared with a vaginal hormonal contraceptive. *Obstet Gynecol* 2005;**106**(1):89–96.

47. Schafer JE, Osborne LM, Davis AR, Westhoff C. Acceptability and satisfaction using Quick Start with the contraceptive vaginal ring versus an oral contraceptive. *Contraception* 2006;**73**(5):488–492.

48. Balkus J, Miller L. Same-day administration of depot-medroxyprogesterone acetate injection: a retrospective chart review. *Contraception* 2005;**71**(5):395–398.

49. Sneed R, Westhoff C, Morroni C, Tiezzi L. A prospective study of immediate initiation of depo medroxypro-

50. gesterone acetate contraceptive injection. *Contraception* 2005;**71**(2):99–103.

50. Murthy AS, Creinin MD, Harwood B, Schreiber CA. Same-day initiation of the transdermal hormonal delivery system (contraceptive patch) versus traditional initiation methods. *Contraception* 2005;**72**(5):333–336.

51. Lesnewski R, Prine L. Initiating hormonal contraception. *Am FamPhysician* 2006;**74**(1):105–112.

52. Ott MA, Adler NE, Millstein SG, Tschann JM, Ellen JM. The trade-off between hormonal contraceptives and condoms among adolescents. *Perspect Sex Reprod Health* 2002;**34**(1):6–14.

53. Harel Z, Riggs S, Vaz R, Flanagan P, Dunn K, Harel D. Adolescents' experience with the combined estrogen and progestin transdermal contraceptive method Ortho Evra. *J Pediatr Adolesc Gynecol* 2005;**18**(2):85–90.

54. Rubinstein ML, Halpern-Felsher BL, Irwin CE Jr. An evaluation of the use of the transdermal contraceptive patch in adolescents. *J Adolesc Health* 2004;**34**(5):395–401.

55. LaGuardia KD, Fisher AC, Bainbridge JD, LoCoco JM, Friedman AJ. Suppression of estrogen-withdrawal headache with extended transdermal contraception. *Fertil Steril* 2005;**83**(6):1875–1877.

56. Burkman RT. The transdermal contraceptive system. *Am J Obstet Gynecol* 2004;**190**(4, suppl 1):S49–S53.

57. Sibai BM, Odlind V, Meador ML, Shangold GA, Fisher AC, Creasy GW. A comparative and pooled analysis of the safety and tolerability of the contraceptive patch (Ortho Evra/Evra). *Fertil Steril* 2002;**77**(2 suppl 2):S19–26.

58. Zieman M, Guillebaud J, Weisberg E, Shangold GA, Fisher AC, Creasy GW. Contraceptive efficacy and cycle control with the Ortho Evra/Evra transdermal system: the analysis of pooled data. *Fertil Steril* 2002;**77**(2 suppl 2): S13–18.

59. Holt VL, Cushing-Haugen KL, Daling JR. Body weight and risk of oral contraceptive failure. *Obstet Gynecol* 2002;**99**(5 Pt 1):820–827.

60. Jick SS, Kaye JA, Russmann S, Jick H. Risk of nonfatal venous thromboembolism in women using a contraceptive transdermal patch and oral contraceptives containing norgestimate and 35 microg of ethinyl estradiol. *Contraception* 2006;**73**(3):223–228.

61. Mishell DR, Edelman AB, Schnare S. *Hormonal Contraception: Separating Myth from Reality. Safety and Efficacy: Evaluating the Data and Promoting Adherence. A CME/CE Initiative.* Veritas Institute for Medical Education, 2006: 2.

62. Courtney K. The contraceptive patch. Latest developments. *AWHONN Lifelines* 2006;**10**(3):250–254.

63. van den Heuvel MW, van Bragt AJ, Alnabawy AK, Kaptein MC. Comparison of ethinylestradiol pharmacokinetics in three hormonal contraceptive formulations: the vaginal

ring, the transdermal patch and an oral contraceptive. *Contraception* 2005;**72**(3):168–174.

64. Novak A, de la Loge C, Abetz L, van der Meulen EA. The combined contraceptive vaginal ring, NuvaRing: an international study of user acceptability. *Contraception* 2003;**67**(3):187–194.

65. Roumen FJ, op ten Berg MM, Hoomans EH. The combined contraceptive vaginal ring (NuvaRing): first experience in daily clinical practice in The Netherlands. *Eur J Contracept Reprod Health Care* 2006;**11**(1):14–22.

66. O'Connell KJ, Osborne LM, Westhoff C. Measured and reported weight change for women using a vaginal contraceptive ring vs. a low-dose oral contraceptive. *Contraception* 2005;**72**(5):323–327.

67. Graham S, Fraser IS. The progestogen-only mini-pill. *Contraception* 1982;**26**(4):373–388.

68. McCann MF, Potter LS. Progestin-only oral contraception: a comprehensive review. *Contraception* 1994;**50**(6 suppl 1):S1–195.

69. Clark LR. Will the pill make me sterile? Addressing reproductive health concerns and strategies to improve adherence to hormonal contraceptive regimens in adolescent girls. *J Pediatr Adolesc Gynecol* 2001;**14**(4):153–162.

70. Perheentupa A, Critchley HO, Illingworth PJ, McNeilly AS. Effect of progestin-only pill on pituitary-ovarian axis activity during lactation. *Contraception* 2003;**67**(6):467–471.

71. Broome M, Fotherby K. Clinical experience with the progestogen-only pill. *Contraception* 1990;**42**(5):489–495.

72. Hussain SF. Progestogen-only pills and high blood pressure: is there an association? A literature review. *Contraception* 2004;**69**(2):89–97.

73. Cromer BA, Smith RD, Blair JM, Dwyer J, Brown RT. A prospective study of adolescents who choose among levonorgestrel implant (Norplant), medroxyprogesterone acetate (Depo-Provera), or the combined oral contraceptive pill as contraception. *Pediatrics* 1994;**94**(5):687–694.

74. Westhoff C. Depot-medroxyprogesterone acetate injection (Depo-Provera): a highly effective contraceptive option with proven long-term safety. *Contraception* 2003;**68**(2):75–87.

75. Thomas AG, Klihr-Beall S, Siqueira L, Horing I, Zhang J. Concentration of depot medroxyprogesterone acetate and pain scores in adolescents: a randomized clinical trial. *Contraception* 2005;**72**(2):126–129.

76. Stevens-Simon C, Kelly L, Kulick R. A village would be nice but . . . it takes a long-acting contraceptive to prevent repeat adolescent pregnancies. *Am J Prev Med* 2001;**21**(1):60–65.

77. Hubacher D, Goco N, Gonzalez B, Taylor D. Factors affecting continuation rates of DMPA. *Contraception* 1999;**60**(6):345–351.

78. Kaunitz AM. Depo-Provera's black box: time to reconsider? *Contraception* 2005;**72**(3):165–167.

79. Cromer B. In favor of continued use of depot medroxyprogesterone acetate (DMPA, Depo-Provera) in adolescents. *J Pediatr Adolesc Gynecol* 2005;**18**(3):183–187.

80. Rager KM. No bones about it – depot medroxyprogesterone acetate remains an excellent contraceptive option for adolescents. *J Pediatr Adolesc Gynecol* 2005;**18**(3):187–188.

81. Cromer BA, Scholes D, Berenson A et al. Depot medroxyprogesterone acetate and bone mineral density in adolescents – the Black Box Warning: a Position Paper of the Society for Adolescent Medicine. *J Adolesc Health* 2006;**39**(2):296–301.

82. Pelkman CL, Chow M, Heinbach RA, Rolls BJ. Short-term effects of a progestational contraceptive drug on food intake, resting energy expenditure, and body weight in young women. *Am J Clin Nutr* 2001;**73**(1):19–26.

83. Thomas AG Jr, LeMelle SM. The Norplant System: where are we in 1995? *J Fam Pract* 1995;**40**(2):125–128.

84. Darney PD. Hormonal implants: contraception for a new century. *Am J Obstet Gynecol* 1994;**170**(5 Pt 2):1536–1543.

85. Polaneczky M, Slap G, Forke C, Rappaport A, Sondheimer S. The use of levonorgestrel implants (Norplant) for contraception in adolescent mothers. *N Engl J Med* 1994;**331**(18):1201–1206.

86. Berenson AB, Wiemann CM. Use of levonorgestrel implants versus oral contraceptives in adolescence: a case-control study. *Am J Obstet Gynecol* 1995;**172**(4 Pt 1):1128–1135; discussion 1135–1137.

87. Shoupe D, Mishell DR. Norplant: subdermal implant system for long-term contraception. *Am J Obstet Gynecol* 1989;**160**(5 Pt 2):1286–1292.

88. Shulman LP, Nelson AL, Darney PD. Recent developments in hormone delivery systems. *Am J Obstet Gynecol* 2004;**190**(4, suppl 1):S39–S48.

89. Darney PD, Atkinson E, Tanner S, MacPherson S, Hellerstein S, Alvarado A. Acceptance and perceptions of NORPLANT among users in San Francisco, USA. *Stud Fam Plann* 1990;**21**(3):152–160.

90. Berenson AB, Wiemann CM. Patient satisfaction and side effects with levonorgestrel implant (Norplant) use in adolescents 18 years of age or younger. *Pediatrics* 1993;**92**(2):257–260.

91. Beerthuizen R, van Beek A, Massai R, Makarainen L, Hout J, Bennink HC. Bone mineral density during long-term use of the progestagen contraceptive implant Implanon compared to a non-hormonal method of contraception. *Hum Reprod* 2000;**15**(1):118–122.

92. Harrison-Woolrych M, Hill R. Unintended pregnancies with the etonogestrel implant (Implanon): a case series from postmarketing experience in Australia. *Contraception* 2005;**71**(4):306–308.

93. Zheng SR, Zheng HM, Qian SZ, Sang GW, Kaper RF. A randomized multicenter study comparing the efficacy and

bleeding pattern of a single-rod (Implanon) and a six-capsule (Norplant) hormonal contraceptive implant. *Contraception* 1999;**60**(1):1–8.

94. Funk S, Miller MM, Mishell DR Jr et al. Safety and efficacy of Implanon, a single-rod implantable contraceptive containing etonogestrel. *Contraception* 2005;**71**(5):319–326.

95. Biswas A, Viegas OA, Roy AC. Effect of Implanon and Norplant subdermal contraceptive implants on serum lipids – a randomized comparative study. *Contraception* 2003;**68**(3):189–193.

96. Burkett AM, Hewitt GD. Progestin only contraceptives and their use in adolescents: clinical options and medical indications. *Adolesc Med Clin* 2005;**16**(3):553–567.

97. Trussell J, Ellertson C, Stewart F, Raymond EG, Shochet T. The role of emergency contraception. *Am J Obstet Gynecol* 2004;**190**(4, suppl 1):S30–S38.

98. Glasier A. Emergency postcoital contraception. *N Engl J Med* 1997;**337**(15):1058–1064.

99. Ellertson C, Webb A, Blanchard K et al. Modifying the Yuzpe regimen of emergency contraception: a multicenter randomized controlled trial. *Obstet Gynecol* 2003;**101**(6):1160–1167.

100. Trussell J, Ellertson C, Dorflinger L. Effectiveness of the Yuzpe regimen of emergency contraception by cycle day of intercourse: implications for mechanism of action. *Contraception* 2003;**67**(3):167–171.

101. Trussell J, Rodriguez G, Ellertson C. New estimates of the effectiveness of the Yuzpe regimen of emergency contraception. *Contraception* 1998;**57**(6):363–369.

102. Webb A, Taberner D. Clotting factors after emergency contraception. *Adv Contracept* 1993;**9**(1):75–82.

103. Ellertson C, Evans M, Ferden S et al. Extending the time limit for starting the Yuzpe regimen of emergency contraception to 120 hours. *Obstet Gynecol* 2003;**101**(6):1168–1171.

104. *FDA News*. FDA Approves Over-the-Counter Access for Plan B for Women 18 and Older. Prescription Remains Required for Those 17 and Under. 2006. Available at: www.fda.gov/bbs/topics/NEWS/2006/NEW01436.html.

105. Task Force on Postovulatory Methods of Fertility Regulation. Randomised controlled trial of levonorgestrel versus the Yuzpe regimen of combined oral contraceptives for emergency contraception. *Lancet* 1998;**352**(9126):428–433.

106. Arowojolu AO, Okewole IA, Adekunle AO. Comparative evaluation of the effectiveness and safety of two regimens of levonorgestrel for emergency contraception in Nigerians. *Contraception* 2002;**66**(4):269–273.

107. von Hertzen H, Piaggio G, Ding J et al. Low dose mifepristone and two regimens of levonorgestrel for emergency contraception: a WHO multicentre randomised trial. *Lancet* 2002;**360**(9348):1803–1810.

108. Raymond EG, Goldberg A, Trussell J, Hays M, Roach E, Taylor D. Bleeding patterns after use of levonorgestrel emergency contraceptive pills. *Contraception* 2006;**73**(4):376–381.

109. Raine TR, Harper CC, Rocca CH et al. Direct access to emergency contraception through pharmacies and effect on unintended pregnancy and STIs: a randomized controlled trial. *JAMA* 2005;**293**(1):54–62.

110. Harper CC, Cheong M, Rocca CH, Darney PD, Raine TR. The effect of increased access to emergency contraception among young adolescents. *Obstet Gynecol* 2005;**106**(3):483–491.

111. Belzer M, Sanchez K, Olson J, Jacobs AM, Tucker D. Advance supply of emergency contraception: a randomized trial in adolescent mothers. *J Pediatr Adolesc Gynecol* 2005;**18**(5):347–354.

112. Korcok M. Plan B available to women 18 and older in US. *CMAJ* 2006;**175**(8):862.

113. Trussell J, Koenig J, Ellertson C, Stewart F. Preventing unintended pregnancy: the cost-effectiveness of three methods of emergency contraception. *Am J Public Health* 1997;**87**(6):932–937.

114. McNaught J, Jamieson MA. Barrier and spermicidal contraceptives in adolescence. *Adolesc Med Clin* 2005;**16**(3):495–515.

115. Riddle JM. *Contraception and Abortion from the Ancient World to the Renaissance*. Cambridge, MA: Harvard University Press, 1992.

116. Winer RL, Hughes JP, Feng Q et al. Condom use and the risk of genital human papillomavirus infection in young women. *N Engl J Med* 2006;**354**(25):2645–2654.

117. de Vincenzi I. A longitudinal study of human immunodeficiency virus transmission by heterosexual partners. European Study Group on Heterosexual Transmission of HIV. *N Engl J Med* 1994;**331**(6):341–346.

118. Weller S, Davis K. Condom effectiveness in reducing heterosexual HIV transmission. *Cochrane Database of Systematic Reviews*, 2002, 1:CD003255.

119. Weinstock H, Berman S, Cates W Jr. Sexually transmitted diseases among American youth: incidence and prevalence estimates, 2000. *Perspect Sex Reprod Health* 2004;**36**(1):6–10.

120. Sulak PJ. Adolescent sexual health. *J Fam Pract* 2004;**suppl**:S3–4.

121. Woods JL, Shew ML, Tu W, Ofner S, Ott MA, Fortenberry JD. Patterns of oral contraceptive pill-taking and condom use among adolescent contraceptive pill users. *J Adolesc Health* 2006;**39**(3):381–387.

122. Cates W Jr, Stone KM. Family planning, sexually transmitted diseases and contraceptive choice: a literature update – Part I. *Fam Plan Perspect* 1992;**24**(2):75–84.

123. Cates W Jr, Stone KM. Family planning, sexually transmitted diseases and contraceptive choice: a literature update – Part II. *Fam Plan Perspect* 1992;**24**(3):122–128.

124. Walsh TL, Frezieres RG, Peacock K, Nelson AL, Clark VA, Bernstein L. Evaluation of the efficacy of a nonlatex condom: results from a randomized, controlled clinical trial. *Perspect Sex Reprod Health* 2003;**35**(2):79–86.

125. Frezieres RG, Walsh TL. Acceptability evaluation of a natural rubber latex, a polyurethane, and a new non-latex condom. *Contraception* 2000;**61**(6):369–377.

126. Gallo MF, Grimes DA, Lopez LM, Schulz KF. Non-latex versus latex male condoms for contraception. *Cochrane Database of Systematic Reviews*, 2006, 1:CD003550.

127. Shervington DO. The acceptability of the female condom among low-income African-American women. *J Natl Med Assoc* 1993;**85**(5):341–347.

128. Haignere CS, Gold R, Maskovsky J, Ambrosini J, Rogers CL, Gollub E. High-risk adolescents and female condoms: knowledge, attitudes, and use patterns. *J Adolesc Health* 2000;**26**(6):392–398.

129. Trussell J, Strickler J, Vaughan B. Contraceptive efficacy of the diaphragm, the sponge and the cervical cap. *Fam Plan Perspect* 1993;**25**(3):100–105, 135.

130. Hubacher D, Cheng D. Intrauterine devices and reproductive health: American women in feast and famine. *Contraception* 2004;**69**(6):437–446.

131. Arias RD. Compelling reasons for recommending IUDs to any woman of reproductive age. *Int J Fertil Womens Med* 2002;**47**(2):87–95.

132. www.teenpregnancy.org/default.asp

133. Trussell J, Koenig J, Stewart F, Darroch JE. Medical care cost savings from adolescent contraceptive use. *Fam Plan Perspect* 1997;**29**(6):248–255, 295.

CHAPTER 29

Contraception in Adolescence

George Creatsas & Efthimios Deligeoroglou
University of Athens Aretaieion Hospital, Athens, Greece

Introduction

Adolescence is a landmark in every woman's life. A number of important events are observed during the transition from childhood to reproductive age, such as the menarche, the acceleration of body development, and the appearance of female body (secondary sexual) characteristics. Lack of knowledge, experience and counseling, along with the exploration of sexuality, may give rise to serious health-related problems, such as unintended pregnancies or infection with sexually transmitted pathogens (sexually transmitted diseases, STDs), including human immunodeficiency virus (HIV). Current rates of sexual activity, pregnancy, and STDs among adolescents remain a public health concern. The safest way to prevent unwanted pregnancy and STDs is to abstain from intercourse or to postpone sexual relationships. Nevertheless, the age at which first sexual intercourse takes place has recently decreased. Also, the percentage of adolescents who are sexually active has increased considerably in recent years [1]. It is reported that 56% of girls and 73% of boys have had sexual intercourse before the age of 18 [2].

Every year, 75 million unwanted pregnancies arise worldwide because of nonadoption of any contraceptive method. Additionally, in at least 8 million cases per year, the applied contraceptive method fails. It is estimated that 350 million couples around the world have inadequate information about contraceptives. Twelve to fifteen million unmarried women do not use any contraceptive method, and 120–150 million married women who want to confine future pregnancies lack the means to do so. In every single

day, 55,000 unsafe abortions are being performed (95% of them in developing countries) and 200 deaths occur, along with an unreported number of disabilities resulting from these unsafe procedures. Adolescents are susceptible to unwanted pregnancies, which push them into unwanted marriages or limit their opportunities for further education or employment, predisposing them to long-term welfare dependence. Adolescents are often non- or misinformed about sexuality or the risks associated with early and unprotected sexual activity. It is estimated that a percentage from 7.5% to 10% of adolescent women get pregnant in developed countries (rising to 27% worldwide) [3]. Approximately 51% of adolescent pregnancies end in a live birth, 35% of them result in an abortion with several complications, while 14% of them end in stillbirth or miscarriage [2,4]. It is estimated that 52% of adolescents use noneffective contraception [2]. In contrast to the general decrease in births in the USA, the frequency of pregnancy increases for ages between 14 and 17 years. Approximately 31% of adolescents reported that they did not use any contraceptive method at first intercourse; mostly these were people who had just met their sexual partner [5].

In Sweden, teenage abortion rates have gone up from 17/1000 in 1995 to 22.5/1000 in 2001, a 25% increase. Genital chlamydial infections have increased from 14,000 cases in 1994 to 22,263 cases in 2001, with 60% of them occurring among young people, and mostly among teenagers [6].

For families, healthcare professionals, educators, government officials, and young people themselves, adolescent contraception continues to be a perplexing and complicated issue. Widespread efforts are made to increase contraceptive use, and especially that of condoms, aiming to prevent not only unwanted pregnancies but also STDs

Pediatric, Adolescent, & Young Adult Gynecology. Edited by A. Altchek and L. Deligdisch. © 2009 Blackwell Publishing, ISBN: 978-1-4051-5347-8.

among sexually active teenagers. Recent studies have reported that, by allowing access to sexual knowledge or birth control in school-based clinics, the rates of sexual activity or intercourse at a younger age are not affected but the use of condoms is increased [7].

In another study, it is reported that most of parents believe that sex education should contain information on birth control methods, including condoms, it should be provided by the family and supplemented by schools before students reach the seventh grade, and that receiving a regular newsletter regarding teen sexual issues could be of great help in communication with their children [8]. In order to be most effective, sex education programs should be developed through a process of co-operation between community, parental organizations, school, media and governmental institutions.

Adolescent sexuality: the role of mass media

Currently, the average American child or adolescent spends 17–21 hours weekly viewing television, not including the time spent on listening to music, watching movies or music videos, playing video games, or surfing the Internet for leisure purposes [9]. On average, children between 9 and 17 years old use the Internet four times per week and spend approximately two hours online each time [10]. By the time adolescents graduate from high school, they will have spent 15,000 hours watching television, as compared with the 12,000 hours spent in the classroom [11].

Advertising and programming media seem to be highly sexualized in their content. In fact, the average young viewer is exposed to 14,000 sexual references each year, with just 165 of these dealing with responsible sexual behavior, accurate information on birth control matters, abstinence or the risks of pregnancy and STDs [12]. Although early sexual activity may be the result of a variety of factors, it is believed that the media play an important role. The media represent the easiest mode of influence on young people, their sexual attitudes and behaviors [13]. There are numerous studies representing television's powerful influence on adolescents' sexual attitudes, beliefs, and values [14]. It is suggested that the media should provide messages that encourage and support the delay of first coitus and should also present information on the

> **Box 29.1 Contraceptive methods**
>
> Abstinence
> Oral contraceptives
>   Combined (estrogen and progestin)
>   Mini-pills (progestin-only pills; POPs)
> Emergency contraceptive methods
> Injectable contraceptives
>   Depot medroxyprogesterone acetate (Depo-Provera)
>   Levonorgestrel implant (Norplant)
> Barrier contraceptive methods
>   Diaphragm
>   Vaginal sponge
>   Cervical cap
>   Vaginal spermicides
>   Female condom
>   Male condom
> IUDs (hormonal/nonhormonal)
>   Progestasert IUD (with progesterone)
>   ParaGard (Copper T380A IUD)
> Periodic abstinence

use of methods to avoid unwanted pregnancies and STDs (Box 29.1).

The male condom

More than 333 million new cases of the four common STDs (gonorrhea, chlamydia, trichomoniasis, and syphilis) occur annually, mostly in the developing world. Combined oral contraceptives (COCs) should be regularly used in combination with the condom as a unique contraceptive method providing a complete protection against unwanted pregnancy as well as STDs. Unfortunately, the combined use of condoms and hormonal contraceptives by adolescents seems to be very low [15]. In COC users, the incidence of chlamydial and mycoplasmal cervical infections is slightly increased, even though the incidence of pelvic inflammatory disease (PID) shows more than 50% decrease. Unfortunately, the pill offers no protection against viral infections, such as HIV. It is estimated that in the US, approximately three million adolescents contract an STD every year, including bacterial (e.g. gonorrhea, chlamydia) and viral infections (e.g. herpes, HIV). The rate of STDs among adolescents is increasing. It is reported that 21% of American adolescents have had more than four partners [16].

Most condoms on the market are made of latex. Condoms which are made of polyurethane have recently become available for use. Natural condoms (made of lamb intestine) may be permeable to micro-organisms. Spermicides, especially nonoxynol-9, have been recommended as a method for improving the effectiveness of condom use [17], with some studies reporting that their simultaneous use is effective in killing or inactivating not only sperm but also a great number of other common pathogens, but no studies have proven the effectiveness of spermicides on STDs or HIV transmission. Furthermore, spermicides have been accused of causing vaginal irritation in some studies [18].

Despite recent trends towards increased use by adolescents, consistent condom use is reported by less than half of all sexually active adolescents [19]. Breakage, slippage, and failure to use throughout intercourse are the most important faults that result in clinical failure. Although rates vary among the various studies as well as according to the user's experience, breakage and slippage rates of the male condom have each been estimated to be less than 2% [20]. When compared with adults, teenagers report condom failure ten times more frequently [21].

So condoms are not 100% effective, with a theoretic annual failure rate of around 2%. Actual failure rates range from 5% to 20% [17]. Goldman et al [22] reported first-year failure rates as low as 2–4% in adolescents. In real life, the use of condoms can be expected to decrease the rates of unwanted pregnancy, STDs and HIV acquisition among those who are sexually active, including adolescents, especially if used consistently and correctly. According to the literature, condom use appears to decrease but not fully eliminate the rate of most STD transmission. The consistent and correct use of reliable contraception and condoms is a responsibility of both male and female adolescents. In the interest of public health, restrictions and barriers should be removed and schools should be considered as appropriate sites for the availability of condoms.

Combined oral contraceptives

The combined oral contraceptive is a popular contraceptive method around the world, as it guarantees the highest contraceptive protection. More than 150,000,000 users are under 30 years old. In some European countries the pill is used by 50% of women and it is considered as an appropriate contraceptive method for adolescents as well.

For a young woman on the pill, hormonal contraception is an important issue. Since 1950, when Pincus started his research on the pill, pharmaceutical researchers have succeeded in creating contraceptive pills with low estrogen and progestogen concentration, with practically no side effects, overcoming issues such as weight gain or bone growth arrest. Other advantages of the pill's use during adolescence include decrease of menorrhagia [23] (blood loss during menses, which is very important when anemia coexists), reduction of benign breast disease, suppression of ovarian functional cysts, lowering the severity of endometriosis and PID, decrease of ovarian and endometrial cancer [24], and reduction of the incidence of ectopic pregnancy. Furthermore, regulation of menstruation, relief from dysmenorrhea [25], and improvement of polycystic ovarian syndrome and acne represent extra important positive effects of hormonal contraception. Moreover, the pill may postpone menstruation over a certain period of time, such as school exams or during holidays, when dysmenorrhea or bleeding can create problems. Taking the pill about the same time every day (every morning just after awakening or every night before going to bed) is recommended in order to create a habit and increase compliance. The maximum contraceptive protection is obtained when the pill is correctly used.

The undesirable side effects of COCs depend on the dose of estrogen and/or the quality of progestogen and can include irregular vaginal bleeding (mainly for pills with low estrogen dose), depression in young girls, especially when other psychologic problems coexist, galactorrhea or amenorrhea (in less than 1% of users) after the interruption of COC use. Hormonal contraception should not be prescribed in the following cases: cardiovascular disorders, venous thrombosis [26], liver disease, depression, focal migraine, breast mass of undefined diagnosis, and excessive obesity.

During adolescence, clinical tests relating to metabolism and lipid profiles are rarely necessary. In some cases, blood coagulating factors and liver function tests are occasionally needed. The incorrect perception that hormonal contraceptive methods are dangerous may originate from breast and pelvic examination during the first consultation, which may cause psychologic problems. The only absolutely necessary fields of investigation are the medical history and measurement of blood pressure. For most women, no further assessment is necessary [27].

A higher rate of COC failure is noted during adolescence compared to older women, and this is due to the greater frequency of sexual relationships and the ideal fertility conditions but, most of all, to the lower compliance with the method or inappropriate use.

Depot medroxyprogesterone acetate

Among the highly effective methods of reversible contraception, DMPA offers the longest duration of contraceptive activity, with a single injection every 13 weeks, which can be reversed simply by discontinuation. DMPA is given in a standard dose of 150 mg intramuscularly every three months and yields a rate of 0–5.2 pregnancies per 1000 women-years [21]. DMPA suppresses the preovulatory surge of luteinizing hormone and follicle-stimulating hormone and thereby inhibits ovulation. It is the most appropriate method of pregnancy prevention for many women, such as adult and adolescent women who have experienced dissatisfaction or contraceptive failures with other methods. Although it has excellent safety and efficacy profiles, the method has failed to achieve its potential for widespread use, mainly as a result of negative publicity and litigation concerning side effects. Preinsertion counseling seems to play an important role in satisfaction and side-effect tolerance.

Emergency contraception

For many years, in any case of need for emergency contraception such as rape or condom rupture, a high dose of estrogens was commonly used but this was associated with a high frequency of side effects, such as nausea and vomiting. The Yuzpe regimen is effective and much better tolerated. Among other proposed methods, danazol is not so highly effective, whereas mifepristone has an adverse-effect profile similar to that of the Yuzpe regimen. Furthermore, there is no extended experience on the use of mifepristone (RU-486) [21]. During recent years, the effectiveness of the progestogen-only pill levonorgestrel, when used as an emergency contraceptive method, has been studied. Levonorgestrel has better results with fewer side effects than the previously mentioned methods. A 0.75 mg levonorgestrel pill which is taken as soon as possible after the insecure intercourse and a second one, 12 hours later, seems to be efficient. The effectiveness

depends on the time span between coitus and pill administration (95% for the first 24 hours, 85% if taken 24–48 hours later, 58% between 48–72 hours later, and nearly no efficacy if more than 72 hours have passed). Knowledge of specific details, such as the recommended time window of effectiveness, is poor among school-age students, while awareness of emergency contraception is high. Appropriate use of emergency contraception could prevent up to 75% of unplanned pregnancies [28,29]. However, lack of knowledge is responsible for the failure of the method.

Debate regarding whether emergency contraception should be available to teens without a prescription is of great interest. Sexually active women, especially the teens, seeking emergency hormonal contraception find that a special family planning unit for adolescents, inside or independent from community hospitals, offers convenience and confidentiality [30]. On the other hand, emergency contraception should not be considered as an alternative regular contraceptive method. The clinician should strongly advise the woman to use an effective contraceptive thereafter.

Female condom

A new contraceptive method, which is not popular with adolescents, is the female condom. This method can be used as an alternative by those reporting latex allergy, as the female condom is made of polyurethane. The device is promoting healthy behaviors and increases sexual self-confidence and autonomy. Unfortunately, the attitudes of healthcare providers and the disposition of regulatory agencies have reduced access to this method.

Vaginal sponge

Another alternative barrier method is the contraceptive vaginal sponge which is made of polyurethane and releases 125 mg of the spermicide nonoxynol-9 over 24 hours of use. It can be used for more than one consecutive intercourse within 24 hours without changing or adding spermicide and does not require a prescription or fitting from a healthcare provider. Other advantages of this method include its control by the woman rather than her partner, the lack of side effects, its antibacterial and antiviral properties, including protection from HIV [21], as well as fewer medical contraindications. Unfortunately,

Table 29.1 Contraceptive methods (%) used during adolescence in European countries, age 12–18 years[35]

Country	PA/CI	COCs	IUD	Barrier	Other/no prophylaxis
Belgium	4.0	61.0	0	12.0	23.0
Denmark	NA	64.0	2.0	19.0	15.0
Finland	NA	32.0	0	50.0	18.0
France	NA	17.3	0.1	NA	NA
Germany	50.0	40.0	0	10.0	NA
Greece	30.5	40.5	3.8	20.7	4.5
Hungary	60.0	35.0	0	5.0	NA
Italy	39.2	7,9	0	31.2	NA
The Netherlands	7.0	56.0	0	29.0	8.0
UK	3.0	43.0	1.0	5.0	48.0

PA/CI, periodic abstinence/coitus interruptus; COCs, combined oral contraceptives; IUD, intrauterine device; NA, information not available.

the sponge is less effective in preventing pregnancy [31]. Similarly, high discontinuation and allergic-type reaction rates have been reported [32].

Implants and patches

Implants which release progestins are made of two types of polymer. Immediately after insertion, they begin to release the progestin in a steady mode. Their effectiveness duration varies from six to 84 months, and the pharmaceutical industry is experimenting on extending this recommended maximum duration of use [33]. This long-term high contraceptive protection makes implants a suitable alternative method for many women.

The transdermal contraceptive patch delivers ethinylestradiol and norelgestromin over seven days, and results in an efficacy similar to COCs. Excessive body weight is associated with lower efficacy. Cycle control and side-effect profile are similar to oral contraceptives. A major advantage of this method compared to other methods, even oral contraceptives, is that it offers nearly 90% perfect compliance to the dosing schedule across all ages. Attachment of the patch is not affected by warm humid climates, vigorous exercise or exposure to saunas or water baths.

Male hormonal contraception

Options for male hormonal fertility control could improve family planning. New methods will come into practice probably within the next few years. Spermatogenesis is dependent on the pituitary gonadotropins. Administration of high-dosage testosterone suppresses gonadotropins and spermatogenesis with an efficacy comparable to female oral contraceptives, resulting in reversible azoospermia in normal men. Combined administration of lower-dosage testosterone similar to physiologic replacement doses plus a progestin or a GnRH agonist has demonstrated further suppression. Most of these male hormonal contraceptives have been associated with modest weight gain and suppression of serum high-density cholesterol levels [34]. The method has not been tested for adolescents.

Other contraceptive methods

Intrauterine devices are not in common use during adolescence. Unless a pregnancy has proceeded, other barrier methods, such as caps or diaphragms, are not in use during adolescence. Unfortunately, many adolescents have unprotected intercourse or use ineffective methods such as periodic abstinence (coitus interruptus or withdrawal prior to ejaculation) (Table 29.1). The Pearl index of these methods may be as high as 16. This is why abortion remains so frequent during adolescence.

Legal and ethical aspects of abortion in adolescence

Current evidence suggests that at least in some European countries, improved access to sexual health information and services leads to better sexual health outcomes. The teen pregnancy, teen birth and teen abortion rates (per 1000 women aged 15–19 years) were respectively estimated to be 8.7, 4.5, 4.2 in The Netherlands, 16.1, 12.5, 3.6 in Germany, and 20.2, 10.0, 10.2 in France, whereas these rates in the United States were 79.8, 48.7, 27.5, showing a 8–11-fold increase [36–39].

In 1999, the International Federation of Gynecology and Obstetrics (FIGO) published eight recommendations concerning the performance of induced abortion for "nonmedical" reasons. The outline recommendation was that "after appropriate counselling, a woman has the right to have access to medical or surgical induced abortion, and that healthcare services have an obligation to provide such services as safely as possible" [40]. In 2003, the World Health Organization (WHO) published the *Technical and Policy Guidance on Safe Abortion* [41] in order to help health systems in making legal abortion safe and accessible.

The WHO typifies unsafe abortion by the lack of skilled providers, safe techniques, and/or sanitary facilities. Even though legality is not necessarily accompanied by safety, it is obvious that illegal abortions are too often also unsafe – performed by unskilled providers in concealed, often risky circumstances. The WHO estimated that 30 million legal abortions and 20 million clandestine abortions occurred throughout the world each year between 1995 and 2000 [42]. In the developing world, the deaths of 64% of the 687,000 women who died as a result of *unintended* pregnancy between January 1995 and December 2000 were attributed to dangerous, usually concealed abortions [43]. In less developed countries, the mortality rate due to unsafe abortion was 330 per 100,000 abortions: more specifically, the above rate was 680 in Africa, 283 in southern and south-eastern Asia, and 119 in Latin America. In contrast, mortality due to legal induced abortions in developed countries is devastatingly reduced when compared to that due to illegal abortions; per 100,000 legal abortions, the USA reported less than one death (0.6), Canada 0.1, The Netherlands 0.2, England and Wales 0.4, Denmark 0.5, Finland 0.7, and Scotland 1.0 [44].

The ideal target for any health service in the modern world would be the elimination of abortions, particularly in adolescents, due to their serious health, social and psychologic consequences in this sensitive age group. If this cannot be achieved, it would be equally crucial to eradicate at least the illegal abortions. The most frequent obvious reason for an adolescent to ask for an illegal abortion seems to be her desire to withhold such a painful, fearful and shameful situation from her family and close relatives. For this particular reason, legislation regarding consent for abortions may play a key role in reducing the unsafe illegal procedures.

In the USA, 43 States require that a woman under age 18 should get consent or notification from one or both of her parents before she can have an abortion. Not surprisingly, it has been reported that parental notification laws had almost no actual effect on an adolescent's decision to talk with her parent or guardian about her decision before having an abortion, whereas the principal factor determining whether a teen consulted her parents was the quality of her relationship with them [45]. In addition, adolescents' excuses for not consulting their parents included their fear for emotional and/or physical abuse, even eviction from their homes. Finally, the Supreme Court requires States with parental consent or notification laws to allow teens to have an abortion by appealing to another adult, such as a judge, doctor or minister; even though this opportunity may be somewhat protective, forcing pregnant teens to apply to a court, physician or other authority figure could have significant, adverse physical and emotional effects.

In Great Britain current abortion legislation is based on the Abortion Act 1967 [46], with modifications introduced by the Human Fertilization and Embryology Act 1990 [47] and, for England and Wales, on further amendments made in 2002 [48]. Legal requirements apply to certification and notification of abortion procedures. Regarding competent adult women (aged over 18 years), for consent to be valid it must be given voluntarily, on the basis of appropriate information, and the woman must have the capacity to consent to the intervention in question [49].

Regarding competent young women aged 16–17 years, they are entitled to consent to their own medical treatment. However, unlike adults, the refusal of a competent person aged 16 or 17 years may, in certain circumstances, be overridden by a person with parental responsibility or by a court. In order to establish whether a young person aged 16 or 17 years has the necessary capacity to consent to an intervention, the same criteria as for adults must be used. If the requirements for legitimate consent are fullfilled, it is not legally necessary to obtain consent from a person with parental responsibility. However, it is good practice to engage the adolescent's family in decision making, unless the adolescent wishes to exclude them.

Regarding young women aged less than 16 years, the legal position is stated as "any competent young person, regardless of age, can give valid consent to medical treatment", and the same criteria as for adults can be used for establishing capacity to consent to treatment. Lord Fraser provided the Fraser criteria [50] to guide doctors when providing contraception for girls aged less than 16 years who refuse to engage their parents. Doctors are justified in proceeding without the parent's consent or knowledge if:

- the girl will understand their advice
- the girl is likely to begin or to continue having sexual intercourse with or without contraceptive advice
- the doctor cannot persuade her to inform her parents or to allow the doctor to inform the parents that she is seeking contraceptive advice
- unless she receives contraceptive advice or treatment her physical or mental health, or both, are likely to suffer
- her best interests require the doctor to give her contraceptive advice, treatment, or both, without parental consent.

Doctors have a responsibility to try to persuade an adolescent to involve her family in treatment decisions but generally should not override the patient's views. Only in the most exceptional cases, e.g. when the pregnancy is thought to have resulted from child abuse, incest or exploitation, may a breach of confidentiality be understandable. In such cases, the adolescent must be informed that confidentiality cannot be guaranteed and offered all the necessary help and support.

Conclusion

Whenever a young girl has an unwanted pregnancy, psychologic and social problems arise. Parents, teachers, physicians, the media, etc., have a responsibility to inform young people about contraception. The theory that sex education and promotion of contraception use encourages sexual activities is incorrect. Due to communication problems between parents and children, teenagers identified friends and the media as the main sources of information relating to contraception. In Sweden, family and sex education are taught in schools and abortions are legal on demand, and free contraceptive counseling is easily available at well-organized family planning units and youth health centers. Condoms and COCs are available at low cost and emergency contraception is sold over the counter. This has resulted in a low teenage child-bearing rate.

If the adolescent chooses to continue her pregnancy, the clinician should remain available for further discussion during the pregnancy. If the adolescent chooses to place the child for adoption or to terminate her pregnancy, the clinician should be available to provide ongoing healthcare and emotional support together with a psychologist. In either case, the clinician should be available to help the adolescent to identify appropriate community programs, and to encourage her to continue her education. The organization of family planning centers for adolescents is without doubt necessary and must become a government priority.

References

1. Haffner DW (ed). *Facing Facts: Sexual Health for America's Adolescents. The Report of the National Commission on Adolescent Sexual Health.* New York: Sexuality Information and Education Council of the United States, 1995.
2. American Academy of Pediatrics, Committee on Adolescence. Adolescent pregnancy – current trends and issues. *Pediatrics* 1999;**103**(2):516–520.
3. Paukku M, Quan J, Darney P, Raine T. Adolescents' contraceptive use and pregnancy history: is there a pattern? *Obstet Gynecol* 2003;**101**(3):534–538.
4. Ventura SJ, Mosher WD, Curtin SC, Abma JC, Henshaw S. Trends in pregnancies and pregnancy rates by outcome: estimates for the United States, 1976–96. *Vital Health Stat* 2000;**56**:1–47.
5. Manning WD, Longmore MA, Giordano PC. The relationship context of contraceptive use at first intercourse. *Fam Plan Persp* 2000;**32**(3):104–110.
6. Edgardh K. Adolescent sexual health in Sweden. *Sex Trans Infect* 2002;**78**(5):352–356.
7. Schuster MA, Bell RM, Berry SH, Kanouse DE. Impact of a high school condom availability program on sexual attitudes and behaviors. *Fam Plan Persp* 1998;**30**:67–72, 88.
8. Jordan TR, Price JH, Fitzgerald S. Rural parents' communication with their teenagers about sexual issues. *J Sch Health* 2000;**70**(8):338–344.

9. Roberts DF, Foehr UG, Rideout VJ, Brodie M. *Kids and Media at the New Millennium: A Comprehensive National Analysis of Children's Media Use*. Menlo Park, CA: Henry J. Kaiser Family Foundation, 1999.

10. Roper Starch Worldwide Inc. The America Online/Roper Starch Youth Cyberstudy. Available online at: http://corp.aol.com/press/study/youthstudy.pdf, 1999.

11. Strasburger VC. Adolescents and the media: five crucial issues. *Adolesc Med* 1993;**4**:479–493.

12. American Academy of Pediatrics, Committee on Public Education. Sexuality, contraception and the media. *Pediatrics* 2001;**107**(1):191–194.

13. Creatsas G. Improving adolescent sexual behavior: a tool for better fertility outcome and safe motherhood. *Int J Gynecol Obstet* 1997;**58**:85–92.

14. Brown JD, Greenberg BS, Buerkel-Rothfuss NL. Mass media, sex, and sexuality. *Adolesc Med* 1993;**4**:511–525.

15. Ott MA, Adler NE, Millstein SG, Tschann JM, Ellen JM. The trade-off between hormonal contraceptives and condoms among adolescents. *Persp Sex Reprod Health* 2002;**34**(1):6–14.

16. Institute of Medicine, Committee on Prevention and Control of Sexually Transmitted Diseases. *The Hidden Epidemic.* Washington, DC: National Academy Press (Centers for Disease Control and Prevention), 2000.

17. Hatcher RA, Trussell J, Stewart F et al. *Contraceptive Technology*, 17th edn. New York: Ardent Media, 1998.

18. Van Damme L. Advances in topical microbicides. Paper presented at the XIII International AIDS Conference, Durban, South Africa, 2000.

19. Sonenstein FL, Ku LC, Lindberg LD, Turner CF, Pleck JH. Changes in sexual behavior and condom use among teenage males: 1988 to 1995. *Am J Public Health* 1998;**88**:956–959.

20. Spruyt A, Steiner MJ, Joanis C et al. Identifying condom users at risk for breakage and slippage: findings from three international sites. *Am J Public Health* 1998;**88**:239–244.

21. Creatsas G. Contraception for adolescents. In: Sultan C (ed) *Pediatric Adolescent Gynecology: Evidence-Based Clinical Practice.* Basel: Karger, 2004: 225–232.

22. Goldman JA, Dicker D, Feldberg D, Samuel N, Resnik R. Barrier contraception in the teenager: a comparison of four methods in adolescent girls. *Pediatr Adolesc Gynecol* 1985;**3**:59–76.

23. Deligeoroglou E. Dysfunctional uterine bleeding. *Ann NY Acad Sci* 1997;**816**:158–164.

24. Deligeoroglou E, Michailidis E, Creatsas G. Oral contraceptives and reproductive system cancer. *Ann NY Acad Sci* 2003;**997**:199–208.

25. Deligeoroglou E. Dysmenorrhea. *Ann NY Acad Sci* 2000;**900**:237–244.

26. Creatsas G, Kontopoulou-Griva I, Deligeoroglou E et al. Effect of the monophasic and triphasic (gestodene-ethinylestradiol) oral contraceptives on natural inhibitor and other haemostatic variables. *Eur J Contraception Reprod Health Care* 1997;**2**(1):31–38.

27. Stewart FH, Harper CC, Ellertson CE, Grimes DA, Sawaya GF, Trussell J. Clinical breast and pelvic examination requirements for hormonal contraception: current practice vs evidence. *JAMA* 2001;**285**(17):2232–2239.

28. Wanner MS, Couchenour RL. Hormonal emergency contraception. *Pharmacotherapy* 2002;**22**(1):43–53.

29. Ellertson C, Trussell J, Stewart F, Koenig J, Raymond EG, Shochet T. Emergency contraception. *Semin Reprod Med* 2001;**19**(4):323–330.

30. Heard-Dimyan J. Issue of emergency hormonal contraception through a casualty department in a community hospital. *Br J Fam Plan* 1999;**25**(3):105–109.

31. Creatsas G, Guerrero E, Guilbert E et al. A multinational evaluation of the efficacy, safety and acceptability of the Protectaid contraceptive sponge. *Eur J Contraception Reprod Health Care* 2001;**6**:172–182.

32. Kuyoh MA, Toroitich-Ruto C, Grimes DA, Schulz KF, Gallo MG. Sponge versus diaphragm for contraception (Cochrane Review). *Cochrane Library*, Issue 1, 2004.

33. Croxatto HB. Progestin implants for female contraception. *Contraception* 2002;**65**:15–19.

34. Anawalt BD, Amory JK. Advances in male hormonal contraception. *Ann Med* 2001;**33**(9):587–595

35. Creatsas G, Vekemans M, Horejsi J et al. Adolescent sexuality in Europe. Multicentric study, International Federation of Infantile and Juvenile Gynecology. *Adolesc Pediatr Gynecol* 1995;**8**:59–63.

36. Ventura SJ et al. Trends in pregnancy rates for the United States, 1976–97: an update. *National Vital Statistics Reports* 2001;**49**(4):1–10.

37. Singh S, Darroch JE. Adolescent pregnancy and childbearing: levels and trends in developed countries. *Fam Plan Persp* 2000;**32**(1):14–23.

38. Rademakers J. Sex Education in the Netherlands. Paper presented to the European Study Tour, Utrecht, Netherlands: NISSO, 2001.

39. Martin JA et al. Births: preliminary data for 2000. *National Vital Statistics Reports* 2001;**49**(5):1–20.

40. McKay HE, Rogo KO, Dixon DB. FIGO society survey: acceptance and use of new ethical guidelines regarding induced abortion for non-medical reasons. *Int J Gynaecol Obstet* 2001;**75**:327–336.

41. World Health Organization. *Safe Abortion: Technical and Policy Guidance for Health Systems*. Geneva: World Health Organization, 2003.

42. World Health Organization. *Unsafe Abortion: Global and Regional Estimates of Incidence of and Mortality Due to Unsafe Abortion*. Geneva: World Health Organization, 1998.

43. Daulaire N et al. *Promises to Keep: The Toll of Unintended Pregnancy on Women's Lives in the Developing World*. Washington, DC: Global Health Council, 2002.

44. Alan Guttmacher Institute. *Sharing Responsibility: Women, Society and Abortion Worldwide*. New York: Alan Guttmacher Institute, 1999.

45. Blum RW et al. The impact of a parental notification law on adolescent abortion decision-making. *Am J Public Health* 1987;**77**:619–620.

46. Abortion Act 1967. London: HMSO, 1967.

47. Human Fertilisation and Embryology Act 1990. London: HMSO, 1990.

48. Statutory Instrument 2002 No. 887. The Abortion (Amendment) (England) Regulations 2002. London: HMSO, 2002.

49. General Medical Council. *Seeking Patients' Consent: The Ethical Considerations*. London: GMC, 1998.

50. Medical Defence Union. *Consent to Treatment*. London: Medical Defence Union, 1996.

CHAPTER 30

Labor in the Adolescent

Emanuel A. Friedman
Harvard Medical School, Boston, MA, USA

Introduction

In addition to the host of special needs that the adolescent gravida has merely because she is a teenager, she often comes to her pregnancy with additional risk factors that put her and her fetus in potential jeopardy. It is clear that she is not merely a small pregnant adult. She is physically, functionally and emotionally immature. Of particular relevance to her obstetric performance, she has important nutritional needs for her own growth and continued development that are simultaneously competing with those of her fetus. Further, depending on how close she is to her menarche, her pelvic architecture is still incompletely formed. As a result, her pelvic capacity may be inadequate to accommodate the birth of her fetus safely.

Not uncommonly, the adolescent indulges in high-risk behavior and exposures. She often has inadequate social support and care systems. She may use tobacco, alcohol, and illicit drugs. Sexually transmitted diseases are encountered. Physical, sexual, and emotional abuse occurs. Prenatal care may be insufficient or even nonexistent. The pregnancy is frequently unwanted. It may cause her own personal disintegration as well as that of her family, her economic status, and her education. These are all burdens she will bear for the rest of her adult life.

The consequences of these adverse circumstances are the complications that are reported to be so much more frequent among these young women. Consistently shown are increased frequencies of spontaneous abortion, iron deficiency anemia, intrauterine fetal growth restriction, preterm labor and delivery, pregnancy-induced hypertension and perinatal-infant morbidity and mortality. Less consistently encountered problems include early vaginal bleeding, preterm premature rupture of the membranes, post-term pregnancy, gestational diabetes, congenital malformations, fetal macrosomia, operative interventions for delivery, and maternal morbidity.

This chapter will focus primarily on issues of pelvic bony development and reproductive performance. We will demonstrate that pregnancy outcome in immature mammals, including human beings, is generally poor and probe for its causes. We will detail the pathophysiology of bone in adolescents and the impact of pregnancy on bony development in teenagers. We will deal with the incomplete development of pelvic architecture and capacity in these youngsters. We will describe the sequential anatomic adaptation of the pelvis during pubertal growth. We will show how immature pelvic development affects the course of labor, and in turn how the labor impacts on outcome. Management principles will be formulated for the obstetric care of young gravidas based on this evidence.

Reproductive performance and bone changes in immature mammals

There is a wealth of veterinarian literature confirming that when conception occurs before full maturity among laboratory animals (mice, rats, rhesus monkeys, for example), livestock (pigs, cattle, and horses) and domesticated pets (dogs and cats), they have frequent pregnancy losses and premature births [1]. The most important determinants of outcome for them are their nutritional status prior to conception and during the pregnancy, and the interval of time since maturation first began. Those with good nutrition and almost complete physical development tend

Pediatric, Adolescent, & Young Adult Gynecology. Edited by A. Altchek and L. Deligdisch. © 2009 Blackwell Publishing, ISBN: 978-1-4051-5347-8.

to do well in pregnancy, as do their fetuses. The longer the interval of time that has elapsed from the beginning of puberty to the conception, the better the outcome. Conversely, the closer to puberty, the greater the complication rates and adverse results to both mother and fetus.

Extensive studies have been carried out on bone structure and how it changes in the adolescent macaque monkey [2]. It has been determined that whole-body mineral content increases in early pregnancy, but drops markedly in late pregnancy and with lactation. Simultaneously, vertebral and pelvic mineral density falls during pregnancy. This decline accelerates during the entire period of postpartum lactation. In well-nourished young animals, calcium, phosphate, 23-hydroxyvitamin D, and osteocalcin increase from midpregnancy to postdelivery weaning. No such increase occurs if there is poor nutrition. Bone formation decreases in midpregnancy, compounded by an increase in the resorption of cancellous bone. During lactation, both cortical and cancellous bone is lost, weakening bone strength and depleting calcium stores. After weaning, partial restoration of bone mineral occurs. Importantly, gravid monkeys who begin pregnancy with calcium deficiency and inadequate bone mineral stores risk the development of osteopenia.

Parallel changes occur in pregnant adolescent girls [3]. The still-growing pubertal gravida has a threefold decrease in bone density, for example, compared to mature women. Nulliparous adolescents have a much greater bone loss in pregnancy than multiparous teenagers. Teenagers with higher bone density in early pregnancy lose more bone than those with lower initial density. The identifiable risk predictors for bone loss in pregnant adolescents are low pregravid weight, poor weight gain during pregnancy, early age at menarche, and low gynecologic age (as defined by the number of years from the menarche to conception). Of special interest, this accelerated bone loss is not fully compensated for by the physiologic increase in calcium absorption that normally occurs in pregnancy. It can be safely concluded that bone loss reflects continuing unmet maternal skeletal needs during pubertal growth, magnified by the demands for fetal mineralization.

Bone deficiency states follow among affected gravidas [4]. Osteoporosis, which occurs far more often in postmenopausal women, can also develop among teenagers. It is associated with reduced bone mass with diminished cortical thickening and decreased numbers and size of cancellous bone trabeculae, but with normal chemical composition. An idiopathic juvenile form is rarely encountered or it may result from chronic exposure to steroids or heparin. It is not uncommon among young women with long-standing anorexia nervosa and bulimia. Secondary bone loss may also occur from prolonged immobilization or debilitation from a neurologic or orthopedic disorder or other chronic disease, most especially in puberty. Pelvic contracture and deformity may result in such cases. Osteomalacia with softening and bending of bones develops because bones containing osteoid tissue fail to calcify due to lack of calcium and vitamin D or, less often, due to renal dysfunction. Osteomalacia is seen among older gravidas whose pregnancies are frequent and closely spaced. In adolescents, it can begin in pregnancy. It is more often encountered among those who conceive before their bone mass is fully matured. Osteopenia is associated with decreased calcification or density of bone, the reduced bone mass resulting from inadequate osteoid synthesis. Osteopenia is rather frequently seen in pregnant teenagers [4]. Again, it is a reflection of the increased unmet calcium needs, enhanced by inadequate intake of calcium and vitamin D. Those who are affected are at high risk of bone demineralization. Bone deficiencies, such as osteopenia, serve to delay, distort or arrest the processes of bony adaptation and development in puberty. These conditions thus adversely affect concurrent and future pregnancies [5].

Changing pelvic architecture and capacity in puberty

Bones adapt to mechanical loading by altering their geometry. Bony adaptation is a continuous process, responsive to physical stresses and changing over time. It occurs in conjunction with and in response to skeletal and muscular growth. The increase in size and strength of bone is age dependent. During puberty, this process is facilitated by the deposition of large amounts of calcium in bones. Since calcium deposition occurs more among young girls than boys, it is logically postulated that it serves to better prepare them for the future demands of pregnancy and lactation [5].

Prior to puberty, all children have a small, sexually undifferentiated justominor pelvis [5]. Pelvic shape is thus

Justominor pelvis
Age 9

Early puberal pelvis
Age 12

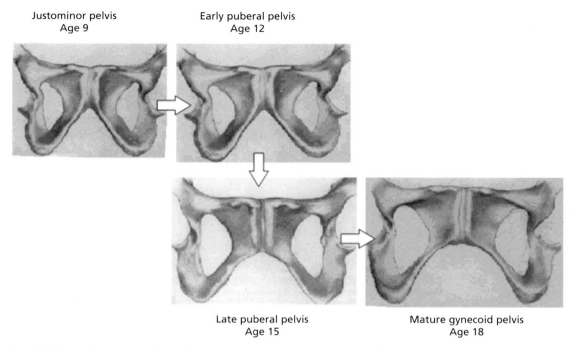

Late puberal pelvis
Age 15

Mature gynecoid pelvis
Age 18

Figure 30.1 Sequential remodeling of the pelvic outlet, frontal views. Beginning with the undifferentiated justominor pelvis of childhood, the inferior pubic rami elongate to produce enlargement of the transverse dimension of the outlet at the intertuberous diameter. Later, the subpubic arch rounds out to change the pointed arch of the immature pelvis to the rounded arch of the mature gynecoid pelvis.

characteristically gynecoid-anthropoid with a rounded posterior segment and a narrowed anterior component. Growth in stature begins early in puberty, usually years before the onset of pelvic growth. Pelvic growth and reshaping begin just prior to menarche and continue until full maturation is reached several years later. The first change in the remodeling of the pelvis in girls, starting just prior to menarche, is lengthening of the anteroposterior diameter. This makes the pelvis decidedly more anthropoid, although it remains small in capacity. With advancing maturity, there is transverse widening of the pelvis. This occurs in an orderly sequence starting first at the outlet, then the inlet and finally at the midplane. The pelvic outlet is affected first by the elongation of the inferior pubic rami. This enlarges the distance between the ischial tuberosities – the intertuberous diameter (Fig. 30.1). In time this is followed by transverse enlargement at the pelvic inlet to begin the rounding process that makes the inlet less anthropoid and more gynecoid in shape (Fig. 30.2). The

last phase prior to full maturation is straightening of the pelvic side wall at the midplane to remodel the acetabular notch so that it no longer encroaches on the midpelvis; this widens the midpelvis transversely (Fig. 30.3). At full maturation, the pelvic shape rounds out to take its typical adult gynecoid shape. The entire process takes at least 3–5 years, nearly all of which occurs after menarche (Fig. 30.4) [6].

Thus, the young adolescent gravida is likely to have an incompletely developed, small-capacity, transversely narrowed anthropoid pelvis. Inadequate pelvic architecture exposes her to bony dystocia. The limited pelvic capacity, however, may be counterbalanced by the aforementioned incomplete calcification and reduced bone density (with resulting osteomalacic softening) due to the unmet intrinsic needs of maternal growth and superimposed fetal demands. Reduced fetal growth is yet another counterbalancing factor that may help avert cephalopelvic disproportion among these young gravidas.

Justominor pelvis
Age 9

Early puberal pelvis
Age 12

Late puberal pelvis
Age 15

Mature gynecoid pelvis
Age 18

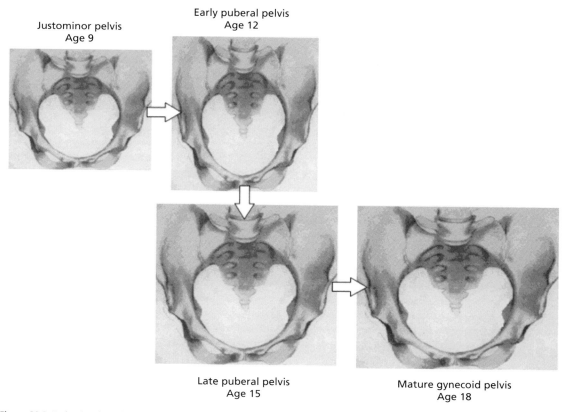

Figure 30.2 Reshaping the pelvic inlet during puberty, inlet view. This process lags behind the enlargement of the outlet. At first, the inlet enlarges to become more anthropoid in shape. Then transverse growth progresses to transform the inlet into a rounded mature gynecoid shape.

Labor in the adolescent

The progress of labor in teenagers has been shown to be slower on average than that of more mature women (Fig. 30.5) [7]. In a large observational study of labor in adolescents compared with that of older gravidas, all measurable aspects of the cervical dilation and the fetal descent patterns are significantly delayed. The latent phase is longer (6.1 ± 0.09 h vs 5.4 ± 0.05 h, p < 0.01); the active phase duration longer (5.5 ± 0.10 h vs 3.9 ± 0.09, p < 0.01); the maximum slope of dilation slower (3.3 ± 0.05 cm/h vs 4.1 ± 0.03 cm/h, p < 0.01); the deceleration phase longer (0.80 ± 0.01 h vs 0.65 ± 0.01 h, p < 0.01); the maximum slope of descent slower (4.0 ± 0.09 cm/h vs 5.3 ± 0.07 cm/h, p < 0.01); and the second stage longer (0.86 ± 0.04 h vs 0.59 ± 0.03h, p < 0.01).

While these slow labor patterns are consistently found in adolescents, one has to consider how teenagers differ from more mature women in other attributes – that is, other than age alone – that might affect their labor course. They are more likely, for example, to go into preterm labor (18.2% vs 12.4%, p < 0.01) and deliver prematurely (10.5% vs 6.3%, p < 0.01) than older gravidas (Fig. 30.6) [8]. Furthermore, the younger the adolescent is in terms of gynecologic age, the higher the rate of preterm labor and delivery [8]. Those who are within three years of menarche delivered prematurely in 12.8% of cases. By contrast, those with gynecologic age greater than five years delivered prematurely only 6.3% of the time, for a significant odds ratio – adjusted for ethnicity, smoking, weight gain, height, diabetes and pregnancy-induced hypertension – of 2.64 (confidence intervals 1.2–5.7, p < 0.01). It follows that teenagers have more small fetuses as a result of preterm

Justominor pelvis
Age 9

Early puberal pelvis
Age 12

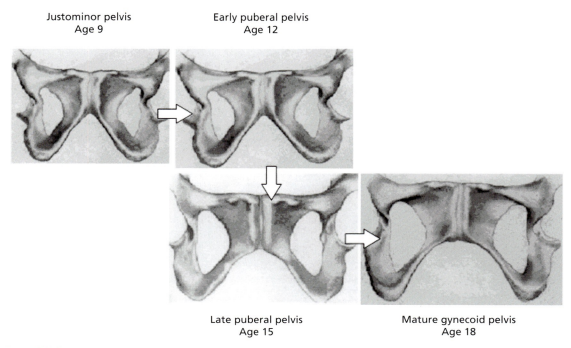

Late puberal pelvis
Age 15

Mature gynecoid pelvis
Age 18

Figure 30.3 The final stage in adaptation for full pelvic maturation occurs in the midpelvis, shown in frontal view. Constriction at the acetabular notch is relieved by bony remodeling and the pelvic side walls at the midplane become parallel, thereby maximizing the midpelvic capacity.

birth. Moreover, their offspring are also more likely to suffer intrauterine growth restriction (13.2% vs 8.0%, p < 0.01) [8]. There do not appear to be any more abnormal labor patterns among teenagers, yet they are definitely exposed to more uterotonic agents in the course of their labors (33.4% vs 13.0%, p < 0.01) [9]. Whereas fewer adolescents are diagnosed with cephalopelvic disproportion (2.0% vs 7.7%, p < 0.01) and fewer require cesarean

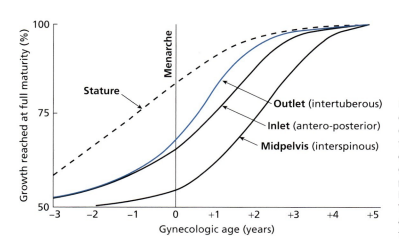

Figure 30.4 Graphic representation of changing pelvic size over time during puberty compared with earlier growth in stature. Note that stature increases long before pelvic change begins. The pelvic outlet begins its growth and grows faster than the rest of the pelvis; then the inlet dimensions follow; and lastly, the midpelvis increases its diameters. The major growth of the pelvis takes 3–5 years and occurs mostly after menarche. Modified from reference 5, with permission.

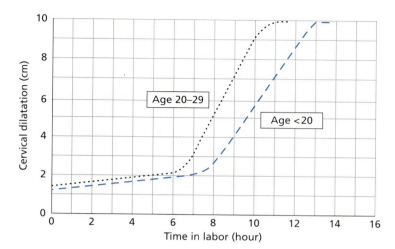

Figure 30.5 Plot of cervical dilation against elapsed time in labor for adolescents (age <20 years, dashed line) vs older gravidas (age 20–29 years, dotted line). Teenage labor is characterized by slower rates of dilation and descent, longer latent, active and deceleration phases, and longer second stages. Adapted from reference 7, with permission.

delivery (4.3% vs 6.5%, p < 0.01), many more are delivered vaginally by forceps (9.4% vs 3.8%, p < 0.01) [9]. These aggressive labor and delivery practices are inexplicable and counterintuitive, suggesting that some obstetricians use them without clinical justification.

Only a small minority of teenagers deliver macrosomic infants, but the labor course in those who do is markedly different from those who do not. Labors associated with macrosomic fetuses are characterized by significantly longer active phase durations (7.4 ± 0.16 h vs 5.5 ± 0.10 h, p < 0.01); longer deceleration phases (1.11 ± 0.04 h vs 0.80 ± 0.01 h, p < 0.01); slower maximum slopes

of dilation and descent (2.0 ± 0.09 cm/h vs 3.3 ± 0.05 cm/h and 2.4 ± 0.12 vs 4.0 ± 0.09, p < 0.01 for both); and longer second stages (1.14 ± 0.07 h vs 0.86 ± 0.04 h, p < 0.01); but latent phase duration is unaffected [7].

Given that teenage gravidas are so dissimilar in substantive ways from older women, the dilatory labor course might be accounted for on the basis of one or more of these confounding factors instead of their age per se [7]. To help distinguish the impact of age from that of other concurrent factors, corrections have been applied for such relevant factors as parity (because adolescents tend to be nulliparous more often), prematurity (so common among

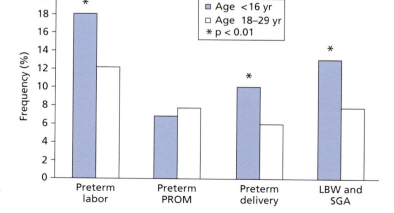

Figure 30.6 Comparative data for the incidence of preterm labor and delivery, preterm premature rupture of the membranes (PROM) and low birth weight (LBW) and small-for-gestational age (SGA) babies among young teenagers and older gravidas. Data from reference 8, with permission.

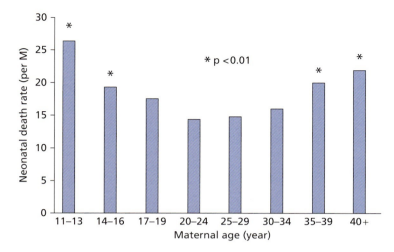

Figure 30.7 Neonatal mortality by maternal age, demonstrating a significant increase among offspring of teenagers and elderly gravidas. The younger the adolescent, the worse the results. From reference 10, with permission.

them), cephalopelvic disproportion (infrequently seen except in association with fetal macrosomia), growth restriction (frequently seen), oxytocin (give often, as noted earlier), analgesia, and anesthesia. The data obtained after all these corrections are made raise doubts that labors in adolescents are necessarily slower than among older women [7]. There is no longer any objective evidence supporting that contention. In fact, the mean latent and deceleration phase durations are actually shorter (5.1 ± 0.56 h vs 7.1 ± 0.28, p < 0.01, and 0.52 ± 0.05 h vs 0.70 ± 0.05, p < 0.01, respectively). Other details of the labor course show no differences. Based on these findings, one can confidently state that the problems facing the adolescent gravid are not necessarily related to her age, but instead reflect the pre-existing or concurrent problems she brings to her pregnancy and the complications that arise as her pregnancy advances. Her age, therefore, can be considered to be merely a marker for those problems and complications.

The overall impact of teenage pregnancy, all adverse factors considered collectively, is nonetheless reflected in associated mortality rates. There is a consistently higher frequency of deaths among offspring of teenagers – and, to a lesser extent, among elderly gravidas as well – to yield a U-shaped curve when mortality is plotted against maternal age (Fig. 30.7) [10]. Moreover, the younger the adolescent (and the lower her gynecologic age relative to menarche), the greater the rate of fetal and infant losses. Compared with the neonatal mortality

among those infants born to women aged 20–24 years, for example, significantly more deaths occurred in those aged 14–16 years (19.6 per 1000 vs 14.6 per 1000, p < 0.01), and still more in the 11–13 year group (26.8 per 1000, p < 0.010). High fetal/infant death rates illustrate the serious problem confronting healthcare providers and public health and social workers who are called upon to deal with pregnancies among these very young women.

Obstetric management considerations

While there are many diverse issues we must face collectively as a society and individually as obstetricians and midwives in regard to adolescents who are exposed to pregnancy or become pregnant, we are perforce limited in what we can accomplish. The spectrum of issues has been well outlined by James et al [11]. They divided their list into preconceptional, antepartum, labor and delivery, and postnatal for convenience, recognizing considerable overlap. Preconceptional issues deal with exploring and developing social supports and educating teenagers about lifestyle, sexual behavior, and family planning. Antepartum needs cover encouraging referral for early and regular prenatal care, providing nutritional and social service expertise, stressing proper diet and lifestyle habits, and mobilizing social supports. These patients also need to be watched carefully during their prenatal course for the development of common complicating disorders, such as anemia, intrauterine growth restriction, pregnancy-induced hypertension, gestational diabetes, and preterm labor. Intrapartum considerations include providing them with specialty care in a high-risk tertiary care obstetric unit and observing for (and dealing with) the expected complications of labor and delivery, such as premature birth, fetal macrosomia, and bony dystocia. Postnatal care objectives encompass education about and the provision of supervision for infant feeding and baby care, guidance about social, financial and educational support services, and reinforcement of contraceptive practices.

We may conclude by re-emphasizing that the adolescent pelvis is immature and incompletely developed during the first several years of pubertal development. This is reflected in both its small capacity and anthropoid architecture, which is especially constrictive at the midplane until near full maturity. Pregnancy in adolescents is often complicated by preterm birth and intrauterine growth restriction. The small size of the fetus in most adolescents counterbalances the potentially adverse labor/delivery impact of the underdeveloped maternal bony pelvis. However, there are some teenagers who are at special risk because of excessive weight gain from chronic dietary excesses or because they have gestational diabetes, resulting in a macrosomic fetus. When fetal macrosomia occurs before full pelvic maturation, there is risk of labor progression abnormalities and cephalopelvic disproportion, often necessitating cesarean delivery. Obstetric healthcare providers should be alert to these problems, astutely evaluate for them, and manage the labor and delivery accordingly.

References

1. Sukanich AC, Rogers KD, McDonald HM. Physical immaturity and outcome of pregnancy in primiparas younger than 16 years of age. *Pediatrics* 1986;**78**:31–36.
2. Ott SM, Lipkin EW, Newell-Morris L. Bone physiology during pregnancy and lactation in young macaques. *J Bone Miner Res* 1999;**14**:1779–1788.
3. Sowers MF, Scholl T, Harris L, Jannausch M. Bone loss in adolescent and adult pregnant women. *Obstet Gynecol* 2000;**96**:189–193.
4. Lyritis GP, Schoenau E, Skarantavos G. Osteopenic syndromes in the adolescent female. *Ann NY Acad Sci* 2000;**900**:403–408.
5. Moerman ML. Growth of the birth canal in adolescent girls. *Am J Obstet Gynecol* 1982;**143**:528–532.
6. Aiman J. X-ray pelvimetry of the pregnant adolescent: pelvic size and the frequency of contraction. *Obstet Gynecol* 1976;**48**:281–286.
7. Friedman EA, Neff RK. *Labor and Delivery: Impact on Offspring*. Littleton, MA: PSG Publishing, 1987:57–58.
8. Hediger ML, Scholl TO, Shall JI, Krieger PM. Young maternal age and preterm labor. *Ann Epidemiol* 1997;**7**:400–406.
9. Friedman EA. *Labor: Clinical Evaluation and Management*, 2nd edn. New York: Appleton-Century-Crofts, 1978:146–152.
10. Friedman EA, Neff RK. *Labor and Delivery: Impact on Offspring*. Littleton, MA: PSG Publishing, 1987:216.
11. James DK, Steer PJ, Weiner CP, Gonik B (eds). *High Risk Pregnancy: Management Options*. Philadelphia, PA: WB Saunders, 1994:37.

CHAPTER 31

The Polycystic Ovary Syndrome – Challenges and Opportunities in Adolescent Medicine

Nathan Kase

Mount Sinai School of Medicine, New York, NY, USA

Introduction

The polycystic ovary syndrome (PCOS) is a common endocrine disorder affecting from 5% to 8% of reproductive women [1]. For decades it was best known as a prevalent cause of anovulatory oligoamenorrhea and infertility, complicated by dysfunctional uterine bleeding, acne, and hirsutism [2]. However, PCOS is now understood as a factor in promoting progressive lifetime health burdens for some affected women. These include the consequences of hyperandrogenemia, central visceral fat accumulation, induced insulin resistance (Ins Res), and a cluster of metabolic risk factors collectively known as the metabolic syndrome (MetS) [3]. As a result, PCOS is no longer entirely within the clinical purview of the gynecologist/infertility specialist. It is now a concern for all physicians, particularly those caring for adolescent women.

Challenges and opportunities of the polycystic ovary syndrome

Challenges

PCOS imposes variable risks for progressive disabilities requiring sustained long-term follow-up. In addition, the salient presenting feature, anovulation, can

be a consequence of any one of a broad range of etiologic possibilities, each of which requires identification and specific treatment. The final common pathway for these endocrine disruptors is the conversion of the oscillating peptide/steroid (ovarian) and peptide/glycoprotein (CNS-pituitary) ovulatory interactions into a chronic, endocrinologically dampened normogonadotropic, normoestrogenic but hyperandrogenic anovulatory state. Meticulous initial differential diagnosis must exclude specific disorders and diseases which interrupt cyclic ovarian function. These "rule out" diagnoses include functioning and nonfunctioning pituitary neoplasms (particularly prolactinoma), nonclassic congenital adrenal hyperplasia, Cushing syndrome, thyroid dysfunction, as well as local ovarian disease such as ovarian endometrioma or chronic pelvic inflammatory disease.

Beyond differential diagnosis, PCOS challenges the physician caring for adolescents to identify, evaluate, and treat early. PCOS affects the young, with symptoms emerging at puberty implicating a developmental basis for the syndrome. PCOS runs in families, hence there is a genetic basis. More than 50% of PCOS women are obese, some morbidly so. There is an environmental acquired basis, and with the "epidemic" of obesity amongst adolescents the incidence/prevalence of PCOS is likely to rise accordingly. Finally, there is that particular adolescent pain, not just reproductive impairment or disease risks, but the immediate cosmetic stigma of acne and hirsutism compounding the ungainly dimensions of the obese teenage girl.

Pediatric, Adolescent, & Young Adult Gynecology. Edited by A. Altchek and L. Deligdisch. © 2009 Blackwell Publishing, ISBN: 978-1-4051-5347-8.

Opportunities

There are challenges but real opportunities exist for interception, modification and even the reversal of the burdens of PCOS. Despite the heterogeneity of presentation, a comprehensive definition of the spectrum of the condition is being formulated. Differential diagnostic algorithms are in place to exclude treatable conditions to which PCOS is secondary. Widely available, reliable methods can identify and assess the risk levels of various metabolic and vascular consequences of PCOS. Finally, effective management strategies can be applied to control and reverse the gynecologic, dermatologic and metabolic manifestations of the syndrome.

Clinical definition and diagnosis

Clinical definition

As important issues of differential diagnosis and management confront the physician, no single clinical, biochemical or genetic marker has been identified that unequivocally defines the syndrome. Nor is there agreement on a single "best practice" starting point for analysis. Even in the seminal report of Stein and Leventhal [4], the heterogeneity of the syndrome was evident: of the seven women with PCOS and amenorrhea, three were obese, four hirsute (one obese) and one had acne. Evidence of recent ovulation was also present in some specimens removed at wedge resection. PCOS is a cluster of symptoms, signs and biochemical features resulting from variable degrees of confluence of genetic and acquired (environmental) factors which emerge over time in various combinations.

Two consensus conferences have been convened to formulate a uniform definition of PCOS. The first (NIH, 1990) and a second revised criteria were formulated at a 2003 joint meeting of the European Society for Human Reproduction and Embryology/American Society for Reproductive Medicine (ESHRE/ASRM) – the "Rotterdam Criteria." The NIH group [5] defined PCOS by three criteria: 1) clinical hyperandrogenism and/or hyperandrogenemia; 2) oligo-ovulation, and 3) exclusion of other known disorders. In the Rotterdam proposal [6], PCOS is defined, after exclusion of other conditions that cause irregular menstrual cycles and androgen excess, when at least two of three features are present: 1) oligo-ovulation or anovulation, usually expressed as oligoamenorrhea or amenorrhea; 2) clinical and/or biochemical signs of hyperandrogenism; and 3) polycystic ovaries as defined by strict ultrasonographic parameters. These differ from the more restrictive NIH criteria in two contentious areas: the new criteria define a wider spectrum of a dysfunctional condition, i.e. polycystic ovaries need not be present to make the diagnosis and conversely their presence alone does not establish the diagnosis. As a result, the new criteria add two new categories of women: a) those with hyperandrogenism, PCO morphology but regular cycles (presumably ovulatory), and b) women with anovulatory oligoamenorrhea and polycystic ovaries by ultrasound but who do not display androgen excess.

This expansion of the PCOS phenotype has not received widespread acceptance [7,8]. While all sides in the debate agree that universal adoption of specific subcategories of the PCOS phenotype would benefit ongoing clinical, epidemiologic, therapeutic outcomes research, and finer delineation of genetic and developmental precursors of PCOS, serious concerns over excessive potentially unnecessary healthcare costs derive from inclusion of women with unproven long-term health consequences and realistic prospects for spontaneous reversibility. Furthermore, premature, incorrect categorization of "at-risk" populations imposes unwarranted adverse effects on healthcare insurability.

Whether these definitions are overly narrow or unjustifiably broad, they are not particularly meaningful in the diagnosis of PCOS in the individual adolescent or the approach of her healthcare provider. Most pubertal adolescents have periodic anovulation/amenorrhea and acne (if not frank hirsutism) and, if examined, ultrasound evidence of "multicystic" ovarian morphology. Finally, the inherent physiology of puberty normally involves increased insulin and leptin levels and an increase in caloric reserve in expanded adiposity.

In this author's opinion, the "solution" to defining the at-risk PCOS subpopulation in adolescence rests on the following:
• the emergence and persistence of the classic combination – hyperandrogenism and oligoamenorrhea
• signals of increased risk of insulin resistance and elements of the metabolic syndrome as displayed by family history and developmental history as well as by increased markers of metabolic dysfunction found at initial evaluation or in follow-up assessments.

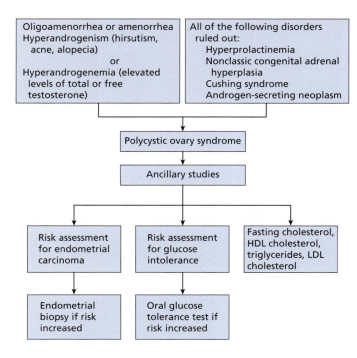

| Oligoamenorrhea or amenorrhea Hyperandrogenism (hirsutism, acne, alopecia) or Hyperandrogenemia (elevated levels of total or free testosterone) | All of the following disorders ruled out: Hyperprolactinemia Nonclassic congenital adrenal hyperplasia Cushing syndrome Androgen-secreting neoplasm |

Figure 31.1 Diagnostic algorithm for the polycystic ovary syndrome. Single measurements of serum prolactin TSH and 17-hydroxyprogesterone are sufficient to rule out hyperprolactinemia, hypothyroidism and nonclassic congenital adrenal hyperplasia due to deficiency of 21-hydroxylase. Measure the 17-hydroxyprogesterone level in an early morning blood sample. Alternatively, 17-hydroxyprogesterone can be measured in response to a single dose of exogenously administered corticotropin. Risks for metabolic syndrome include an elevated BMI, an increased waist circumference, a history of gestational diabetes, a family history of type 2 diabetes. HDL, high-density lipoprotein; LDL, low-density lipoprotein. Reprinted with the permission of *The New England Journal of Medicine* from reference 3.

In summary, to identify the subpopulation of adolescents at risk, not only the presenting symptoms and signs but evidence of the presence of precursors and/or emerging consequences of PCOS is required (Fig. 31.1).

Diagnosis of PCOS in adolescents

Using this adolescent phenotype, the diagnosis of PCOS is achieved through clinical history, physical exam and confirmative laboratory findings. The principal features are: a) persistent anovulation and menstrual dysfunction, and b) clinical features of hyperandrogenism. In addition, adolescent girls with PCOS frequently present with obesity (over 50%). Premature pubarche (even precocious puberty) can herald the onset of the syndrome. Any one of these findings may be the sole presenting feature but usually a variable combination of these elements is present. Diagnostic sensitivity is heightened by the family history of metabolic dysfunction such as insulin resistance and the metabolic syndrome.

Anovulation [9]

Approximately two-thirds of adolescents with PCOS display symptoms of chronic anovulation. These manifestations vary but include:

- amenorrhea, either primary (despite normal growth, pubarche and thelarche) or secondary (lasting > one year)
- oligomenorrhea, which persists beyond two years after menarche often punctuated by episodes of dysfunctional uterine bleeding.

The presence of hyperandrogenemia or hirsutism helps to distinguish PCOS menstrual dysfunction from the physiologic spontaneously reversible anovulatory amenorrhea of early adolescence.

Hyperandrogenism [10]

Clinical hyperandrogenism in PCOS includes facial hirsutism (terminal hair in male distribution), acne and rarely androgenic alopecia. These manifestations are present to varying degrees in approximately two-thirds of hyperandrogenic females. However, although elevated testosterone (T) levels (primarily free T) are identified in similar proportions (60–80%) of PCOS patients, not all hirsute girls show increased T concentrations and not all hyperandrogenemic women demonstrate clinical androgen excess. These disparities reflect the wide excursions of serum T in the adolescent, the difficulties in performing the assays (free T) reproducibly, and variable sensitivity of the pilosebaceous unit among populations. For diagnostic purposes any evidence of androgen excess, whether clinical or biochemical, supports the diagnosis of PCOS providing other criteria are also present.

The presence of polycystic ovary morphology (PCOM) by ultrasound [11]

Although the Rotterdam criteria accept inclusion of PCOM as one of the diagnostic criteria for PCOS, practically speaking this position cannot be applied to the adolescent. It is unlikely that a sophisticated study as required by Rotterdam is uniformly achievable in the community setting. The finding of PCOM in ovulatory, nonandrogenized healthy women (even those on steroid contraception) further limits the authenticity of such a study. In the author's opinion, PCOM can be assumed to be present if both hyperandrogenism and amenorrhea exist. This is good news – the possibility of performing a meticulous transvaginal ultrasound in a pubertal, probably obese virginal young woman is too remote for inclusion in valid diagnosis.

Obesity [12]

While neither set of criteria defining adult PCOS includes obesity, there is little question of the relationship of visceral obesity in the development of PCOS in the adolescent (even as the initiating sign). Obesity is at once a cause as well as a consequence of PCOS. It is typically visceral, indicated by a waist circumference ≥88 cm (about 35"), which is approximately the 85th percentile for American girls age 13 years or older. A crucial point: visceral adiposity may exist in girls with normal body mass index (BMI). A clinical "pearl": normal waist size essentially rules out PCOS as a diagnosis.

There is a difference in sequential appearance of PCOS criteria suggesting at least two categories of provocative dysfunction: a) amenorrheic young women who are normal or moderately overweight who display early and progressive androgenization; b) primarily obese adolescents with amenorrhea but later onset and modest degrees of androgenization.

Premature pubarche and precocious puberty

Premature pubarche, the appearance of sexual hair before eight years of age, seems to be a risk factor for, or predecessor of, PCOS. One subphenotype of PCOS [13]

includes SGA at birth, rapid weight gain and overshoot in infancy, premature pubarche and early appearance of PCOS.

Summary

Neither the NIH nor the Rotterdam criteria fully address the complicated problem of diagnosing PCOS in adolescents. Even in girls without PCOS, anovulation occurs in approximately one-half of menstrual cycles in the first two years after menarche. The multifollicular ovary of the normal adolescent also may be confused with the polycystic ovary of an adult woman with PCOS. In addition, the full spectrum of established PCOS may not emerge for several years after the initial presenting elements. As a result of these considerations, in the adolescent girl the presence of any evidence of hyperandrogenism rises to defining importance.

Differential diagnosis of polycystic ovary syndrome in adolescents [9,14]

PCOS accounts for more than 90% of the syndromes of androgen excess in adolescent females. But as a syndrome, other potential etiologies exist and must be identified. That anovulatory amenorrhea is common in puberty adds to the complexity of differential diagnosis. However, practically speaking, the presence of normal waist circumference, normal androgen levels and the absence of cutaneous hyperandrogenization not only effectively rules out the diagnosis of PCOS in adolescence but also excludes other sources of hyperandrogenism such as Cushing syndrome, nonclassic congenital adrenal hyperplasia or the rare androgen-secreting neoplasms of adrenal or ovary. On the other hand, if androgen excess is evident (biochemically and/or on physical diagnosis) additional clarifying steps must be undertaken. These include evaluation of androgen status by total testosterone (extremely high levels suggest androgen-producing tumors), DHAS (3β-ol-dehydrogenase adrenal defect), a morning 17α-OH progesterone (21α-hydroxylase deficiency) and random serum cortisol levels ($<10\ \mu g/dL$ is evidence against endogenous Cushing disease). Any abnormality in these tests requires clarification by imaging, dexametasone suppression and ACTH testing. With regard to imaging, the limits of transvaginal ultrasound have been mentioned. But the possibility of intrasellar tumors in amenorrheic adolescents requires a prolactin level and, if elevated, imaging of the sella is indicated. TSH levels are useful to rule out primary hypothyroidism.

A word of caution; it is essential to identify the "best practice" laboratory and their normal ranges established for each test in adolescent age groupings.

In summary, the differential diagnosis of PCOS in adolescents proceeds by exclusion of known causes of androgen excess or amenorrhea and is relatively straightforward. More difficult is differentiating PCOS from the variations inherent in physiologic puberty.

Pathophysiology of polycystic ovary syndrome

PCOS, as a syndrome, is not a specific disease but a dysfunctional state, induced by multiple potential etiologies, often interactive and synergistic, with variable clinical presentations and a range of clinical consequences affecting reproductive and nonreproductive systems. Given this complexity, in order to develop informed management strategies to counter the burdens it may impose, a thorough understanding of the pathophysiology of PCOS is necessary.

A comprehensive model of PCOS

Construction of any valid model of PCOS dysfunction, its antecedents and consequences, must integrate the following observations.
• PCOS is a state of normogonadotropic, normoestrogenic, oligoanovulation representing a conversion of oscillating to dampened nonoscillating endocrine interactions linking the ovary and the CNS/anterior pituitary.
• In most instances, PCOS gradually emerges as a distinct clinical entity in pre- and peripubertal and adolescent girls and evolves into its full form in late adolescence or early adulthood.
• There is a genetic basis: the prevalence of PCO morphology and PCOS in first-degree relatives as well as the family history of diabetes, cardiovascular disease and/or elements of the metabolic syndrome suggest a genetic basis for the syndrome.

• A relationship exists among PCOS (anovulatory amenorrhea and hyperandrogenization), visceral fat accumulation and metabolic consequences such as insulin resistance.
• The morphology of the polycystic ovary depicts a variable rate of activation and recruitment but otherwise normal follicle development and progression, which is arrested at the early antral stage. Normal numbers of primordial "reserve" follicles, normal numbers of primary and secondary follicles, and a normal rate of atresia emphasize the inherent "normalcy" of these follicles other than the pace of their development and their failure to proceed to dominant follicle maturation [15].
• Finally, regardless of what therapy is applied – weight loss, exercise, insulin sensitizers, gonadotropin enhancement with human menopausal gonadotrophin (HMG) or recombinant human follicle-stimulating hormone (FSH) or modulation with estrogen agonists/antagonists or aromatase inhibitors – the PCO is capable of surprising resiliency with swift recovery of normal, albeit therapeutically induced cyclic oscillations and ovulation.
In summary, the PCO ovary in most instances is inherently physiologically normal. It is inhibited by imposed intra- and extragonadal factors. When this inhibition is eliminated or reversed, normal function is restored.

Genesis and pathophysiology of anovulation

Abnormal androgen production
As Marshall has noted, "Elevated plasma androgens influence several physiologic systems with generally negative implications for the normal regulation of female reproduction and metabolism" [16] (Fig. 31.2). While under normal circumstances theca cell testosterone is an essential precursor for estrogen synthesis by FSH-induced aromatase in the granulosa, excess androgen limit progression of follicle maturation by inhibition of aromatase activity and the production of nonaromatizable dihydrotestosterone (Fig. 31.3). Furthermore, elevated secretion of ovarian testosterone acts centrally to increase gonadotropin-releasing hormone (GnRH) and luteinizing hormone (LH) pulse frequencies resulting in relative elevation of circulating LH. As LH increases, theca cells are stimulated to even higher testosterone concentrations. As a result, a positive feed-forward interplay between ovary and CNS/pituitary is engaged, yielding

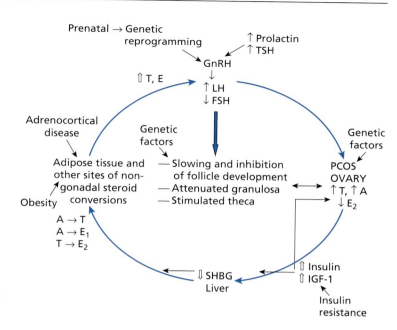

Figure 31.2 Model of the synergistic, self-perpetuating, interactive cycle of anovulatory amenorrhea and hyperandrogenemia in PCOS. Induction and perpetuation of chronic anovulation and hyperandrogenemia by which any one of a variety of initiating factors, e.g. genetic (insulin action, follicle maturation, steroid synthesis and activity) and/or environmental (obesity, insulin resistance, acquired disease), can initiate/accelerate the PCOS. T, testosterone; E, total estrogen; E_2, estradiol; A, androstenedione; SHBG, sex hormone-binding globulin; IGF-1, insulin-like growth factor-1; FSH, follicle-stimulating hormone; LH, luteinizing hormone; GnRH, gonadotropin-releasing hormone; ↑, increase; ↓, decrease.

increased secretion and sustained overall excess production of testosterone. The androgen-induced reduction of sex hormone-binding globulin (SHBG) serves to aggravate this condition further by increasing circulating concentrations of free unbound biologically active testosterone (reviewed in reference 16).

Elevated androgens also modify adipose cell function through androgen receptors primarily expressed on abdominal preadipocytes [17]. Androgen exerts a unique dimorphic effect in women, increasing visceral fat accumulation by this mechanism [18]. In addition, hyperandrogenemia adversely modulates adipocyte production of cytokines such as TNF-α, IL-6 and plasminogen activator inhibitor-1, factors which induce Ins Res and the MetS [17]. In support of this thesis, Coviello et al [19] have provided evidence that adolescents with PCOS suffer a higher incidence of metabolic syndrome and that hyperandrogenemia is an additive risk factor for metabolic syndrome independent of obesity and insulin resistance.

The role of hyperinsulinemia and obesity
(Fig. 31.4)

While some anovulatory women with polycystic ovary syndrome who are not overweight may be insulin resistant, overweight women, especially those with anovula-

tion and polycystic ovaries, generally are insulin resistant [20]. The resulting hyperinsulinemia may initiate or aggravate the anovulatory polycystic syndrome. Speroff [9] has summarized the findings supporting the incremental effect of hyperinsulinemia in PCOS.

1 The administration of insulin to women with polycystic ovaries increases circulating androgen levels.

2 The administration of glucose to hyperandrogenic women increases the circulating levels of both insulin and androgens.

3 Weight loss or insulin-sensitizing therapy decreases the levels of both insulin and androgens and the levels of IGF-binding proteins.

4 Acting as a co-gonadotropin, insulin stimulates theca cell androgen production *in vitro*.

5 After normalization of androgens with GnRH agonist treatment, the insulin response to glucose challenge (OGTT) remains abnormal in obese women with polycystic ovaries.

6 Correction of hyperandrogenism with oral contraceptive treatment, surgical wedge resection or laparoscopic ovarian cautery does not restore insulin sensitivity or abnormal lipoprotein levels to normal in obese PCOS.

7 Insulin levels are higher, while SHBG and IGF-1 are lower in obese women with polycystic ovary syndrome compared with nonobese anovulatory women.

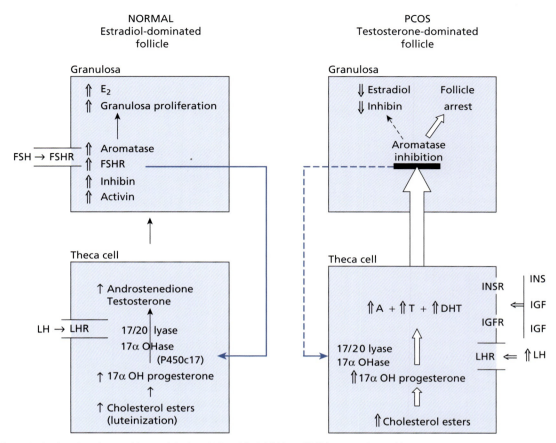

Figure 31.3 Altered ovarian steroidogenesis in the PCOS and the inhibition of follicle maturation and function. Increased testosterone and DHT (nonaromatizable active androgen) theca cell synthesis and delivery to granulosa inhibits granulosa cell proliferation and differentiation by reducing aromatase activity, estrogen synthesis, inhibins and activin synthesis and FSHR number and/or activity. Compounding these changes, hyperinsulinemia, increased IGF-1 and increased LH drive excess androgen availability and effects.

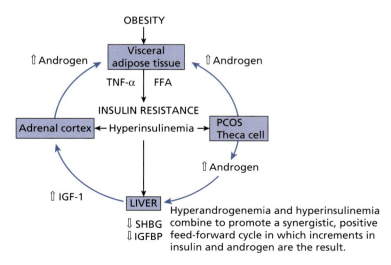

Figure 31.4 Insulin resistance and the pathogenesis of PCOS.

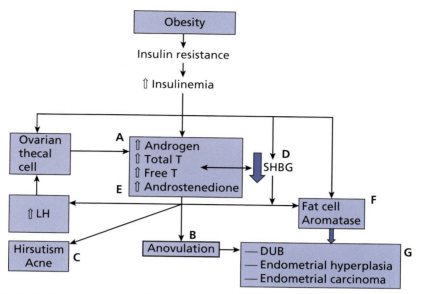

Figure 31.5 How the double stimulus of obesity and increased LH leads to PCOS and its major long-term clinical burdens. The effects of obesity and its attendant insulin resistance combined with the increased LH associated with PCOS induce self-sustaining and accelerating positive feed-forward and feed-back interactions among a variety of systems. The combination of increased LH and IGF leads to increased synthesis of theca cell androgens (**A**). These androgens act locally to inhibit follicle development (anovulation) (**B**), circulating hyperandrogenemia induces cutaneous masculinization (**C**) and, with insulin-induced reduction of SHBG (**D**), higher concentrations of "free" bioavailable steroids (**E**). The increased aromatase capacity of obesity-expanded fat cell resources (**F**) results in increased levels of estrogen which with anovulation results in unrestricted endometrial proliferation (**G**).

Synergism between hyperinsulinemia and hyperandrogenemia (Fig. 31.5)

In normal adult menstruating women, about 50% of plasma testosterone is derived in equal proportions from ovarian and adrenal cortical secretions. The remaining 50% is produced from conversion of androstenedione to testosterone in "nonendocrine" peripheral tissues, notably fat cells. Because the ovary remains sensitive to the actions of insulin, in obese individuals with insulin resistance, the associated hyperinsulinemia acts as a "cogonadotropin" with LH to increase androgen production by ovarian theca cells. Insulin significantly adds to the already suppressed hepatic synthesis of SHBG and hepatic production of IGF-1. As a result, free testosterone levels increase still further. Given the androgen effect on the GnRH generator and LH secretion, a double stimulus of elevated LH and hyperinsulinemia results in increased velocity and intensity of the self-sustaining cycle of hyperandrogenicity and anovulation (reviewed in reference 16).

In summary, adolescent PCOS may be divided into two groups: 1) those with primary hyperandrogenemia and secondary insulin resistance, and 2) those with primary insulin resistance and secondary hyperandrogenicity. In clinical practice, regardless of the degree to which adolescents with polycystic ovary syndrome share these elements, unfortunately all are at potential risk for major disease later in life.

Genetic basis of PCOS [20]

This section addresses two questions. Not all adolescents with hyperinsulinemia are hyperandrogenic. Why? Not all obese diabetics are anovulatory and infertile. Why? Although the answers remain elusive, interest has turned to examination of genetic susceptibilities leading to a) altered folliculogenesis, b) genetic variation of androgen availability and/or activity, or c) genetic alteration of insulin dynamics (insulin secretion or insulin action). A description of possible genetic bases for these proclivities is warranted.

Genes regulating androgen synthesis and function [21,22]

The key initial observation that women with a history of 2lα-hydroxylase deficiency demonstrate hypersecretion of LH and polycystic ovaries lent support to the hypothesis that exposure to androgen excess (in this instance not ovarian) pre- and/or postnatally could "program" the system to develop PCO morphology. Intriguingly, a genetic association with PCOS has also been found in altered androgen availability involving neither the adrenal cortex nor ovarian theca cells. Mutations in the 11β-hydroxysteroid dehydrogenase (11β-HSD) gene results in low 11β-HSD expression and nicotinamide adenine dinucleotide phosphate (NADPH) generation. The resulting loss of 11β-HSD activity results in accelerated metabolic clearance of cortisol and feedback "demand" for adrenocorticotropic hormone (ACTH)-stimulated additional cortisol secretion. As a result excess androgen (similar to compensated 21-OH deficiency) is secreted and PCO morphology is induced [23].

These observations also prompted consideration of candidate genes encoding steroid synthesis enzymes in the etiology of ovarian hyperandrogenism in PCOS (reviewed in references 3, 22). Almost all initial candidates encoding 17α-OHase, 17/20 lyase (P450c 17) and cholesterol side chain cleavage (P450 scc) enzymes have failed to show association or linkage to the PCOS phenotype. One exception is deficiency in the aromatase enzyme system by which a genetic variation in CYP19 may contribute to prenatal androgenization. A common genomic variant (an intronic single nucleotide polymorphism (SNP50)) of the CYP19 produces a hyperandrogenic state by both increased secretion of unutilized substrate and reduced metabolic clearance of testosterone. It is associated with early adrenarche, pubertal hyperandrogenism and PCOS [24].

In addition, hyperandrogenism may reflect genetic variation in androgenic receptor (AR) sensitivity. Clinical hyperandrogenism and androgen levels were increased in girls with shorter AR (CAG)n repeat alleles. Thus high AR sensitivity is associated not only with greater target tissue (including visceral adipocytes) impact but through a series of positive feed-forward mechanisms with increased overall androgen production.

Evidence exists that reduction in SHBG in PCOS, independent of hyperinsulinism or hyperandrogenism, may also be genetically determined. Women with PCOS were more frequently carriers of longer allele genotypes (TAAAA)n in the promoter of the SHBG gene, leading to lower SHBG levels, than controls.

In summary, genetic variation in androgen availability and activity at target tissues (shorter AR (CAG)n repeat alleles, longer SHBG (TAAAA)n repeats and polymorphic variants of the aromatase gene) may contribute to the prenatal "androgenization" of the hypothalamus (programming the GnRH generator), and visceral adipocytes.

Genes regulating folliculogenesis

The activin/inhibin system plays an important role in normal follicle development. Disregulation of this system has been implicated in PCOS [25]. Activin promotes granulosa cell proliferation, enhances FSH receptor expression, decreases LH-induced androgen production, and increases pituitary FSH secretion – all factors that promote follicular growth. Inhibin antagonizes these actions. Decreased activin has been reported in women with PCOS but depiction of either overexpression of the inhibin gene or defective expression of activin has not been established.

Genes regulating insulin actions (reviewed in references 3, 26)

The association of PCOS with insulin resistance and resulting hyperinsulinemia is well documented. The mechanism by which hyperinsulinemia induces androgen excess proceeds by insulin (and IGF) enhancement of LH stimulation of ovarian testosterone synthesis. Accordingly, the search to identify abnormalities of genes regulating insulin action in the pathogenesis of PCOS has been undertaken.

Although environmental factors including physical inactivity and excess caloric intake play important roles in the development of obesity and insulin resistance, epidemiologic and family studies show that there are genetic influences in the development of insulin resistance. Using a variety of tests for insulin resistance, the heritability of insulin resistance is estimated at 30–40%.

Ins Res is thought to be due to the inheritance of a number of mutations in a variety of genes [27,28]. These mutations have been categorized (Class 2 to 5) in which missense mutations lead to reduced amounts of receptor

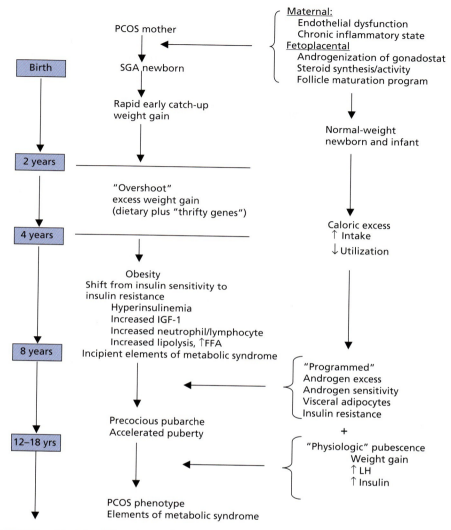

Figure 31.6 Hypothetic model relating SGA newborn and emergence of PCOS phenotype at puberty. Whether by genetics, intrauterine environment, catch-up weight gain and overshoot (SGA) or excess weight gain in AGA throughout infancy and childhood, obesity (BMI >30) leads to early and accelerated pubescence and the PCOS phenotype. The normal physiologic rise in LH and insulin at puberty compounds the vulnerabilities of obesity and pre-programming.

on the cell surface, impaired insulin binding to the receptor, impaired tyrosine kinase activity of the insulin receptor or accelerated degradation of IR protein. Whole-genome scans have identified both the calpain 10 SNP-43 variant and membrane glycoprotein PC-1 overexpression (with decreased tyrosine kinase activity in the insulin receptor/IRS complex) as possibilities (see also references 71, 72, 73, 74).

PCOS: a syndrome of developmental origin with peripubertal adolescent expression [22,29,30] (Fig. 31.6)

The "thrifty" phenotype thesis posits that a fetal protective metabolic adaptation to an unfavorable intrauterine milieu leads to reprogramming that has lifelong adverse effects in adult life (e.g. insulin resistance).

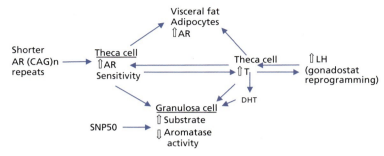

Figure 31.7 Androgen receptor "hypersensitivity" as a factor in fetal programming of PCOS by androgen excess. As a result of increased AR sensitivity, a positive feed-forward cycle is entrained in which enhanced intrauterine androgen leads to visceral fat sensitization, theca cell androgen dominance, aromatase inhibition, and "androgenization" of GnRH control of LH secretion at puberty. Each element is activated and the entire cycle synergistically accelerated by increments in LH, insulin, IGF-1 and weight gain with establishment of PCOS. AR, androgen receptor; T, testosterone; LH, luteinizing hormone; DHT, dihydrotestosterone; ↑, increase; ↓, decrease).

In the case of PCOS, untimely and/or excess androgen exposure of the female fetus and/or deficient intrauterine nutritional state (small for gestational age – SGA) may separately or together lead to expression of such permanent maladaptive "rewiring." In some children low birth weight is linked to the development of premature pubarche followed by hyperandrogenism, insulin resistance and PCOS during adolescence. SGA girls show an increased risk of developing central obesity, insulin resistance, type II diabetes and hypertension, all elements of the MetS. Two potential mechanisms for this fetal reprogramming are considered.

Prenatal androgenization (Fig. 31.7)

As has been discussed, genetic variation in intrauterine androgen activity and availability to target tissues contributes to prenatal androgenization – one feature underlying the "fetal origin" of PCOS. In this thesis androgens program the hypothalamic gonadostat generator along male lines at a critical time in fetal development. Because body fat distribution is sexually dimorphic, the visceral fat accumulation in PCOS may reflect a fetal programming of central preadipocytes along male lines. The extent to which pregnancy levels of HCG affect these early programming vulnerabilities is a plausible but unproven factor.

However, with this pre-program in place, the normal developmental changes in puberty "unmask" their adverse reproductive and metabolic potential. Accordingly, the pubertal rise in LH induces hypersecretion of androgen. Similarly, the physiologic increase in serum concentrations of insulin throughout puberty and adolescence, necessary for energy availability and growth, may promote androgenization and anovulation and induce the metabolic consequences of insulin resistance. Obese adolescent PCOS girls demonstrate increased insulin concentrations and reduced insulin sensitivity compared to weight-matched (equally obese) control subjects [31–33].

Fetal "undernutrition"

The frequency of SGA infants born to PCOS mothers is higher than non-PCOS mothers matched by age and weight [34]. Whether this outcome reflects maternal vascular dysfunction or epigenetic effects on androgen receptor sensitivity imposed by maternal overnutrition is unclear. On the other hand, the various elements leading to androgenic hyperactivity and central fat accumulation and the later association of PCOS with the metabolic syndrome could have been conferred by a metabolic genotype or phenotype which favors the economic use and storage of energy, conferring a survival advantage for the newborn. While such an advantage might apply to periods of undernutrition, in developed societies where food is plentiful and exercise limited, this intrauterine protection is maladaptive in the pubertal adolescent.

In this respect, while most SGA newborns have achieved equal weight to appropriate for gestational age (AGA) infants by puberty, some SGA fetuses face a less positive outlook [35]. Following catch-up weight gain between birth and two years, at which time SGA children have similar body composition to AGA, between two and four years SGA children begin to accumulate more abdominal adiposity and less lean mass than AGA children. Thereafter an inflammatory state (increased neutrophil counts) emerges. Later these SGA girls, after weight acceleration, begin to show a cluster of metabolic risk factors by age eight, including dyslipidemia and impaired glucose tolerance. This dramatic transition from central adiposity to insulin resistance and later precocious pubarche (androgenization) demonstrates the maladaptive consequences of fetal programming in PCOS. However, as we will see, it also presents a window of opportunity for prevention and correction.

How PCOS induces insulin resistance

Insulin "resistance" is a transient and appropriate physiologic reaction, which preserves glucose in support of brain function in threatening circumstances such as starvation, environmental stress and acute infection. In pregnancy, it preserves a positive glucose transfer gradient to the fetus regardless of variation in maternal feeding practice and nutrition. What converts this benefit (usually in the context of obesity) into the driving force for the metabolic syndrome and conditions that threaten the quality and duration of human life such as type 2 diabetes mellitus and atherosclerotic cardiovascular disease? In short, what factors convert an acute benefit into a chronic burden (reviewed in references 36–38).

Adipose tissue is an endocrine organ that communicates with all body tissues by secretion of various proteins which regulate metabolism (Table 31.1) [36]. These functions are modulated by the location of the adipose tissue (visceral), by the size of the average adipocyte (obesity), by adipocyte receipt and metabolism of glucose, lipids, corticosteroids and gonadal steroids and the amount and type of secreted proteins these factors provoke. Insulin resistance arises when pathologic levels of adipose-derived proinflammatory factors disrupt insulin signaling locally by autocrine and paracrine mechanisms and later, in distant tissues by circulating humoral mechanisms. One exception is fat-derived adiponectin which at normal concentrations enhances insulin action locally and peripherally but circulates at reduced levels in obesity, compounding insulin resistance. In overnutrition and visceral obesity, adipose tissue is in a chronic state of metabolic stress resulting in activation of the inflammatory response and accumulation of macrophages. In this state adipocytes release cytokines, adipokines and nonesterified fatty acids

Table 31.1 Proteins secreted by adipose tissue that play a role in obesity-associated insulin resistance and diabetes

Adipose-derived protein	Effect on insulin sensitivity	Other tissue sources
Leptin	Improvement	None
Adiponectin	Improvement	None
Adipsin/ASP	Decline	None
Resistin	Decline	None (rodent) Macrophage (human)
TNF-α	Decline	Macrophage
IL-6	Decline	Macrophage
MCP-1	Decline	Macrophage
Visfatin (PBEF)	Improvement	Liver, lymphocytes
PAI-1	Decline	Liver
Angiotensinogen	Decline	Liver
Serum amyloid A	Not known	Liver
α1-acid glycoprotein	Not known	Liver

From reference 36. Reprinted with permission from *Science*.

which amplify the proinflammatory state within adipose tissue, inducing localized insulin resistance. In time these proinflammatory factors travel to the liver and muscle and produce systemic insulin resistance [39,40] (Fig. 31.8).

Independent of adipose tissue-derived factors, inflammatory signals can arise in circulating macrophages. As can be seen in Table 31.1, many proteins that may be adipose derived but are not adipose specific play a role in innate immunity, and in the chronic activated state convert a primitive defense mechanism, usually aligned against both infection and starvation, into sustained deleterious insulin resistance. How?

The molecular mechanism by which proinflammatory pathways lead to insulin resistance (reviewed in references 41, 42) (Fig. 31.9)

Proinflammatory proteins, from circulating activated macrophages and in stressed adipocytes
• induce TNF-α serine phosphorylation of IRS-1 which prevents normal tyrosine phosphorylation of the insulin receptor with interference in insulin signal transduction
• IL-6 and TNF-α induce suppressor of cytokine signaling-3 (SOC-3), an intracellular signaling molecule that interferes with tyrosine phosphorylation of insulin

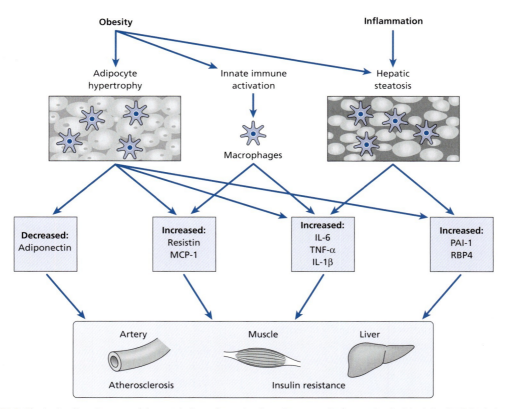

Figure 31.8 Obesity, insulin resistance and the metabolic syndrome. Insulin resistance results from pathophysiologic levels of circulating factors derived from several different cell types. The potential roles of adipocytes, macrophages (in adipose tissue, liver and elsewhere), hepatocytes and the secreted factors which modulate insulin action at the cellular level are shown. Reprinted with the permission of Macmillan Publishing from reference 37.

Figure 31.9 Model of the pathogenesis of the metabolic syndrome. The combination of excess food intake, established obesity (visceral) and genetic factors induces a localized and general state of oxidative stress and inflammation which leads to insulin resistance. The resulting release of circulating free fatty acids (FFA) intensifies the insulin resistance and both combine to promote further oxidative stress and inflammation. Reprinted with the permission of Lippincott, Williams and Wilkins from reference 41.

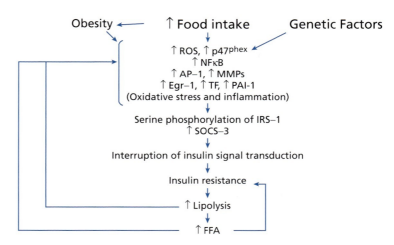

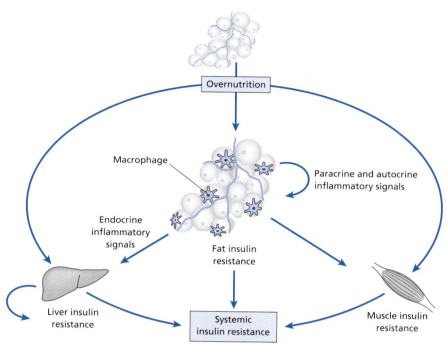

Figure 31.10 The development of systemic insulin resistance in overnutrition-induced inflammation and stress. In obesity, adipose tissue, particularly visceral fat, is under constant metabolic stress resulting in the activation of stress and inflammatory responses leading to the accumulation of macrophages. Adipocytes release cytokines, adipokines and free fatty acids, which act in a paracrine or autocrine fashion to amplify the proinflammatory state within adipose tissue and cause localized insulin resistance. Adipose tissue also serves as an endocrine organ whereby these cytokines, adipokines and free fatty acids travel to liver and muscle, further decreasing insulin sensitivity. In addition to the adipose tissue-derived factors, stress and inflammatory signals can arise independently within liver and muscle, and result in local insulin resistance within these organs. Reprinted with the permission of Lippincott, Williams and Wilkins from reference 39.

receptor and IRS-1 as well as promoting proteosomal degradation of IRS-1

• with diminished insulin transduction, activation of Akt (protein kinase B) is reduced, thereby attenuating translocation of the insulin-responsive glucose transporter Glut-4 to the plasma membrane

• reduced Akt is also responsible, in part, for reduced nitric oxide synthase (NOS) activity and diminished generation of nitric oxide (NO)

• in the absence of Akt there is greater formation of NADPH oxidase complex with increased superoxide generation. Reactive oxygen species (O_2-) and their companion peroxynitrites (reactive ONOO- species) scavenge and entrap nitric oxide, thereby limiting vasodilation but also decreasing prostacyclin and increasing the vasoconstrictor endothelin-1.

Proinflammatory mediators produced in adipose cells (primarily visceral and, as will be seen, hepatic fat) and associated immune cells lead to a systemic inflammatory process, resulting in glucose intolerance and atherogenesis [41] (Fig. 31.10). Entrainment of this entire process is exemplified in the reaction of a single organ, the liver [38,43,44].

Portal delivery of visceral fat-derived proinflammatory cytokines and free fatty acids, and absorption of the tide of dietary lipids and carbohydrates accompanying chronic macronutrient overnutrition ("fast food") places the liver as the first target organ prior to systemic distribution. In the liver hepatocytes and Kupfer cells (liver macrophages) are activated and cell adhesion molecules are induced on hepatic endothelial cells, compounding macrophage entry. As nutrient stores increase, nonalcoholic fatty

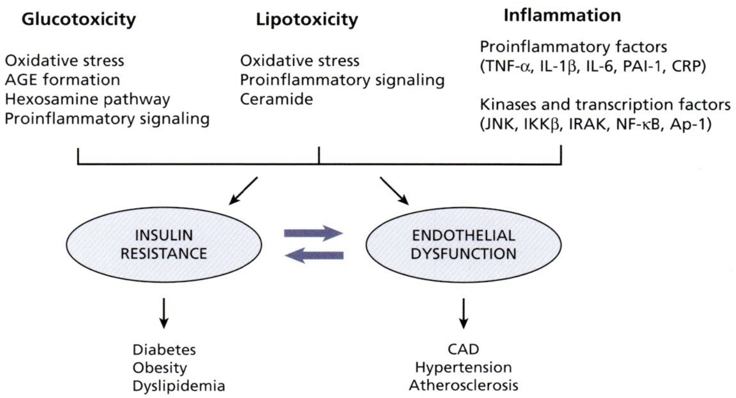

Figure 31.11 Combined "toxic" effects on general cell function. Shared and interacting mechanisms of glucotoxicity, lipotoxicity, and inflammation underlie reciprocal relationships between insulin resistance and endothelial dysfunction that contribute to the linkage between metabolic and cardiovascular diseases. CAD, coronary artery disease. Reprinted with the permission of Lippincott, Williams and Wilkins from reference 45.

liver steatosis develops, adding to the local and eventually to the circulating proinflammatory feed-forward process.

Excess visceral adiposity compounded by macronutrient overnutrition is the primary link between the polycystic ovary syndrome and the induction of systemic insulin resistance.

But not all metabolic effects of insulin resistance are due to activation of the inflammatory pathway [45]. The systemic excess delivery of glucose and lipids at the intracellular level disrupts homeostasis at key organelles, leading to mitochondrial, genomic and endoplasmic reticulum (ER) stress dysfunction [46]. Increased, saturating fuel flow leads to excessive generation of reactive oxygen species and mitochondrial dysfunction [47,48]. Similarly, the nuclear genome may be adversely affected by the accumulation of intracellular lipids as well as oxidative modifications to transcriptional damage–repair mechanisms. Finally, excessive demand on the ER induces intracellular stress responses and local inflammation in all cells. As Quon has pointed out [45], these maladaptive reactions ultimately lead to cellular dysfunction and genomic instability. With continued nutrient saturation at the cellular level, inflammatory stress but also glucotoxicity and lipotoxicity are the result (Fig. 31.11).

Box 31.1 Clinical consequences and burdens of polycystic ovary syndrome

Anovulation
- Oligoamenorrhea
- Dysfunctional bleeding
- Endometrial hyperplasia and cancer

Hyperandrogenemia
- Hirsutism
- Acne
- Alopecia

Metabolic derangements
- Visceral adipocyte hypertrophy *plus*
- Endothelial dysfunction *plus*
- Chronic inflammatory state *leading to*:
  - insulin resistance
  - hepatic steatosis
  - β-cell dysfunction
  - impaired fasting, 2-h glucose tolerance
  - gestational diabetes
  - type 2 diabetes mellitus
  - dyslipidemia
  - procoagulant state
  - hypertension
  - pre-eclampsia
  - cardiopulmonary dysfunction
  - obstructive sleep apnea
  - SGA fetus

Management of adolescents with polycystic ovary syndrome

The goals of management and therapy of adolescents with PCOS can be categorized in three groupings (Box 31.1).

Hyperandrogenemia

Goal: reduce the secretion, production, bioavailability and activity of androgens whether there is clinical evidence (biologic expression) or biochemical evidence (testosterone concentration elevations).

Anovulation

Goal: avoid the progressive proliferation of endometrial tissue (hyperplasia, adenomatous hyperplasia) which underlies dysfunctional uterine bleeding and polymenorrhea. In addition, protect the endometrium from further progression to atypical adenomatous hyperplasia and possible endometrial carcinoma.

Metabolic derangements

Goal: recognize, control, and reverse the existing or emerging markers of insulin resistance and the metabolic syndrome, thereby preventing progressive glucose intolerance and retarding atherogenesis.

Several important principles must be emphasized in any management scheme:
• the approach must be comprehensive and multifaceted, not limited to one identified pathophysiologic feature
• as a clinical syndrome, PCOS may present with one dominant element such as amenorrhea, but over time will progress to androgenization or insulin resistance
• sustained effective lifestyle initiatives such as increased exercise and caloric restriction will modify all aspects of the syndrome even in those without elevated BMI.

Therefore, the overall goals of treatment are as follows.

Control of androgenization (reviewed in reference 17)

Low-dose combined steroid oral contraceptives will modify the excess androgen stimulation of the pilosebaceous unit associated with hirsutism and acne or alopecia [49].
• Reduction of secretion and production of androgens: combined OCs induce negative feedback and suppress circulating LH levels. As a result, theca cell synthesis of testosterone is reduced and ovarian secretion of testosterone diminished. OCs also affect production (extragonadal) of testosterone. Since androstenedione, secreted by both adrenal cortex and the activated theca of polycystic ovaries, is converted to testosterone in adipose tissue and returned to circulation as T, the parallel reduction of ovarian androstenedione secretion via OCs also diminishes overall production of testosterone.
• Reduction of biologic availability and target tissue activity of testosterone: the combination of elevated testosterone and insulin decreases SHBG production by 50%.

The pharmacologic levels of estrogen in OCs reverse that deficiency. Decreasing the free testosterone reduces stimulation of androgen receptors directly and limits the available substrate for 5α-reductase conversion to the more locally active dihydrotestosterone. The progestin content of the OC may also provide beneficial target organ effects. Depending on the progestin involved, it may competitively reduce substrate availability for AR and/or diminish activity of the 5α-reductase system. In addition, when added to OCs, spironolactone provides incremental effects if required [50]. Spironolactone exerts multiple actions in the treatment of hirsutism: reduction of androgen synthesis in both the adrenal and the ovary, competitive inhibition at the AR and inhibition of 5α-reductase activity. Like OCs, its effect is slow, often requiring several months for any observed clinical results.

Insulin and IGF (as co-gonadotropins) increase synthesis of androgen and reduce SHBG concentrations. Reducing hyperinsulinemia with an insulin sensitizer such as metformin decreases androgen concentrations and increases SHBG. However, the effect of metformin on established hirsutism is limited [51]. Ablative procedures may be necessary for cosmetic effect in established hirsutism.

Combinations of OCs containing drosperinone, metformin and/or an antiandrogen such as flutamide control androgenization in young PCOS girls [52]. Flutamide is a nonsteroidal compound with antagonistic effects on androgen receptors and inhibition of androgen synthesis. Added to metformin, the combination results in reduced insulin resistance and reduced body fat, particularly visceral fat. OCs with drosperinone do not counter these benefits and add, as a relatively "pure" progestin, antimineralocorticoid and antiandrogenic properties [53]. These tactics may have important applications in the "normal weight, metabolically obese" subphenotype cohort of PCOS patients.

One important caveat: any suspicion of nonalcoholic fatty liver such as elevated ALT levels should contraindicate the use of flutamide.

For adolescents in whom administration of pharmacologic estrogen at any level is considered risky, Depo-Provera may be employed. The progestin impact is twofold: reduction of LH-driven androgen synthesis and competitive inhibition at the AR. Contraceptive efficacy and compliance are additional advantages of this therapeutic tactic.

Recommendations

In nonsmoking, nonhypertensive adolescents the recently introduced low dose (20–30 μg ethinyl estradiol) preparations which reduce or eliminate the hormone-free interval or reduce cycle frequency are recommended for stabilization and modification of hirsutism and control of acne (as well as providing the added benefit of contraception). The addition of spironolactone at 100–200 μg daily is useful in severe accelerating cases of cutaneous androgenization. In this regard rapidly progressive virilization or failure to control testosterone levels with standard therapy demands evaluation for an androgen-secreting tumor.

Control of endometrial dysfunction and disease [3,9]

Chronic anovulation/amenorrhea

The prolonged amenorrhea typical of PCOS does not reflect inactivity or atrophy of the endometrium. Rather, in contrast to the organized predictable pattern of sequential estrogen-progesterone stimulation and withdrawal menses characteristic of the ovulatory menstrual cycle, the anovulatory PCOS woman is always in the proliferative estrogen phase without the modulating structural and growth-restraining influences of corpus luteum progesterone. Furthermore, in the absence of the programmed duration of a corpus luteum, there is no regularity of tissue shedding. Over a period of time (and by definition, in adolescents with PCOS this may be in excess of one year), unrestrained estrogen-stimulated growth yields a thickened, glandular, highly vascularized unstable tissue which is prone to intermittent, sometimes heavy and prolonged recurrent vaginal bleeding (dysfunctional uterine bleeding). As can be predicted from this mitogenic stimulus, there is an increased prevalence of adenomatous endometrial hyperplasia and even carcinoma in adult women with PCOS. The additional growth stimulation associated with obesity and hyperinsulinemia at the endometrium accelerates the progression to neoplasia [54].

The therapeutic imperative is to reinstitute the benefits of progesterone before dysfunctional uterine breakthrough bleeding occurs, let alone prior to the emergence of cancer precursors. Progestins at adequate doses and duration are antimitotic and antiestrogenic at the endometrium. They stimulate conversion of estradiol to the weaker rapidly cleared estrone sulfate. Progestin also antagonizes estrogen action by inhibiting estrogen in-

duction of its own receptor and estrogen-abetted transcription of oncogenes. In addition, the progestin effect on the endometrial stroma – the pseudodecidual reaction – converts an unstable, easily fragmented tissue to a mechanically rigid endometrium which resists the asynchronous random breakdown underlying dysfunctional uterine bleeding. Furthermore, prolonged progestin use virtually eliminates development of endometrial cancer not only during use but for a prolonged period after discontinuation. These goals can be achieved by administering either cyclic progestins or combined monophasic OC.

Recommendations

Two considerations direct therapeutic decisions in this area: 1) the patient's desire for contraception, and 2) the willingness of the adolescent to adhere to efficacious therapy. As the method of choice, any monophasic combined oral contraceptive provides contraception, reduces androgenization, and protects and heals the endometrium. Less patient-dependent methodologies such as the combined steroid vaginal contraceptive ring or patch are useful alternatives. When contraception is not required, oral medroxyprogesterone acetate, 5–10 mg daily for two weeks of every month, is effective in achieving endometrial control. Whatever method the adolescent will reliably use is the determining issue, because all progestin-containing strategies are effective.

One note of caution: the longer the duration of anovulatory amenorrhea, the greater the possibility of occult endometrial malignancy. This can occur early in the third decade. When and how should that assessment be made? In the face of prolonged amenorrhea, prior to starting any therapy, either a transvaginal ultrasound assessment of endometrial thickness or an endometrial biopsy by an experienced gynecologist should be undertaken. Furthermore, if there is any question of delinquent utilization or recurrent bleeding despite standard therapy, then biopsy is in order.

Control of metabolic derangements (Box 31.2)

While the adolescent's (and her parents') motivation to seek medical evaluation is oligoamenorrhea or hirsutism and acne, the associated complications of PCOS (obesity, dyslipidemia, insulin resistance and hypertension) are the

---

Box 31.2 Core metabolic risk factors and the expression of their underlying components comprising the metabolic syndrome

Central obesity (↑ waist circumference, ↑ waist:hip ratio)
↑ circulating FFA
↓ adiponectin
↑ proinflammatory cytokines
↑ TNF-α
↑ IL-1, IL-6, IL-8, IL-10, IL-18
↑ acute phase reactants: ↑ CRP, sialic acid
↑ plasminogen activator inhibitor 1 (PAI-1)

Atherogenic dyslipidemia
↑ triglycerides (TGs)
↑ apolipoprotein B (apoB)
↑ small low-density lipoprotein particles (LDL)
↓ high-density lipoproteins (HDL)

Insulin resistance and hyperglycemia
↑ fasting insulin
↑ fasting glucose
impaired glucose tolerance
type 2 diabetes mellitus

Vascular dysfunction and inflammation
hypertension
endothelial dysfunction – atherogenesis
↑ carotid intima – media thickness (IMT)
↑ coronary artery calcium (CAC)
↑ left ventricular hypertrophy

---

more important indices of the child's long-term health prospects. The metabolic derangements associated with PCOS cluster about lipid and nonlipid factors associated with increased risk of cardiovascular disease and diabetes mellitus. In the former are included dyslipidemia, a procoagulant state, hypertension and endothelial dysfunction. Insulin resistance, β-cell dysfunction, and progressive impairment of glucose tolerance are hallmarks of the latter. The core "metabolic risk factors" are atherogenic dyslipidemia, elevated blood pressure, elevated plasma glucose, a prothrombotic state and a proinflammatory state. Each of these risk factors has several components (see Box 31.2).

The presence of the metabolic syndrome in a particular individual can be reliably identified by a set of simple, widely available easily applied criteria. For adolescents, these include hypertension (greater than 95th percentile) which is roughly equal to or greater than blood pressure 130/85 for most height, weight and age groups be-

tween 12 and 18, triglyceride levels equal to or greater than 110 μg /L, HDL-cholesterol less than 40 μg/dL, abdominal obesity greater than 35 inches waist circumference, and fasting glucose equal to or greater than 100 μg/dL or IGT (2-h plasma glucose of 140–199 mg/dL) or type 2 diabetes (2-h glucose of at least 200 μg/dL) [16]. Three of these five criteria are sufficient to capture the clustering risk phenomenon. This aggregation is also associated with nonalcoholic fatty liver disease and sleep apnea, the "uncommon manifestations of a common disease, i.e. obesity." As noted, there are two major acquired causes of metabolic syndrome (MetS): obesity (especially abdominal obesity) and insulin resistance. These are closely interrelated through the common linkage of a chronic systemic and cellular inflammatory state expressed in generalized endothelial microvascular (diabetes) and macrovascular (atherosclerosis) dysfunction. Physical inactivity and/or accelerating obesity aggravates the syndrome.

With regard to recognition and management of MetS, four critical clinical issues inform responsive strategies.

Time

MetS may begin insidiously with minimal increase of abdominal girth or impaired glucose tolerance and progresses over time. On the other hand, risk factor clustering may appear at first diagnosis of PCOS in early adolescence and unless intercepted will accelerate rapidly. For example, in one study the prevalence of MetS in an adolescent cohort was three times higher than a local reference population [55]. In another study as many as one-third of nondiabetic women with PCOS had MetS, usually before the end of their third decade of life [56]. This prevalence exceeds by several multiples those reported in NHANES III for similar age groups. Indeed, the prevalence reported "approached that seen in women who are usually between the ages of 50 and 60 years" [56].

Obesity

Data from the National Health and Nutritional Examination Survey (NHANES III 1999–2002) provide evidence of the marked increase in obesity over the past 30 years [57]. The prevalence of being overweight (>95th percentile BMI for age) has increased 4–5-fold in children and adolescents between the ages of six and 19 years so that 16% of both 6–11 year olds and 12–19 year olds met these BMI obesity criteria in 2002. Coincident with this increase in obesity has been a marked increase in the finding of elements of the metabolic syndrome and type 2 diabetes mellitus in this age group. Extrapolating from the NHANES sample, a total of 39,000 US adolescents have type 2 diabetes mellitus and close to 2.8 million have impaired fasting glucose levels. In obese (by BMI) children, the prevalence of specific components of the metabolic syndrome compared with US children in general is striking: hypertension doubles and dyslipidemia (by triglycerides and HDL-C) doubles. Relatively uncommon findings in adolescents such as obstructive sleep apnea and evidence of fatty liver disease (inflammation by ALT or steatosis by ultrasound) reach prevalences ten times higher in clinically obese children than the overall age comparable findings (reviewed in reference 59). PCOS as a disorder of pre- and peripubertal onset and commonly associated with obesity and complicated by early markers of the MetS demands early recognition and vigorous efforts to reduce body weight and increase exercise.

Androgens

Hyperandrogenemia, predominantly of ovarian origin, is a common consequence of obesity and, although the associated emergence of MetS in PCOS was thought to be entirely a reflection of visceral obesity, evidence is now in hand that demonstrates the independent additive as well as synergistic impact of excess testosterone on the prevalence of MetS in PCOS [19]. Adolescent girls with PCOS show double the prevalence of MetS (63%) compared to that seen in obese girls in the overall NHANES data (32%). Importantly, even after adjusting for BMI, girls with PCOS were four times more likely to show MetS and the odds for finding MetS features were higher for each quartile increment in elevated unbound free testosterone. Adolescents with PCOS have a higher prevalence of MetS and hyperandrogenemia independent of obesity and insulin resistance. It is a risk factor for MetS which requires correction.

Metabolic syndrome risk subphenotypes [60]

Elevated BMI has consistently been associated with adverse health outcomes. However, subphenotypes have been recognized that deviate from the apparent dose–response relationship between BMI and its consequences. Metabolically obese but normal weight by BMI (MONW) individuals have been identified who demonstrate the metabolic syndrome characteristics typical of BMI-defined obese individuals. In addition, metabolically healthy but obese (MHO) by BMI (>30 kg/m^2) individuals have also been described who are insulin sensitive and lack the other elements of the MetS. These subphenotypes, MONW and MHO, dissect obesity from its usual metabolic consequences and enable identification of the core risk factor(s) for MetS that are independent of overall BMI-defined obesity. In one large community-based study with follow-up for up to 11 years [60], 7% of the entire cohort were MONW, displaying insulin resistance or metabolic syndrome, and with a relative risk rate of diabetes at 3.97 (1.35–11.6) and cardiovascular disease (CVD) of 3.01 (1.68–5.41). Among obese individuals, 37% were MHO and did not have metabolic syndrome or increased risk of events. As expected, obese subjects with MetS have higher relative risk for diabetes and for CVD than MONW individuals. These subphenotypes are not uncommon in adult populations; whether a similar distribution exists in adolescents is not known. However, ascertainment of insulin resistance and/or MetS in all PCOS adolescents independent of obesity-defined BMI is essential.

Recommendations (Box 31.3)

The metabolic syndrome is evident at an early age in PCOS and appears irrespective of race and ethnicity. Hyperinsulinemia is both a central factor in the "vicious cycle" pathogenesis of PCOS and the critical link between PCOS-associated MetS and the long-term risks of diabetes mellitus and cardiovascular disease. Strategies that attenuate insulin resistance are useful for both PCOS and metabolic syndrome and are likely to reduce progression of endothelial dysfunction, atherogenesis, fatty liver disease, β-cell dysfunction and the prothrombotic state. These include the use of insulin sensitizers, individual or combination therapies for MetS or its individual elements, and for all patients lifestyle changes which include weight loss, exercise and, even for those adolescents without PCOS, smoking cessation [3] (reviewed in reference 69).

Pharmacological therapies targeting insulin resistance

Metformin, at daily doses of 1500– 2000 μg or in generic extended-release single dose formulations, has profound impact on two major PCOS elements: insulin sensitivity and free testosterone levels. Glucose tissue uptake and

Box 31.3 Polycystic ovary syndrome in adolescence: monitoring for and early detection of metabolic consequences

Family history
- parents with DM, CVD, HTN
- Met syndrome in either parent
- gestational diabetes, gestational hypertension
- PCOS, androgenicity or PCOM in first-degree relatives

Personal history
- anovulation, amenorrhea
- androgenization
- low birth weight
- childhood obesity

Physical exam
- hirsutism, acne, alopecia, acanthosis
- hypertension
- abdominal obesity (>90% >35 inch waist)
- BMI ≥30 kg/m²

   Laboratory
- for insulin resistance
- fasting insulin (where reliably available)
- fasting and 2-h glucose
- SHBG, triglycerides
- WBC (neutrophil/lymphocyte ratio)
- liver function tests
- for metabolic syndrome
- fasting cholesterol, HDL-C, LDL-C
- triglycerides

CHECK ANNUALLY FOR EMERGING ⊕ RESULTS
TREAT ⊕ FINDINGS IMMEDIATELY

cious gradual escalation of metformin dosage from low to higher doses will minimize the burden of side effects. Any question of renal or liver disease contraindicates metformin usage. Metformin is the first choice in all PCOS adolescents who display insulin resistance. However, although testosterone is reduced, the impact on clinical hirsutism is minimal.

Other insulin-sensitizing therapy options include thiazolidinediones (TZDs-synthetic PPAR-γ ligands) which induce the full range of beneficial metabolic effects on adipose tissue, skeletal muscle and the liver similar to those seen with metformin. Unfortunately, current formulations are associated with edema and weight gain and are not useful in the adolescent PCOS [9,66]. The utility of angiotensin-converting enzyme (ACE) inhibitors and angiotensin receptor blockers (ARBs) has not been studied in the adolescent population, though theoretically their efficacy in diminishing adult MetS, as well as endothelial dysfunction, suggests a possible application [67,68]. Taken together, drugs that improve insulin sensitivity through mechanisms that include enhancing insulin PI3 kinase-dependent signaling (particularly on the endothelium), increased adiponectin and reduced systemic proinflammatory state significantly attenuate the risk of insulin resistance and MetS.

Nonpharmacologic lifestyle interventions

Lifestyle interventions including diet, weight loss and physical exercise have beneficial effects on the health status of all populations studied. These measures decrease insulin resistance, improve endothelial function, decrease the acute and chronic systemic inflammatory state and have relevance to all adolescents, particularly PCOS youngsters. In all populations studied, the combination of a high-fiber Mediterranean-style diet and moderate daily physical exercise results in weight loss (reduced visceral adiposity as well as decreased BMI), decreased systemic inflammatory markers, and improved cardiovascular endothelium-based function [41,42,45].

But as all of us know too well, not only in our professional but also personal lives, the difficulty of sustaining these beneficial measures is very real. This is particularly true in adolescents given peer pressures, dietary abuse, preoccupation with video games and television (sedentary behavior) and the widespread availability of fast food, sugar-rich drinks and nutritionally empty, high-caloric snacks.

utilization is increased while at the same time glucose production is decreased (decreased hepatic gluconeogenesis and decreased intestinal absorption of glucose) with resulting reduction of β-cell insulin secretion and reduced insulinemia. At the same time, insulin target tissue sensitivity is increased by enhanced insulin receptor binding, greater glucose transporter expression and increased insulin receptor tyrosine kinase activity [61]. Not only are insulin levels reduced but basal and GnRH-stimulated LH, free testosterone concentrations, PAI-1 and endothelin 1 are also diminished. An antilipolytic effect is seen in lower free fatty acids [62]. A greater than 5% weight loss is experienced, and occurs independent of side effects [63] (nausea and vomiting or diarrhea). Interestingly, the metabolic benefits occur in both normal weight and obese individuals [63,64]. Forty to fifty percent of recipients ovulate on metformin, so contraception is mandatory [65]. Judi-

Two publications, one describing an individual case of extreme adolescent obesity [59] and a report of a task force [70] seeking solutions to cope with this problem as a global challenge, emphasize the utility and limitations of all levels of intervention. The need to mobilize individuals, parents, families, schools and communities by sustained realistic weight loss programs, trainers, drug therapy for appetite appeasement, and even bariatric surgery may be necessary. The pediatrician is in a position to identify and react to emerging obesity from infancy through young adulthood and has the opportunity, indeed the responsibility, to intervene in the otherwise relentless progression and deleterious effects of all obesity phenotypes.

Will the bright future that is predicted for genome-wide applications to common diseases and the evolution of "personalized medicine" include an early and accurate risk assessment prediction for a PCOS family and/or child? Recent genome-wide association studies have yielded robust, previously unpredicted information on several genetic markers for common chronic diseases such as diabetes and heart disease [71], obesity [72] and cancer [73]. Furthermore, epigenetics, the study of non-DNA sequence-related heredity, is beginning to explain the interaction between the individual's unchanging genetic background and the environment (from embryogenesis to aging) that results in dysfunction and disease [74]. Clearly, PCOS is suitable for similar assessment. It is a very common disorder which features an inherent genetic "proclivity" upon which an adverse environmental impact is overlaid which over time combines to yield a syndrome of significant clinical consequence. Not only might generalizable and specific individual clues for risk assessment/predictions emerge, but unique preventive, interceptive even corrective measures as well.

Summary

Adolescent girls with PCOS are at substantially increased risk for MetS relative to adolescent girls in the general population. Hyperandrogenemia, obesity and insulin resistance are important risk factors for development of MetS and its consequences in PCOS. These defects can be targeted with traditional therapies such as low-dose OCs, diet and exercise, as well as with novel interventions using insulin sensitizers. Since PCOS women may undergo asymptomatic adverse metabolic alterations at an early age well before the appearance of frank clinical disease, the appropriate clinical management strategy must not only address the immediate symptoms and concerns but also undertake appropriate counseling and surveillance regarding their risks. Early identification and intervention is the key in adolescent girls with PCOS and will mitigate the associated metabolic effects and reduce the risks of developing diabetes and cardiovascular disease.

Conclusion

PCOS causes pain and impairment. It is syndromal, characterized by the presentation of a cluster of signs and symptoms and without a single identified lesion or causation. However, it progresses in the fashion of a disease. Untreated, the burdens of PCOS become more diverse and less responsive to treatment. On the other hand, inexplicably, for some the syndrome disappears with time. It affects the young, runs in families and is found in every culture. It can affect multiple systems – reproductive and nonreproductive. But despite the many causes and effects that exist in PCOS, the central organ from which it derives its name – the polycystic ovary – returns to practically normal function once relieved of the stultifying stresses that inhibit it. We are not talking here about assisted reproductive therapeutics or technologies – just weight loss and exercise! The ovary is resilient and can become "unstuck." But if the ovary is resilient, the metabolic consequences of the syndrome are not. The role of the physician is to identify and intercept these processes before irreversibility takes hold. What is needed is recognition; the corrective strategies are waiting to be implemented.

References

1. Azziz R, Woods KS, Reyna R, Key TJ, Knockenhauer ES, Yildiz BO. The prevalence and features of the polycystic ovary syndrome in an unselected population. *J Clin Endocrinol Metab* 2004;**89**:2745–2749.
2. Buggs C, Rosenfield RL. Polycystic ovary syndrome in adolescence. *Endocrinol Metab Clin North Am* 2005;**34**:679–705.
3. Ehrmann DA. Medical progress. Polycystic ovary syndrome. *N Engl J Med* 2005;**352**:1223–1236.
4. Stein IF, Leventhal ML. Amenorrhea associated with bilateral polycystic ovaries. *Am J Obstet Gynecol* 1935;**29**:181–191.
5. Zawadski JK, Dunaif A. Diagnostic criteria for polycystic ovary syndrome: towards a rational approach. In: Dunaif A,

Gwens JR, Haseltine, FP, Merriam GR (eds) *Polycystic Ovary Syndrome.* Boston: Blackwell Scientific Publications, 1992; 377–384.

6. ESHRE/ASRM. Revised 2003 consensus on diagnostic criteria and long-term health risks related to polycystic ovary syndrome. *Fertil Steril* 2004;**81**:19–25.

7. Franks S. Controversy in clinical endocrinology: diagnosis of polycystic ovarian syndrome: in defense of the Rotterdam criteria. *J Clin Endocrinol Metab* 2006;**91**:786–789.

8. Azziz R. Controversy in clinical endocrinology: diagnosis of polycystic ovary syndrome: the Rotterdam criteria are premature. *J Clin Endocrinol Metab* 2006;**91**:781–785.

9. Speroff L, Fritz MA. Anovulation and the polycystic ovary. In: *Clinical Gynecologic Endocrinology and Infertility*, 7th edn. Philadelphia: Lippincott, Williams and Wilkins, 2005; 465–498.

10. Rosenfield RL. Clinical practice: hirsutism. *N Engl J Med* 2005;**353**:2578–2588.

11. Polson DW, Adams J, Wadsworth J, Franks S. Polycystic ovaries – a common finding in normal women. *Lancet* 1988;**1**:870–872.

12. Ehrmann DA, Barnes RB, Rosenfield RL, Cavaghan MK, Imperial J. Prevalence of impaired glucose tolerance and diabetes in women with polycystic ovary syndrome. *Diabetes Care* 1999;**22**:141–146.

13. Ibanez L, Potau N, Francois I, de Zegher F. Precocious pubarche, hyperinsulinism and ovarian hyperandrogenism in girls: relation to reduced fetal growth. *J Clin Endocrinol Metab* 1998;**83**:3558–3562.

14. Chang RJ. A practical approach to the diagnosis of polycystic ovary syndrome. *Am J Gynecol* 2004;**191**:713–717.

15. Maciel GA, Baracat EC, Benda JA et al. Stockpiling of transitional and classic primary follicles in ovaries of PCOS. *J Clin Endocrinol Metab* 2004;**89**:5321–5327.

16. Marshall JC. Editorial: obesity in adolescent girls: is excess androgen the real bad actor? *J Clin Endocrinol Metab* 2006;**91**:393–395.

17. Pasquali R. Obesity and androgens: facts and perspectives. *Fertil Steril* 2006;**85**;1319–1340.

18. Dieudonne MN, Pecquery R, Boumediene A, Lenevue MC, Guidicelli Y. Androgen receptors in human preadipocytes and adipocytes: regional specificities and regulation by steroids. *Am J Physiol* 1998;**274**:C1645–C1652.

19. Coviello AD, Legro RS, Dunaif A. Adolescent girls with polycystic ovary syndrome have an increased risk of metabolic syndrome associated with increasing androgen levels independent of obesity and insulin resistance. *J Clin Endocrinol Metab* 2006;**91**:492–497.

20. Legro RS, Spielman R, Urbanek M, Driscoll D, Strauss JT, Dunaif A. Phenotype and genotype in polycystic ovary syndrome. *Recent Prog Horm Res* 1998;**53**:217–256.

21. Legro RS, Driscoll D, Strauss JF, Fox J, Dunaif A. Evidence for a genetic basis for hyperandrogenemics in polycystic ovary syndrome. *Proc Natl Acad Sci USA* 1998;**95**:14956–14960.

22. Xita N, Tsatsoulis A. Review: fetal programming of polycystic ovary syndrome by androgen excess: evidence from experimental clinical and genetic association studies. *J Clin Endocrinol Metab* 2006;**91**:1660–1666.

23. Draper N, Walker EA, Bujalska IJ et al. Mutations in the genes encoding 11 beta-hydroxysteroid dehydrogenase type 1 and hexose-6-phosphate dehydrogenase interact to cause cortisone reductase deficiency. *Nat Genet* 2003;**34**:434–439.

24. Petry CJ, Ong KK, Michelmore KF et al. Association of aromatase (CYP19) gene variation with features of hyperandrogenism in two population of young women. *Hum Reprod* 2005;**20**:1837–1843.

25. Eldar-Geva T, Spitz IM, Groome ND, Margalioth EJ, Hamburg R. Follistatin and activin A serum concentrations are lower in PCOS. *Hum Reprod* 2001;**16**:668–672.

26. Franks S, McCarthy M. Genetics of ovarian disorders: PCOS. *Rev Endocr Metab Disord* 2004;**5**:69–76.

27. Stern MP. Genetics of insulin resistance syndrome. *Endocr Pract* 2003;**9**:S35–S38.

28. Groop L. Genetics of visceral obesity and insulin resistance: relationships to non-insulin-dependent diabetes mellitus. *Growth Horm IGF Res* 1998;**8**:9–14.

29. Barker DJP. In utero programming of chronic disease. *Clin Sci (Lond)* 1998;**95**:115–128.

30. Abbott DH, Barnett DK, Bruns CM, Dumesic DA. Androgen excess fetal programming of female reproduction: a developmental aetiology for polycystic ovary syndrome? *Hum Reprod Update* 2005;**11**:357–374.

31. Palmert MR, Gordon CM, Kartashov AI, Legro RS, Dunaif A. Screening for abnormal glucose tolerance in adolescents with polycystic ovary syndrome. *J Clin Endocrinol Metab* 2002;**87**:1017–1023.

32. Arslanian SA, Levy VD, Danadian K. Glucose intolerance in obese adolescents with polycystic ovary syndrome: roles of insulin resistance and β-cell dysfunction and risk of cardiovascular disease. *J Clin Endocrinol Metab* 2001;**86**:66–71.

33. McCartney CR, Prendergast KA, Chhabra S et al. The association of obesity and hyperandrogenemia during the pubertal transition in girls. Obesity as a potential factor in the genesis of postpubertal hyperandrogenism. *J Clin Endocrinol Metab* 2006;**91**:1714–1722.

34. Sir-Petermann T, Hitchsfeld C, Malequeo M et al. Birth weight in offspring of mothers with polycystic ovary syndrome. *Hum Reprod* 2005;**20**:2122–2126.

35. Ibanez L, Ong K, Dunger DB, deZegher F. Early development of adiposity and insulin resistance after catch-up weight gain in small-for-gestational-age children. *J Clin Endocrinol Metab* 2006;**91**:2153–2158.

36. Lazar MA. How obesity causes diabetes: not a tall tale. *Science* 2005;**307**:373–375.

37. Lazar MA. The humoral side of insulin resistance. *Nat Med* 2006;**12**:43–44.

38. Shoelson SE, Lee JL, Goldfine AB. Inflammation and insulin resistance. *J Clin Invest* 2006;**116**:1793–1801.

39. deLuca C, Olefsky JM. Stressed out about obesity and insulin resistance? *Nat Med* 2006;**12**:41–42.

40. Neels JG, Olefsky JM. Inflamed fat: what starts the fire? *J Clin Invest* 2006;**116**:33–35.

41. Dandona P, Aljada A, Chaudhuri A, Mohanty P, Garg R. Metabolic syndrome: a comprehensive perspective based on interactions between obesity, diabetes and inflammation. *Circulation* 2005;**111**:1448–1454.

42. Grundy SM. Drug therapy of the metabolic syndrome: minimizing the emerging crisis in polypharmacy. *Nat Rev: Drug Discovery* 2006;**5**:295–309.

43. Setji TL, Holland ND, Sanders LL, Pereira KC, Deihl AM, Brown AJ. Nonalcoholic steatohepatitis and nonalcoholic fatty liver disease in young women with polycystic ovary syndrome. *J Clin Endocrinol Metab* 2006;**91**:1741–1747.

44. Franzese A, Vajro P, Argenziano A. Liver involvement in obese children: ultrasonography and liver enzyme levels at diagnosis and during follow-up in an Italian population. *Dig Dis Sci* 1997;**42**:1428–1432.

45. Kim J, Montagnani M, Koh KK, Quon MJ. Reciprocal relationships between insulin resistance and endothelial dysfunction. *Circulation* 2006;**113**:1888–1904.

46. Semenkovich CF. Insulin resistance and atherosclerosis. *J Clin Invest* 2006;**116**:1813–1822.

47. Houstis N, Rosen ED, Lander ES. Reactive oxygen species have a causal role in multiple forms of insulin resistance. *Nature* 2006;**440**:944–948.

48. Gonzalez F, Rote NS, Minium J, Kirwan JP. Reactive oxygen species-induced oxidative stress in the development of insulin resistance and hyperandrogenism in polycystic ovary syndrome. *J Clin Endocrinol Metab* 2006;**91**:336–340.

49. Deplewski D, Rosenfeld RL. Role of hormones in pilosebaceous unit development. *Endocr Rev* 2000;**21**:363–392.

50. Spritzer DM, Lisboa KO, Mattiello S, Lhullier F. Spironolactone as a single agent for long term therapy of hirsute patients. *Clin Endocrinol (Oxf)* 2000;**52**:587–594.

51. Lord JM, Flight IH, Norman RJ. Insulin sensitizing drugs (metformin, troglitazone, rosiglitazone, pioglitazona D-chiro-inositol) for polycystic ovary syndrome. *Cochrane Database Syst Rev* 3: CD003053, 2003.

52. Ibanez L, deZegher F. Ethinyl estradiol-drospironone, flutamide-metformin or both for adolescents and women with hyperinsulinemic hyperandrogenism: opposite effects on adipokines and body adiposity. *J Clin Endocrinol Metab* 2004;**89**:1592–1594.

53. Krattenmaker R. Drosperinone: pharmacology and pharmacokinetics of a unique progestogen. *Contraception* 2003;**62**:129–138.

54. Hardiman P, Pillay OC, Atiomo W. Polycystic ovary syndrome and endometrial carcinoma. *Lancet* 2003;**361**:1810–1812.

55. Liebel NI, Baumann EE, Kocherginsky M, Rosenfield RL. Relationships of adolescent polycystic ovary syndrome to parental metabolic syndrome. *J Clin Endocrinol Metab* 2006;**91**:1275–1283.

56. Ehrmann DA, Liljenquist DR, Kasza K, Azziz R, Legro RS, Ghazzi MN. Prevalence and predictors of the metabolic syndrome in women with polycystic ovary syndrome. *J Clin Endocrinol Metab* 2006;**91**:48–53.

57. Hedley AA, Ogdon CL, Johnson CL, Carroll MD, Curtin LR, Flegal KM. Prevalence of overweight and obesity amongst US children-adolescents and adults 1999–2002. *JAMA* 2004;**291**:2847–2850.

58. Duncan GE. Prevalence of impaired fasting glucose levels among US adolescents: National Health and Nutrition Survey, 1999–2002. *Arch Ped Adol Med* 2006;**160**:523–528.

59. Hoppin AG, Katz ES, Kaplan LM, Lauwers GY. Case 31-2006: a 15-year-old girl with severe obesity. *N Engl J Med* 2006;**355**:1593–1602.

60. Meigs JB, Wilson PWF, Fox CS et al. Body mass index, metabolic syndrome, and risk of type 2 diabetes or cardiovascular disease. *J Clin Endocrinol Metab* 2006;**91**:2906–2912.

61. Bailey CJ, Turner RC. Metformin. *N Engl J Med* 1996;**334**:574–579.

62. Velazquez EM, Mendoza S, Hamer T, Sosa F, Glueck CJ. Metformin therapy in polycystic ovary syndrome reduces hyperinsulinemia, insulin resistance, hyperandrogenemia, and systolic blood pressure, while facilitating normal menses and pregnancy. *Metabolism* 1994;**43**:647–654.

63. Haupt E, Knick B, Koschinsky T. Oral antidiabetic combination therapy with sulphonylureas and metformin. *Diabetes Metab* 1991;**17**:224–232.

64. Pasquali R, Gambineri A, Biscotti D et al. Effect of long term treatment with metformin added to hypocaloric diet on body composition, fat distribution, and androgen and insulin levels in abdominally obese women with and without polycystic ovary syndrome. *J Clin Endocrinol Metab* 2000;**85**:2767–2774.

65. Nestler JE, Jakubowicz DJ, Evans WS, Pasquali R. Effects of metformin on spontaneous and clomiphene induced

ovulation in polycystic ovary syndrome. *N Engl J Med* 1998;**338**:1876–1880.

66. Fonseca VA, Valiquett TR, Huang SM. Troglitazone monotherapy improves glycemic control in patients with type 2 diabetes mellitus: a randomized, controlled study. *J Clin Endocrinol Metab* 1998;**83**:3169–3176.

67. DREAM (Diabetes REeduction Assessment with ramipril and rosiglitazone Medication) Effect of ramipril on the incidence of diabetes. *N Engl J Med* 2006;**355**:1551–1562.

68. Kurtz TW. New treatment strategies for patients with hypertension and insulin resistance. *Am J Med* 2006;**119**(suppl 1):524–530.

69. Guzik DS. Cardiovascular risk in PCOS. *J Clin Endocrinol Metab* 2004;**89**:3694–3695.

70. Speiser PW for the Obesity Consensus Working Group. Consensus statement: childhood obesity. *J Clin Endocrinol Metab* 2005;**90**:1871–1887.

71. Wellcome Trust Case Control Consortium. Genome-wide association study of 14,000 cases of seven common diseases and 3,000 shared controls. *Nature* 2007;**447**:661–678.

72. Emilsson V, Thorleifsson G, Zhang B et al. Genetics of gene expression and its effect on disease. *Nature* 2008;**452**:423–428.

73. Easton DF, Pooley KA, Dunning AM et al. Genome-wide association study identifies novel breast cancer susceptibility loci. *Nature* 2007;**447**:1087–1093.

74. Feinberg AP. Epigenetics at the epicenter of modern medicine. *JAMA* 2008;**299**:1345–1350.

CHAPTER 32

Acute Abdominal and Pelvic Pain

Jeremy T. Aidlen[1] *& Stephen E. Dolgin*[2]

[1] The Warren Alpert Medical School of Brown University, Hasbro Children's Hospital, Providence, RI, USA
[2] Schneider Children's Hospital, North Shore-Long Island Jewish Hospital, New York, NY, USA

Introduction

The evaluation of a child with abdominal pain should be prompt and systematic since delay in effectuating proper care may lead to progressively more serious consequences. Most diagnoses can be made correctly using a combination of careful history and physical examination. Clinical features of the individual patient and knowledge of the pathophysiology usually allow the clinician to determine which children require intervention and which organ is crying for help. This chapter surveys some of the common causes of acute abdominal pain in young females. Without being exhaustive, some principles are emphasized that help provide effective care. The clinician is well served by an understanding of the pathophysiologic basis of the pain that is grounded in organogenesis and anatomy.

The sensory nerve fibers from the organs themselves, the visceral fibers, generally course along the arteries whose anatomic distribution is established early in the development of the organ systems. Intra-abdominal organs that derive from the embryonic foregut (stomach, proximal duodenum, biliary tree and pancreas) receive blood supplied by branches of the celiac artery and refer pain when distension stimulates their visceral nerves to the epigastric region. Midgut structures (distal duodenum, small intestine, appendix, cecum, ascending and proximal transverse colon) are all supplied by the superior mesenteric artery. The organs derived from the midgut refer pain when their visceral nerves are stimulated to the mid abdomen. Structures derived from the hindgut (distal

transverse colon, descending colon, and rectum), supplied by branches of the inferior mesenteric artery, elicit lower abdominal or pelvic pain. The intestines themselves are insensitive to touch and to inflammation that does not affect the enclosing peritoneum. However, severe pain can emanate from any part of the intestine when it is severely distended or when its muscle contracts violently [1].

It might be of particular interest to readers of this text to emphasize the distinction between children with acute pain who suffer from intestinal illness as compared to pathology of the ovaries or Müllerian structures. Associated symptoms may suggest if the involved organ is gastrointestinal or otherwise. Minimal symptoms of gastrointestinal dysfunction, such as nausea, vomiting, obstipation or diarrhea, with no sign of gastrointestinal dilation on exam will warn the clinician that the cause of the abdominal pain may not be intestinal. Pain of severe acute onset localizing to one side of the pelvis suggests ovarian or adnexal pathology.

Appendicitis and the assessment of peritonitis

The value of understanding the pathophysiology is well illustrated by considering the patient with acute appendicitis. The classic history is of vague midabdominal pain that then migrates to the right lower quadrant and becomes progressively more severe. The evolution of peritoneal signs in the right lower quadrant on physical exam has been the time-honored indication for appendectomy. What is the pathophysiologic basis of this scenario? Appendicitis arises from obstruction of the appendix whether from lymphoid hyperplasia or an obstructing fecalith. Since the appendix is part of the midgut, when it

Pediatric, Adolescent, & Young Adult Gynecology. Edited by
A. Altchek and L. Deligdisch. © 2009 Blackwell Publishing,
ISBN: 978-1-4051-5347-8.

Table 32.1 Anatomic basis of symptoms

	Primary blood supply	Organs affected	Site of referred pain
Foregut	Celiac trunk	Stomach, proximal duodenum, biliary tree, pancreas	Epigastric region
Midgut	Superior mesenteric artery	Distal duodenum, small intestine, appendix, right and proximal transverse colon	Mid abdomen, periumbilical area
Hindgut	Inferior mesenteric artery	Distal colon and rectum	Lower abdomen, pelvis

is distended its visceral nerves refer pain to the periumbilical region, as would distension of any organ derived from the midgut. Therefore the initial pain is vague and mid abdominal. With bacterial proliferation and mucosal secretions, inflammation progresses through the wall of the appendix and stimulates somatic (or parietal) nerve fibers in the parietal peritoneum. This causes migration of the pain to the site of the appendix (usually the right lower quadrant). The localized pain is accompanied by tenderness and peritoneal signs.

To further illustrate this pathophysiology, consider a person whose appendix rests elsewhere, such as the right upper quadrant. That patient would also present with periumbilical pain since distension of the appendix stimulates visceral fibers that refer to the mid abdomen no matter where the appendix resides. That initial pain, arising from distension, transmitted by visceral or splanchnic fibers, reflects the embryonic origin of the appendix. As inflammation progresses and extends to the overlying parietal peritoneum, the local parietal or somatic nerves would send pain to the right upper quadrant where tenderness, guarding, and peritoneal signs would ensue.

Peritoneal signs usually lead a surgeon to advise operation and the results are rewarding for the patient.

Which of the young patients with acute abdominal pain have peritonitis? How is that determined? The presence of often mentioned "rebound tenderness" has the same physiologic basis as the other more discerning signs of peritoneal irritation. Rapid movement of the body wall stimulates the parietal nerves and elicits sharp pain. However, eliciting rebound tenderness on physical exam is not a refined maneuver and can frighten a child. Observation is a useful opening salvo for the clinician. Young patients with peritonitis walk haltingly or lie still in bed. They refuse to jump or suffer pain when they try. The Rovsing sign is the diagnostician's friend. When a child complains of right lower quadrant pain, listen with the stethoscope to the left side of the abdomen. Gently press increasingly deeply and ask where it hurts. Tenderness in the right lower quadrant from pressure applied on the left side (a positive Rovsing sign) is a clear demonstration of right-sided peritoneal irritation.

Although modern imaging has lessened the reliance on these clinical tools, unnecessary exposure to the tests and inaccurate interpretations are avoided if the clinician's skills are refined. A child who walks briskly and jumps up on a bed with no discomfort and is without Rovsing, psoas, obturator or other tests for peritonitis usually does not need to be rushed to the CT scanner. Just a few conditions are the exception to the rule that peritonitis warrants an operative intervention. These include pelvic inflammatory disease, primary peritonitis, and pancreatitis. Usually the clinical context allows suspicion of these conditions. Pancreatitis should not be overlooked in childhood. Although the common causes of the condition in adults, alcohol toxicity and gallstones, are not thought of as childhood afflictions, gallstone pancreatitis is in fact not rare in children, and there are other causes of pancreatic inflammation such as trauma, medications, and anatomic abnormalities. If pancreatitis is suspected, the addition to the blood tests of serum amylase and lipase determinations will help establish that diagnosis.

Primary peritonitis typically occurs in the setting of ascites. It can be the clinical announcement of nephrotic syndrome. A urinalysis showing significant proteinuria should not be misconstrued as a lab error. In a child with peritoneal signs, proteinuria strongly points to nephrotic syndrome with primary peritonitis.

The focus of this chapter is on those conditions that do require operative intervention. The clinical history and physical exam will be strikingly different in the patient with appendicitis as compared to the young lady who suffers adnexal torsion, ovarian cyst rupture or pelvic inflammatory disease. Acute onset of severe localizing pain directs the clinician to these possibilities and especially when symptoms of intestinal dysfunction are not prominent.

Appendicitis remains the most common acute surgical condition of the abdomen and accurate diagnosis can be problematic. The lifetime risk for appendicitis is 7% for women, about one-third of whom are younger than 18 years of age when afflicted [2]. The peak incidence occurs between ages 11 and 12. Diagnostic accuracy for appendicitis is lower among young women than young men because of the variety of gynecologic conditions that can cause low abdominal pain.

While the presentation of acute appendicitis is widely variable, classically the patient recounts a story of vague, central abdominal pain that gradually increases in severity as it migrates towards the right lower quadrant. Anorexia, nausea, and vomiting are common but any severe gastrointestinal symptoms that precede the onset of pain cast some doubt on the diagnosis. Once the inflammatory exudate from the appendiceal wall contacts the parietal peritoneum, somatic pain fibers are triggered and the pain localizes near the appendiceal site, most typically at McBurney's point [3]. If the physical findings are not pathognomic, admission to the hospital for serial abdominal examinations to increase diagnostic accuracy is a safe alternative to immediate appendectomy [4].

Increasingly, imaging has been utilized to identify the inflamed appendix. Since the use of the CT scan to determine who has appendicitis was prominently propagated, it has become commonplace [5,6]. A skilled sonographer can frequently recognize a distended appendix. Sonography is particularly useful if an ovarian cyst or tumor is suspected. The downsides of the extremely popular CT scan include the radiation exposure [7], the need for GI contrast which if taken by mouth can be time consuming and quite unappealing for the nauseated child, and the incidence of erroneous interpretations.

Local peritoneal inflammation from appendicitis may cause irritation of adjacent structures, including bladder and rectum. Subsequent dysuria and frequent diarrhea of low volumes are often associated symptoms of the advanced, inflamed pelvic appendix. Pyuria and microscopic hematuria commonly accompany appendicitis. The obturator sign can help identify the inflamed appendix lying low in the pelvis, especially since the usual findings on the anterior abdominal wall may be absent when the appencis lurks in that site. Pain elicited from cervical motion during pelvic exam performed to rule out

other causes may be misleading [8]. Pain from a retrocecal appendix may localize in the flank or back. In such cases the psoas sign is helpful. When the appendix is not near the anterior abdominal wall, such as when it lies retrocecal or in the pelvis, the expected signs on the anterior abdominal wall may not be present. In such patients useful signs of peritonitis include the hop test (the patient is asked if it hurts when she jumps), psoas and obturator. Ultimately, complete appendiceal obstruction leads to congestion and loss of venous outflow with resultant tissue ischemia and necrosis. Appendiceal wall erosion leads to spillage of infected contents and localized abscess formation, or generalized peritonitis. Traditional teaching is that appendicitis evolves from luminal obstruction to perforation over a 24–48 hour period. Younger patients are far more likely to present with perforation due to their inability to give an accurate history, and perhaps because of a lower index of suspicion by physicians [9,10]. Signs of perforation include diffuse tenderness, palpable right lower quadrant mass, fever greater than 101.5°F, and leukocyte count greater than 14,000/mm^3 [11].

If perforation has occurred, intravenous fluid and antibiotics are the first therapeutic steps. The best timing of the appendectomy is individualized. An abscess warrants drainage and initial nonoperative management has become a standard approach.

The effect of perforated appendicitis on tubal infertility is an unresolved issue. One retrospective study of 389 females treated for perforated appendicitis over an 18-year period reported that complicated appendicitis before puberty plays little if any role in the cause of tubal infertility [12]. Another study of 279 patients who had been diagnosed with tubal infertility and had a history of perforated appendicitis reported that the associated risk is increased fourfold [13]. Regardless, it is clear that all patients benefit from swift diagnosis and treatment of appendicitis.

Intussusception

Intussusception is the invagination of one portion of the intestine into another. It is the second most common cause of acute abdominal pain in infants and preschool children after constipation [14]. The incidence of intussusception is 1 in 2000 children [15], with a typical age at presentation between three months and three years. At that age intussusception is usually ileocecal and idiopathic (as opposed to intussusception caused by an anatomic lesion serving as a lead point). The presence of two classic symptoms (abdominal pain, vomiting) and two classic signs (abdominal mass, rectal bleeding) helps make the diagnosis in an infant or child. It is important to recognize, however, that all four are only present in 30% of cases [16].

The pain of intussusception is colicky, intermittent, and severe. Children often draw their legs up towards their belly with pain, and become lethargic as it recedes. This is the pain of distal small bowel obstruction. Listlessness and irritability are expected. Sometimes they dominate the clinical picture. If a child is happy, laughing and interactive, intussusception is unlikely. Vomiting occurs as a reflex or as bowel wall edema with progressive intussuception obstructs the intestinal lumen. The sausage-like abdominal mass of intussusception is not a subtle finding in the dehydrated, lethargic child. It can, however, be difficult to appreciate in a vigorous child. Rectal bleeding, often described as "redcurrant jelly", is a result of colonic mucosal irritation from prolonged ischemia. This is a late finding and one should not wait for the appearance of bloody stools to diagnose or treat intussusception. Other associated symptoms may be highly variable. A viral-type prodrome of upper respiratory illness or gastroenteritis is particularly common. The robust immune response in an otherwise healthy child with viral illness leads to mesenteric lymphadenopathy. Right lower quadrant lymph nodes or perhaps lymphoid hyperplasia may promote the typical idiopathic ileocolic intussusception. Postoperative intussusception is a poorly understood condition encountered most frequently after gastrointestinal surgery and more often in children than in adults.

The diagnosis of intussusception can be confirmed by ultrasonography.

Ileocolic intussusception is most often treated successfully by air or water-soluble contrast enema reduction. An operation is required if nonoperative reduction is not successful. Small bowel–small bowel intussusceptions and those associated with a pathologic lead point (such as Meckel's, hemangioma, polyp) are less likely to escape operative intervention.

Intestinal malrotation with volvulus

The cost of delayed treatment for midgut volvulus from malrotation is high since resulting infarction means the loss of the critical absorptive surface from mid duodenum to mid transverse colon. During organogenesis and the early fetal period the midgut creates a midsagittal loop that herniates into the exocoelom and rotates 270° counterclockwise as it returns to the coelom and fixes in place. The midgut includes the evolving intestine that receives its blood supply from the superior mesenteric artery and its branches. That artery is the axis of rotation for the midgut loop.

With malrotation, the midgut loop returns to the coelom without rotating so the duodenojejunal junction is to the right of the spine and the ileocecal junction is nearby in the mid abdomen. Therefore, the mesentery, extending from the duodenojejunal junction to the ileocecal junction, forms an abnormally narrow pedicle as opposed to the normal longer oblique course from left upper quadrant to right lower quadrant forming a wide-based anchor. The narrow mesentery of malrotation puts the midgut at risk of torsion, known as volvulus. This is a lifelong and life-threatening risk for a person with midgut malrotation, but a more common event in the younger age group. Because of acute obstruction, bilious vomiting is the clinical hallmark that accompanies abdominal pain when a child suffers midgut volvulus and alerts the clinician that the patient needs prompt attention. Abdominal flat plate and upright views may show a paucity of air or signs of obstruction. Sonogram or CT scan can provide evidence of malrotation by revealing a reverse of the usual anatomic relation of the superior mesenteric artery and vein [17]. Upper gastrointestinal series (UGI) is the most direct study, showing an abnormal position of the duodenojejunal junction. Volvulus can be missed on UGI but the presence of malrotation by UGI in a patient with acute abdominal pain dictates a prompt operation. The operative intervention is called the Ladd procedure and includes detorsing the volvulus, dividing any pathologic bands that cross the duodenum, and widely separating the two ends of the mesentery, leaving the midgut in the malrotated position and removing the appendix.

Constipation

Constipation is the most common cause of childhood emergency room visits for abdominal pain. While pain may be acute, a thorough history of bowel habits usually reveals the chronic nature of this problem. Colonic obstruction with impacted feces can lead to pain that is diffuse, severe, and disabling. Discomfort is often greatest in the right lower quadrant, where the cecum distends. Abdominal exam usually reveals a distended abdomen. The abdomen is often mildly tender. Stool within the colon may be palpable as an abdominal mass in the thin, nondistended patient.

Constipation is not expected to cause marked leukocytosis and fever. Fever or an elevated white blood cell count makes the diagnosis suspect. If an enema gives significant relief, the diagnosis of constipation is supported. Parents should be encouraged to supplement their child's diet with fiber. Oral hydration is inadequate therapy for the chronically constipated child.

Meckel's diverticulum

Meckel's diverticulum is the most common congenital anomaly of the gastrointestinal tract, a vitelline duct abnormality occurring with an incidence of 1–2% in the general population. Usually it causes no symptoms and remains unrecognized for the life of the patient. The most common presentation is hemodynamically significant painless rectal bleeding. This bleeding results from ectopic gastric mucosa within the lumen that secretes acid and causes a nearby ulcer of the ileum. Alternatively, a diverticulum may present with bowel obstruction (internal hernia, volvulus, intussusception). Inflammation (Meckel's diverticulitis) and perforation are less common. When symptomatic, the diverticulae should be removed, either by intestinal resection and anastomosis or by diverticulectomy.

The management of the incidentally discovered asymptomatic Meckel's diverticulum is a bit controversial. While not universal, most surgeons agree that the lifetime risk to a young child of complications related to the presence of Meckel's diverticulum warrants resection. The argument for resection is stronger in the younger patient. The indications are less convincing in the adult population.

Mittelschmerz

The physiologic trauma of ovulation may cause midmenstrual cycle pain. The clinical clues are acute lateralizing pain of sudden onset. Ultrasonographic evidence of pelvic free fluid at ovulation represents follicular rupture with hemorrhage [18]. The hemoperitoneum leads to focal lower abdominal tenderness and might be quite misleading, especially around the time of menarche.

Adnexal torsion

An ovarian tumor or cyst can promote adnexal torsion, causing pain and the risk of ischemia and infarction. The most common ovarian neoplasia of childhood, ovarian teratoma, often announces itself with pain from adnexal torsion. Interestingly, ovarian teratomas are not seen in newborn patients. The pain may be intermittent or unremitting. Imaging usually establishes the presence of a teratoma. If pain is severe, torsion can be assumed. A preoperative serum AFP and HCG are indicated and would be useful if elevated and the pathology reveals an immature teratoma. The very large teratoma presenting with torsion in the child can be managed with ovariectomy without incrimination. The other ovary must be examined to exclude bilateral disease and lifelong screening sonograms are appropriate.

Ovarian cysts are common in the fetus and the newborn because of the hormonal influences stimulating the fetal ovary. Most resolve spontaneously. Torsion and infarction can occur, especially from large follicular cysts. Some advocate intervention in the neonate when a cyst is more than 25 cc in volume calculated from ultrasonographic measurements, or 5 cm in any dimension by sonography. The danger of torsion in this setting is infarction with hemorrhage, peritonitis, gastrointestinal or genitourinary obstruction or a wandering tumor [19].

Idiopathic adnexal torsion

Torsion of the uterine adnexa causes abdominal pain and can lead to necrosis. Prompt diagnosis and treatment has obvious advantages but has been regarded as difficult because the symptoms are described as nonspecific. These include abdominal pain, nausea, vomiting, and fever. The signs usually mentioned in the literature are no more specific, including abdominal tenderness and guarding.

When a tumor is present, resection is appropriate but when the torsion is idiopathic, ovarian salvage may be a more sensible approach. The best management of idiopathic adnexal torsion with apparent necrosis has generated controversy. Although, as the name suggests, the

Table 32.2 Classic presentation

	History	Physical	Associated signs and symptoms
Appendicitis	Midabdominal pain progressing to right lower quadrant pain	Right lower quadrant tenderness with guarding	Nausea, vomiting, dysuria. High fever, diffuse peritonitis and palpable mass are associated with perforation
Intussusception	Severe intermittent, colicky pain with lethargy	Palpable mass	"Redcurrant jelly" stools
Malrotation with midgut volvulus	Midabdominal pain and bilious vomiting	Nonspecific, progresses to shock	Bilious vomiting
Constipation	Intermittent pain and chronic symptoms	Abdominal distension, palpable fullness, right-sided tenderness not uncommon	Nausea, vomiting
Meckel's diverticulum	Painless rectal bleeding, self-limiting	Nonspecific	Hemodynamic instability
Mittelschmerz	Midcycle lower abdominal pain	Lower abdominal tenderness	Nausea, vomiting
Adnexal torsion	Sudden, severe lateralizing lower abdominal pain	Tenderness, guarding	Nausea, vomiting

cause of idiopathic torsion is unknown, the physiologically active ovary is at particular risk.

Series of children with idiopathic adnexal torsion are retrospective and extend over many years. So the description of the clinical picture may not be refined. The clinical presentation is often likened to appendicitis but it is worth emphasizing some differences. A history of vague midabdominal pain that migrates to the right lower quadrant predicts the likelihood of appendicitis [4]. Adnexal torsion is more likely to cause pain of sudden onset. One study of 14 girls with adnexal torsion observed that all patients presented with lower abdominal pain, and onset of pain was abrupt in all cases [20].

Historically, the diagnosis of adnexal torsion has been missed or discovered at laparotomy for appendicitis. Sonography is the single best modality to recognize adnexal torsion. The torsed adnexus appears as a large heterogenous ovary. The complete and diagnostic sonographic picture is of a large heterogenous ovary with peripheral cysts and fluid in the pelvis. The contralateral ovary appears normal. Unfortunately, the sonogram may not be that clear and may fail to determine that torsion is responsible. Doppler ultrasound has a mixed track record with reports of many false positives and negatives.

When a large ovarian neoplasm causes adnexal torsion, the presence of the tumor is thereby unearthed. When

adnexal torsion is due to a large ovarian tumor, both the cause and treatment are usually clear. Ovariectomy is often performed and raises few questions. When torsion affects a normal ovary (idiopathic adnexal torsion), a different approach can be considered. It has become increasingly clear that when the surgeon encounters a large, edematous, blue-black ovary from idiopathic torsion, the adnexa can safely be untwisted and the ovarian function may be preserved. Although some patients with idiopathic adnexal torsion treated this way have experienced a few days of fever and pain, the long-term outcome has generally been good [20–22]. Despite apparent necrosis, ovarian function has often been maintained when the torsed adnexa is untwisted. To avoid missing a tumor, a sonogram can be obtained about six weeks after recovery. Interestingly, the absence of flow on a Doppler sonogram after the operation may not predict future ovarian failure, since the ovary may appear normal in examinations done much later [20].

The fear that untwisting a torsed adnexus causes catastrophic embolism has been debunked [23]. There is no role for pexy of the ipsilateral or contralateral side when adnexal torsion is due to underlying unilateral pathology. If adnexal torsion results from an ipsilateral tumor, excision does not leave the patient at significant risk for future torsion. However, if torsion is idiopathic, pexy of

Quick Take 32.1

A few exceptions to the rule that peritonitis warrants an operative intervention

- Pelvic inflammatory disease
- Primary peritonitis
- Pancreatitis

Acute onset of severe localizing pain directs the clinician towards nonintestinal pathology

- Adnexal torsion
- Ovarian cyst rupture

Downsides to the abdominal CT scan to diagnose appendicitis

- Radiation exposure
- Need for intestinal contrast
- Delay to diagnosis or treatment
- Expense
- Erroneous interpretations

Young patients are most likely to present with signs of perforated appendicitis

- High fever
- Diffuse abdominal tenderness
- Palpable right lower quadrant mass
- Markedly elevated leukocyte count

both the ipsilateral and contralateral side has advocates since ipsilateral recurrence and contralateral occurrence are known to happen [20,22].

References

1. Silen W. *Cope's Early Diagnosis of the Acute Abdomen*, 18th edn. Oxford: Oxford University Press, 1991.
2. Addiss DG, Shaffer J, Fowler BS, Tauxe RV. The epidemiology of appendicitis and appendectomy in the United States. *Am J Epidemiol* 1990;**132**:910.
3. Grosfeld J (ed). *Pediatric Surgery*, 6th edn. St Louis: Mosby Elsevier, 2006: 1502.
4. Dolgin SE, Beck AR, Tartter PI. The risk of perforation when children with possible appendicitis are observed in the hospital. *Surg Gynecol Obstet* 1992:**175**:320–324.
5. Rao PM, Rhea JT, Novelline RA et al. Effect of computed tomography of the appendix on treatment of patients and use of hospital resources. *N Engl J Med* 1998:**338**(3):141–146.
6. Novelline RA, Rhea JT, Rao PM, Stuk JL. Helical CT in emergency radiology. *Radiology* 1999;**213**(2):321–339.
7. Brenner DJ, Elliston CD, Hall EJ, Berdon WE. Estimated risks of radiation-induced fatal cancer from pediatric CT. *Am J Roentgenol* 2001;**176**:289–296.
8. Rothrock SG, Green SM, Dobson M. Misdiagnosis of appendicitis in nonpregnant women of childbearing age. *J Emerg Med* 1995:**13**(1):1–8.
9. Grosfeld J. Appendicitis in the first two years of life. *J Ped Surg* 1973;**8**:285.
10. Huang CB, Yu HR, Hung GC, Huang SC, Chuang JH. Clinical features and outcome of appendicitis in children younger than three years of age. *Chang Gung Med J* 2001;**24**:27–33.
11. Samelson SL, Reyes HM. Management of perforated appendicitis in children revisited. *Arch Surg* 1987;**122**:691.
12. Puri P, McGuinness EPJ, Guiney EJ. Fertility following perforated appendicitis in girls. *J Ped Surg* 1989;**24**:547.
13. Meuller BA, Daling JR, Moore DE. Appendectomy and the risk of tubal infertility. *N Engl J Med* 1986;**315**:1506.
14. Grosfeld J. Intussusception. In: *Pediatric Surgery*, 6th edn. St Louis: Mosby Elsevier, 2006.
15. Ravitch MM. Intussusception. In: Grosfeld J (ed) *Pediatric Surgery*, 4th edn. St Louis: Mosby Yearbook Medical, 1986.
16. Ein SH, Stephens CA, Minor A. The painless intussusception. *J Ped Surg* 1976;**11**:563.
17. Aidlen JT, Anupindi SA, Jaramillo D, Doody DP. Malrotation with midgut volvulus: CT findings of bowel infarction. *Pediatr Radiol* 2005;**35**:529–531.
18. Hann LE. Mittelschmerz. Sonographic demonstration. *JAMA* 1979;**241**(25):2731–2732.
19. Dolgin SE. Ovarian masses in the newborn. *Semin Pediatr Surg* 2000;**9**:121–127.
20. Celik A, Ergun O, Aldemir H et al. Long-term results of conservative management of adnexal torsion in children. *J Ped Surg* 2005;**40**:704–708.
21. Aziz D. Ovarian torsion in children: is oophorectomy necessary? *J Ped Surg* 2004; **39**:750–753.
22. Dolgin SE. Maximizing ovarian salvage when treating idiopathic adnexal torsion. *J Ped Surg* 2000;**35**:624–626.
23. Roday A. The conservative management of adnexal torsion – a case report and review of the literature. *Eur J Obstet Gynecol Reprod Biol* 2002;**101**:83–86.

33

CHAPTER 33

Acute Gynecologic Pain

Charles J. Ascher-Walsh & Michael Brodman

Mount Sinai School of Medicine, New York, NY, USA

Introduction

Acute pelvic pain in children and adolescents may have many causes. A thorough history is the most important first step in attempting to determine its cause. Usually, when girls of this age group have acute pain, their evaluation begins in the emergency room or in the pediatrician's office. By the time a gynecologist is called in, an initial evaluation has already been performed, frequently by both a pediatrician and a pediatric surgeon. While much important and helpful information can be achieved by tapping these resources, it is important for the gynecologist to be as thorough as possible to avoid missing the correct diagnosis.

Different age groups have their own challenges in acquiring a thorough history. Because infants have very limited ability in communicating the symptoms related to their pain, much of the history is dependent on the parent or caregiver. Young children can often give a better explanation of their pain and the circumstances surrounding it. It is frequently helpful to consult the parent as well to achieve a more complete understanding of the child's complaints. In older adolescents, it may actually be difficult to achieve a complete history with the parent present. It is frequently very difficult to balance the patient's right to privacy with the parents' rights to be involved in the care of their child. At times it may feel that these conflicts actually interfere with the care of the child. In cases such as this, it may be helpful to involve a social worker or other child advocates to mediate in the best interests of the child.

Pediatric, Adolescent, & Young Adult Gynecology. Edited by
A. Altchek and L. Deligdisch. © 2009 Blackwell Publishing,
ISBN: 978-1-4051-5347-8.

Box 33.1 lists some of the potential causes of acute pelvic pain in pediatric and adolescent patients. Some are clearly more common in specific age groups but thorough evaluation should be performed for each patient. As surgical intervention is often required for some of the potential causes of acute pain, and the diagnosis is frequently delayed due to challenges in acquiring a complete history and physical, it is important to be as comprehensive as possible in the initial evaluation.

In addition to a general history of the problem and a medical and surgical history of the patient, the doctor should acquire a complete menstrual and sexual history, including use of contraceptives and known history of recent contacts. The doctor should also acquire any previous medical documentation that may be pertinent to the patient's current condition.

The physical exam is obviously an important part of the evaluation but it may not be tolerated by all patients. For younger children, it is very important to make them feel comfortable and in control of the situation. The exam can be completed while the child is sitting on the lap of one parent. As with adults, talking to the child during the exam and explaining each step makes it more tolerable to the child. Visual examination of the vulva and perineum is important, especially if trauma or sexual abuse is suspected. An intravaginal exam may not always be possible, especially in children with an intact hymenal membrane. If inspection of the vagina is thought to be important, it can be accomplished with an otoscope. Pelvic organs may be difficult to palpate in very young children. If an exam is deemed to be necessary, a rectal exam is an alternative to an intravaginal exam that can often yield similar information. Some young patients may prefer to be evaluated without their parents in the room while others may be more comfortable with a family member present. Older adolescents should be questioned concerning what makes

Box 33.1 Potential causes of acute pelvic pain

Nongynecologic
   Trauma/Abuse
      Accidents
      Sports injury
      Sexual abuse
      Physical abuse
   GI
      Gastroenteritis
      Appendicitis
      Crohn disease
      Intestinal obstruction
      Volvulus
   GU
      Urethritis
      Cystitis
      Pyelonephritis
      Renal calculus
   Nongynecologic malignancies with bone metastasis
   Psychologic/psychosomatic
Gynecologic
   Normal physiology
      Dysmenorrhea
      Follicular/corpus luteum cysts
      Ovulation
   Abnormal physiology
      Pregnancy
         Ectopic
         Spontaneous abortion
      Nonfunctional ovarian cysts
         Rupture
         Internal hemorrhage
         Adnexal torsion
      Tumors
         Degeneration
         Infection
         Torsion
      Vaginitis
      Pelvic inflammatory disease
      Congenital malformations

and the appropriate testing is imperative. Blood and urine analysis is also important for differentiating between multiple causes of pain.

Of the possible radiologic tests, ultrasound has become the most frequently used for diagnosis of pelvic pathology. It is a minimally invasive method that gives reliable information about the female pelvis. It is relatively inexpensive compared to CT scan or MRI and is readily accessible in most gynecology offices and in the emergency room. The study is best when performed vaginally but can also give useful information when done through the perineum, rectally or abdominally.

When available testing is exhausted and the diagnosis is still unclear, diagnostic laparoscopy is a potential tool for managing the pediatric patient. Certainly with signs of an acute abdomen such as rebound tenderness and guarding, a diagnostic laparoscopy may lead to the earlier diagnosis and treatment of a serious problem. It would also be appropriate in patients in whom an ectopic pregnancy cannot be excluded. If the pain is getting progressively worse or is recurrent without a clear source, then laparoscopy may be warranted to achieve a diagnosis. Many patients undergoing diagnostic laparoscopy for pelvic pain will be found to have a normal abdomen and pelvis. While this is frustrating for both the patient and clinician, it is reassuring that a major pathologic condition does not exist.

The potential causes of acute pelvic pain in the pediatric patient are many and the ability to achieve a complete history may be limited. It is therefore important to maximize the amount of available information by using all possible means to achieve this information. This will include the information acquired by others examining the patient previously as well as information from other reliable sources such as family members and from objective laboratory and radiologic tests.

them most comfortable. Some time alone with the patient may enable her to give information about sexual abuse that she is not comfortable giving around a family member.

Radiologic and laboratory tests may be helpful in achieving the correct diagnosis in these patients. Any patient who has been sexually active or has any findings on exam that indicate the possibility of sexual activity or sexual abuse should be tested for sexually transmitted diseases. In cases where sexual abuse is possible, a rape kit

Early pregnancy complications

When a pediatric patient presents to the doctor's office or emergency room with new-onset pelvic pain, the first test that should be performed is one for pregnancy. Given the potential for sexual abuse in any pediatric patient, even patients denying any history of sexual activity should still be evaluated for pregnancy. While abnormal vaginal bleeding can be a clue that pelvic pain may be secondary to an abnormal pregnancy, the absence of this or even a history of regular menses occurring within the last month should not exclude evaluation for pregnancy. Urine pregnancy tests are readily available and give almost immediate results. These are now sensitive down to a β-hCG level of 50. Hormonal levels less than this in patients who have not already been treated in this pregnancy are unlikely to be the source of pelvic pain. If the urine test for pregnancy is positive then the patient must be thoroughly assessed for pregnancy outside the uterus – an ectopic pregnancy. The patient may have a normal intrauterine pregnancy or may be spontaneously aborting the pregnancy; however, because an ectopic pregnancy has the greatest risk to the patient, its existence must be determined.

Of all pregnancies, 1.6% are located outside the uterus. Of these, 95% are located in the fallopian tube, usually in the ampulla. Ectopic pregnancies can also be found in the interstitial portion of the fallopian tube. While these are often called cornual pregnancies, their correct name is interstitial pregnancy. The only place to find a truly pathologic cornual pregnancy is in women with a rudimentary uterine horn where the pregnancy implants. Women with normal uteri who have implantation in the cornua will go on to have normal pregnancies. In rare cases the pregnancy can implant on the peritoneal surface in the abdomen or into the cervix after passing through the tubes and fundus of the uterus. Pregnancies have also been found on the ovary and in the broad ligament – a ligamentous pregnancy. In rare cases, a woman may have a twin gestation with one pregnancy in the uterus and one outside it – a heterotopic pregnancy. This occurs in one in 30,000 spontaneous pregnancies but is greatly increased to one in 5000 in pregnancies from assisted reproduction.

Ectopic pregnancies carry significant risk of morbidity and mortality. In addition to the risks to future fertility, women with ectopic pregnancies frequently require surgical care with the concomitant risks of surgery and anesthesia. If unrecognized, a ruptured ectopic pregnancy frequently requires transfusion and the infectious risks associated with this; 15% of maternal deaths are due to ectopic pregnancies [1]. The risk of death is greatest in teenagers with the risk being five times greater in African-American women compared to white women. After having one ectopic pregnancy, the patient has a significantly increased risk of future ectopic pregnancy. Reviews of women with ectopic pregnancies have found that 50–

Box 33.2 Risk factors for ectopic pregnancy

Previous pelvic infections such as pelvic inflammatory disease
Tubal sterilization
Advanced maternal age
Prior ectopic pregnancy
Pregnancy secondary to assisted reproduction
Pelvic surgery, especially tubal reconstruction
Smoking
Pregnancy with intrauterine device in place
Progestin-only contraceptive

80% have intrauterine pregnancies in the next pregnancy, while 10–15% have an ectopic pregnancy again and the rest are infertile [2].

Ectopic pregnancies most frequently develop as the result of abnormally functioning fallopian tubes. This can either be the result of injury from previous surgery or infection or hormonal effects on the tubes. Normal tubal function is dependent on normal action of the fine cilia within the tube. Implantation of the egg by the sperm typically occurs within the fallopian tube. The cilia are required to bring the impregnated egg into the uterine cavity for implantation. These cilia are easily damaged. Box 33.2 is a list of factors associated with ectopic pregnancies. The majority of these may have a direct effect on the functionality of the fallopian tubes and it can clearly be seen why they increase the risk of ectopic pregnancy. Others such as assisted reproduction and cigarette smoking are not so clear. Epidemiologic studies undoubtedly demonstrate a connection. Women with assisted reproduction have ectopic pregnancy rates as high as 4.6% [2] and smokers of at least a pack per day have a 2.5 times greater risk of an ectopic pregnancy than nonsmokers [3].

Unfortunately, there are no findings that specifically rule in or out the existence of an ectopic pregnancy. The clinician must use all tools available to appropriately treat the patient. Occasionally this includes a diagnostic laparoscopy when all other tests are inconclusive and the fear of rupture of the fallopian tube is high. While the risk of complications during a diagnostic laparoscopy in a young woman is low, the risk of an untreated ruptured ectopic pregnancy includes death, making the occasional negative laparoscopy justified.

After a positive urine pregnancy test, the next step in evaluation is a thorough history and physical exam. Information pertinent to evaluating early pregnancy includes the regularity of the menstrual cycle and when and how the last menstrual cycle occurred, a complete sexual history, and a history of birth control use. The patient should be questioned for other risk factors for ectopic pregnancy including previous abdominal or pelvic surgery or infection and previous ectopic pregnancy. Early physical complaints including amenorrhea, vaginal spotting, and pelvic cramping are also commonly found in normal intrauterine pregnancies. The degree of pain is typically greatly increased in patients with a ruptured ectopic pregnancy but as many studies on pain mapping in the pelvis have demonstrated, pain from one site in the pelvis can be referred to other areas and is not always reliable in localizing the problem. As ectopic pregnancies are located on one side of the pelvis, pain would be thought to be unilateral; however, bilateral pelvic pain is found in many patients with ectopic pregnancies. Patients with normal intrauterine pregnancies can also have significant pain from hemorrhagic or ruptured ovarian cysts. Hence, pain is not pathognomonic of an ectopic pregnancy.

The same is true for the findings on physical exam. Tenderness on exam can be found in patients with an ectopic pregnancy as well as a normal intrauterine pregnancy. The same is true with the palpation of an adnexal mass which could be an ectopic pregnancy or a functional ovarian cyst. Vital signs usually only aid in the diagnosis of an ectopic pregnancy once the pregnancy has ruptured. At that point, the patient will likely first become tachycardic. This is followed by hemodynamic instability and then persistent hypotension. As the bleeding increases peritoneal signs and cervical motion tenderness will likely develop. Most patients present before rupture, however, and the physical exam has limited diagnostic ability.

The most helpful tests in diagnosing an ectopic pregnancy are laboratory and radiologic tests, specifically the quantitative β-hCG and pelvic ultrasound. The single value of the quantitative β-hCG is often not helpful in differentiating between an intrauterine and an ectopic pregnancy, but serial measurements are invaluable in this determination. Viable pregnancies with quantitative β-hCG measurements greater than 2000 mIU/mL should be seen by vaginal ultrasound. Measurements greater than 6000 mIU/mL should be seen by abdominal ultrasound. However, if the pregnancy is not seen, this does not mean that the pregnancy is definitely ectopic. It does typically mean that the pregnancy is not normal. Here the history

is important in attaining a diagnosis. If the patient has a quantitative β-hCG above the discrimination zone and complains of significant bleeding, possibly passing blood and tissue vaginally, and the ultrasound and exam are negative, then the likely diagnosis is a complete abortion. If the patient is bleeding and her cervix is dilated and there is tissue still seen in the uterine cavity on ultrasound with normal adnexae, then the likely diagnosis is an incomplete abortion. In this case the patient may need to go to the operating room to complete the abortion in order to stop the bleeding. If the patient has a quantitative β-hCG above the discrimination zone with no history of vaginal bleeding or just a small amount of spotting, and nothing is seen in the uterus on ultrasound, then the possibility of an ectopic pregnancy greatly increases.

The best use of quantitative β-hCG is in serial measurements. Many patients present with the quantitative β-hCG below the discrimination zone. Others may have a quantitative β-hCG above the discrimination zone but the diagnosis is still unclear. These patients will require serial measurements of quantitative β-hCG. Kadar and Romero demonstrated that its level has an approximate doubling time of 1.98 days in early pregnancy [4]. However, there is a significant variability to this time which overlaps with the abnormal increase typically found in ectopic pregnancies; 15% of all normal pregnancies will show less than a 66% increase over two days while the same percentage of ectopic pregnancies will demonstrate a greater than 66% increase over the same time period. In their review, none of the patients whose initial quantitative β-hCG was less than 2000 mIU/mL and increased less than 50% over two days had viable intrauterine pregnancies. The most predictive finding for an ectopic pregnancy is a quantitative β-hCG that has plateaued [5]. When a patient presents with abnormal bleeding or pelvic pain and the initial pregnancy test is positive, an initial quantitative β-hCG is drawn and a pelvic ultrasound is performed. If the quantitative β-hCG is below 2000 mIU/mL and the ultrasound does not identify a pregnancy, as long as the patient is only minimally symptomatic, the quantitative β-hCG should be drawn every two days till it is above 2000 mIU/mL. At this point another ultrasound should be performed. If a pregnancy is not found in the uterus, the patient should be treated as if she has an ectopic pregnancy until proven otherwise. The same is true if the value never reaches 2000 mIU/mL but plateaus instead of falling.

Ultrasound has significantly increased the percentage of patients correctly diagnosed with an ectopic pregnancy and decreased the need for diagnostic surgery. Gynecologists and various physicians working in the emergency room should be trained in vaginal sonography. While additional experience in vaginal sonography may be necessary to be able to see an ectopic pregnancy, most physicians should be able to find the uterus and evaluate for the presence of an intrauterine pregnancy. If the quantitative β-hCG is above 2000 mIU/mL and the endometrial cavity is clearly seen to be vacant, an abnormal pregnancy must be suspected. The presentation of an ectopic pregnancy may be confused by the presence of a pseudosac within the endometrial cavity. This is an accumulation of fluid, presumably blood, in the cavity. It differs from a true gestational sac as the latter is eccentric because it implants into the endometrium and will not be seen in the middle of the cavity. The finding of a yolk sac or even a fetal pole with heartbeat within the endometrial cavity is obviously even more reassuring of an intrauterine pregnancy. The same would be true of diagnosing an ectopic pregnancy if the yolk sac or fetal pole were to be seen within a gestational sac within the adnexa. The classic ultrasonographic finding of an ectopic pregnancy is a bagel sign, where the trophoblastic tissue of the pregnancy within the tube resembles a bagel on ultrasound.

Another blood test used to diagnose abnormal pregnancies is that for serum progesterone. It is not as helpful as the quantitative β-hCG but, in a few cases, it can determine immediately whether the pregnancy is viable or not. Stovall demonstrated that a value below 5 ng/mL was found in only 0.67% of normal pregnancies while a value greater than 25 ng/mL had a positive predictive value for normal pregnancy of 98% [6]. It does not help with determining the location of the abnormal pregnancy and there is no value in serial measurement. There is also little value to results between 5 ng/mL and 25 ng/mL. Because of this, it is frequently not used in the assessment of ectopic pregnancy.

The last step in the diagnosis of ectopic pregnancy is surgery. In this case, diagnosis may be partnered with treatment. In cases where the diagnosis is still unclear after laboratory and radiologic testing and the suspicion for an ectopic pregnancy is high, the patient should proceed to the operating room. A simple D&C may be all that is required to achieve a diagnosis and avoid a more significant surgery or treatment with potentially toxic medications.

The tissue attained from a curettage should be floated in normal saline to evaluate for chorionic villi. The villi have a lacy appearance that floats in the saline. If available, the specimen may also be examined by a pathologist to evaluate for the presence of gestational tissue. If chorionic villi are found then it is extremely likely that the pregnancy was an abnormal intrauterine pregnancy and will have been terminated by the procedure. This technique is not fool-proof as a pregnancy may be missed if it is extremely early or by poor technique. If no pregnancy is found then treatment for an ectopic pregnancy is warranted.

While laparoscopy is considered the gold standard for diagnosis of an ectopic pregnancy, it is not perfect as very early pregnancies may not be seen. It involves all the adherent risks of a surgical procedure. If done, it should be performed with the intention to treat if an ectopic pregnancy is found. Surgical treatment typically consists of either opening the tube, removing the pregnancy and leaving the tube in place, called a salpingostomy, or removing the tube with the pregnancy inside, called a salpingectomy. The reason for leaving the tube in place would be to attempt to maintain future fertility. Because of the risk that the entire pregnancy may not be removed when performing a salpingostomy, if the patient does not desire future fertility, a salpingectomy should be performed. Ory et al followed patients after an ectopic pregnancy and did not find a difference in fertility rates in patients having undergone a salpingostomy versus a salpingectomy [7]. If the contralateral fallopian tube is normal it may actually be in the patient's best interest to remove the tube as Ory demonstrated that patients with a history of infertility actually had a higher incidence of ectopic pregnancy in future pregnancies if the tube is left *in situ*. This can be left up to the judgment of the surgeon.

The laparoscopic approach has become the standard of care for surgically treating the stable patient with an ectopic pregnancy. Unstable patients are still frequently treated via laparotomy. With the appropriate equipment, including a 10 mm suction to quickly remove blood clots, a ruptured ectopic can often be managed quickly laparoscopically by a skilled surgeon even if the patient is unstable, as long as the equipment is readily available. Appropriate patient selection is the most important variable in choosing the laparoscopic route. An unstable patient with a history of previous pelvic surgery that could delay locating the bleeding tube would likely benefit from a laparotomy to facilitate dissection. This should left to the discretion of the surgeon.

Medical treatment has become increasingly more popular in the treatment of patients with an ectopic pregnancy. Numerous medications have been used, some injected directly into the pregnancy either sonographically or laparoscopically. Intramuscular methotrexate has emerged as the standard for medical treatment of ectopic pregnancies. Numerous treatment regimens of methotrexate exist but our protocol has become commonly used around the country. It involves first confirming the presence of or at least having a high suspicion of an ectopic pregnancy. The methods for this have previously been described. Methotrexate is contraindicated in patients with significant liver disease or pre-existing bone marrow suppression. It should obviously not be used in patients where a ruptured tube is suspected; however, any pain is a relative contraindication. This is because there is always a risk that medical treatment will fail and tubal rupture may occur. The first indication that this may occur is pelvic pain, so patients already in pain make this assessment difficult. Other findings that have demonstrated a decrease in the success rate of this medical treatment include an adnexal mass greater than 4 cm, quantitative β-hCG greater than 15,000 mIU/mL, and fetal cardiac activity.

Before initiating treatment, blood should be drawn to assess renal and liver function (SGOT, BUN, creatinine). The patient should have a complete blood count demonstrating a white blood cell count above 2000/mL and platelets above 100,000. A quantitative β-hCG and blood type should also be drawn on the day of treatment. If the patient is Rh-negative she should receive $Rh_o(D)$ immune globulin although the risks of isoimmunization are extremely low in early pregnancy. The patient should be thoroughly counseled about the risks, especially about the risk of failure, which is approximately 5%, and tubal rupture. The more common side effects of methotrexate include leukopenia, thrombocytopenia, bone marrow aplasia, ulcerative stomatitis, diarrhea and hemorrhagic enteritis. They are related to the medication's inhibition of folate synthesis. The side effects occur in less than 1% of patients treated with a one-dose regimen for ectopic pregnancy. Patients should avoid folic acid which can counteract the effects of the medication. The patient should also be told to refrain from sexual intercourse and strenuous physical activity. Crampy pain is common

with methotrexate treatment but the patient should be told to report any excessive or prolonged pain or vaginal bleeding.

Once counseled and with the consent signed, the patient may receive the medication. Multiple dosing regimens have been used, the most common being a one-dose treatment of 50 mg/m^2 given intramuscularly. The patient then returns on the fourth day after treatment for a repeat quantitative β-hCG. This value is then repeated on the seventh day after treatment along with a repeat of the other pretreatment blood tests. It is not unusual to see a rise in the level from the day of treatment to the fourth day after treatment; however, the level is expected to drop at least 15% from the fourth to the seventh day after treatment. If it does not and the patient is still without significant symptoms or laboratory abnormalities, a repeat dose of the methotrexate may be given. An ultrasound should also be repeated on the seventh day to assure no significant increase in the size of any adnexal mass. If the level drops more than 15%, it should be checked weekly until it reaches 0. If the patient is retreated, the quantitative β-hCG should be checked again in a week. If this level also does not drop by at least 15%, the patient should be treated as a medical treatment failure and proceed to the operating room.

Methotrexate may also be used for a persistent ectopic pregnancy after salpingostomy. Because the risk of a persistent ectopic pregnancy is approximately 15%, patients should receive weekly testing of quantitative β-hCG after a salpingostomy until the level reaches 0. If the level plateaus or rises after the surgical procedure, methotrexate may be used as described previously as treatment. The other alternative would be to return to the operating room and remove the fallopian tube.

On rare occasions, the ectopic pregnancy will occur outside the tube. The most common locations include the cervix, ovary and within the abdominal cavity. Each of these is potentially more serious than a tubal ectopic pregnancy. Ultrasound is the primary tool for diagnosis for each.

A cervical ectopic pregnancy can be treated either surgically with a D&C or medically with the injection of methotrexate. The surgical risks are great in these cases as transfusion and hysterectomy are a serious possibility as well as maternal death. Embolization has been used to attempt to control bleeding. Methotrexate is now preferred to try and avoid the surgical risks. Risk factors for cervical pregnancy include previous elective pregnancy termination, prior cesarean section, *in utero* exposure to diethylstilbestrol, fibroids and assisted reproduction [8]. If a cervical pregnancy is expected, a referral to a high-risk center is appropriate as the management is often very difficult.

The same is true for abdominal pregnancies. While ovarian pregnancies are usually treated in a similar fashion to tubal pregnancies, abdominal pregnancies, whether formed initially in the abdomen or the result of a persistent tubal abortion, have a significant risk of major maternal morbidity and death. It must be treated surgically; however, unless a solitary blood supply to the placenta can be identified and ligated, it is better to leave the placenta in place. The abdomen frequently must simply be packed to control the bleeding. The risk of complications to all abdominal organs is great as well as the risk of subsequent infection. Again, if recognized, the patient should be managed at an institution with the availability of intensive care.

Spontaneous abortion of the pregnancy can present with symptoms similar to an ectopic pregnancy. The diagnostic steps would be similar to those patients being evaluated for ectopic pregnancy. Patients are more likely to complain of midline, cramp-like pain and greater vaginal bleeding and are more likely to report significant vaginal bleeding while the ultrasound may demonstrate tissue or blood within the uterine cavity.

Any vaginal bleeding in patients with an intrauterine pregnancy gives a diagnosis of threatened abortion. Thirty percent of all normal pregnancies that proceed to term have some bleeding in the first trimester so the patient should not be alarmed by early bleeding as long as an ectopic pregnancy has been ruled out. Because of the risk of genetic abnormalities to the fetus, very little is done to preserve pregnancies which are threatening to abort in the first trimester. If the rest of the exam is normal, patients should be reassured but told that if the pregnancy progresses to abortion, the patient may stay at home unless the bleeding becomes profuse and a curettage becomes necessary.

A viable pregnancy within the uterine cavity that has some vaginal bleeding but a closed cervical os is called a threatened abortion. If the patient has begun to actually pass tissue and presents with an open cervical os and tissue remaining in the uterine cavity on ultrasound, this is called an incomplete abortion. If the bleeding is light, these patients may be managed expectantly. Many physicians will give these patients misoprostol vaginally or methergine orally to complete the abortion although these techniques have not been well studied. If the patient is actively bleeding or has a significant amount of tissue in the uterus, she may require a suction D&C to complete the abortion.

Patients who present after significant bleeding at home with an empty cavity and a closed cervical os are likely to have had a complete abortion. Unless they present with the aborted tissue and pregnancy is confirmed, these patients must be treated as if they have a potential ectopic pregnancy and have serial quantitative β-hCG measurements. A precipitously dropping value supports the diagnosis of complete abortion.

Pelvic inflammatory disease

Pelvic inflammatory disease (PID) is an infection that begins on the cervix and ascends within the female genital tract, first causing an endometritis within the uterus, a salpingitis within the fallopian tubes and then, potentially, a generalized infection within the pelvic cavity and/or infection including the ovary, called a tubo-ovarian abscess. It is thought to be initiated by sexual transmission of either *Chlamydia trachomatis* or *Neisseria gonorrhoeae*, although these organisms are not always found in a culture of the infected area. Because of its higher incidence in sexually active adolescents and it serious sequelae, including infertility, it should be considered in the differential of all adolescents presenting with a complaint of new pelvic pain.

Adolescents and young women seem to be at the greatest risk of acquiring a sexually transmitted disease and having it progress to PID. There are approximately 9.5 million cases of sexually transmitted diseases in the United States each year among women and adolescents, 15–24 years of age [9]. Since *Chlamydia trachomatis* and *Neisseria gonorrhoeae* have the closest relationship to PID, the trends in infection with these organisms are related to PID diagnosis trends. In 2005, the CDC reported an increase of 5.2% in the incidence of chlamydia infections. While the national rate of chlamydia infection is 332.5 per 100,000 people, the number is highest in girls aged 15–19 where the incidence is 2796.6 per 100,000. African-American females had an incidence that was seven times that of white females and twice that of Hispanic females. Part of the increase in reported infections in the past few years is thought to be due to more widespread screening, but this is unlikely to account for the entire increase as the incidence of presentation to the emergency room for PID has also risen in recent years. The CDC last reported on incidence of PI in 2002. At that point it had dropped steadily from the 1980s till 2000 but had risen slightly in the last two years reported. In 2002, approximately 200,000 women were diagnosed with PID at the initial visit in the doctor's office and an additional 80,000 were diagnosed with PID in the hospital [10].

Along with the incidence of PID, the cost of treating STDs is increasing. The estimated annual cost reported by the CDC in 2005 was $14.1 billion [11]. This does not take into account the secondary costs from an estimated 100,000 women that become infertile every year as a result of PID. In addition to infertility, PID can lead to chronic pelvic pain and ectopic pregnancy due to pelvic and tubal adhesions and nonfunctional tubal cilia required to transport the fertilized egg through the tube and into the uterus. This also results in significant future medical costs in these female patients.

PID is thought to start as an asymptomatic cervical infection. It is unclear how long *C. trachomatis* and *N. gonorrhoeae* can exist on the cervix without causing symptoms or ascending into the uterus and above. It is also unclear what finally triggers the ascension of the infection. There are clear risk factors for PID which include multiple sexual partners, drug use, lack of barrier contraception, and partners or patient with a history of STD. It is not clear how these risk factors translate into ascension of an asymptomatic cervical infection.

Although the inciting infection of PID is thought to be either *C. trachomatis* or *N. gonorrhoeae*, PID is a multiorganism infection. The abscess formation around the tubes and ovaries typically includes anaerobic bacteria as well, although it is not clear what the source of these organisms is. It is also theorized that involvement of the ovary in this abscess requires a disruption of the ovarian cortex, as occurs with ovulation. The ascension of a cervical infection and progression to PID is an area which warrants further study.

Patients with PID typically present with complaints of recent-onset pelvic pain. This may be unilateral but is more often generalized to the entire pelvis. Dyspareunia is also a frequent complaint as well as vaginal discharge.

Patients may give a prolonged history of postcoital bleeding as evidence of a history of cervicitis. Recent midcycle spotting may also be reported as a result of endometritis as the infection ascends into the uterus. In advanced cases, the patient may report elevated temperatures and complain of chills as well as nausea and vomiting. A thorough sexual history is an important part of this initial evaluation to determine if the patient is at risk for PID.

PID can present with a variety of signs on examination. Lower abdominal pain is a typical finding. With generalized peritonitis, the exam may even demonstrate significant guarding and rebound tenderness. On pelvic exam, the cervix will typically appear inflamed and bleed easily on palpation. Mucopurulent discharge from the cervix is also a common finding on speculum exam and a sample of this fluid should demonstrate many white blood cells on microscopic culture. Cultures should be sent specifically looking for *C. trachomatis* and *N. gonorrhoeae*. If midcycle spotting is the chief complaint, an endometrial biopsy may be performed. Endometrial carcinoma is exceedingly rare in the adolescent population but the sample may be sent for evaluation for pathologic organisms and the histology may demonstrate signs of infection.

The pelvic exam will demonstrate adnexal tenderness, usually bilateral, and cervical motion tenderness. As other causes of pelvic pain such as ovarian cysts will also present with pelvic pain, the presence of cervical motion tenderness is very telling for infection. If the exam is not done carefully, patients will frequently report cervical motion tenderness with any cause of pelvic pain. The patient should be distracted with unrelated questions while the cervix is moved; true cervical motion tenderness will not be missed by this technique and may be differentiated from other types of pelvic pain.

Laboratory and radiologic tests should also be performed, including a complete blood count to evaluate the number of white blood cells and their differential. The patient may also demonstrate an elevated C-reactive protein and erythrocyte sedimentation rate. Ultrasound should be performed to evaluate for other cause of acute pelvic pain such as an ovarian cyst. The presence of a tubo-ovarian abscess (TOA) can also be determined to aid in the appropriate treatment. Ultrasound is important in the rare presentation of a ruptured TOA which can present with a pelvic complex on ultrasound as well as free fluid in the abdomen and pelvis that has the consistency of pus. This is potentially a surgical emergency. PID is often confused on presentation with acute appendicits. A CAT scan with contrast can often differentiate between the two, but occasionally a diagnostic laparoscopy is needed to make the diagnosis.

PID may be treated as either an outpatient or inpatient depending on the severity of the infection. The main risk of outpatient treatment is progression of the infection. It should only be offered to patients who are thought to be compliant with taking the medication and willing to return for follow-up evaluation within the following three days. If the patient is nauseated and vomiting, she is unlikely to tolerate oral medication and should be admitted to hospital for intravenous antibiotics. Also, a temperature greater than 101°F, symptoms of peritonitis, significantly elevated white blood cell count and adnexal complex are considered to be evidence of more advanced infection and the patient should be initially treated as an inpatient with intravenous antibiotics. Because of the significant risk of infertility due to tubal damage from the infection, many physicians believe that adolescents should be treated as inpatients to assure appropriate use of and response to the medications.

Because infection that has spread to the upper genital tract has been found to involve not only the inciting organisms, *N. gonorrhoeae* and *C. trachomatis*, but also Gram-negative, Gram-positive facultative and anaerobic bacteria, treatment should cover infection with all these types of organism. Typical outpatient treatment includes cefoxitin 2 g IM with probenecid 1 g then doxycycline 100 mg by mouth twice a day for two weeks. An alternative treatment may include levofloxacin 500 mg daily and metronidazole 500 mg three times per day, both for two weeks. Inpatient treatment options include cefoxitin 2 g IV every 6 h or cefotetan 2 g IV every 12 h, both with oral or intravenous doxycycline 100 mg every 12 h. Another option is clindamycin 900 mg intravenous every 8 h plus gentamicin 1.5 mg/kg every 8 h. For TOA, McNeeley et al reported an increased rate in successfully treating women medically when ampicillin 2 g every 6 h was added to gentamicin and clindamycin [12].

Tubo-ovarian abscesses may complicate the management of PID, most significantly because an abscess may lead to sepsis and death in rare untreated cases. Historically, the treatment of tubo-ovarian abscesses that were not responsive to medications was surgery. While this still may become the best option for some patients, the intermediary step of drainage via interventional radiology is more frequently utilized. Because the blood supply to an abscess cavity is limited, which in turn may limit the ability to treat the infection by antibiotics, the old principle of incising and draining abscesses as primary treatment may apply in these cases as well. Via interventional radiology, the abscess cavity may frequently be incised either vaginally, usually with ultrasound guidance, or abdominally with CAT scan guidance. Once incised, a catheter should be left in place to allow continued drainage until the abscess cavity empties. This technique may be limited if the abscess cavity is separated from the vagina or abdominal wall by bowel. Also, if the abscess has multiple loculations, complete drainage may not occur. Both Perez-Medina et al [13] and Goharkhay et al [14] demonstrated more rapid improvement and greater avoidance of surgical management with percutaneous drainage and antibiotics as compared to antibiotics alone. Kumar et al demonstrated that patients with abscess cavities greater than 6.5 cm and a temperature greater than 101.2°F were more likely to fail conservative management with antibiotics alone and require percutaneous drainage [15]. Goharkhay also demonstrated a more rapid time to recovery and therefore shorter hospital stay with drainage. When a tubo-ovarian abscess is discovered by radiologic testing, drainage of the cavity should always be considered as an option for treatment and should be attempted prior to progressing to surgery in a stable patient.

Surgery should be used as the last method of choice for treating tubo-ovarian abscesses, especially when treating teenagers and young women. This is because the surgery frequently results in a unilateral and occasionally bilateral salpingo-oophorectomy. These cases are frequently some of the more difficult surgeries that a gynecologist or pediatric surgeon can face. This is because of the blurred surgical planes and friable surfaces caused by the inflammation due to the infection. It is often very difficult to control the bleeding in the surgical field when simply attempting to lyze the adhesions forming the tubo-ovarian complex. The tube must typically be removed, but because the ovary is usually densely adherent in the complex, it must often be removed with the specimen to maintain hemostasis.

The route of surgery depends on the training of the surgeon. Minimally invasive surgery is preferred to minimize recovery time but may not allow for the most appropriate management of the infection due to the technical limitations of laparoscopy and the skill of the surgeon. If a laparotomy is performed, a vertical incision allows for the best exposure as well as giving the surgeon the ability to extend the surgical field into the upper abdomen when necessary. A culture of the infected cavity should be attained to assure the appropriate use of antibiotics after the procedure. Fallopian tubes enlarged due to infection should be removed as the resulting hydrosalpinx will not be functional and may have actual negative effects on assisted reproduction in the future, should this become necessary. The abdomen should be irrigated profusely with saline and surgical drains should be left in place to continue to drain any remaining infected areas after the procedure is concluded. Postoperatively, the patient should be continued on antibiotics and monitored closely to assure continued improvement.

PID can have serious long-term consequences in young women. Long-term infertility is a serious risk, especially when tubo-ovarian abscesses have developed. Although early PID may be confused with pain from hemorrhagic ovarian cysts, if there is any doubt in the diagnosis, it is in the best interest of the patient to treat for PID even if the diagnosis has not been confirmed, as this often may not occur until the infection has progressed and more damage to her pelvis has occurred. While there is risk in unnecessarily treating with antibiotics, this risk is outweighed by the risk to the patient if PID exists and is not treated.

Ovarian torsion

Another important cause of acute pelvic pain in adolescents and young women is ovarian torsion. Because of the anatomic structure of the female pelvis, a twisting of either adnexa can lead to a decrease in blood supply to the ovary and fallopian tube. This decreased blood supply due to twisting is called torsion. If untreated, it can lead to necrosis and permanent loss of function of the ovary.

Much of the epidemiologic information on adnexal torsion comes from a review by Hibbard of 128 cases at the University of Southern California Medical Center [16]. He found that the average age of the patient presenting with adnexal torsion was the mid 20s but it occurred in all ages from childhood to the postmenopausal years. Pregnant women seem especially susceptible to torsion, comprising 20% of the total presenting population. Sixty percent of patients have an ovarian tumor, the most common being the dermoid. Ovarian cancer was found in only 2.5% of

the patients with tumors. Hibbard also found that the torsion involved the right ovary 60% of the time.

Patients typically present to the emergency room complaining of acute onset of severe pelvic pain, usually localized to one side of the pelvis. It is not uncommon for the pain to be so severe that it is accompanied by nausea and vomiting which may confuse the presentation with a pathologic condition of the bowel. The patient frequently complains of intermittent pain as the adnexa twists and untwists which may have been occurring for hours or days; 90% of patients have a palpable mass in the adnexa. Even if a tumor is not present, the patient usually has a functional cyst of the ovary that may be felt. Even in the rare normal ovary that twists, the increased venous and lymphatic compression over arterial compression leads to edema and enlargement of the ovary. If the condition progresses, the ovary will become hypoxic and eventually necroses. At this stage the patient may present with a low-grade fever and elevated white blood cell count.

The patient with adnexal torsion frequently presents with significant enough symptoms that explorative surgery is warranted. However, if examined between episodes of torsion, the diagnosis might be missed. Ultrasound may aid in the diagnosis if scanned during a period of torsion as decreased or no blood flow may be seen in the ovary with a Doppler study. Occasionally the ovary will appear enlarged due to the edema even if it is not currently twisted.

The most common condition that presents similarly to the twisted ovary is a hemorrhagic corpus luteum. In this case surgery is not warranted unless the ovary is bleeding and the patient is becoming unstable, a very rare event. Pain from a hemorrhagic corpus luteum is much more common than torsion, typically occurring in the second half of the menstrual cycle. Unfortunately the two conditions are difficult to distinguish from each other, and if there is concern for torsion then the patient should be taken for a diagnostic laparoscopy.

During laparoscopy, in a premenopausal patient, the goal is to save the ovary if possible. While it has been theorized that an untwisted, infarcted ovary may lead to dissemination of the clot within the ovarian vein, this has not been found to be the case. Untwisting is therefore always warranted to assess for return of normal coloring in the adnexa. Only if the ovary is completely necrotic should it be removed. Any mass on the ovary should be removed both to achieve a pathologic diagnosis and to attempt to assure that the ovary will not twist again. If the adnexa has sufficient laxity to twist again, it can be stabilized with sutures. Because there is a 10% incidence of torsion of the contralateral ovary, it should also be evaluated and stabilized as well if any laxity is present. This procedure should usually be performed laparoscopically as pelvic adhesions from previous surgery or other conditions of the pelvis that would make a surgeon less likely to feel comfortable with laparoscopy would also make torsion very unlikely.

In the adolescent or young woman presenting with acute, intermittent pelvic pain, torsion must always be considered. When the pain is right sided, the condition needs to be differentiated from an acute appendicitis; however, the treatment for this is also surgical and the diagnosis can be made in the operating room. Left-sided pelvic pain in a child is more likely to be adnexal in origin and has a higher risk of being from torsion. Given the low morbidity of a diagnostic laparoscopy, progressing to the operating room rapidly for a diagnosis may make the difference in the patient being able to keep both ovaries.

Conclusion

Acute pelvic pain in female children and adolescents is a common reason for presentation to the emergency room. Pregnancy is often responsible for this pain and its presence should be immediately evaluated with a urine pregnancy test. A thorough history and physical must be attained. In the young patient all resources, including recruiting the caregiver of the child, should be utilized to achieve this goal. Laboratory and radiologic tests are often crucial for reaching the correct diagnosis. Although pregnancy, infection and adnexal torsion are the most common causes for acute pelvic pain, all possible etiology must be addressed to assure proper care for the patient.

Assessing pain in a child or adolescent can be very difficult and only by using all available resources may a clinician be successful in the care of the young female patient.

References

1. National Center for Health Statistics. *Annual Summary of Births, Marriages, Divorces and Deaths: United States, 1989.* Hyattsville, MD: US Dpartment of Health and Human Services, Public Health Service, 1990, vol 38, p. 23.

2. Chow WH, Daling JR, Cates W Jr et al. Epidemiology of ectopic pregnancy. *Epidemiol Rev* 1987;**9**:70–94.

3. Coste J, Job-Spira N, Fernandez H. Increased risk of ectopic pregnancy with maternal cigarette smoking. *Am J Public Health* 1991;**81**:199–201.

4. Kadar N, Romero R. Further observations on serial human chorionic gonadotropin patterns in ectopic pregnancies and spontaneous abortions. *Fertil Steril* 1988;**50**:367–370.

5. Kadar N, Caldwell BV, Romero R. A method of screening for ectopic pregnancy and its indications. *Obstet Gynecol* 1981;**58**:162–165.

6. Stoval TG, Ling FW, Carson SA et al. Serum progesterone and uterine curettage in differential diagnosis of ectopic pregnancy. *Fertil Steril* 1992;**57**:456–458.

7. Ory SJ, Nnadi E, Herrmann R et al. Fertility after ectopic pregnancy. *Fertil Steril* 1993;**60**(2):231–235.

8. Parent JT, Ou CS, Levy J et al. Cervical pregnancy analysis: a review and report of five cases. *Obstet Gynecol* 1983;**62**:79–82.

9. Weinstock H, Berman S, Cates W Jr. Sexually transmitted diseases among American youth: incidence and prevalence estimates 2000. *Perspect Sex Reprod Health* 2004;**36**:6–10.

10. Centers for Disease Control and Prevention. *National STD Surveillance Reports.* Available at www.cdc.gov/std.

11. Chesson HW, Blandford JM, Gift TL, Tao G, Irwin KL. The estimated direct medical cost of STDs among American youth, 2000. Paper presented at the 2004 National STD Prevention Conference, Philadelphia, PA, March 8–11, 2004.

12. McNeeley SG, Hendrix SL, Mazzoni MM, Kmak DC, Ransom SB. Medically sound, cost effective treatment for pelvic inflammatory disease and tuboovarian abscess. *Am J Obstet Gynecol* 1998;**178**(6):1272–1278.

13. Perez-Medina T, Huertas MA, Bajo JM. Early ultrasound-guided transvaginal drainage of tubo-ovarian abscesses: a randomized study. *Ultrasound Obstet Gynecol* 1996;**7**(6):398–400.

14. Goharkhay N, Verma U, Maggiorotto F. Comparison of CT- or ultrasound-guided drainage with concomitant intravenous antibiotics vs. intravenous antibiotics alone in the management of tubo-ovarian abscesses. *Ultrasound Obstet Gynecol* 2007;**29**(1):65–69.

15. Kumar RR, Kim JT, Haukoos JS et al. Factors affecting the successful management of intra-abdominal abscesses with antibiotics and the need for percutaneous drainage. *Dis Colon Rectum* 2006;**49**(2):183–189.

16. Hibbard LT. Adnexal torsion. *Am J Obstet Gynecol* 1985;**152**:456.

CHAPTER 34

Vulva Disorders in Children

Raymond H. Kaufman
The Methodist Hospital and Baylor College of Medicine, Houston, TX, USA

Introduction

This chapter will focus on diseases involving the vulva, and not include those related to the vagina.

There are many disease processes that can involve the vulva in the child and adolescent. Berenson has suggested a breakdown of these conditions into four major categories. These include infectious disorders, ulcerations, dermalogic disorders, and urethral disorders. I have added a fifth – tumors. Some of the disease processes which will be discussed are listed in Box 34.1.

Infectious disorders

Candidiasis

Candidiasis is not a common problem seen in the child. It is generally seen in infants under the age of three and may present as an erythematous rash. Satellite pustules are often present. It is associated with pruritus of the vulvar skin.

Treatment consists of the application of any of the potent antifungal creams that are available both over the counter and by prescription.

Human papillomavirus infections

HPV infections may be passed on to the newborn by vertical transmission through the birth canal or by sexual molestation. Transmission from mother to infant can occur but is very uncommon. Condyloma can be seen in young children secondary to infection during the course of delivery; however, even in the presence of overt condyloma in the mother, the frequency of this occurring in the child is probably less than one in 100. Infection transmitted to the newborn from the mother usually presents in the form of genital warts within one to two years of birth. When examining the infant with condyloma acuminata, careful attention should be paid looking for evidence of sexual molestation. If no evidence of this is found, the likelihood of transmission through sexual contact is remote.

The diagnosis of condyloma acuminata can usually be made quite easily by visual inspection (Fig. 34.1a) It is rarely necessary to obtain a biopsy to confirm the diagnosis.

There are several options available for the management of the infant or child with vulvar condyloma acuminata. The first would be observation if the child is asymptomatic. Over the course of one to two years, spontaneous regression will occur in approximately 75% of cases. When the child is symptomatic (pruritus, pain, discharge) and/or the family is apprehensive about these they can be removed.

Treatment

If treatment is required, there are several options available, none of which is ideal since the recurrence rate following treatment is quite high. The application of bichloroacetic acid or trichloroacetic acid topically to the warts can be done in the office but extreme care should be taken to avoid contact with the adjacent normal skin. Likewise, a 15–20% solution of podophyllin in benzoin can be applied topically. Both of these treatments often result in local burning which soon subsides. If podophyllin is used it should be washed off in approximately eight hours. Cryotherapy utilizing liquid nitrogen or a carbon dioxide

Pediatric, Adolescent, & Young Adult Gynecology. Edited by
A. Altchek and L. Deligdisch. © 2009 Blackwell Publishing,
ISBN: 978-1-4051-5347-8.

probe can be performed but often it is a difficult approach in the office in the young child. Eradication of the lesions with the carbon dioxide laser is effective (Fig. 34.1b). This should be done in the operating room under general anesthesia. Imiquimod has not been extensively utilized in managing condyloma in the child, as this does require application three times weekly and results in considerable vulvar irritation.

Molluscum contagiosum

Molluscum contagiosum is a proliferative process of the skin resulting in the formation of multiple papules, frequently with umbilicated surfaces (Fig. 34.2). In adults it is usually sexually transmitted but in children it may be obtained by close proximity of the child to an infected individual or by autoinoculation from lesions elsewhere on the child's body. It is caused by a pox virus that produces self-limiting tumors of the genital and perianal tissues.

Following the inoculation of the virus there may be an incubation period extending for many months. Lesions not uncommonly will regress but this usually takes place over a course of 9–12 months. If the child is asymptomatic, they are probably best left alone in the genital area. However, they can be removed by curettage after the application of a topical local anesthetic.

Ulcerations

The most common ulcerative disease seen in the child is herpes simplex virus (HSV) infection. This can be transmitted to the infant via direct contact with an individual who has this infection, especially if sexual molestation has taken place. In the infant or young child diagnosed with a HSV infection, the possibility of sexual molestation should be investigated and the proper authorities notified.

Herpes presents in the child and adolescent in a fashion similar to that seen in the adult. Often there are

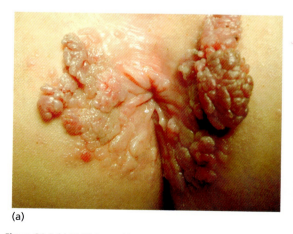

(a)

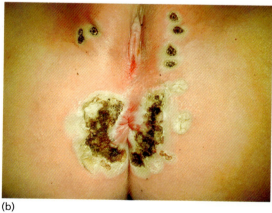

(b)

Figure 34.1 (a) Multiple condyloma acuminata noted on the perineum and perianal region in a child. (b) Condyloma acuminata after treatment with the carbon dioxide laser in the operating room (courtesy of Dr Robert Zurawin, Houston, TX).

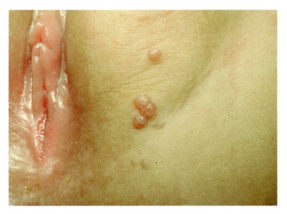

Figure 34.2 Molluscum contagiosum in a child. Slight umbilication is noted in the lower papules (courtesy of Dr Robert Zurawin, Houston, TX).

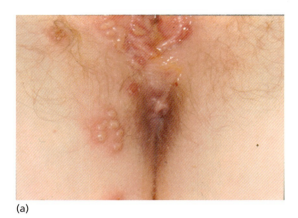

(a)

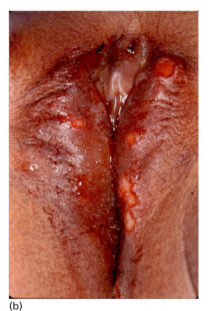

(b)

Figure 34.3 (a) Primary herpes genitalis. This five-year-old child had been sexually molested. A cluster of vesicles is noted lateral to the anus on the right as well as scattered superficial ulcers above. (b) Primary herpes. This is a 17-year-old adolescent demonstrating the presence of numerous superficial painful ulcers scattered over the vulva.

prodromal symptoms of pain and burning in the vulvar area followed by the development of multiple vesicles on a red base. These vesicles soon rupture, leading to shallow painful ulcerations (Fig. 34.3) which, in the instance of a primary infection, may take 10–20 days to completely resolve. Cultures should always be taken from the lesions to verify the diagnosis. Both HSV I and HSV II can involve the genitalia, as they do in the adult.

Treatment of primary infection is similar to that provided to the adult. Aciclovir, valaciclovir or famciclovir can be utilized. If aciclovir is used, it is given orally in a dose of 200 mg five times a day for 7–10 days for primary infection.

The recurrent disease can occur and, as in the adult, it is much milder in its clinical course than is the primary infection. This also develops as vesicles on a red base that are painful and rapidly rupture, leaving shallow and painful ulcers. The recurrent infection will usually resolve spontaneously within a week; however, the course of the infection and symptoms of pain can be shortened by the use of the medications listed above. If aciclovir is used, 200 mg are given orally five times daily for a period of five days.

Apthous ulceration

Apthous ulceration can be seen in the child and adolescent but it is most common in the adolescent girl. It may present as a minor or major form. The minor form presents as shallow ulcerations that may last for days before spontaneously regressing. Similar shallow ulcerations can be seen in the mouth as well. These are frequently referred to as apthous ulcers. The major variety of apthous results in the development of a large deep ulcer that is often similar in appearance to the ulcerations seen in the patient with Behçet disease (Fig. 34.4). One of the

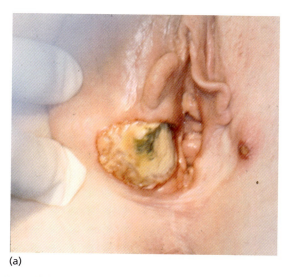
(a)

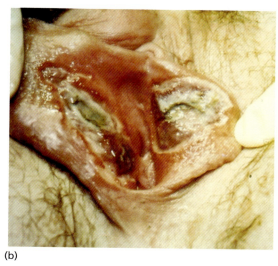
(b)

Figure 34.4 (a) Apthous ulceration. A large necrotic-appearing ulcer is noted in this child. Treatment with infiltration of Kenalog suspension beneath the ulcer resulted in rapid disappearance. (b) Behçet disease. Several deep necrotic ulcers are noted in this 13-year-old child.

major differences between this and Behçet disease is the fact that the individual with apthousis rarely if ever has systemic manifestations of the disease such as arthritis, renal or central nervous system abnormalities.

The apthous ulcers begin as small vesicles or papules that ulcerate, become craterous, and are usually covered by a necrotic slough. They vary from a few millimeters in diameter in the minor variety to several centimeters in the major variety (Fig. 34.4a). These tend to occur and recur at irregular intervals and are associated with extensive pain. When the ulcers of apthousis major ultimately heal, the healing process may be followed by significant scarring and labial perforation. These individuals have significant pain. Oral lesions are also frequently seen in association with this.

The management of apthousis minor usually consists of warm sitz baths and, if the lesions are painful, the application of a topical lidocaine ointment or gel. The management of apthousis major is somewhat more complicated and difficult. Several approaches have been suggested, including injection of 10 mg of triamcinolone acetonide diluted to 2 mL with 1% lidocaine under the base of the ulcer. Systemic steroids can also be used to treat this. Usually with injection of the steroids the ulcers will slowly heal but may very well recur in time.

The Epstein–Barr virus rarely involves the vulva. When it does, there is the development of shallow ulcerations that are difficult to distinguish from those of herpes genitalis. The diagnosis is made on the basis of culture.

Dermatologic disorders

Lichen sclerosus

Lichen sclerosus is probably the most frequently seen dermatosis involving the vulva in children. Powell and Wojnarowska found a prevalence of approximately one case of lichen sclerosus in 900 children in their community in England [1]. They noted an increase in referral of children with lichen sclerosus through their pediatric vulvar clinic over time, possibly due to increased recognition by practicing physicians that lichen sclerosus may involve the genital area of children.

Lichen sclerosus must be distinguished from the vulvar changes associated with sexual abuse. Ecchymotic areas, erosions, and fissures may sometimes be seen in lichen sclerosus and following sexual abuse. One of the distinguishing features between the two is the fact that with lichen sclerosus the hymen is usually intact and has not been traumatized. However, it must be kept in mind that

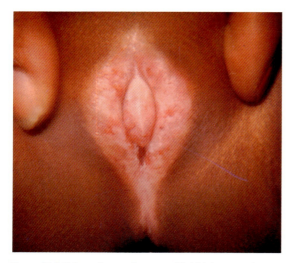

Figure 34.5 Lichen sclerosus. Four-year-old child demonstrating changes of lichen sclerosus extending around the anal opening.

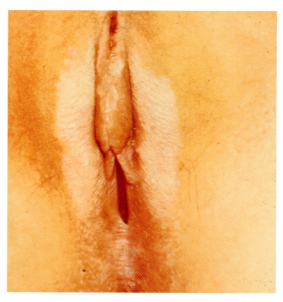

Figure 34.6 Lichen sclerosus. This ten-year-old child complained of intense vulvar pruritus. Typical changes of lichen sclerosus are noted involving primarily the labia majora.

sexual abuse and lichen sclerosus can occasionally be seen in the same child.

The etiology of lichen sclerosus is unknown, but it appears to be an autoimmune disease and individuals with lichen sclerosus have been found to have an increased presence of other autoimmune disease, such as thyroid disease, vitiligo, and rheumatoid arthritis. There may be a genetic component to the disease since it is not uncommonly found in other members of the family and has been reported in twins. Children with lichen sclerosus have an increased prevalence of atopy as do members of their family. A study of 70 children with lichen sclerosus by Powell and Wojnarowska found that, in all patients, the mean onset of development of symptoms was five years and the mean age of diagnosis was 6.7 years [1].

As in the adult, the most common presenting symptoms are itching and soreness. Other presenting symptoms and complaints include genital erosion, extragenital lichen sclerosus, constipation, and pain on defecation.

Lichen sclerosus presents with findings similar to those seen in the adult. There is a white discoloration of the skin of the labia majora, which may be relatively localized or may be diffuse and extend down around the rectum in a figure-of-eight fashion (Figs 34.5, 34.6). The tissue has a white crinkled appearance and often focal areas of ecchymosis and telangiectasia are seen. This is occasionally

noted as well as abrasions if the child has been scratching the tissue. Often the labia minora have been absorbed into the labia majora and are no longer visible. Phimosis may be present. Up to 8–10% of the children may have evidence of extragenital lichen sclerosus. The histopathology is the same as that seen in the adult. There is thinning of the lining squamous epithelium with flattening of the epithelial folds, and hyperkeratosis. The underlining dermis has a relatively acellular appearance and deep to this there is an inflammatory infiltrate of lymphocytes and some plasma cells. Follicular plugging is often seen (Fig. 34.7).

Treatment

New approaches to the treatment of lichen sclerosus in the child or adolescent have been utilized over recent years. For many years it was thought that in time the changes of lichen sclerosus would spontaneously regress, especially after the child had passed through the menarche. This is not true and current studies have demonstrated that lichen sclerosus will persist in most young girls well after menarche. Powell and Wojnarowska followed 18 patients who presented through puberty [1]. Only two showed complete resolution of the symptoms and signs of lichen sclerosus. In many of these, mild symptoms persisted and

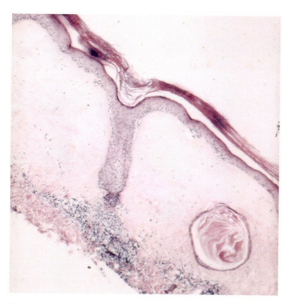

Figure 34.7 Lichen sclerosus. The biopsy of the vulva of this three-year-old child demonstrates all the features associated with lichen sclerosus – thinning of the epithelium, flattening of the epithelial folds, hyperkeratosis, and acellular pink staining zone beneath the epithelium, follicular plugging, inflammatory infiltrate in the deeper portion of the dermis.

in approximately 30% of adults treated with clobetasol [3]. In the child and adolescent, complete remission occurred in about 20–25% of patients. Clobetasol ointment resulted in disappearance of the pruritus and soreness in this group of patients. It has no influence whatsoever on persistence of the disease when the young woman goes through the menarche. Pimecrolimus 1% cream has recently been used for treatment of lichen sclerosus in childhood. Boms et al reported on four prepubertal girls treated with this medication twice daily [4]. After three to four months, all four patients had complete remission of symptoms of itching, pain, and inflammation. Only minor change was noted in the white appearance of the vulva. Tacrolimus 0.1% cream used once daily has also been found to be effective in a small group of prepubertal girls. One of the problems with both tacrolimus and pimecrolimus is that they often result in local burning and youngsters find this difficult to tolerate.

Contact dermatitis

Contact dermatitis can be either allergic or irritant in nature. In most cases of allergic contact dermatitis signs and symptoms develop 48 hours after contact with the allergen. An example of this is poison ivy. In most instances, contact irritant dermatitis is a result of some irritating substance or chemical that comes in contact with the vulva. Several examples of this include soaps, perfumed toilet paper, topical antibiotic ointments, and bubble baths. The symptoms usually begin shortly after the vulva comes in contact with these substances. The symptoms of pruritus and burning rapidly develop. The areas affected become erythematous, at times edematous, and small vesicles may develop that rupture and exude fluid. Secondary pustules may also develop. This should be distinguished from atopic dermatitis and generally the fact that it is restricted to the vulva and developed after contact with an irritant allows the diagnosis to be made.

Treatment consists of removal and no further use of the contact irritant that provoked the symptoms. The use of moderate level topical corticosteroids is of help in alleviating the symptoms of pruritus and burning.

Psoriasis

This is a multifactorial genetic disorder and may be seen in childhood. When it involves the vulva, disease is usually present elsewhere. It presents as red plaques that are

others were asymptomatic. It appears that the presence of persistent lichen sclerosus does not interfere with the ability to engage in sexual intercourse or have an uneventful vaginal delivery.

One of the ultra-potent corticosteroids is recommended for the treatment of lichen sclerosus in the child and adolescent. Clobetasol propionate ointment 0.05% has been used successfully in this age group [2]. Our approach is to recommend application of the ointment twice daily for a period of two weeks, at bedtime for two weeks, and then every other day for one month. At the end of that time, the child is re-evaluated for both the presence of symptoms and regression of the vulvar changes of lichen sclerosus. Smith and Quint reported a 93% improvement in symptoms and skin appearance within four to seven weeks after treatment in 15 girls [2]. In a small series of cases with long-term follow-up of 11 cases, two had no further vulvar symptoms after the initial treatment, five had one or two total flares, three had three to eight flares per year, and one was unresponsive to therapy. We have found complete regression of the lichen sclerosus

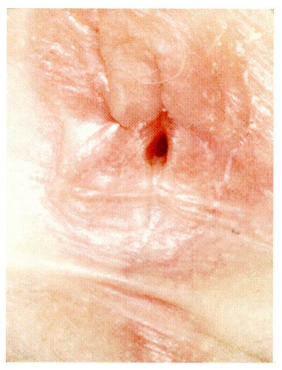

Figure 34.8 Labial agglutination, demonstrating fusion of the labia minora in the midline. A small opening is still present so that urination was not impeded in this child (courtesy of Dr Robert Zurawin, Houston, TX).

well defined and often covered by silvery scales. If one lifts the scales off, small pinpoint areas of bleeding are noted. Psoriasis may be associated with intense pruritus of the vulva. The diagnosis can usually be substantiated by looking for and identifying other areas of the body that have lesions characteristic of psoriasis. The management of this disorder is best left to a dermatologist.

Labial agglutination

Labial agglutination involves the adherence of the labia minora in the midline (Fig. 34.8). This most commonly occurs in the posterior portion of the vulva but at times may extend up to and literally obliterate the introitus of the vulva. When this occurs urinary retention is likely to develop. When the agglutination is extensive but not complete, urine may collect behind the labial skin and dribbling of urine occurs. It must be emphasized that

separation of the labia manually should not be attempted in the office.

The appropriate treatment is the application of conjugated estrogen in small amounts directly to the line of adhesion twice daily. It is important not to overuse the estrogen since a small percentage is absorbed and can result in breast budding and development. The child should be checked again in a period of two to four weeks to determine progress and also to observe whether or not any secondary effects have developed from use of the topical estrogen. In most instances, the labia will completely separate but recurrence is reasonably high. To help prevent this, the use of an ointment such as Desitin or A&D ointment applied to the edges of the lips can be of value. When recurrence occurs or the condition does not respond well to the topical estrogen, it may be necessary to surgically separate the labia. This should be done in the hospital under anesthesia. Here again recurrence is quite high and the parents must be instructed to separate the labia on a daily basis and apply an emollient ointment to the edges to help prevent this recurrence.

In most instances, where the patient is totally asymptomatic and has only a partial labial agglutination, no therapy is necessary. Once the child begins to produce her own endogenous estrogen, the labia will spontaneously separate.

Urethral disorders

Prolapse of urethral mucosa

Prolapse of urethral mucosa is in essence a sliding out of the urethral mucosa through the external meatus. It is seen most often in the premenarchal female and may be related to lack of estrogen. There are other theories that have been suggested regarding its etiology but none has been conclusively confirmed.

A urethral prolapse usually presents as an edematous red ring of tissue surrounding the external urethral meatus (Fig. 34.9). Ulceration and necrosis may occur and, not uncommonly, abnormal bleeding can be attributed to it. In most instances, there is little in the way of pain or discomfort associated with prolapse of the urethral mucosa but some patients may have difficulty in urinating, especially if there is significant edema of the tissue. The diagnosis can be established by locating the urethral meatus in relation to the presenting mass.

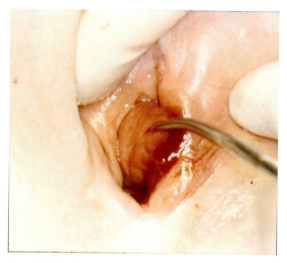

Figure 34.9 Prolapse of urethral mucosa. The clamp points to the opening into the urethra.

Treatment

Hot sitz baths to ease congestion and edema often will result in decrease of the size of the mass; however, usually it will not spontaneously disappear. The use of topical estrogen to the lesion may be of some help, especially if there is only a small area of urethral prolapse. The preferred method of treatment is excision. This should be done under anesthesia with a catheter in place. The redundant tissue is excised and the mucosa of the urethra is then attached to the mucosa of the vestibule using interrupted 4-0 absorbable sutures. Complications rarely occur but may consist of urethral stricture with stenosis, urinary incontinence, urinary retention, and recurrence of prolapse.

Simple ligation of the prolapsed mucosa over a Foley catheter has also been effective. A purse-string suture is passed around the prolapsed mucosa at the level of the external meatus around the Foley catheter. The balloon is then deflated and as the tissue undergoes necrosis, the catheter and necrotic tissue are spontaneously discharged. This usually takes two to five days and is certainly not a preferred approach to management.

Paraurethral cyst

Paraurethral cysts may occasionally be seen and present as small cystic structures most often in the region of the opening of Skene's duct in the vulvar vestibule. They are of little clinical significance and unless they enlarge and cause problems, such as difficulty urinating or discomfort, they are best left alone.

Tumors

Hemangioma

Hemangioma of the vulva is not at all uncommon in the child and adolescent. The hemangioma is actually a malformation of blood vessel origin and is not considered a true neoplasm by many. The most common type seen in childhood is the strawberry hemangioma. This gets its name from its resemblance to a strawberry and is most often observed shortly after birth. It is seen as an elevated bright red to dark red soft tumor mass measuring in diameter from a few millimeters to several centimeters (Fig. 34.10a). It may grow rapidly in early infancy and then usually undergoes spontaneous regression over several years. Andrews and co-workers followed 153 untreated children with strawberry hemangioma and in 63% of cases there was involution or improvement of the tumors within a five-year period [5]. However, strawberry hemangiomas often will ulcerate and result in bleeding and this is intolerable both for the child and for the parents.

Treatment

The most effective treatment for vulvar lesions is cryosurgery (Fig. 34.10b). A probe is selected to cover the entire surface of the lesion or different segments of the tumor can be treated separately. The probe should be held in contact with the hemangioma for approximately 30 seconds or until an ice ball is produced. This treatment may be repeated after four to six weeks and often two to four applications are necessary. The argon laser has also been used to treat these lesions.

Congenital venous malformation (cavernous hemangioma)

Vascular abnormalities are usually classified on the basis of the type of vessel involved and the flow characterized. They are separated into slow-flow lesions that encompass capillary, lymphatic, and venous malformations and fast-flow lesions that include arterial malformations, arteriovenous fistulas and arteriovenous malformations. The most common are the venous malformations

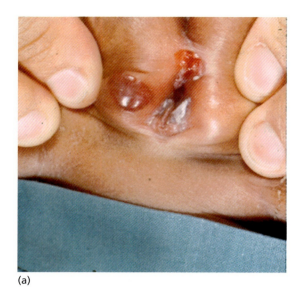

(a)

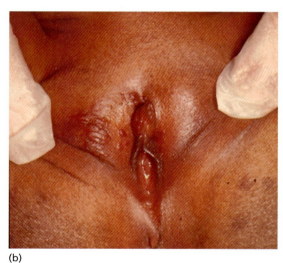

(b)

Figure 34.10 (a) Strawberry hemangioma on the lower right labium majus in a 4-month-old child. (b) Several months after treatment with cryocautery the hemangioma has disappeared.

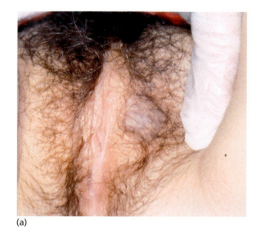

(a)

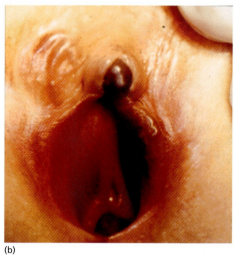

(b)

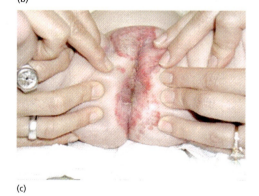

(c)

Figure 34.11 (a) Hemangioma, multilobular purplish hemangioma in a 14–year-old girl. (b) Hemangioma, involving the clitoris. (c) Extensive hemangioma extending from the mons pubis down and around the anus.

accounting for over two-thirds of congenital vascular malformations. Involvement of the external genitalia is relatively rare. Ultrasonography using Doppler flow imaging and magnetic resonance imaging are two diagnostic techniques that can be used to establish a correct diagnosis. These approaches will usually reveal the extent of tissue involvement and distinguish the fast-flow from slow-flow

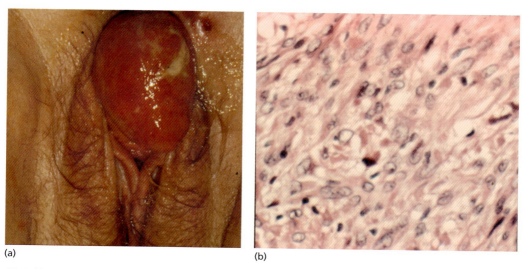

(a)

(b)

Figure 34.12 (a) Leiomyoma has prolapsed from the lower inner vaginal wall out past the introitus in this 13-year-old child. (b) The leiomyoma had grown rapidly resulting in anoxic change. This is demonstrated by variability in size and shape of some nuclei and hyperchromasia. This was a benign lesion.

anomalies. These lesions often appear during the first few months of life and increase in size until the child reaches the age of 18 months, following which they remain static or may grow larger in relation to the growth of the individual.

Clinical features

Lesions of the vulva are frequently purplish and multilobular in appearance (Fig. 34.11). They may vary in size and shape from a few millimeters to several centimeters. The tumor masses may extend into the vagina or bulge from beneath the vaginal mucosa into the vaginal canal. They may be lobulated, nodular, flat or round. They usually are asymptomatic but ulceration and bleeding associated with pain may occur. Rarely, hemorrhage will develop.

Treatment

Treatment is usually expectant and conservative unless ulceration and bleeding occur or unless the tumor continues to grow rapidly and distorts the surrounding tissue. If the hemangioma should grow rapidly, become ulcerated and hemorrhage profusely, this may threaten the life of the child. Under these circumstances aggressive treatment may be advisable and several approaches can be taken. Small isolated lesions can be injected with sclerosing

solution at intervals of two to four weeks. This is done in the operating room under general anesthesia. Rarely the tumors require surgical removal, but this can be treacherous since branches of the hemangioma may extend deep into the tissue and the surgical procedure can be accompanied by severe blood loss and risk to the child. Argon laser therapy has proven to be effective in treating selected hemangiomas.

Leiomyoma

Rarely, leiomyoma may involve the vulvovaginal area. These usually present as solid masses of varying size which at times may grow quite rapidly (Fig. 34.12a). They are managed by excision. If the growth has been rapid, anoxic changes may occur within the cells of a benign tumor that may mislead the pathologist into thinking this represents leiomyosarcoma (Fig. 34.12b).

Developmental cysts

The most common developmental cyst seen on the vulva, which is usually located in the vestibule, is the mucous cyst. It is lined by a mucous columnar epithelium and derived from the urogenital sinus. These are usually small and unless symptomatic are best left untreated.

Paramesonephric (Müllerian) and mesonephric duct cysts (Gartner's duct) are rarely identified in the child since they are located primarily within the vagina.

References

1. Powell J, Wojnarowska F. Childhood vulvar lichen sclerosus: an increasingly common problem. *J Am Acad Dermatol* 2001;**44**:803–806.

2. Smith YR, Quint EH. Clobetasol propionate in the treatment of premenarcheal vulvar lichen sclerosus. *Obstet Gynecol* 2001;**98**:588–591.

3. Lorenz B, Kaufman RH, Kutzaner SK. Lichen sclerosus: therapy with clobetasol propionate. *J Reproduct Med* 1998;**43**:790–794.

4. Boms S, Gambichler T, Freitag M, Altmeyer P, Kreuter A. Pimecrolimus 1% cream for anogenital lichen sclerosus in childhood. *BMC Dermatol* 2004;**4**:14.

5. Andrews GC, Domonkos AN, Torres-Rodriguez VM et al. Hemangioma – treated and untreated. *JAMA* 1957;**165**:114–117.

CHAPTER 35

Dermatology – The Dermatologist's View of Diagnosis and Treatment of Vulvar Conditions

Jennifer Aranda & K. Robin Carder

Department of Dermatology, University of Texas Southwestern Medical Center, Dallas, TX, USA

Introduction

The dermatologic conditions that affect the vulva are broad and have multiple etiologies. Medical training in primary care or in the specialties of dermatology and gynecology rarely addresses these conditions in depth, and vulvar clinics exist in very few institutions. In addition, the dermatoses of the genitalia, by virtue of the unique anatomic environment, do not appear as they would on other areas of the skin. Finally, medical conditions of the genitalia are often a cause of anxiety or embarrassment for the patient and/or their parents. Because of these and other factors, patients are often misdiagnosed or mismanaged.

General approach to diagnosis and management

The clinical diagnosis of vulvar dermatoses is greatly assisted by thorough history taking. Along with an extensive family and personal history, a detailed menstrual and sexual history should be performed in older children and adolescents when appropriate. A complete list of previously used prescriptions and over-the-counter products, as well as cleansers, bath products or feminine hygiene products, should be obtained.

When examining the perineum, it is important to keep in mind that the appearance of dermatoses may be altered in this location. In particular, due to moisture and occlusion by clothing or diapers, many conditions lack the scale or well-defined borders commonly seen on nonoccluded skin. In addition, recognizing confounding factors that may contribute to irritation, both innate (urine, feces) and extrinsic (creams, wipes), can aid diagnosis and treatment. Examining the skin on the rest of the body, along with the hair, nails, and other mucosal sites, can provide clues to conditions that may be difficult to distinguish from one another.

Examination of the skin should be done gently, remembering that many of these conditions can be painful. Knowledge of the normal appearance of the vulva during the different stages of development is essential. Determining if the condition involves the vulvar skin alone or if there is concomitant vestibular mucosal involvement can aid in making the diagnosis.

If a biopsy is needed for diagnosis, a topical lidocaine anesthetic cream applied 30 minutes before can help minimize pain. Anesthetics with prilocaine should be used with caution in younger children, as cases of methemoglobinemia have been reported, particularly following use on large surface areas or for prolonged periods of time. Additional studies, such as KOH preparations, cultures, and saline wet preps, can be performed when appropriate without much discomfort.

Treatment regimens need to be tailored to the disease condition, the chronicity, the site of involvement, and the age of the patient. Monitoring for side effects,

Pediatric, Adolescent, & Young Adult Gynecology. Edited by A. Altchek and L. Deligdisch. © 2009 Blackwell Publishing, ISBN: 978-1-4051-5347-8.

of topical steroids in particular, is an important part of management. Familiarity with the topical steroid potency classification assists in choosing an appropriate strength. In general, the lower the class number, the higher the strength and the potential for side effects. The mildest topical steroids comprise classes 6 and 7 (e.g. desonide and hydrocortisone 1%, respectively); the most potent steroid creams comprise class 1 (e.g. clobetasol propionate). With rare exceptions, which will be discussed later, mid- to high-potency topical steroids should be avoided in the perineum.

Topical calcineurin inhibitors, tacrolimus and pimecrolimus, are currently FDA approved for children above two years of age with atopic dermatitis. Several off-label uses are mentioned in this chapter. When using these medications in the perineum, caution should be used since increased systemic absorption has been reported following mucosal application and in younger children.

Patient and parent education regarding gentle cleaning, with avoidance of over-the-counter irritants (soaps) and allergens (benzocaine, neomycin), is an important part of the healing process.

The diagnosis and management of vulvar skin diseases in young patients require special attention to certain important points. Infants by nature are more prone to skin irritation and maceration from stool and urine and are therefore at increased risk for secondary infections. The preadolescent, nonestrogenized genitalia is more fragile and easily subject to trauma or irritation. Treatment options are limited by the potential pain or irritation that some therapies may cause and by the fact that they are rarely systematically studied in young individuals and/or approved by the US Food and Drug Administration (FDA) for pediatric use, much less for genital use. Many patients and/or parents are understandably anxious and need appropriate counseling. Finally, the care of adolescents may be complicated by the need for privacy and confidentiality.

We will limit our discussion to some of the most common vulvar skin conditions and briefly mention rarer and sometimes more challenging conditions. The conditions have been divided into three broad categories to aid in the formation of a differential diagnosis, although it must be realized that some conditions vary in appearance and may fit into more than one category.

Eczematous diseases

Diaper dermatitis

Diaper dermatitis is very common in infancy, with a prevalence of 7–35%. The peak incidence occurs at 9–12 months of age when infants are sleeping through the night and have less frequent diaper changes. Exposure to urine and feces along with friction from diapers leads to chronic irritation. This may occur within a single day if diarrhea is present. Damage to the skin barrier then predisposes to superinfection with candida and bacteria.

The diagnosis of diaper dermatitis is made clinically. The skin is erythematous with a glazed appearance and sharp borders, and the erythema spares the skin folds. In some cases there may be papules with erosions, referred to as Jacquet's erosive dermatitis. Use of potent topical steroids predisposes infants to granuloma gluteale infantum, which is more nodular and is considered by some to be a variant of Jacquet's erosive dermatitis.

The differential diagnosis includes allergic contact dermatitis, seborrheic dermatitis, and psoriasis. It should be noted that atopic dermatitis typically spares the diaper area.

Disposable diaper technology has significantly limited the occurrence of diaper dermatitis. Newer wipes do not contain ethanol or isopropanol as they did in the past, but some may contain preservatives that could aggravate diaper dermatitis. Treatment includes frequent diaper changes and the use of barrier creams, such as petrolatum or zinc oxide. For severe or recalcitrant cases, the skin inflammation may benefit from a short course of a mild topical steroid, such as hydrocortisone. A more potent topical steroid or a potent topical steroid/antifungal combination product in the diaper area would be inappropriate for this condition. Candida superinfection may be treated with miconazole nitrate ointment 0.25%, ciclopirox oral or topical 0.77%, clotrimazole or nystatin cream. Bacterial superinfection can be treated with an appropriate oral antibiotic based on culture results.

Atopic dermatitis

Atopic dermatitis (AD) typically presents with scaly, erythematous, pruritic plaques. The condition has a chronic, fluctuating course. There may be an associated family history of atopic dermatitis and a family or personal history of asthma or allergic rhinitis.

The diagnosis is based on the history and clinical features. In the acute setting, lesions may appear more exudative (weepy), whereas in the chronic stages they appear more lichenified (thickened). There is usually cheek, scalp, and extensor limb involvement in infants and neck, eyelid, and flexural limb involvement (e.g. the antecubital fossae) in older children. Involvement of the genital mucosa is rare, but buttock or labial involvement in children no longer wearing diapers is common.

AD may often be exacerbated by secondary infections with *Staphylococcus aureus* or by contact dermatitis. Treatment of genital atopic dermatitis includes avoidance of irritant or allergic components, gentle washing with water and soap-free cleansers, use of fragrance-free emollients or barrier creams, and a mild topical steroid or calcineurin inhibitor.

Psoriasis

Psoriasis is a chronic inflammatory skin condition that occurs in 1–3% of the population. Most patients develop psoriasis as adults, but it is estimated that 10% develop skin manifestations in childhood. The younger onset is seen predominantly in those with a family history of psoriasis.

The classic psoriatic lesion is an erythematous sharply demarcated plaque with silvery-white scales. However, in the vulvar or perianal area, the scale may only be present peripherally (Fig. 35.1). There are several clinical variants of psoriasis. The "inverse type" has predilection for skin-

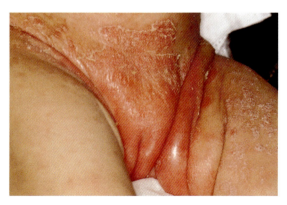

Figure 35.1 Bright red confluent plaques with peripheral scale typical of psoriasis.

folds, including the anogenital area. There may be other sites of skin involvement including the scalp, elbows, knees and nails that may provide clues to the diagnosis. The management of genital psoriasis consists of mild topical steroids or calcineurin inhibitors.

Seborrheic dermatitis

Seborrheic dermatitis is characterized by nonpruritic erythema with a yellow-white ("greasy") scale. The pattern of involvement varies with age. Infants have prominent scalp involvement ("cradle cap") which may be quite thick, as well as generalized plaques on the body and diaper area. Moist or macerated red intertriginous plaques are also common. Onset is around 4–6 weeks of age with resolution around 6–8 months. Adolescents have the adult pattern of flaky scalp ("dandruff") and red scaly plaques on the eyebrows and nasal folds.

The differential diagnosis includes psoriasis and atopic dermatitis. The involvement of scalp and lack of other features associated with atopy, such as pruritus, may help in making the diagnosis. In infants, histiocytosis may closely resemble seborrhea in both distribution and appearance.

Treatment is generally with topical ketoconazole (or other antiyeast) cream or hydrocortisone cream.

Langerhans cell histiocytosis

Langerhans cell histiocytosis (LHC), formerly called histiocytosis X, results from the abnormal accumulation of a class of dendritic cells (Langerhans cells) normally found in the epidermis. LCH primarily affects infants and children, but has been reported in all ages. It may be limited to one organ, such as the skin, or may be disseminated. Common sites of skin involvement include the scalp, postauricular and inguinal creases. Typical lesions are skin-colored to pink scaly plaques, closely resembling seborrheic dermatitis, with petechiae, crusted papules or ulcerations (Fig. 35.2).

To determine the extent of disease and subsequent treatment plan, additional investigation is required including complete blood count (CBC), electrolytes, urine specific gravity, liver function tests and possibly bone marrow biopsy and cranial magnetic resonance imaging (MRI). The percentage of LCH patients that develop diabetes insipidus is around 30%. In some cases, the disease will regress without any treatment at all. In others, radiation therapy or chemotherapy may be indicated.

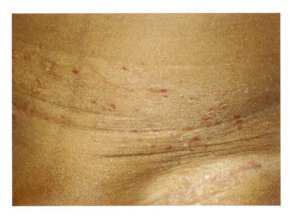

Figure 35.2 Histiocytosis, characterized by petechial papules, has a predilection for the intertriginous areas.

Acrodermatitis enteropathica

Acrodermatitis enteropathica (AE) occurs as a result of zinc deficiency. Classic AE is caused by an inherited autosomal recessive defect in zinc absorption and is indistinguishable from the acquired forms (e.g. due to zinc-deficient total parenteral nutrition or breast milk). The presentation is that of an irritable infant with diarrhea, alopecia (hair loss), and skin lesions affecting acral and periorificial sites.

Cutaneous features range from erythematous and eczematous to denuded/erosive plaques around the diaper area, eyes, mouth, and extremities. Care should be taken to monitor for and treat secondary skin infections, since sepsis in these infants is a common cause of death.

New-onset cystic fibrosis (CF) can appear identical to AE and these patients also have low zinc levels, but often do not respond as quickly to zinc replacement. A sweat chloride test or genetic studies can determine the presence of CF. The differential diagnosis also includes hypovitaminosis, epidermolysis bullosa, and glucagonoma.

The diagnosis can be confirmed by low levels of plasma zinc and low urinary zinc excretion. Low levels of serum alkaline phosphatase, a zinc-dependent metalloenzyme, are suggestive of zinc deficiency and may be obtained from the lab in less time.

Treatment is elemental zinc supplementation, starting with an oral dose of 5–10 mg/kg/day, then maintenance at 1–2 mg/kg/day.

Erosive, blistering, and scarring diseases

Lichen sclerosus

Lichen sclerosus is a chronic inflammatory skin disorder of unknown origin that has been associated in some patients with antibodies to extracellular matrix protein 1. It has also been reported in association with a variety of autoimmune diseases.

Lichen sclerosus affects predominantly females. This disorder typically involves the genital skin, although lesions may also occur on extragenital sites. The incidence is bimodal, clustering around the prepubertal and postmenopausal ages. Patients may be asymptomatic or may present with complaints of pruritus, pain, constipation or dysuria. Skin changes usually involve the labia majora, perianal region and clitoris, forming what is often described as a figure-of-eight or hourglass pattern. The affected skin is characteristically white, atrophic (thinned), with a smooth, shiny appearance. The occasional presence of hemorrhage within the lesions (Fig. 35.3) is common and should not be confused with sexual abuse, keeping in mind that these conditions are not mutually exclusive. Complications may include introital narrowing, burying of the clitoris, and resorption of the labia minora.

The prognosis for pediatric lichen sclerosus is unknown. It was once believed to resolve at puberty, but observations of persistence into adulthood have been made. Similarly, the long-term risk of squamous cell carcinoma in the pediatric group is not well established, but the risk in adults is estimated to be 4%. For this reason, close follow-up for the development of vulvar malignancy, as well as for scarring or the development of corticosteroid side effects, is recommended.

Most cases with the typical hypopigmentation and "cigarette paper" skin texture can be diagnosed clinically. Diagnosis is more challenging in early stages in which only mild erythema is present, in more erosive variants or in late-stage scarring. When the features are not obvious, skin biopsy can be helpful for diagnosis.

Management consists of superpotent topical steroids, such as clobetasol proprionate 0.05% ointment applied qhs for 6–12 weeks, then decreased based on improvement to 2–3 times per week. Close monitoring and patient education are needed to prevent perianal or inguinal atrophy and striae. Other treatment options include the calcineurin inhibitors (tacrolimus and pimecrolimus). There

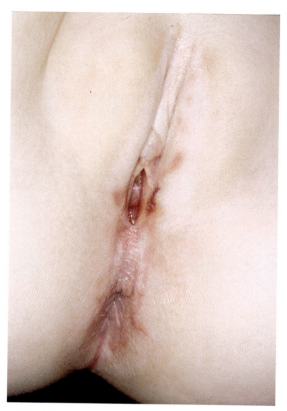

Figure 35.3 Lichen sclerosus. White, atrophic perivaginal and perianal plaques forming a "figure of eight" pattern. The central areas of hemorrhage are a common finding.

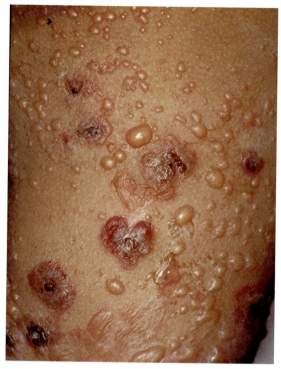

Figure 35.4 Multiple blisters, some forming ring-like clusters, in a child with chronic bullous dermatosis of childhood.

is no indication for the use of testosterone cream. Data are limited regarding the efficacy of estrogen and progesterone creams. Surgery is reserved only for the complications of scarring.

Chronic bullous disease of childhood

Chronic bullous disease of childhood (CBDC), also called linear IgA bullous disease, is an autoimmune disease with onset typically by age ten years. The characteristic "clusters" of bullae most commonly appear on the groin and buttocks, but may be widespread (Fig. 35.4).

The differential diagnosis includes herpes, bullous impetigo, bullous pemphigoid, and linear IgA bullous disease secondary to medications. The diagnosis is confirmed by biopsy with direct immunofluorescence revealing linear IgA deposition at the basement membrane zone.

Most cases of CBDC respond to treatment with oral dapsone. Dapsone therapy is often required for a period of one to a few years, after which many attain a clinical remission.

Behçet disease

Behçet disease is a multisystem disorder of unknown origin that is mainly observed in young adults with only rare reports in children. It is classically characterized by recurrent aphthous ulcers of the oral and genital mucosa, along with possible articular, cutaneous, ocular, gastrointestinal, pulmonary, vascular, and neurologic manifestations.

In order to meet criteria, patients must have at least three episodes of oral ulcers in a 12-month period along with two of the following: recurrent genital aphthae, ocular findings (typically uveitis), cutaneous lesions (erythema nodosum, pustular skin eruptions), and a positive pathergy test (pustule formation at injection sites). Biopsy

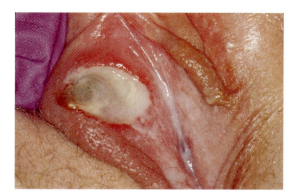

Figure 35.5 Exquisitely tender aphthous ulcer of the inner labia in a girl with major aphthosis. This patient did not meet criteria for Behçet disease.

findings are nonspecific and histopathologic confirmation is not part of the diagnostic criteria.

Oral ulcers most frequently occur on the buccal mucosa, gingiva, lips, and tongue. The vulvar ulcerations are most likely to occur on the labia majora (Fig. 35.5). These lesions begin as red macules that rapidly progress to form 3–20 mm sharply marginated ulcers. They present with pain, particularly with voiding, and may heal with scarring. It is important to realize that the presence of recurrent oral and genital aphthae ("major aphthosis") alone is not uncommon and should not be considered Behçet's. The differential diagnosis also includes herpes simplex, which can be ruled out by viral culture or PCR.

The treatment of aphthae can be with local application of topical lidocaine for pain and topical steroids. Oral steroids at starting doses of 1 mg/kg/day, tapering over several weeks, and colchicine 0.02–0.06 mg/kg/day may be used for more recalcitrant cases. Additional systemic therapies include sulfasalazine, methotrexate, cyclosporin, dapsone, and thalidomide. These medications should only be used by physicians familiar with their use and potential adverse effects (e.g. thalidomide is a known teratogen and has also been associated with thromboembolic events).

Benign familial pemphigus

Benign familial pemphigus, also known as Hailey–Hailey disease, is a dermatosis with an autosomal dominant mode of inheritance. The age of onset is variable but usually occurs after puberty, in the 20s and 30s, with rare reports in children.

Hailey–Hailey is characterized by lesions in the intertriginous areas, especially the axillae and groin, but can also appear on the lateral neck creases and the antecubital and popliteal fossae. The primary lesion is a very superficial vesicle that is not perceived clinically due to its fragility. The most common clinical picture is of maceration or crusted erosions. Chronic lesions can become thick, with central fissures, and may become malodorous due to bacterial or fungal superinfection. The differential includes psoriasis, which tends not to be erosive or crusted, and pemphigus (mostly the vegetans type), which has a positive direct immunofluorescence, as opposed to Hailey–Hailey. The family history, especially in early lesions, can be helpful in distinguishing these conditions.

Treatment characteristically comprises wearing loose-fitting clothes to minimize friction; treating superinfections with topical antimicrobials, cleansers or oral medications; and topical steroids. Recalcitrant cases can be treated topically with calcineurin inhibitors or calcipotriol (limited by irritation) or orally with prednisone, retinoids or dapsone. The use of laser ablation has been successful in several case reports. Management should also include long-term follow-up for the development of squamous cell carcinoma.

Lichen planus

Lichen planus (LP) is an inflammatory skin disorder of unknown etiology with several different clinical manifestations. LP is rare in infancy and childhood. The most common presentation is the classic papular variant, consisting of flat-topped, pruritic, pink-purple papules and plaques with lacy, white surfaces involving the ankles and wrists.

Although cases affecting the nails, scalp, and other cutaneous sites have been described, mucosal involvement is rare and vulvar lesions are typically an extension of widespread skin lesions. Primary vulvar or vaginal LP has been reported rarely in adolescents, including descriptions of the vulvovaginal-gingival syndrome. Symptoms vary from itching to burning and pain. In sexually active adolescents there may be a complaint of dyspareunia and postcoital bleeding.

Diagnosis is confirmed in most cases by exam alone, especially if accompanied by classic findings elsewhere on the body. To meet criteria for vulvovaginal-gingival syndrome, vulvar, vaginal and gingival sites (all three) must be involved, and such patients are at risk for esophageal, eye, and external auditory canal involvement. In the case of erosive vulvar LP, the white reticulated (lacy) border at the edge of the erosion can be helpful, but a biopsy can help to differentiate between this and other erosive disorders, such as cicatricial pemphigoid (CP) or erosive lichen sclerosus (LS). The scarring caused by LP may be indistinguishable from that of CP and LS.

Genital lesions are historically the most refractory to therapy. Cutaneous papular or erosive lesions on the vulva can be treated with topical steroids of mild to medium potency, tacrolimus or pimecrolimus.

Oral treatment regimens should be reserved for extensive cutaneous involvement, recalcitrant vulvar or vaginal LP, in particular to prevent scarring. Systemic therapy has included dapsone, oral corticosteroids, oral retinoids, cyclosporin, hydroxychloroquine, azathioprine, and mycophenolate mofetil. Surgical procedures may be performed for the scarring. To prevent progression resulting in pain or loss of sexual function due to scarring, recalcitrant or severe cases should be promptly referred to a dermatologist familiar with the systemic management of LP.

Cicatricial pemphigoid

Cicatricial pemphigoid (CP), also known as mucous membrane pemphigoid, usually presents with erosions in mucosal areas (mouth, eyes, nose or genitalia). It has been reported in children with vulvar involvement as the only manifestation, but is rare in this age group. It may lead to severe scarring with fusion of the labia and narrowing of the introitus.

Differentiation from erosive lichen planus can be achieved by biopsy and immunofluorescence that shows linear IgG and/or C3 (less commonly IgA or IgM) along the basement membrane which is characteristic of CP.

Treatment is traditionally with dapsone and/or oral corticosteroids. In mild cases, topical steroids alone may be beneficial and there are reports of efficacy with topical tacrolimus. In more progressive cases, azathioprine, cyclophosphamide, methotrexate, mycophenolate mofetil, daclizumab, etanercept, and intravenous immunoglobulin therapy have been used.

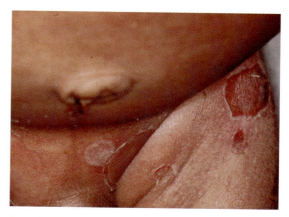

Figure 35.6 Scattered crusted erosions with collarettes of scale typical of bullous impetigo. The intertriginous distribution is most common in infants.

Infections and infestations

Bullous impetigo

Bullous impetigo is caused by *Staphylococcus aureus*, phage 2, type 71. This strain produces an endotoxin that leads to the intraepidermal cleavage. This condition is most frequently seen in infants and young children and favors the intertriginous areas, such as the groin and axillae. The characteristic early lesions are cloudy fluid-filled vesicles and bullae with erythema of the surrounding skin. Older ruptured lesions leave a characteristic collarette ("ring") of scale and erosions with crusting (Fig. 35.6). The diagnosis is generally made clinically, but may be assisted by skin culture of the affected areas.

Treatment may be with mupirocin ointment 2%, if there are few lesions, or with oral antibiotics, such as the β-lactamase resistant antibiotics (cephalexin, amoxicillin/clavulanate). For cases of methicillin-resistant *Staph. aureus* (MRSA) it should be based on cultures (commonly rifampin and trimethoprim/sulfamethoxazole or clindamycin). Infants should be monitored for signs of bacteremia.

Perineal streptococcal cellulitis

Perineal streptococcal infection may vary in presentation. Most commonly, well-demarcated, beefy red erythema is present on the vulvar or perianal areas (Fig. 35.7), but fissuring or erosions may occur. Constipation (due to painful defecation) or dysuria may be the presenting

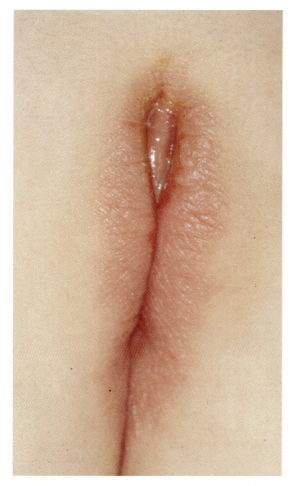

Figure 35.7 Tender, bright red, well-demarcated plaque in a girl with perineal streptococcal cellulitis.

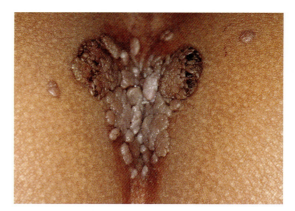

Figure 35.8 Cauliflower-like clusters of verrucous papules typical of condyloma (genital warts).

penicillin or erythromycin 40 mg/kg/d divided every 8 h for ten days. Efficacy with topical mupirocin 2% ointment has also been reported.

Genital warts

Genital warts, caused by human papilloma virus (HPV), present as clustered, skin-colored papules, most often on the perianal and vulvar areas. Lesions may vary from smooth 1–3 mm papules to larger cauliflower-like plaques (Fig. 35.8).

The diagnosis is not usually a clinical challenge, but there is often the question of sexual transmission. There is evidence suggesting that cases of genital warts can be transmitted congenitally from the mother or after birth via contact with common warts on the hands of caregivers. In some instances of perinatal infection, papillomas may also develop in the child's respiratory tract. The incubation period has been described to be as long as 9–20 months.

At this time, sexual abuse is always a concern for children of any age with anogenital HPV infections. Every case needs a medical evaluation and thorough social history to determine whether enough concern for abuse exists to merit additional investigations. Another unanswered question is the issue of potential cervical cancer in the future and whether to initiate screening Pap smears and at what age. Screening for oncogenic types of HPV is not routinely performed, since it has not been shown to assist in determining the mode of transmission. The differential diagnosis includes molluscum and the condyloma lata lesions of syphilis.

symptom. Streptococcal vulvovaginitis presents as a red, tender and edematous vulva. There may be an accompanying milky discharge in cases of vaginal involvement.

Vulvar and perianal involvement may occur separately or together in the same person and are caused by group A β-hemolytic streptococci (*Streptococcus pyogenes*). Throat cultures may also be positive for streptococci. Like streptococcal pharyngitis, perineal streptococcal cellulitis has also been associated with subsequent genital or guttate psoriasis.

The source of the infection may be the gastrointestinal tract, throat or hands. Treatment is with oral amoxicillin,

Treatment is based on the extent of the lesions and the age of the patient. It is important to note that none of these treatments have been FDA approved in children. Some clinicians may advocate nonintervention, since genital warts resolve on their own in 54% of children within five years.

Nonpainful options should be considered first-line therapy, since more than one treatment session is often required. Patient- or parent-applied treatments such as imiquimod cream or podofilox gel are generally painless, but can lead to irritation. The application of imiquimod is generally three times each week at night, then washed off the next morning. Treatment should be discontinued if irritation occurs. The podofilox gel is applied twice a day for three consecutive days, followed by four days of no therapy. In children, it is best to start podofilox once weekly and then increase by one application per week, stopping if irritation develops. Healthcare providers can administer topical treatments such as podophyllin 25% (apply to lesions, let dry, then wash off after 4–6 hours).

Destructive therapies, such as cryotherapy, laser, curettage, and electrosurgery can also be used but are poorly tolerated by children, including some adolescents, and general anesthesia may be required. Because of the increased risk of pain, blistering, discoloration, and scarring, these procedures should only be performed by experienced clinicians.

Molluscum contagiosum

Molluscum contagiosum is caused by a poxvirus and most commonly affects children. It is often distributed on the lower abdomen and thighs and therefore may spread by autoinoculation to the genital areas. Occasionally, it affects the vulva or perianal area alone and this should raise the question of sexual transmission, especially in adolescents. Typically lesions consist of skin-colored to pink, 2–5 mm umbilicated papules with a white central core (Fig. 35.9). Redness and scaling (eczema) of the skin are common features.

The differential diagnosis may include warts but on close inspection, the white core or central umbilication can often be observed. A Giemsa stain of the molluscum bodies can confirm the diagnosis under the microscope.

Some infections will resolve spontaneously in a 6–12-month period. One treatment option is curettage of the lesions after application of a topical anesthetic cream. Lesions can also be treated with imiquimod cream,

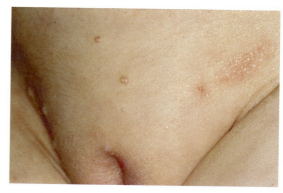

Figure 35.9 Scattered skin-colored to pink umbilicated papules in a child with molluscum contagiosum.

cantharidin, cryotherapy or 25–50% trichloroacetic acid. Cantharidin should not be applied to the face or groin. In general, treatment of eyelid lesions in children should be deferred. Blistering, discomfort, and scarring are potential risks of destructive therapies, so caution should be exercised.

Scabies

Scabies is caused by the mite *Sarcoptes scabiei*, specific to the human host. Transmission occurs through close personal contact. The female mite burrows into the skin, depositing ova and scybala (feces). Pruritus is caused by a hypersensitivity reaction and not by the mite itself, which explains why some people with mites, but without sensitization, are completely asymptomatic.

On physical exam, there are scattered eczematous papules and plaques on the trunk and extremities. The characteristic burrows are mostly found in the finger webs and wrists. Infants and young children may have involvement of the scalp, lower face, palms and soles, including pustular or nodular skin lesions, features not seen in older children or adolescents (Fig. 35.10). The genitalia can be involved at any age but scabetic nodules, which represent a form of granulomatous hypersensitivity response, are mostly seen in infants. Scabetic nodules may persist months after adequate treatment and mite eradication.

The diagnosis can be confirmed by scraping a burrow, vesicle or papule and identifying the mite, eggs or feces microscopically. A relatively painless scraping can be done by applying mineral oil to the area and gently scraping the skin using a No. 15 blade or curette.

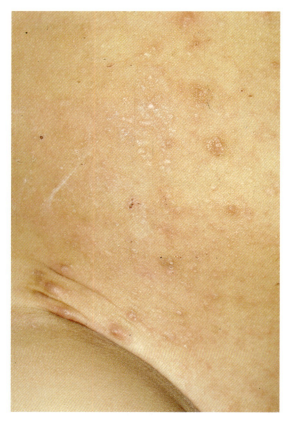

Figure 35.10 Erythematous crusted and eczematous papules in an infant with scabies. The generalized distribution and nodular lesions, as noted in the inguinal fold, are more typically seen in infants.

The recommended treatment is topical permethrin 5% cream. The cream should be applied all over the skin (in infants and young children this includes face and scalp, with avoidance of perioral or periocular sites) for eight hours then washed off; a repeated course may be performed a week later. For pregnant females or infants under two months of age, an older, less pleasant treatment, precipitated sulfur 6% in petrolatum, may be used instead, applied nightly for three consecutive nights. Lindane is not recommended due to decreased efficacy and the potential for neurotoxicity. There are reports of the effective use of oral ivermectin at 200 μg/kg/dose administered once and repeated in two weeks, but it does not have an FDA-approved indication for scabies. The entire family and all close contacts should be treated even if they have no complaints of itching or signs of infestation. It is im-

portant to emphasize that the pruritus may persist for up to two weeks post treatment.

Pediculosis pubis

Pediculosis pubis is caused by *Phthirus pubis*, which is different from the types of lice causing pediculosis capitis or corporis. Due to their anatomic structure (almost as wide as they are long), these lice can adhere to widely spaced pubic hair or eyelashes (pediculosis palpebrarum).

If nits or lice are seen on either pubic hair in adolescents or the eyelashes of children, the possibility of sexual transmission and abuse should be investigated. Other routes of infestation can be passage from the axillary or chest hair of a caretaker.

The diagnosis is made by clinically visualizing the nits or lice. Adolescents with pubic lice may have the characteristic blue macules on the thighs, maculae caeruleae, as a result of the bites.

Management should include screening for other sexually transmitted diseases. In a retrospective analysis, adolescents with pediculosis pubis were twice as likely as uninfested adolescents to have chlamydial and gonorrheal infections. Treatment of the genital area is with application of permethrin 1% cream, washed off after ten minutes. Other topical treatment options are pyrethrins (resistance has been documented and allergic contact sensitivity may occur), lindane (banned in some areas due to neurotoxicity and contraindicated in pregnancy), and malathion (highly pediculocidal, but with an unappealing odor and flammable vehicle). The eyelashes can be smothered with petrolatum twice a day for ten days.

Enterobius vermicularis **(pinworms)**

Pinworms usually present as perianal and/or vulvar itch that worsens at night. The pruritus occurs as the female worm emerges from the anus to deposit eggs at night. Clinically, the presentation is perianal and vulvar erythema with associated excoriations. Although vulvitis is common, vaginitis may occur in the rare instance that the worm moves into the vagina.

The diagnosis can be made by visualizing the ova on a morning tape test (touching a clear piece of tape to the perianal area), since stool cultures may be negative.

Treatment for children older than two years of age is oral mebendazole 100 mg once, and a dose may be repeated two weeks later. Alternative treatments include pyrantel pamoate or pyrvinium pamoate.

Other conditions

Hidradenitis suppurativa

Hidradenitis is a chronic inflammatory condition affecting apocrine gland-bearing skin. It is usually more prevalent in women and the onset is often around or after puberty. The condition occurs in the intertriginous areas of the axilla, groin, and/or under the breasts. Presentation is that of chronic, recurring, tender, red, acne-like nodules and abscesses eventually leading to sinus tract formation, bridged keloidal scars, and double-ended comedones ("blackheads"). Cultures of abscesses and sinus tracts often reveal mixed flora. The association of acne conglobata (a severe form of nodulocystic acne) and dissecting cellulitis of the scalp with hidradenitis suppurativa is well known and this condition is termed the "follicular occlusion triad."

The diagnosis of hidradenitis suppurativa is clinical and is based on the chronic recurrent course, appearance and distribution of skin lesions, and the end-result of scarring and fibrosis. Complications include rectal or urethral strictures, genital edema, fistula formation, and development of squamous cell carcinoma.

The treatment is often not satisfying and mostly consists of topical antibacterial agents and oral antibiotics that may be guided by culture (usually chronic suppressive doses of doxycycline or minocycline). Isolated inflamed lesions may be treated with intralesional steroids. Isotretinoin has been tried with mixed results. There are also successful case reports of the off-label use of biologic agents such as infliximab, etanercept, and adalimumab. Surgery often consists of excision and primary closure for localized disease and wide excision with or without skin grafting for diffuse disease, which can be helpful in select cases, but skin involvement may recur following surgery and significant scarring may result.

Further reading

Allen AL, Siegfried EC. The natural history of condyloma in children. *J Am Acad Dermatol* 1998; **39**:951–955.

Borlu M, Uksal U, Ferahbas A, Evereklioglu C. Clinical features of Behcet's disease in children. *Int J Dermatol* 2006; **45**:713–716.

Byrd JA, Davis MD, Rogers RS 3rd. Recalcitrant symptomatic vulvar lichen planus: response to topical tacrolimus. *Arch Dermatol* 2004; **140**:715–720.

Carder KR. Skin diseases of the neonate, including diaper dermatitis. In: Burg FD, Ingelfinger JR, Polin RA, Gershon AA (eds) *Current Pediatric Therapy*, 18th edn. Philadelphia: Elsevier, 2006.

Edwards L. Dermatologic therapy of chronic genital disease. *Dermatol Ther* 2004; **17**:1–7.

Fischer G. Anogenital warts in children. *Pediatr Dermatol* 2006; **23**:291–293.

Fischer G, Rogers M. Vulvar disease in children: a clinical audit of 130 cases. *Pediatr Dermatol* 2000; **17**:1–6.

Garzon MC, Paller AS. Ultrapotent topical corticosteroid treatment of childhood genital lichen sclerosus. *Arch Dermatol* 1999; **135**:525–528.

Mengesha YM, Holcombe TC, Hansen RC. Prepubertal hidradenitis suppurativa: two case reports and review of the literature. *Pediatr Dermatol* 1999; **16**:292–296.

Moresi JM, Herbert CR, Cohen BA. Treatment of anogenital warts in children with topical 0.05% podofilox gel and 5% imiquimod cream. *Pediatr Dermatol* 2001; **18**:448–452.

Perafan-Riveros C, Franca LF, Fortes Alves AC, Sanches JA. Acrodermatitis enteropathica: case report and review of the literature. *Pediatr Dermatol* 2002; **19**:426–431.

Powell J, Wojnarowska F. Childhood vulvar lichen sclerosus. The course after puberty. *J Reprod Med* 2002; **47**:706–709.

Scheinfeld N. Diaper dermatitis: a review and brief survey of eruptions of the diaper area. *Am J Clin Dermatol* 2005; **6**:273–281.

Setterfield JF, Neill S, Shirlaw PJ et al. The vulvovaginal gingival syndrome: a severe subgroup of lichen planus with characteristic clinical features and a novel association with the class II HLA DQB1*0201 allele. *J Am Acad Dermatol* 2006; **55**:98–113.

Strittmatter HJ, Hengge UR, Blecken SR. Calcineurin antagonists in vulvar lichen sclerosus. *Arch Gynecol Obstet* 2006; **274**:266–270.

Wendel K, Rompalo A. Scabies and pediculosis pubis: an update of treatment regimens and general review. *Clin Infect Dis* 2002; **35**(suppl 2):S146–151.

CHAPTER 36

Management of Ovarian Cysts in the Adolescent and Young Adult

Leslie R. Boyd, Khush Mittal, & John P. Curtin
New York University School of Medicine, New York, NY, USA

Introduction

Appropriate management of an ovarian cyst in the adolescent and young adult requires an understanding of the normal physiologic changes and the common pathologic states encountered in this age group. We will review the most commonly found adnexal masses, as well as ways to distinguish between benign and malignant disease. Accurate assessment by physical and radiographic examinations allows for correct determination of when conservative versus operative management is required and, when necessary, can inform the type and approach of the surgical procedure.

- Adolescents and young adults undergoing surgery for an adnexal mass are most likely to have physiologic (functional) cysts.
- In adolescents with tumors, benign cystic teratoma is the most common lesion.
- In simple-appearing cysts, observation for 3–6 cycles is appropriate. Surgery should be reserved for symptomatic patients or those with persistent cysts following the observation period.
- Given the relatively low incidence of malignancy and the need to preserve fertility, cystectomy is generally the procedure of choice if surgery is warranted.
- Pelvic or abdominal ultrasound can provide a diagnosis with a high positive predictive value; this should aid in guiding the treatment plan.

- A laparoscopic approach should be strongly considered in most cases, as complication rates between laparoscopy and laparotomy are comparable, while laparoscopy yields multiple patient and economic benefits.
- In cases of torsion, untwisting and leaving the affected adnexa (with possible oophoropexy) is usually sufficient treatment.
- When malignancy is suspected, the patient's care should be managed with the help of a gynecologic oncologist, who can balance the need to optimize resection for curative intent with the desire to preserve fertility when feasible.

Epidemiology

Adolescents have a low risk of malignancy in the presence of an adnexal mass. In one series, children 15 years old or younger had a rate of malignancy of 11%, as compared to 4.4% in children over age 15 [1,2]. Young adults (age 20–29) have an even lower risk of malignancy due to the rarity of both germ cell and epithelial neoplasms in this age group [3]. Several large series have elucidated the most common ovarian cysts encountered in adolescents and young adults. We will review the most common of these in the following paragraphs.

Functional cysts

Ovulatory dysfunction is common in the period immediately following menarche. In a study of healthy, asymptomatic adolescents, 16% developed cysts over the course of one year [4]. Enlarged (unruptured) follicles as well as corpora lutea (in some cases hemorrhagic) make up the

Pediatric, Adolescent, & Young Adult Gynecology. Edited by
A. Altchek and L. Deligdisch. © 2009 Blackwell Publishing,
ISBN: 978-1-4051-5347-8.

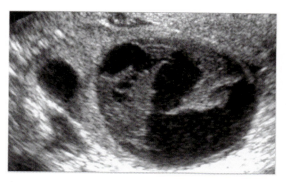

Figure 36.1 Ultrasound image of a hemorrhagic corpus luteum. Although the cyst is thin walled, the hypoechoic debris (consistent with clotted blood) could be confused with a solid lesion or thick septae (courtesy of Dr Ilan E. Timor-Tritsch).

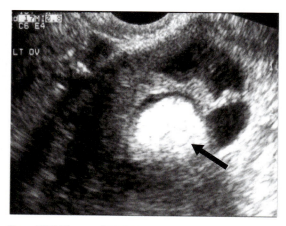

Figure 36.2 Ultrasound image of a benign cystic teratoma. Note the septate, cystic structure with a hypoechoic area representing Rokitansky's protuberance (*black arrow*) (courtesy of Dr Ilan E. Timor-Tritsch).

majority of these cysts. In most cases, they resolve without treatment within the first three months after detection.

Pathologic cysts

Neoplasms

Germ cell tumors

Germ cell tumors are the most common neoplastic tumors in adolescents and young adults (Table 36.1). These tumors are derived from various parts of the primordial germ cell of the ovary. In general, the most malignant subtypes are more common in young children, but all have been reported in adolescents and young adults. Table 36.2 gives a short description of the most common germ cell neoplasms.

Benign cystic teratoma, or dermoid tumor, is the most common neoplasm in women of reproductive age. The tumor may include ectodermal, mesodermal and endodermal elements, most often including skin, hair,

teeth and mucin. Mature teratomas are bilateral in 15–25% of cases, although this propensity is skewed towards older patients.

In comparison to the well-differentiated tissues found in dermoids, immature teratomas are characterized by poorly differentiated elements. The most significant of these from a prognostic standpoint is the finding of immature neural cells. Although immature (malignant) elements are only present in 1–2% of ovarian teratomas overall, in children under age 18 the percentage may be as high as 14% [5]. This can present a challenge in clinical practice in those instances where the malignant teratoma appears cystic on imaging, thereby mimicking the benign lesion.

Table 36.1 Ovarian neoplasms by type in children aged 15–17 years

	n (%)
Germ cell	126 (49)
Common epithelial	71 (28)
Sex cord stromal	40 (16)
Miscellaneous	20 (08)
Total	257

From Breen and Maxson [1].

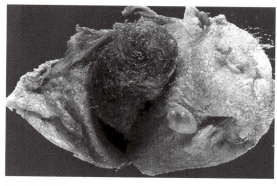

Figure 36.3 Benign cystic teratoma on gross inspection. Prominent elements in this specimen include a ball of hair and skin-like lining.

Table 36.2 Neoplasms described in adolescents and young adults

Cell type	Description
Germ cell tumors	
Mature teratoma (benign cystic teratoma)	Benign, bilateral in 15–25%; contents may be derived from ecto-, endo- and mesodermal layers with skin, hair, teeth and mucin predominating. Median age at diagnosis, 15 years.
Immature teratoma	Malignant, solid-appearing tumor. Usually poorly differentiated histology; poor prognosis secondary to rapid growth, early metastasis. Median age at diagnosis, 11 years.
Dysgerminoma	Resemble primordial germ cells of the ovary, bilateral in 10–20% of cases. May be associated with LDH or hCG production, sexual precocity, rarely androgenization. Usually presents as stage I disease, and is generally radiation and chemosensitive. Median age at diagnosis, 13 years.
Endodermal sinus	Form large, friable solid masses with solid and cystic areas. Extraembryonic differentiation noted microscopically. Associated with AFP production. Aggressive tumor with improved prognosis noted with use of multiagent chemotherapy. Median age at diagnosis, 18–25 years.
Mixed germ cell	Contains a combination of elements; clinical course dependent upon the most aggressive histology present. Most common combination is dysgerminoma and endodermal sinus tumor.
Epithelial tumors	
Serous cystadenoma (-carcinoma)	Generally unilocular with clear cyst fluid, bilateral in approximately 20% of cases. On inspection, the epithelium lining the cyst wall resembles that lining the fallopian tube. Serous adenocarcinomas usually exhibit obvious invasion on histology.
Mucinous cystadenoma (-carcinoma)	Can grow very large, with cysts over 30 cm not uncommon. It is important to sample these tumors thoroughly as they may have variable morphology in different parts of the tumor, with benign- and malignant-appearing areas in the same tumor. Of mucinous cysts, approximately 5% are found to be malignant. When malignant, close to 50% are bilateral.
Clear cell carcinoma	Benign counterpart is rare. Bilateral in less than 15% of cases. Clear and hobnail cells present on histologic examination. Young age at diagnosis may represent a poor prognostic indicator.
Sex cord stromal tumors	
Granulosa cell	Juvenile type found in majority of cases in young adults; secrete estradiol, inhibin; often present with abdominal fullness secondary to ascites or vaginal bleeding. Usually well encapsulated. Almost all present as stage I disease, with infrequent extraovarian spread.
Theca cell	Lipid-laden stromal cells. Bilateral in 2% of cases. Present with increasing abdominal girth, frequently hormonally active. Usually benign, extraovarian spread is rare.
Sertoli–Leydig cell	Similar to tumors found in testis. Solid tumor with gray-yellow coloration. Ranges from well to poorly differentiated. Androgenization noted in 50% of patients. Extraovarian spread is rare (2–3% of patients). Median age at diagnosis, 25 years.

Epithelial tumors

While they represent 70–80% of all ovarian tumors, in young patients only 16% of neoplasms are of epithelial origin [6]. The most common types found among adolescents and young adults are serous cystadenomas, mucinous cystadenomas, serous cystadenocarcinoma, mucinous cystadenocarcinoma, and clear cell carcinoma. (Serous cystadenoma is the most common benign lesion in postmenopausal women, which is consistent with the increased incidence noted with age.) Serous and mucinous cystadenomas generally have a round, uniform appearance, with a watery content in serous tumors and thicker mucinous material in mucinous tumors. On histology serous cysts have cuboidal or low columnar cells lining the cyst wall, as compared to the tall columnar epithelium with goblet cells visualized in mucinous tumors. Seven to 15% of cystadenomas in this age group are malignant (cystadenocarcinoma) [1,5]. It is unclear if these malignant tumors carry the same prognosis in adolescents as they do in postmenopausal patients due to the small numbers of applicable patients in each reported series.

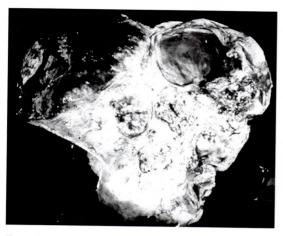

Figure 36.4 Gross specimen of an immature teratoma. Note the appearance of both solid and cystic areas with pronounced necrosis.

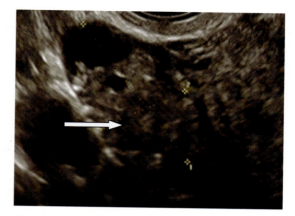

Figure 36.6 Ultrasound image of a granulosa cell tumor. The calipers outline the overall ovarian dimensions. The large white arrow points to a small, solid-appearing mass which on final pathology was determined to be a granulosa cell tumor (courtesy of Dr Ilan E. Timor-Tritsch).

Sex cord stromal tumors

These are relatively uncommon neoplasms, which include the granulosa cell, theca cell and Sertoli–Leydig cell tumors. Granulosa cell tumors are divided into adult and juvenile subtypes, and the juvenile type comprises 90% of the tumors diagnosed in women aged 30 and under. These tumors secrete estrogen and are the most common cause of isosexual precocious puberty. Theca cell tumors are composed of lipid-laden stromal cells and are often hormonally active. Clinical manifestations of androgenization are noted in up to 50% of patients with Sertoli–Leydig cell tumors, with menstrual disorders and virilization common prior to diagnosis.

Other pathologic cysts

In sexually active women, the differential diagnosis for an ovarian mass includes ectopic pregnancy, theca lutein cysts, and sequelae from pelvic inflammatory disease. Pregnancy tests should be performed irrespective of stated sexual history to exclude any pregnancy-related pathology. Whenever the clinical presentation suggests an infectious process, hydrosalpinx and tubo-ovarian abscess should be considered in the differential diagnosis.

Endometriosis has been documented in patients as young as eight years old, and is a common cause of pelvic pain in adolescents. However, an endometrioma is generally rare in the youngest age groups. Not surprisingly, the incidence of endometriomas increases markedly with age amongst premenopausal women, and is not uncommon in young adults. Endometriosis has been associated with patients with Müllerian anomalies leading to outflow obstruction, presumably due to an increase in retrograde menstruation. In these patients, the stigmata of endometriosis, including endometriomas, may be present at an earlier age.

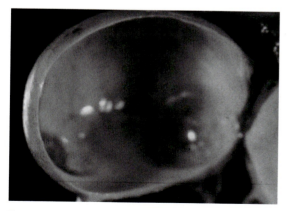

Figure 36.5 Serous cystadenoma on gross inspection. The smooth cyst walls visible here are characteristic of these lesions.

Evaluation

History and physical

As with any clinical problem, the first step in diagnosis remains a thorough history and physical examination. The

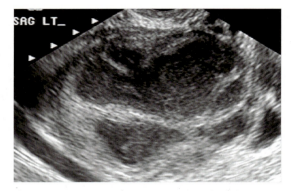

Figure 36.7 Ultrasound image of a tubo-ovarian abscess. Important elements include: thickened and edematous walls; inability to discern the ovary from the fallopian tube; confluent, loculated fluid collections (courtesy of Dr Ilan E. Timor-Tritsch).

patient's menstrual and reproductive history should be reviewed. Consideration should be given to ruling out pregnancy even in those adolescents who deny sexual activity, given known barriers to open communication in this age group. The review of systems should include questions on abdominal pain, fullness, vaginal bleeding, nausea and/or vomiting. Constitutional symptoms such as weight loss should be reviewed. On physical exam, speculum and bimanual examination should not be neglected, because palpation alone is generally inadequate to rule out adnexal disease. For the adolescent, the physical should include documentation of Tanner stages for breast and sexual hair development. Any signs of virilization should be noted.

Imaging

Since its introduction, transvaginal ultrasound has been validated for the evaluation of ovarian anatomy. Several groups have developed scoring methods to discriminate between benign and malignant cysts using their appearance on gray-scale ultrasound. These evaluate the wall structure, shadowing, septae and echogenicity [7]. In addition to routine gray-scale, the vessels associated with lesions may be assessed using color Doppler technology. Blood vessels in neoplastic tumors have decreased smooth muscle as compared to normal vessels. This leads to predictable differences in resistance and pulsatility of the measured blood flow. Timor-Tritsch et al [8] reported a positive predictive value of 94% when gray-scale and color

Doppler evaluation was combined to differentiate benign from malignant ovarian masses.

Scoring systems consistently show low negative predictive values due to the high number of false positives in their data sets. Several common benign structures (including mature teratoma and endometrioma) contain "complex" attributes. For these reasons, a skilled sonographer using learned pattern recognition often outperforms strict scoring guidelines when assessing adnexal masses.

The benefit of these studies to the practitioner lies in the ability to reliably rule out malignancy in certain situations. In a large, multicenter trial evaluating ultrasonographic parameters of adnexal masses, less than 1% of uniloculated masses were malignant on final histology [9]. If the cyst is also less than 5 cm in size, the risk of malignancy drops even further. These findings allow us to comfortably advise expectant management in patients whose lesions are in this category.

In virginal patients in whom a transvaginal probe cannot be inserted, due to either cultural or anatomic constraints, transabdominal or transperineal sonography may be utilized. Alternatively, a standard transvaginal probe can be placed in the rectum. This approach is generally well tolerated by patients, and improves visualization in comparison to either the transabdominal or transperineal views.

Ultrasound will likely remain the first line in diagnostic imaging for ovarian lesions because it is relatively inexpensive, readily available in most settings, and noninvasive. However, computed tomography (CT) and magnetic resonance imaging (MRI) with their associated contrast agents are often useful adjuncts, particularly regarding associated abdominal findings such as ascites and lymphadenopathy, where applicable.

Tumor markers

Serum markers may be helpful in diagnosing certain neoplasias in this age group. Tumors with yolk sac or chorionic elements secrete AFP or hCG, respectively (Table 36.3). Estradiol and inhibin levels are often elevated in patients with granulosa cell tumors. When positive, an informative marker also provides valuable information regarding response to treatment and recurrence of disease.

The most commonly used serum marker, CA-125, is elevated in most processes involving the coelomic, tubal, endometrial or endocervical epithelium. As a result it has poor specificity to detect cancer among young patients,

Table 36.3 Serum markers in malignant germ cell tumors

Histology	AFP	hCG
Dysgerminoma	−	+/−
Endodermal sinus tumor	+	−
Immature teratoma	+/−	−
Mixed germ cell tumor	+/−	+/−
Choriocarcinoma	−	+
Embryonal carcinoma	+/−	+

as it is elevated in many benign processes, including endometriosis and pelvic inflammatory disease.

Management

The appropriate management algorithm takes into consideration two important points: 1) the low rate of malignancy in cysts found in this age group, and 2) the importance of preserving normal ovarian function.

Simple cysts: incidental finding

The incidental finding of an ovarian mass is not uncommon in this age group, as discussed earlier. The majority of these cysts will be physiologic and should appear as enlarged (unruptured) follicular cysts on ultrasound. In these cases, there is ample evidence to support observation for several cycles, followed by repeat ultrasound to confirm spontaneous resolution. Porcu et al [4] performed monthly ultrasounds on 139 healthy adolescents for the course of one year. In that time 16% developed ovarian cysts, the majority of which (74%) resolved spontaneously within the first three months after detection. In a retrospective analysis of 119 girls with ovarian cysts diagnosed on ultrasound, time to cyst resolution was an average of 4.5 weeks in those in whom observation only was performed [10]. These patients need to be counseled regarding the possibility of ovarian torsion, and should have a good understanding of the symptoms heralding the need for immediate attention.

Although combined oral contraceptives are often prescribed to hasten cyst resolution, this practice has not been supported by the evidence. In addition to a multitude of retrospective analyses, Grimes et al [11] published a meta-analysis of four randomized controlled trials with a total of 227 women in whom treatment with combined oral contraceptives was initiated for ovarian cysts. Treatment did not improve resolution of physiologic cysts; most cysts resolved without treatment within a few cycles.

Repeat ultrasound at three to six months is necessary to confirm resolution of the cyst. Persistent cysts likely represent a pathologic process and surgical removal should be considered. The exact procedure and approach should be individualized for each patient, with the information gleaned from both physical findings and ultrasound.

Simple cysts: symptomatic patient

Patients with symptomatic cysts are most likely to complain of pain and/or pressure. In these cases, management is driven by the need to palliate symptoms, as well as the degree of suspicion for a pathologic versus physiologic process.

In those patients with significant symptoms and a benign-appearing cyst on ultrasound, ovarian cystectomy should be offered. A laparoscopic approach should be considered standard of care. Yuen et al [12] randomized patients at a teaching hospital with benign-appearing cysts to laparoscopy or laparotomy. The laparoscopic approach was associated with decreased operative morbidity, analgesic requirement and length of stay, and was comparable to laparotomy in the rate of cyst rupture. An experienced surgeon can avoid uncontrolled rupture during removal of large cysts, using several safe laparoscopic techniques.

Torsion

Adnexal torsion is an emergency condition requiring expedited diagnosis and management, which we will review here separately. Although children presenting with adnexal torsion will generally complain of abdominal pain, this pain is more likely to localize to the pelvis as the child ages. Regardless of age, nausea and vomiting remain two of the most common symptoms. Given the wide differential diagnosis in these cases, maintaining a high index of suspicion is important to make the diagnosis.

On bimanual examination, adnexal fullness with pain on palpation are usually present. Ultrasound is an important diagnostic tool, as in the majority of cases adnexa undergoing torsion are 5 cm in size or larger. The visualization of an enlarged adnexa in the presence of this constellation of symptoms is sufficient to make the presumptive diagnosis of torsion. Many studies have used ultrasound Doppler flow technology to accurately diagnose the lack of blood flow which is the underlying

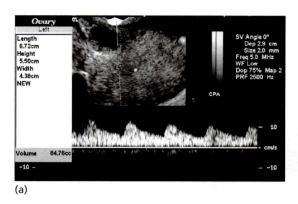

(a)

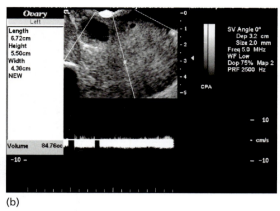

(b)

Figure 36.8 These two transvaginal ultrasound images were taken while evaluating a patient with a clinical history suspicious for adnexal torsion. Both arterial and venous flow were present on Doppler interrogation, yet the diagnosis of torsion was confirmed intraoperatively (courtesy of Dr Ilan E. Timor-Tritsch).

pathology of the condition. There is significant variation in the literature regarding the sensitivity of Doppler ultrasonography for this indication, likely reflecting the operator-dependent nature of the study. As a result, Doppler ultrasonography may be a useful adjunct but should not be relied upon to make the diagnosis.

Management of ovarian torsion requires expedited surgical intervention to untwist the adnexa. Rapid resumption of normal blood flow is considered central to preservation of ovarian function. In the past, unilateral salpingo-oophorectomy was advocated due to theoretic concerns regarding promulgation of clot after untwisting the occluded vessels. Long-standing experience now points to the safety of ovarian conservation. The ovary should be untwisted and closely examined for reperfusion. In general, the ovary will appear dusky, with a bluish hue while flow is occluded. If flow is re-established, the ovary should turn from blue to pink. If any improvement in coloration is noted, the ovary should be left *in situ*. Several authors advocate salpingo-oophorectomy in cases in which no visible improvement is noted after prolonged observation intraoperatively, presumably representing irreversible ischemic injury. However, many groups have reported on successful retention in children and young adults who exhibited complete resolution of what initially appeared to be a nonfunctional ovary [13]. Further, negative sequelae from retention of a nonfunctional ovary are rare. Due to the potential benefits, with few significant drawbacks, we advocate for the maintenance of the

ovary after an episode of torsion as the rule, with salpingo-oophorectomy reserved for exceptional cases.

If a large cyst is present, cystectomy is indicated to reduce the risk of recurrence. However, torsion is often noted in normal ovaries, particularly in this age group. In certain cases oophoropexy may be considered to further reduce the recurrence risk. This may be accomplished by suturing the ovary to the peritoneum overlying the pelvic brim using a permanent suture. Disruption of the ovary's attachments should be kept to a minimum to decrease the risk of ovarian failure. In cases in which there is concern for tissue integrity due to edema or necrosis, this step should be avoided.

Complex adnexal mass

The presence of a complex adnexal mass should always increase the practitioner's suspicion for the presence of malignancy. However, two of the most common cysts in this age group, benign cystic teratomas and endometriomas, have components which may appear concerning on ultrasound. Luckily, both of these cysts have predictable patterns on ultrasound that, when taken as a whole, allow for the correct diagnosis in the vast majority of instances [14].

Benign cystic teratoma

As discussed previously, the diagnosis of benign cystic teratoma carries a 15–20% risk of bilaterality. As a result, both ovaries must be carefully inspected to rule out a

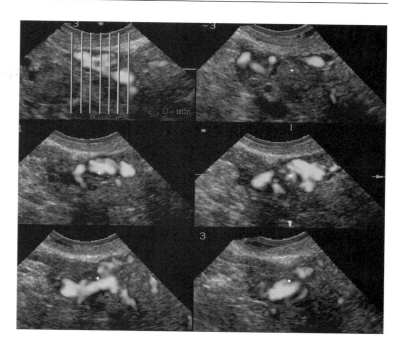

Figure 36.9 Ultrasound imaging of blood flow to a suspicious adnexal mass. The vascularity noted in this mass led to surgical removal. Final pathology revealed a granulosa cell tumor (courtesy of Dr Ilan E. Timor-Tritsch).

lesion in the contralateral ovary. Several researchers have argued for the adoption of intraoperative laparoscopic ultrasound to aid in assessment of the contralateral ovary, but this has not yet gained wide acceptance.

Cystectomy is the treatment of choice. Adoption of the laparoscopic approach has been slower amongst some practitioners due to reports of chemical peritonitis following intraoperative cyst rupture. However in large series, chemical peritonitis has been shown to be a rare event, mitigated by good surgical technique and copious irrigation should incidental rupture occur [15].

Malignant degeneration of the mature elements within the teratoma does rarely occur, but is more often found in patients over the age of 40. While it is appropriate to consider the two entities as separate, the relationship between the mature and immature teratoma is complex. Grossly visible dermoid cysts have been found within 25% of immature teratomas, and are also present in the contralateral ovary in 10% of cases [16]. Therefore, careful intraoperative and pathologic assessment is important to appropriately rule out malignancy.

Suspected malignancy

The complex adnexal mass that is not readily classifiable as a mature teratoma or endometrioma requires further evaluation. Doppler ultrasound can help identify whether suspicious blood flow, indicative of angioneogenesis, is present. Serum markers such as CA-125, AFP and hCG may be helpful in ruling in one of the more uncommon neoplastic diseases.

Ultimately, a persistent mass with suspicious aspects will require removal. The objectives for this surgery include: 1) making a correct diagnosis of the condition; 2) correctly establishing the extent of disease through a staging procedure, if necessary; and 3) preserving fertility whenever possible without compromising the patient's health. When possible, these cases should be planned and performed with the assistance of a gynecologic oncologist. Intraoperative frozen section should be utilized in order to determine the exact pathology and further aid in management decisions.

Once the pathology of the lesion has been determined, decisions regarding the extent of surgery are based on the known behavior of the lesion. Benign lesions should be managed by cystectomy whenever possible. In cases of ovarian cancer, surgical staging is the standard of care. Although routine staging includes bilateral salpingo-oophorectomy and hysterectomy, this may be adapted in certain cases for patients who wish to maintain fertility.

An experienced surgeon can perform the procedure using a laparoscopic approach.

Exhaustive preoperative patient counseling should be undertaken to ensure that the patient and her family understand the range of issues if the intraoperative diagnosis is consistent with malignant disease. In patients in this age group, it may be appropriate to perform the staging procedure as a second operation, after final pathology has been reviewed and the prognosis and extent of surgery needed has been discussed.

Although a detailed discussion of the management algorithm for each malignancy is beyond the scope of this chapter, a brief review by category follows.

Germ cell tumors

The majority of these tumors are almost always unilateral, allowing for the performance of a fertility-sparing staging procedure with preservation of the contralateral ovary and the uterus. Dysgerminomas pose several management issues. As these are often bilateral, the decision of whether or not to biopsy the contralateral ovary poses a question. In those cases where the contralateral ovary has a gross abnormality, biopsy should certainly be performed. However, the role of biopsy to rule out microscopic disease is less clear, given the risks of ovarian failure and adhesive disease secondary to biopsy, which may decrease future fertility. Since dysgerminomas may arise in dysgenetic ovaries, information on karyotype is important; in those patients with abnormal karyotypes, preserving the gonad is associated with a high risk of subsequent cancer. Ideally, a karyotype would be available preoperatively to inform regarding the need for bilateral gonadectomy.

In addition to a staging procedure (either standard or fertility preserving) almost all patients are offered multiagent chemotherapy. The treatment of choice, BEP (bleomycin, etoposide and cisplatin), has demonstrated long-term remissions with increased survival rates in comparison to older therapeutic regimens [17].

Epithelial tumors

Malignant epithelial tumors are rare in this patient group. In patients with overt disseminated disease, a standard staging procedure followed by platinum-based chemotherapy will be required to optimize survival. In the rare patient with stage IA disease (limited to one ovary with no evidence of spread), a fertility-sparing staging procedure is often sufficient therapy.

Sex cord stromal tumors

Similar to epithelial lesions, fertility-sparing surgery can be offered to patients who are found to have disease limited to one ovary. However, in the case of granulosa cell tumor, curettage must be performed to rule out endometrial disease prior to retaining the uterus. In cases with advanced disease, several multiagent chemotherapy regimens have been shown to have activity. The role of radiation therapy is unclear.

Conclusion

Adolescents and young adults with ovarian cysts have an excellent prognosis overall. Using appearance on ultrasound to triage these lesions, conservative management can be offered to the majority of patients. In the remainder, fertility-preserving surgery is often appropriate. A cautious approach, in consultation with an experienced gynecologic oncologist when necessary, can optimize outcomes for these young patients.

References

1. Breen JL, Maxson WS. Ovarian tumors in children and adolescents. *Clin Obstet Gynecol* 1977;**20**(3):607–623.
2. Templeman C, Fallat ME, Blinchevsky A et al. Noninflammatory ovarian masses in girls and young women. *Obstet Gynecol* 2000;**96**(2):229–233.
3. Koonings PP, Campbell K, Mishell DR Jr. et al. Relative frequency of primary ovarian neoplasms: a 10-year review. *Obstet Gynecol* 1989;**74**(6):921–926.
4. Porcu E, Venturoli S, Dal Prato L et al. Frequency and treatment of ovarian cysts in adolescence. *Arch Gynecol Obstet* 1994;**255**(2):69–72.
5. Brown MF, Hebra A, McGeehin K et al. Ovarian masses in children: a review of 91 cases of malignant and benign masses. *J Pediatr Surg* 1993;**28**(7):930–933.
6. Morowitz M, Huff D, von Allmen D. Epithelial ovarian tumors in children: a retrospective analysis. *J Pediatr Surg* 2003;**38**(3):331–335.
7. Lerner JP, Timor-Tritsch IE, Federman A et al. Transvaginal ultrasonographic characterization of ovarian masses with an improved, weighted scoring system. *Am J Obstet Gynecol* 1994;**170**(1 Pt 1):81–85.
8. Timor-Tritsch IE, Lerner JP, Monteagudo A et al. Transvaginal ultrasonographic characterization of ovarian masses by means of color flow-directed Doppler measurements and a

morphologic scoring system. *Am J Obstet Gynecol* 1993;**168**(3 Pt 1):909–913.

9. Timmerman D, Testa AC, Bourne T et al. Logistic regression model to distinguish between the benign and malignant adnexal mass before surgery: a multicenter study by the International Ovarian Tumor Analysis Group. *J Clin Oncol* 2005;**23**(34):8794–8801.

10. Kanizsai B, Orley J, Szigetvari I et al. Ovarian cysts in children and adolescents: their occurrence, behavior, and management. *J Pediatr Adolesc Gynecol* 1998;**11**(2):85–88.

11. Grimes DA, Jones LB, Schulz KF. Oral contraceptives for functional ovarian cysts. *Cochrane Database of Systematic Reviews* (4): CD006134, 2006.

12. Yuen PM, Yu KM, Yip SK et al. A randomized prospective study of laparoscopy and laparotomy in the management of benign ovarian masses. *Am J Obstet Gynecol* 1997;**177**(1):109–114.

13. Templeman C, Hertweck SP, Fallat ME. The clinical course of unresected ovarian torsion. *J Pediatr Surg* 2000;**35**(9):1385–1387.

14. Jermy K, Luise C, Bourne T. The characterization of common ovarian cysts in premenopausal women. *Ultrasound Obstet Gynecol* 2001;**17**(2):140–144.

15. Nezhat CR, Kalyoncu S, Nezhat CH et al. Laparoscopic management of ovarian dermoid cysts: ten years' experience. *J Soc Laparoendosc Surg* 1999;**3**(3):179–184.

16. Yanai-Inbar I, Scully RE. Relation of ovarian dermoid cysts and immature teratomas: an analysis of 350 cases of immature teratoma and 10 cases of dermoid cyst with microscopic foci of immature tissue. *Int J Gynecol Pathol* 1987;**6**(3):203–212.

17. Williams S, Blessing JA, Liao SY et al. Adjuvant therapy of ovarian germ cell tumors with cisplatin, etoposide, and bleomycin: a trial of the Gynecologic Oncology Group. *J Clin Oncol* 1994;**12**(4):701–706.

CHAPTER 37
Pediatric Gynecologic Cancer

William Bradley III & Jamal Rahaman

Mount Sinai School of Medicine and Hospital, New York, NY, USA

Introduction

Although pediatric gynecologic cancers are rare, their evaluation and management has undergone increasing sophistication in recent years. Improvements in each of the treatment modalities have led to superior outcomes in both survival and quality for life. Whereas patients in the past were often treated with life-altering therapy, today's techniques offer better survival with lower morbidity employing minimally invasive surgery, tailored radiotherapy, and targeted chemotherapy.

Ovarian tumors

The ovary is composed of three types of tissue: epithelial, stromal and germ cells. Each of these cell lines is capable of malignant transformation in both the adult and pediatric population. In adult patients epithelial cancer accounts for more than 85% of all ovarian malignancies. Unlike adult patients, ovarian cancer among children usually arises from non-epithelial – components. Germ cell cancers are the most frequent and comprise a histologically diverse and chemotherapeutically sensitive cohort of carcinomas. Stromal cancers are less common and also have a very favorable prognosis. Stromal neoplasms can be hormonally active and typically behave in an indolent fashion. Although they are the second most common gynecologic cancer among adults, invasive epithelial ovarian cancers are very rare among children. Borderline tumors, a subset of epithelial ovarian neoplasm, are more frequent than invasive cancers [1,2].

Pediatric, Adolescent, & Young Adult Gynecology. Edited by A. Altchek and L. Deligdisch. © 2009 Blackwell Publishing, ISBN: 978-1-4051-5347-8.

Similar to the adult population, surgical staging is the cornerstone of treatment for pediatric ovarian cancers. For fertility preservation, a more limited extirpative procedure is typically advocated, with preservation of the uninvolved ovary as well as the uterus [3]. Patients should undergo washings for cytology, peritoneal biopsies, omentectomy, and pelvic and para-aortic lymph node assessment. Adequate staging allows the pediatrician to clearly delineate the extent of disease, quantify the risk of recurrence and determine the need for adjuvant therapy (Box 37.1).

Germ cell tumors

Malignant germ cell tumors of the ovary occur most often in girls and young women. Single institution and intergroup series show the average age to range from 16 to 21, with pediatric patients reported as young as 1.4 years [3–5]. Germ cell tumors can grow to impressive size (up to 45 cm in one reported case), and the most common presentation is a pelvic mass. Other presentations include pain or an acute abdomen. Hormonal manifestations, including precocious puberty, are occasionally seen. The majority of these tumors will have a cystic component, adding to their size.

There are multiple subtypes of germ cell tumor, and histology affects both prognosis and treatment.

Dysgerminoma

The most common germ cell carcinoma is the dysgerminoma, accounting for approximately 50% of cases. Grossly, the tumor appears as a bland, lobulated solid mass, and histologically it resembles primordial germ cells of the ovary. Although as a rule, germ cell cancers are rarely bilateral, dysgerminoma may occur in a contralateral ovary in up to 10% of cases. The tumor may occur

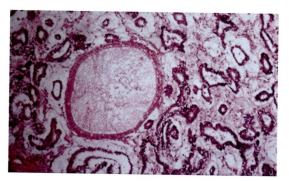

Figure 37.1 Immature teratoma. Immature neuroectodermal tubules surrounding mucin-secreting cystic structure. H&E × 100.

in patients with an XY karyotype or gonadal dysgenesis. If the tumor is diagnosed in patients with gonadoblastoma elements in the specimen or streak ovaries, the contralateral ovary should be removed as these patients are at increased risk of recurrence of gonadoblastoma [6]. For those patients who have been diagnosed with gonadal dysgenesis, bilateral gonadectomy is recommended, as the risk of dysgerminoma or gonadoblastoma reaches 20–30%. Patients with androgen insensitivity syndrome (female phenotype with XY karyotype without testosterone receptors) are recommended to undergo gonadal extirpation after puberty, as the risk for an early carcinoma, while still present, is less than in those patients with gonadal dysgenesis [7].

Immature teratoma

The benign, mature teratoma, also called a benign dermoid, is the most common ovarian mass among pediatric patients. The immature teratoma denotes the presence of a malignant component within the dermoid, and accounts for approximately 20% of all malignant germ cell tumors. Immature teratomas are distinguished by the presence of immature neuroectodermal tissue (Fig. 37.1). Although typically unilateral, these cancers may be associated with a benign teratoma in the contralateral ovary, and therefore

bilateral masses in this setting should be approached with caution. Immature teratomas are composed of components derived from the three germ layers – endoderm, ectoderm and mesoderm. Tumor grade, which is a prognostically important factor, is assigned based on the amount of immature neural tissue present [8].

Immature teratomas may be associated with gliosis – small, scattered implants throughout the peritoneum. These implants are typically formed of mature neural tissue, are not malignant, and do not impact the staging of the patient. Rarely these implants can undergo malignant transformation [8].

Endodermal sinus tumor (EST)/yolk sac tumor

A yolk sac or endodermal sinus tumor component occurs in up to 20% of germ cell cancers. They are composed of primitive epithelial cells that form irregular spaces surrounding a central vessel. These characteristic formations are called Schiller–Duval bodies. Yolk sac tumors can recapitulate primitive liver and gut structures, and α-fetoprotein (AFP) is a consistent marker for these tumors. The level of AFP may be prognostic for recurrence, with patients having a tenfold increase for recurrence with a value >1000 kU/L [9].

Gonadoblastoma

Gonadoblastoma is a rare tumor associated with dysgenic XY chromosome ovaries in phenotypically female patients. Stromal and germ cell elements comprise these tumors, which are surrounded by dense connective tissue. Slightly more than 50% of the time gonadoblastomas

Germ cell/stromal tumor	β-hCG	AFP	LD	Inhibin
Dysgerminoma	+/−	−	++	−
Immature teratoma	+/−	+/−	+/−	−
Yolk sac/endodermal sinus tumor	+/−	++	+/−	−
Choriocarcinoma	++	−	−	−
Juvenile granulosa cell tumor	−	−	−	++
Sertoli–Leydig tumor	−	−	−	++

Table 37.1 Serum markers in germ cell and stromal tumors

are associated with malignant germ cell tumors, typically dysgerminomas or mixed cancers. Although not all gonadoblastomas progress to frank carcinoma, it is recommended to remove ovarian tissue in these patients [7].

Choriocarcinoma

Extremely rare in on its own, nongestational choriocarcinoma may be seen in mixed germ cell tumors. Much as the uterine choriocarcinomas (GTN), the germ cell version is made of cytotrophoblast and intermediate trophoblast as well as syncytiotrophoblast. Occasionally, in both the pure and mixed forms, abundant production of hCG induces sexual precocity with or without irregular vaginal bleeding [1].

Mixed germ cell tumors

Approximately 10% of germ cell cancers will be mixed. Most commonly, the mixture will include a dysgerminoma component. When such histology is present, the risk for bilateral tumors is similar to unmixed dysgerminoma, and should be considered. Considerations for adjuvant treatment should be based on the most malignant histology present (e.g. yolk sac tumor or choriocarinoma) [3].

Presentation

For all germ cell tumors the most common presentation is a pelvic mass, frequently rapidly enlarging, with or without pain. Rarely there may be endocrine manifestations such as precocious puberty. Tumor makers should be evaluated (Table 37.1), as well as imaging of the chest, abdomen, and pelvis via CT or MRI.

The vast majority of patients with germ cell tumors should be offered fertility-sparing surgery with the expectation of good reproductive outcomes [9,10]. Most patients will have unilateral, grossly limited tumors. Adequate staging can be offered to all such patients via a

unilateral salpingo-oophorectomy, omentectomy, biopsies of the peritoneum, and pelvic as well as para-aortic lymph biopsies. If the contralateral ovary appears enlarged or abnormal, cystectomy or biopsy can be considered but should be avoided in the case of a normal-appearing ovary. There are limited data on the appropriate role of any conservative management for bilateral ovarian involvement with a germ cell malignancy. Extrapolating from the testicular literature, it may be possible to resect overt disease from an involved contralateral ovary while still preserving tissue for future fertility. Such surgical decisions must be made in clear consultation with the patient and her family. As techniques such as oocyte preservation become more commonly available, resection with such preservation may be preferred in some cases. Retention of the uterus should also be considered in cases where a bilateral salpingo-oophorectomy has been performed.

Chemotherapy

Given their relative rarity, chemotherapy regimens for gynecology germ cell malignancies have largely been derived from protocols employed for testicular germ cell tumors. Successful early regimens (1970s) comprised vincristine, actinomycin D, and cyclophosphamide (VAC). Although VAC represented an improvement, patients with advanced disease succumbed to disease in approximately 50% of cases. Patients with incomplete resection were even more likely to experience disease progression.

BVP (bleomycin, vincristine, and cisplatin) was the preferred regimen in the 1980s. As the efficacy of etoposide (VP-16) was demonstrated in those patients with testicular germ cell cancers with measurable tumor burden, it began to replace vincristine in the treatment of germ cell tumors. This led to the development of the current regimen, utilizing bleomycin, etoposide, and cisplatin (BEP). A modified BEP protocol is now given every 21 days with 20 units/m^2 of bleomycin given only on day 1 (maximum

30 units per cycle with cumulative total dose of 120 units). Etoposide (75 mg/m^2) and cisplatin (20 mg/m^2) are given on days 1 through 5 [11]. Secondary malignancies including leukemia and myelodysplastic syndrome are now well recognized with cumulative doses of etoposide exceeding 1700–2000 mg/m^2 [11].

Most patients with germ cell tumors are candidates for adjuvant chemotherapy. Treatment with BEP is not recommended for those patients with grade 1, stage 1A immature teratoma, but should be considered for all others. Many authors advocate avoiding adjuvant therapy in grade 2, stage 1A immature teratoma and stage 1A dysgerminoma [12], but these decisions should be made on a case-by-case basis. Close observation must be advocated for both diagnoses, especially given that the risk of recurrence among early dysgerminomas may be as high as 15–20%.

Patients with malignant germ cell tumors can be expected to do well with current surgical and chemotherapy techniques [13,14]. The majority of patients are early stage in which progression-free survival is greater than 90% [15]. Risk factors for failure include advanced disease (stage III and IV), grade 3 immature teratomas, endodermal sinus tumor/yolk sac tumors, and highly elevated tumor markers. Appropriate treatment of these tumors involves fertility-preserving staging, risk stratification, and judicious use of chemotherapy.

Stromal cell tumors

Stromal cell neoplasms account for approximately 5% of ovarian masses in the pediatric population [2]. Fortunately the majority of these tumors are benign. There are two important types that are most commonly seen: juvenile granulosa cell tumors and Sertoli–Leydig tumors.

Juvenile granulosa cell tumor

Adult granulosa cell tumors typically occur in patients 50 years or older. Normally granulosa cells support germ cell follicles and secrete estrogen. The classic adult presentation involves a hemorrhagic mass, abnormal bleeding and, perhaps, endometrial hyperplasia or endometrioid carcinoma. In the juvenile population there is a similar premature estrogen release with precocious puberty. Serum inhibins A and B function as specific tumor markers, useful in detection of recurrence and evaluating response to therapy. A palpable mass is an almost ubiquitous

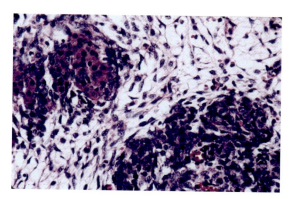

Figure 37.2 Juvenile granulosa cell tumor. Granulosa tumor cells with hyperchromatic nuclei and luteinized cells (upper left). H&E × 400.

finding. The vast majority of the tumors will be stage I, with most of these stage 1A.

Grossly the juvenile granulosa cell tumor appears similar to the adult type with a hemorrhagic cystic and solid appearance. Histologically, there are important differences that will be encountered. The classic Call–Exner bodies will not be seen. Nuclei of adult granulosa cell tumors have a "coffee bean" appearance, which is absent in the juvenile type. The nuclei are rounded and hyperchromatic with classic vacuoles in the cytoplasm (Fig. 37.2).

Prognosis appears to mirror stage. Most patients present with stage I tumors and do not require adjuvant chemotherapy. There are limited data regarding those patients who will need treatment. Most recommendations are based on the adult experience, which favors BEP in advanced (stage III and IV) or recurrent cases. Long-term follow-up is recommended, given the propensity for late recurrence. Alternative salvage chemotherapy regimens include multiagent therapy incorporating combinations including ifosfamide, etoposide, taxanes and other platinum agents. Recent data regarding the use of taxanes in both a salvage and adjuvant role have been encouraging [16].

Sertoli–Leydig tumors

Although extremely rare, the Sertoli–Leydig tumor may present with poorer prognostic features early in life. Generally, they occur after menses and can be associated with significant virilization as well as an abdominal mass. Irregular bleeding may occur due to conversion of peripheral androgenic hormones to estrogen.

These tumors tend to be solid, with a size between 5 and 15 cm. Histologically, the degree of differentiation of the tumor will affect the recapitulation of male seminiferous tubules. Lipid can be observed as well, as the Sertoli or Leydig cells may be manufacturing hormone.

Well over 90% of these tumors will be confined to the ovary at diagnosis, and the majority will not exhibit any malignant features [1]. Malignant tumors are notable for having advanced stage at diagnosis, moderate or poor degrees of differentiation, or heterologous features. The retiform pattern is associated with malignancy as well.

Other stromal tumors

The remainder of the stromal tumors represents a collection of unusual masses. The most common is the thecoma but very few of these are malignant, and even fewer present before the age of 30. Fibromas are likewise more common among older patients but may be seen in patients with Gorlin syndrome (also known as basal nevus syndrome, an inherited group of multiple defects involving the skin, nervous system, eyes, endocrine system, and bones), and may be associated with ascites and pleural effusion in Meig syndrome. Finally, sex cord tumors with annular tubules (SCAT) are associated with Peutz–Jeghers syndrome (PJS; hereditary intestinal polyposis with hyperpigmentation around the mouth and on the hands and feet). Fortunately, almost all patients with PJS have benign SCAT. When discovered in a patient without PJS, malignancy can be diagnosed in approximately 20% of SCAT cases.

Epithelial ovarian tumors

Epithelial tumors of the ovary are rare in the premenstrual population. In a 15-year review from the Children's Hospital of Philadelphia epithelial tumors represented 19 (16.2%) of 240 cases of ovarian masses identified. The majority of these tumors were not malignant, with only three mucinous cystadenocarcinomas and four serous borderline tumors [2].

The mean age at diagnosis for epithelial tumors was 13.9 years with pain and asymptomatic masses being the most common presentation. Historically, epithelial tumors have accounted for approximately 15% of pelvic masses diagnosed.

Although adenocarcinoma is rare in this population, staging and treatment are similar to adult cases. For apparent early-stage disease (stage I and II) fertility preservation is encouraged with unilateral oophorectomy, omentec-

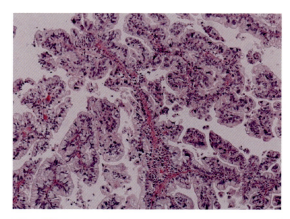

Figure 37.3 Ovarian mucinous tumor of borderline malignancy with glandular crowding and minimal cytologic atypia. H&E × 40.

tomy, biopsies, and retroperitoneal lymph node sampling. Adjuvant therapy guidelines mirror the adult recommendations with taxol (175 mg/m^2) and carboplatin (AUC 5-6) chemotherapy.

Borderline tumors

Although rare in the pediatric population, borderline ovarian tumors can be seen with greater frequency than frank carcinoma. These tumors are more common in the second decade of life and warrant special consideration of their surgical and postoperative management. In this age group mucinous ovarian tumors are more common than serous papillary (Fig. 37.3).

Although the generic term "borderline" has been widely used in the past, currently these neoplasms are dichotomized to delineate those patients who can be safely observed versus those who require adjunctive chemotherapy. The most important and pathologic feature is the presence of implants, either grossly or microscopically. The treating pathologist should label such implants "invasive" or "noninvasive."

Patients with borderline tumors (without invasive implants) tend to have early-stage disease and enjoy excellent outcomes. The vast majority will not recur, nor will they require any treatment. Even in these patients, however, careful surveillance is required, as the median time to recurrence is 5–7 years. Patients who do recur tend to do so with recurrent borderline tumors and occasionally with low-grade carcinomas, which may require adjuvant chemotherapy. For patients who recur without frank carcinoma, re-resection is the treatment of choice. The decision for adjuvant treatment is based on the presence of an invasive component.

Patients with borderline tumors with invasive implants have a 34% risk of death from disease [17] and therefore full surgical staging is required. These patients require adjuvant chemotherapy with taxol and carboplatin and are managed analogously to patients with invasive epithelial ovarian cancer.

Rhabdomyosarcoma

Rhabdomyosarcoma (RMS) is a mesenchymally derived neoplasm notable for occurring in children. The peak incidence is approximately 2–6 years for vaginal RMS and the second decade of life for primary cervical involvement. The tumor is highly malignant and at one time carried a dismal prognosis, with most patients dying of metastatic disease. In the past, attempts to manage this cancer resulted in aggressive, life-altering operations such as pelvic exenteration for vaginal rhabdomyosarcoma. Current management is directed toward multimodal therapy, with chemotherapy given upfront and surgery or radiation reserved for persistent disease.

Gynecologic rhabdomyosarcoma is a rare anatomic site of a very unusual cancer. Only 250 cases of soft tissue RMS of all anatomic sites will be diagnosed annually, and of these only 5–10% will be embryonal subtype "sarcoma botryoides" of the vagina and cervix [18]. Grossly, the tumor has a classic "grape-like" polypoid appearance. Physiologically these cancers resemble skeletal muscle of a 7–10 week fetus (see Chapter 10, Figures 10.1–10.3).

Presentation of vaginal RMS usually involves a mass projecting from the vaginal introitus accompanied by a foul smell and bloody discharge. Initial evaluation involves imaging with a CT scan or MRI of the chest, abdomen, and pelvis. A vaginoscopy with biopsy is necessary for confirmation of the diagnosis.

Chemotherapy is the cornerstone of treatment of vaginal RMS. This represents a major change in treatment from the early 1970s, when pelvic examination was considered primary therapy. Over the intervening years, the Soft Tissue Sarcoma Committee of the Children's Oncology Group has refined treatment protocols to feature upfront therapy primarily with vincristine, dactinomycin, and cyclophosphamide (VAC). Using this modality, the need for surgical excision has dropped from 100% in the years 1972–1978 to 13% in 1999 [19]. Some referral centers have employed different chemotherapy regimens for primary disease. Chemotherapy is generally given over a 12-week period followed by repeat assessment via vaginoscopy with biopsies. For those patients with residual disease who need resection, limited surgical intervention is possible [20]. For patients with residual disease, the recommendation is for external beam pelvic radiation, which invariably compromises future fertility. To preserve ovarian function, tailored radiation via high-dose brachytherapy may be utilized for local control, but can still be associated with late, local complications [21].

With current treatment modalities, excellent outcomes can be expected. Patients with localized disease can be cured in the majority of cases with minimal long-term morbidity. For patients with persistent disease after primary treatment with VAC, either surgery, radiation or a combination is employed. Secondary chemotherapy is often used for those patients with progressive or recurrent disease. Agents utilized include ifosfamide, etoposide, cisplatin, melphalan or doxorubicin [22]. Importantly, an interval biopsy taken during initial therapy may demonstrate conversion to mature rhabdomyoblasts. This is not a sign of treatment failure, but is thought to represent maturation of the malignant cells as an index of chemoresponse. In this setting, further chemotherapy should be employed and the temptation to undertake radical extirpative surgery should be resisted.

Clear cell cervical/vaginal cancer

Historically clear cell cancer of the vagina and cervix was associated with in utero diethylstilbestrol exposure. For the most part, these patients have aged beyond the pediatric population but sporadic, spontaneous cases are still seen. Treatment of localized disease has historically consisted of radical hysterectomy with or without preservation of the ovaries.

For these pediatric patients, the issue of fertility preservation is paramount. Radical trachelectomy in this pediatric population represents a novel approach [23]. Given the limited geometry of the vaginal orifice, an abdominal approach is recommended. Vaginoscopy can help delineate the extent of disease and define margins for excision. Preservation of the gonadal vessels provides adequate blood supply for the uterus. Long-term pregnancy outcomes are lacking, as children treated with radical trachelectomy have not yet reached child-bearing age. There is, however, no reason to assume that fertility and pregnancy outcomes will differ significantly from adults treated with radical trachelectomy. Adjuvant chemotherapy agents employed either for metastastic disease or for improvement of local control include etoposide, cisplatin, taxanes, and anthracyclines [24].

References

1. Gribbon M, Ein SH, Mancer K. Pediatric malignant ovarian tumors: a 43-year review. *J Pediatr Surg* 1992;**27**:480–484.
2. Morowitz M, Huff D, von Allmen D. Epithelial ovarian tumors in children: a retrospective analysis. *J Pediatr Surg* 2003;**38**:331–335; discussion 331–335.
3. Peccatori F, Bonazzi C, Chiari S, Landoni F, Colombo N, Mangioni C. Surgical management of malignant ovarian germ-cell tumors: 10 years' experience of 129 patients. *Obstet Gynecol* 1995;**86**:367–372.
4. Tewari K, Cappuccini F, Disaia PJ, Berman ML, Manetta A, Kohler MF. Malignant germ cell tumors of the ovary. *Obstet Gynecol* 2000;**95**:128–133.
5. Billmire D, Vinocur C, Rescorla F et al. Outcome and staging evaluation in malignant germ cell tumors of the ovary in children and adolescents: an intergroup study. *J Pediatr Surg* 2004;**39**:424–429.
6. Troche V, Hernandez E. Neoplasia arising in dysgenetic gonads. *Obstet Gynecol Surv* 1986;**41**:74–79.
7. Pauls K, Franke FE, Buttner R, Zhou H. Gonadoblastoma: evidence for a stepwise progression to dysgerminoma in a dysgenetic ovary. *Virchows Arch* 2005;**447**:603–609.
8. O'Connor DM, Norris HJ. The influence of grade on the outcome of stage I ovarian immature (malignant) teratomas and the reproducibility of grading. *Int J Gynecol Pathol* 1994;**13**:283–289.
9. Mitchell PL, Al-Nasiri N, A'Hem R et al. Treatment of nondysgerminomatous ovarian germ cell tumors: an analysis of 69 cases. *Cancer* 1999;**85**:2232–2244.
10. Zanetta G, Bonazzi C, Cantu M et al. Survival and reproductive function after treatment of malignant germ cell ovarian tumors. *J Clin Oncol* 2001;**19**:1015–1020.
11. Homesley HD, Bundy BN, Hurteau JA, Roth LM. Bleomycin, etoposide, and cisplatin combination therapy of ovarian granulosa cell tumors and other stromal malignancies: a Gynecologic Oncology Group study. *Gynecol Oncol* 1999;**72**:131–137.
12. Schneider DT, Calaminus G, Wessalowski R et al. Ovarian sex cord-stromal tumors in children and adolescents. *J Clin Oncol* 2003;**21**:2357–2363.
13. Dimopoulos MA, Papadimitriou C, Hamilos G et al. Treatment of ovarian germ cell tumors with a 3-day bleomycin, etoposide, and cisplatin regimen: a prospective multicenter study. *Gynecol Oncol* 2004;**95**:695–700.
14. Kondagunta GV, Bacik J, Donadio A et al. Combination of paclitaxel, ifosfamide, and cisplatin is an effective second-line therapy for patients with relapsed testicular germ cell tumors. *J Clin Oncol* 2005;**23**:6549–6555.
15. Rogers PC, Olson TA, Cullen JW et al. Treatment of children and adolescents with stage II testicular and stages I and II ovarian malignant germ cell tumors: a Pediatric Intergroup Study-Pediatric Oncology Group 9048 and Children's Cancer Group 8891. *J Clin Oncol* 2004;**22**:3563–3569.
16. Brown J, Shvartsman HS, Deavers MT et al. The activity of taxanes compared with bleomycin, etoposide, and cisplatin in the treatment of sex cord-stromal ovarian tumors. *Gynecol Oncol* 2005;**97**:489–496.
17. Seidman JD, Kurman RJ. Ovarian serous borderline tumors: a critical review of the literature with emphasis on prognostic indicators. *Hum Pathol* 2000;**31**:539–557.
18. Crist W, Gehan EA, Ragab AH et al. The Third Intergroup Rhabdomyosarcoma Study. *J Clin Oncol* 1995;**13**:610–630.
19. Andrassy RJ, Wiener ES, Raney RB et al. Progress in the surgical management of vaginal rhabdomyosarcoma: a 25-year review from the Intergroup Rhabdomyosarcoma Study Group. *J Pediatr Surg* 1999;**34**:731–734; discussion 734–735.
20. Solomon LA, Zurawin RK, Edwards CL. Vaginoscopic resection for rhabdomyosarcoma of the vagina: a case report and review of the literature. *J Pediatr Adolesc Gynecol* 2003;**16**:139–142.
21. Nag S, Tippin D, Ruymann FB. Long-term morbidity in children treated with fractionated high-dose-rate brachytherapy for soft tissue sarcomas. *J Pediatr Hematol Oncol* 2003;**25**:448–452.
22. Arndt CA, Donaldson SS, Anderson JR et al. What constitutes optimal therapy for patients with rhabdomyosarcoma of the female genital tract? *Cancer* 2001;**9**:2454–2468.
23. Abu-Rustum NR, Su W, Levine DA, Boyd J, Sonoda Y, Laquaglia MP. Pediatric radical abdominal trachelectomy for cervical clear cell carcinoma: a novel surgical approach. *Gynecol Oncol* 2005;**97**:296–300.
24. McNall RY, Nowicki PD, Miller B, Billups CA, Liu T, Daw NC. Adenocarcinoma of the cervix and vagina in pediatric patients. *Pediatr Blood Cancer* 2004;**43**:289–294.

CHAPTER 38

Cervix Cytology, Dysplasia, and Human Papillomavirus

Ali Mahdavi & Bradley J. Monk
University of California Irvine Medical Center, Irvine, CA, USA

Introduction

Human papillomavirus (HPV) infection is believed to be the most common sexually transmitted infection both in the United States and worldwide [1]. Rates of HPV infections are highest in adolescent populations with cumulative prevalence rates as high as 82% in selected groups. A study of adolescents who were initially HPV negative found that 55% acquired HPV within three years. In another study of college-enrolled women who were HPV negative, and reported never having sexual intercourse at enrollment, approximately 30% acquired HPV within 12 months after initiating intercourse and more than 50% became HPV positive within four years (Fig. 38.1) [2]. These numbers underscore the ease of sexual transmission of HPV in adolescent and young adult women.

Persistent infection with high-risk HPV types (e.g. HPV-16 or -18) is considered necessary for the development of cervical cancer. Since cervical cancer screening with the Papanicolaou (Pap) smear has become widespread, the incidence of invasive cervical cancer in developed countries has dramatically decreased. At the same time, the detection of cervical dysplasia has significantly increased. Diagnosis, management, and follow-up of preinvasive cervical lesions are now a major public health challenge. With teens becoming sexually active earlier, the incidence of cervical dysplasia in adolescents has risen in the past decade. For these young women, the benefits of detecting and eradicating cervical dysplasia must be balanced against the long-term complications of treatment and the low incidence of cervical cancer.

This chapter discusses HPV infection and evaluation and management of abnormal cervical cytology and histology in adolescents and young adults. We also review existing evidence regarding efficacy and tolerance of HPV vaccines and discuss key issues related to HPV vaccine implementation.

Human papillomavirus

More than 40 different HPV types have been identified that infect the anogenital epithelia and other mucosal membranes. Some 13–18 of these types are recognized as high-oncogenic risk HPV types (Fig. 38.2) [3]. It is estimated that HPV-16 accounts for approximately 60% of cervical cancers, with HPV-18 adding another 10–20%. Other high-risk types include 31, 33, 35, 39, 45, 51, 52, 56, 58, 59, 68, and 73.

The HPV genome regulates synthesis of eight proteins. The late L1 and L2 genes code for the viral capsid proteins, the early proteins E1 and E2 are responsible for viral replication and transcription, and E4 seems to aid virus release from infected cells (Fig. 38.3). The early genes of the high-risk HPV types (E6 and E7) encode the main transforming proteins. These genes are capable of immortalization of epithelial cells and are thought to play a role in the initiation of the oncogenic process. The protein products of these early genes interfere with the normal

Pediatric, Adolescent, & Young Adult Gynecology. Edited by A. Altchek and L. Deligdisch. © 2009 Blackwell Publishing, ISBN: 978-1-4051-5347-8.

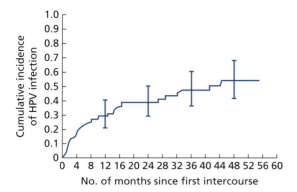

Figure 38.1 Cumulative incidence of HPV infection from time of first sexual intercourse. Adapted from [2].

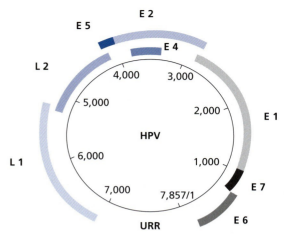

Figure 38.3 Schematic presentation of the HPV genome.

function of tumor suppressor genes. HPV E6 is able to interact with p53, leading to its dysfunction, thereby impairing its ability to block the cell cycle when DNA errors occur. E6 also keeps the telomerase length above its critical point, protecting the cell from apoptosis. HPV E7 binds to retinoblastoma protein (pRb) and activates genes that start the cell cycle, leading to tissue proliferation (Fig. 38.4). To a lesser extent, E5 has also been implicated in cellular transformation.

It is now widely accepted that high-risk (HR) HPV infections are a necessary, but not sufficient, cause of virtually all cases of cervical cancer worldwide (Fig. 38.5) and are a likely cause of a substantial proportion of other anogenital neoplasms and oral squamous cell carcinomas. An estimated 85% of anal cancers, 50% of the cancers of the vulva, vagina, and penis, 20% of oropharyngeal cancers, and 10% of laryngeal and esophageal cancers are attributable to HPV.

Epidemiology and pathogenesis of HPV infection

There are an estimated 6.2 million new cases of HR-HPV infection occurring in the US each year, and approximately 20 million Americans are infected with HPV at any one time [1].

Risk determinants for HPV infection that have been identified in various cross-sectional and prospective cohort studies include the number of sexual partners (lifetime and recent), age at first intercourse, smoking, oral contraceptive (OC) use, other sexually transmitted infections (e.g. chlamydia and herpes simplex virus), chronic inflammation, immunosuppressive conditions including HIV infection, and parity. Nevertheless, the most consistent determinant of HPV infection is age, with most

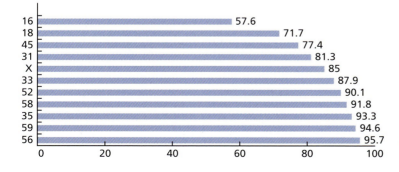

Figure 38.2 HPV types in cervical cancer. Adapted from [16].

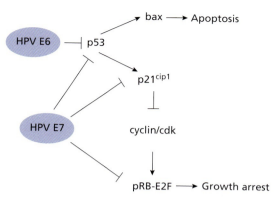

Figure 38.4 Functional abrogation of the p53 and retinoblastoma (pRB) tumor suppressor pathways by high-risk HPV E6 and E7 oncoproteins. E6 and E7 can interact with p53 and pRB, respectively, and induce their proteolytic degradation. HPV E7 can also interfere with the transcriptional activity of p53 and can inactivate the cdk inhibitor p21$^{CIP1/WAF1/SDI1}$, a major mediator of p53-induced growth arrest. The combined inactivation of the pRB and p53 tumor suppressor pathways interferes with the integrity of important cell cycle checkpoints and the cellular apoptosis defense program. See text for details.

studies indicating a sharp decrease in risk after the age of 30. The decrease in risk of HPV infection with increasing age seems to be independent of changes in sexual behavior, suggesting a role for immune response.

Most infections seem to clear spontaneously; cohort studies have consistently found that only a small proportion of women positive for a given HPV type are found to have the same type in subsequent specimens [4]. Whether infections clear completely or the virus remains latent in basal cells at undetectable levels is a matter of debate and cannot be verified empirically. What is clear, however, is the fact that risk of subsequent cervical intraepithe-

lial neoplasia (CIN) is proportional to the number of specimens testing positive for HPV. This suggests that carcinogenesis results from HPV infections that persist productively (i.e. with sustained viral replication within the squamous epithelium) for prolonged periods of time.

In studies of adolescents with newly acquired HPV infection, the average length of detectable HPV is 13 months. In most adolescent patients with an intact immune system, an HPV infection will resolve within 24 months. Further evidence that the HPV infection will resolve without treatment comes from the high rates of resolution of CIN 1 and CIN 2, 70% and 50% respectively.

Human papillomavirus transmission

HPV is transmitted by skin-to-skin contact. For fulminant infection, HPV requires access to basal cells through microabrasions or tears in the squamous or mucosal epithelium that are often produced during sexual activity [5] (Fig. 38.6). Infection of the cervix is generally thought to require sexual intercourse, but HPV can infect other anogenital sites such as the external genitalia. Additionally, HPV can be transmitted through skin-to-skin contact during nonintercourse foreplay and may even be transmissible by fingers or sex toys. HPV infection has been detected in women who have reported never having sexual intercourse with men, which supports the existence of these alternative modes of transmission. As such, adolescents who abstain from sexual intercourse but not other forms of sexual behavior remain at risk of acquiring HPV, and adolescents who use condoms may still acquire HPV infection at epithelial sites outside the area covered by a condom.

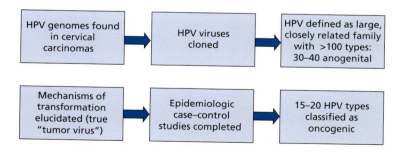

Figure 38.5 Discovery of the link between HPV and cervical cancer [3].

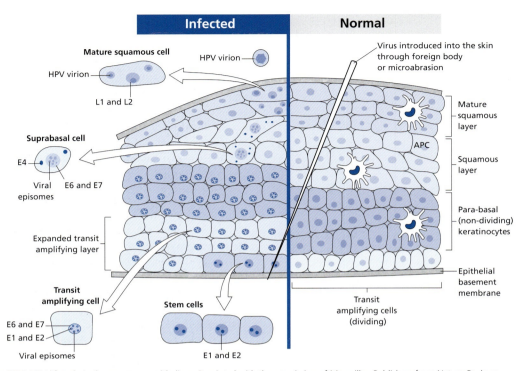

Figure 38.6 HPV lifecycle in the squamous epithelium. Reprinted with the permission of Macmillan Publishers from *Nature Reviews Immunology* 2004;**4**:46–54.

In rare instances, HPV can be transmitted from a mother to her newborn baby during vaginal delivery, resulting in recurrent respiratory papillomatosis, which can be fatal. Moreover, unexplained and extremely rare cases have been reported in newborns delivered by cesarean section; however, the rarity of neonatal transmission does not justify performing a cesarean section delivery for women with genital warts or abnormal cytology.

Cervical dysplasia and cervical cancer

Cervical cancer is the second most common cancer in women worldwide, with more than 500,000 new cases diagnosed each year. In the United States, the American Cancer Society estimates that 11,150 new cases of invasive cervical cancer were diagnosed and 3650 women died from cervical cancer in 2007 [6].

Although often illustrated as a simple progression from CIN 1 to cancer, the spectrum of precursor lesions is quite complex owing to its origins in a site (transformation zone) that supports a wide range of differentiation, including squamous, columnar and metaplastic epithelium (Fig. 38.7). The lowest-grade CIN lesions, including condylomata, most likely do not progress, whereas lesions containing greater degrees of cellular atypia are at greater risk. Not all lesions begin as condylomata or as CIN 1; they may enter at any point in the sequence, depending on the associated HPV type and other host factors. The rates of progression are by no means uniform, and although HPV type is a potential predictor of lesion behavior, it is difficult to predict the outcome in an individual patient. These findings underscore the fact that risk of cancer is conferred only in part by HPV type and may depend on both host–virus interactions and environmental factors to bring about the evolution of a cancer precursor. Most cases of CIN 1 will remit spontaneously; however,

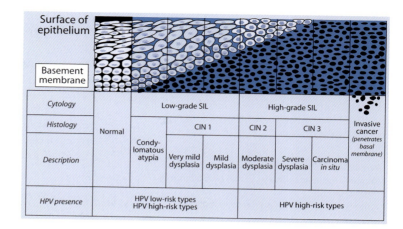

Figure 38.7 HPV-related dysplasia and neoplasia.

untreated CIN 1 in adult women signifies a risk of 13% for diagnosis of CIN 2 or CIN 3 at two-year follow-up. In contrast to CIN 1, CIN 2 and CIN 3 are recognized potential cancer precursors, although CIN 2 is associated with significant spontaneous regression. Evidence from large studies suggests that approximately 40% of CIN 2 cases regressed over two years, whereas regression of CIN 3, if present, was too rare to measure. Predictably, lesions that have completely evolved (CIN 3) constitute the greatest cancer risk. Progression to invasive carcinoma, when it occurs, may develop in a few months to years.

Based on the natural history data and the rarity of cervical cancer in the population of women younger than 21 years, the American Cancer Society (ACS) recommendations for initial Pap testing have changed and the new criteria have been endorsed by the American College of Obstetricians and Gynecologists (ACOG) [7]. Adolescents should undergo their first Pap test approximately three years after the onset of vaginal intercourse or no later than age 21 years.

Cervical cytology

Cervical cytology screening is associated with a reduction in the incidence of and mortality from invasive squamous cancer. Conventional cytology is reported to be 30–87% sensitive for dysplasia. Treatment based on conventional

cytology results does not seem to decrease the incidence of glandular invasive cancers, suggesting that sensitivity for glandular precursors is less than that observed for squamous lesions.

Because the range of sensitivity (30–87%) is so broad, all abnormal cytology results must be evaluated, although the vast majority does not represent underlying CIN 2/3. Reproducibility among observers and among multiple readings by the same observer is quite modest. Therefore, when cytologic testing is selected for follow-up of previous abnormal results, repeat testing at 6–12 month intervals is recommended.

Bethesda classification and screening guidelines

In May 2001, representatives from 44 professional societies endorsed a revised system of terminology, the 2001 Bethesda system, to describe cervical cytology (Box 38.1). The goal was to promote more consistent, comprehensible reporting of findings for clinical management. Two important changes are a new description of specimen adequacy and the designation of a new category of epithelial cell abnormality. The 2001 system eliminates the category of "less than optimal" or "satisfactory but limited by" from descriptions of specimen adequacy, leaving only the options of "satisfactory

Box 38.1 The 2001 Bethesda system

SPECIMEN ADEQUACY

Satisfactory for evaluation (*note presence/absence of endocervical/transformation zone component*)
Unsatisfactory for evaluation

GENERAL CATEGORIZATION (optional)

Negative for intraepithelial lesion or malignancy
Epithelial cell abnormality
Other

INTERPRETATION/RESULT

Negative for Intraepithelial Lesion or Malignancy

Organisms
Trichomonas vaginalis, fungal, bacterial vaginosis

Other nonneoplastic findings
Inflammation, radiation, atrophy

Epithelial Cell Abnormalities

Squamous cell
  Atypical squamous cells (ASC)
  of undetermined significance (ASCUS)
  cannot exclude HSIL (ASC-H)
  Low-grade squamous intraepithelial lesion (LSIL)
  High-grade squamous intraepithelial lesion (HSIL)
  Squamous cell carcinoma
Glandular cell
  Atypical glandular cells (AGC)
  Atypical glandular cells, favor neoplastic (*specify endocervical or NOS*)
  Endocervical adenocarcinoma *in situ* (AIS)
  Adenocarcinoma

Other (*List not comprehensive*)
  Endometrial cells in a woman ≥40 years of age

for evaluation" or "unsatisfactory for evaluation." Adequacy is decided independently of whether endocervical/transformation zone cells are present, so a specimen may be labeled "satisfactory for evaluation" even if there are no endocervical cells present. Bethesda 2001 terminology includes a new category of epithelial cell lesion, "atypical squamous cells, cannot exclude high-grade lesion" (ASC-H). ASC-H specimens, which represent about 5–10% of all ASC specimens, have a positive predictive value for CIN 2 or 3 in between that of atypical squamous cells of undetermined significance (ASCUS) and high-grade squamous intraepithelial lesions (HSIL), and therefore merit particular attention from clinical providers [8].

Management of abnormal cervical cytology in adolescents

New information has prompted different organizations, including ACOG, to modify the guidelines on the management of abnormal cervical cytology in adolescents. Compared to the adult population, management of abnormal cervical cytology in adolescents is more conservative as most low-grade lesions spontaneously resolve in this group of young women.

Atypical squamous cells of undetermined significance (ASCUS)

In the adolescent population, the prevalence of HPV in ASCUS is higher than its prevalence in the older population. The risk of invasive cancer in the adolescents approaches zero and the likelihood of HPV clearance is very high. It is estimated that over two-thirds of adolescents with ASCUS would be referred to colposcopy using a program of "reflex" HPV DNA testing. Therefore, repeat cytology is recommended in adolescents with ASCUS; this approach greatly limits the use of colposcopy in this group of patients [9]. At the 12-month follow-up, only adolescents with HSIL or greater on the repeat cytology should be referred to colposcopy. At the 24-month follow-up, those with an ASCUS or greater result should be referred to colposcopy. HPV DNA testing and colposcopy are unacceptable for adolescents with ASCUS. If HPV testing is inadvertently performed, the results should not influence the treatment [9,10].

Low-grade squamous intraepithelial lesions or atypical squamous cells: cannot exclude high-grade squamous intraepithelial lesions

In adolescents with LSIL, follow-up with annual cytologic testing is recommended. At the 12-month follow-up, only adolescents with HSIL or greater on the repeat cytology should be referred to colposcopy. At the 24-month follow-up, those with an ASCUS or greater result should be referred to colposcopy [9].

Because of a lack of specific evidence and the high rate of CIN 2, CIN 3, and cervical cancer in individuals with ASC-H, the adolescent with ASC-H should undergo immediate colposcopic evaluation [10].

Table 38.1 Differences in cervical cancer screening and management of CIN in adolescents and adults

	Adolescents	Adults
ASCUS LSIL	Repeat cytology twice at 12-month intervals	Colposcopy
CIN 2/3	Repeat colposcopy and cytology at six-month intervals	Ablation or excision

High-grade squamous intraepithelial lesions

High-grade squamous intraepithelial lesion (HSIL) is a significant cytologic abnormality that requires colposcopy and endocervical assessment because of the high rate of histologically confirmed CIN 2, CIN 3 or cervical cancer. The "see and treat approach" should be avoided in the adolescent population. When CIN 2/3 is not identified histologically, observation for up to 24 months using both colposcopy and cytology at six-month intervals is preferred, provided that the colposcopic examination is satisfactory and endocervical sampling is negative [10]. After two consecutive negative results, adolescents without a high-grade colposcopic abnormality can return to routine cytologic screening.

Atypical glandular cells

The prevalence of atypical glandular cells (AGC) cytology in the adolescent population is very low, and most of these abnormalities will arise from the squamous component of the cervix. The adolescent with AGC should undergo a colposcopy and endocervical sampling. Endometrial sampling would not be used in most adolescents unless they are morbidly obese, have abnormal uterine bleeding or there is a suspicion of endometrial cells.

Treatment of cervical dysplasia in adolescents

Management of cervical dysplasia in adolescents differs from that for the adult population. It is important to avoid aggressive management of benign lesions in adolescents because most CIN grades 1 and 2 regress spontaneously.

Cervical intraepithelial neoplasia 1

Depending on the time from HPV exposure to evaluation, the adolescent who is infected may have a normal cervix, mildly abnormal cervix or biopsy-confirmed CIN 1. In the adolescent population, the rate of resolution of

CIN 1 is extremely high (greater than 85%). The ACOG recommends observation as the best approach to CIN 1 in adolescents [10]. Follow-up with annual cytologic assessment is recommended for adolescents with CIN 1 [11]. At the 12-month follow-up, only adolescents with HSIL or greater on the repeat cytology should be referred to colposcopy. At the 24-month follow-up, those with an ASCUS or greater result should be referred to colposcopy.

For those few individuals who require therapy for CIN 1, cryotherapy, laser therapy, and LEEP are equally effective. Care should be taken to remove or ablate the least amount of cervical tissue that is necessary to eradicate the lesion.

Cervical intraepithelial neoplasia 2/3

CIN 2/3 includes lesions previously referred to as moderate dysplasia (i.e. CIN 2) and severe dysplasia/carcinoma *in situ* (i.e. CIN 3). Although CIN 2 lesions are more heterogenous and more likely to regress during long-term follow-up than are CIN 3 lesions, histologic distinction between CIN 2 and CIN 3 is poorly reproducible [11].

For adolescents and young women with a histologic diagnosis of CIN 2/3 not otherwise specified, either treatment or observation for up to 24 months using both colposcopy and cytology at six-month intervals is acceptable, provided colposcopy is satisfactory (Table 38.1). When a histologic diagnosis of CIN 2 is specified, observation is preferred but treatment is acceptable. When a histologic diagnosis of CIN 3 is specified or when colposcopy is unsatisfactory, treatment is recommended. If the colposcopic appearance of the lesion worsens or if HSIL cytology or a high-grade colposcopic lesion persists for one year, repeat biopsy is recommended [11].

Prophylactic human papillomavirus vaccine

As HPV is present in almost all cervical cancer cases, the concept of a vaccine against HPV becomes central in prevention of cervical cancer. When considering prevention on a broad scale, it is important to bear in mind that HPV-6 and -11 are responsible for most cases of genital warts, and that HPV-16 and -18 account for 60–70% of cervical cancers. A vaccine targeted against these four types of HPV would have the greatest potential for decreasing the incidence of HPV-associated disease, as well as decreasing the morbidity and mortality associated with cervical cancer.

In general, prophylactic vaccines induce the generation of neutralizing antibody to the pathogen and thus prevent disease on subsequent exposure [12]. A vaccine generating such responses must contain L1 protein in the correctly folded, tertiary or "native" form. Technically, this was very difficult but a major experimental breakthrough showed that the L1 protein, when expressed by vectors such as recombinant baculovirus or yeast, self-assembled into virus-like particles (VLPs). The L1 VLP is a conformationally correct, empty capsid (i.e. it contains no DNA) that appears morphologically identical to, and contains the major neutralizing epitopes of, the native virion.

The results of a randomized, double-blind placebo-controlled multicenter phase II trial of a quadrivalent VLP vaccine were published recently [13]. The vaccine included four recombinant HPV type-specific VLPs consisting of the L1 major capsid proteins of HPV-6, -11, -16, and -18 adsorbed onto amorphous aluminum hydroxyphosphate sulfate adjuvant (Gardasil®, Merck Research Laboratories, Whitehouse Station, NJ). Two hundred and seventy seven young women (mean age 20.2 years) were randomly assigned to quadrivalent HPV (20 μg type 6, 40 μg type 11, 40 μg type 16, and 20 μg type 18) L1 VLP vaccine and 275 (mean age 20.0 years) to one of two placebo preparations at day 1, month 2, and month 6. In the according-to-protocol cohort, the incidence of persistent HPV-6, -11, -16 or -18 infection or associated disease decreased by 90% (95% CI 71–97) in women who received the vaccine compared with placebo. The results were similar in an intention-to-treat analysis. All women who received vaccine developed HPV antibody to the four HPV types after the series was completed, and antibody titers were substantially higher than in placebo recipients who had had a previous HPV infection. Mean antibody titers at month 36 remained at or above the titers in women who had a natural HPV infection and cleared the virus.

A phase III trial of the quadrivalent vaccine, involving 17,800 women aged 16 to 23 years, has recently been completed. In a subsample of 12,167 women who were randomized to receive quadrivalent HPV-6/11/16/18 recombinant vaccine (Gardasil®) or placebo and who followed the protocol closely, the vaccine was 100% effective in preventing incident HPV-16/18-related CIN 2/3, adenocarcinoma in situ, and cervical cancer during two years of follow-up. The vaccine was well tolerated and there were no vaccine-related serious adverse events. In June 2006, the FDA announced the approval of Gardasil®, the first vaccine developed to prevent cervical cancer, precancerous genital lesions and genital warts due to HPV types 6, 11, 16 and 18 [14]. Gardasil is indicated in girls and women 9–26 years of age. Vaccination with Gardasil does not substitute for routine cervical cancer screening, and women who receive Gardasil should continue to undergo screening per standard of care. The vaccine-related adverse experiences that were observed among recipients of Gardasil at a frequency of at least 1.0% and greater than placebo were pain, swelling, erythema, fever, nausea, pruritus, and dizziness. GlaxoSmithKline has filed for FDA approval of Cervarix®, a bivalent HPV-16/18 VLP vaccine; Cervarix has been approved for use in women and children in 67 countries around the world. Table 38.2 compares the characteristics of the quadrivalent and bivalent VLP HPV vaccines.

There is some evidence that VLP vaccines may induce higher antibody titers in preteens/adolescents compared with adult women. Higher antibody titers in the younger women might result in longer antibody persistence and be particularly advantageous when an HPV vaccine is administered at a young age well before sexual activity.

In the short term, HPV vaccines should have little impact on frequency of cervical cancer screening. Since the vaccines may initially cover only types 16 and 18, one must continue to screen for the other 30% of HPV disease caused by the types not in the first versions of these vaccines. It is possible that screening programs may evolve from a cytopathologic basis to a DNA testing base over time. In the longer term, screening recommendations might be modified based on the field data and cost-effectiveness considerations, but some level of screening is likely to be required for decades [15].

Concerns have been raised about the impact of HPV vaccination on both sexual risk behaviors and screening

Table 38.2 Comparison of quadrivalent and bivalent L1 VLP prophylactic vaccines

	Bivalent vaccine	Quadrivalent vaccine
Design	Randomized double-blind controlled trial	Randomized double-blind controlled
Vaccine type	Bivalent HPV 16/18 VLP, L1 capsid component	Quadrivalent HPV 6/11/16/18 VLP, L1 capsid component
Age (yrs)	15–25	16–23
Trial size	560 vaccinees 553 placebo	277 vaccinees 275 placebo
Site	US, Canada, Brazil	US, Brazil, Europe
Antigen	20 μg HPV-16 20 μg HPV-18	20 μg HPV-6, 40 μg HPV-11 40 μg HPV-16, 20 μg HPV-18
Adjuvant	500 μg aluminum hydroxide 50 μg 3-deacylated monophosphoryl lipid (ASO4)	225 μg aluminum hydroxyphosphate sulfate
Dose and administration	0.5 mL intramuscular	0.5 mL intramuscular
Schedule	0–1–6 months	0–2–6 months
Follow-up	Up to 27 months	Up to 35 months
Clinical outcome	100% efficacy preventing persistent HPV-16/18 infection; 93% efficacy preventing cytologic abnormalities	90% efficacy preventing HPV-6/11/16/18 infections; 100% efficacy preventing cytologic abnormalities
Major adverse effects	None	None

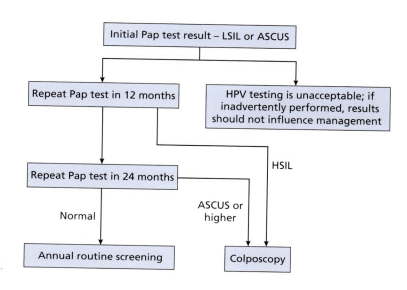

Figure 38.8 Management of LSIL or ASCUS in the adolescent patient. Adapted from [10].

behaviors. Some have expressed concern that adolescents who receive an HPV vaccine may feel less vulnerable to sexually transmitted infections (STI) and thus undertake riskier sexual behaviors; however, there are no published data to support this concern [16]. Vaccinated women should understand that HPV vaccines will not prevent infection with other sexually transmitted diseases, nor will their introduction eliminate the need for cervical cancer screening.

Given the lack of a pharmacologic intervention that can eradicate HPV in infected individuals and the prevalence of cervical cancer secondary to HPV infection across the world, the HPV vaccine represents a significant breakthrough in women's health. It is hoped that with implementation of HPV vaccines worldwide, we will witness a significant decline in incidence and mortality from cervical cancer in the next two decades.

Conclusion

HPV infection is common in young women, but rarely progresses to invasive cervical cancer. For this reason, the management of abnormal cervical cytology and histology in adolescents differs from that for the adult population. Aggressive management of benign lesions in adolescents should be avoided because most CIN 1 and 2 regress. Surgical excision of cervical tissue in a nulliparous adolescent may be detrimental to future fertility and cervical competency. Destruction of normal cervical tissue should be minimized whenever possible.

Prophylactic HPV vaccines may substantially reduce the morbidity and mortality associated with cervical cancer, other oral and genital malignancies, and genital warts. Clinical trials suggest that they are safe, well tolerated, highly immunogenic, and prevent both HPV infection and CIN. The FDA has approved Gardasil®, a quadrivalent vaccine to prevent cervical cancer, precancerous genital lesions and genital warts due to HPV types 6, 11, 16 and 18. Gardasil is indicated in girls and women 9–26 years of age; it does not substitute for routine cervical cancer screening, and women who receive Gardasil should continue to undergo screening per standard of care.

Finally, adolescents should be given appropriate education about HPV and conditions associated with this infection. They should also be encouraged to obtain appropriate gynecologic care after initiating sexual activity.

References

1. Centers for Disease Control and Prevention. *Genital HPV Infection Fact Sheet.* Atlanta, GA: CDC National Prevention Information Network, 2004. Available at: www.cdc.gov/nchstp/dstd/Stats_Trends/1999SurvRpt.htm.
2. Winer RL, Lee SK, Hughes JP et al. Genital human papillomavirus infection: incidence and risk factors in a cohort of female university students. *Am J Epidemiol* 2003;**157**:218–226.
3. Mahdavi A, Monk BJ. Recent advances in human papillomavirus vaccines. *Curr Oncol Rep* 2006;**8**:465–472.
4. Trottier H, Franco EL. The epidemiology of genital human papillomavirus infection. *Vaccine* 2006;suppl 1:S1–15.
5. Moscicki AB. Impact of HPV infection in adolescent populations. *J Adolesc Health* 2005;**37**:S3–9.
6. American Cancer Society. Statistics for 2007. Available online at: www. cancer.org.
7. American College of Obstetricians and Gynecologists. ACOG Practice Bulletin number 66. Management of abnormal cervical cytology and histology. *Obstet Gynecol* 2005;**106**:645–664.
8. Solomon D, Davey D, Kurman R et al. The 2001 Bethesda System: terminology for reporting results of cervical cytology. *JAMA* 2002;**287**:2114–2119.
9. Wright TC Jr, Massad LS, Dunton CJ, Spitzer M, Wilkinson EJ, Solomon D. 2006 American Society for Colposcopy and Cervical Pathology-sponsored Consensus Conference. 2006 consensus guidelines for the management of women with abnormal cervical cancer screening tests. *Am J Obstet Gynecol* 2007;**197**:346–355.
10. American College of Obstetricians and Gynecologists. ACOG Committee Opinion. Evaluation and management of abnormal cervical cytology and histology in the adolescent. Number 330. *Obstet Gynecol* 2006;**107**:963–968.
11. Wright TC Jr, Massad LS, Dunton CJ, Spitzer M, Wilkinson EJ, Solomon D. 2006 American Society for Colposcopy and Cervical Pathology-sponsored Consensus Conference. 2006 consensus guidelines for the management of women with cervical intraepithelial neoplasia or adenocarcinoma in situ. *Am J Obstet Gynecol* 2007;**197**:340–345.
12. Mahdavi A, Monk BJ. Vaccines against human papillomavirus and cervical cancer: promises and challenges. *Oncologist* 2005;**10**:528–538.
13. Villa LL, Costa RL, Petta CA et al. Prophylactic quadrivalent human papillomavirus (types 6, 11, 16, and 18) L1 virus-like particle vaccine in young women: a randomised double-blind

placebo-controlled multicentre phase II efficacy trial. *Lancet Oncol* 2005;**6**:271–278.

14. FDA licenses new vaccine for prevention of cervical cancer and other diseases in females caused by human papillomavirus. Available online at: www.fda.gov/bbs/topics/NEWS/2006/NEW01385.html.

15. Kahn JA. Vaccination as a prevention strategy for human papillomavirus-related diseases. *J Adolesc Health* 2005; **37**:S10–16.

16. Monk BJ, Wiley DJ. Will widespread human papillomavirus prophylactic vaccination change sexual practices of adolescent and young adult women in America? *Obstet Gynecol* 2006;**108**:420–424.

Further reading and Internet resources

www.nccc-online.org
www.asccp.org
www.acog.org
www.cancer.org
www.cdc.gov/cancer
www.cancer.gov
www.ashastd.org
www.wcn.org
www.hpvtest.com

CHAPTER 39

Herpes Simplex Viruses Types 1 and 2

David A. Baker
Stony Brook University Medical Center, New York, NY, USA

Introduction

Herpes simplex viruses types 1 and 2 (HSV-1 and HSV-2) can be differentiated by differences in antigenic composition and biochemical characteristics. Although they are distinct, the degree of sharing of antigenic determinants between the type 1 and 2 viruses results in some cross-reacting immunity. In addition, HSV-1 and HSV-2 can be identified on the basis of different biologic properties.

The principal sites of viral replication are nongenital in the prepuberty years and genital in the postpuberty, adolescence and sexually active young adult years. Modes of dissemination include mouth-to-face/hand for nongenital spread. Initial contact with HSVs usually occurs early in childhood and involves HSV-1. Less than 10% of primary infections with HSV-1 are clinically overt. HSV-1 is the causative agent for most nongenital herpetic lesions: herpes labialis, gingivostomatitis, and keratoconjunctivitis.

In adolescents and young adults genital tract infection by HSV-1 is by the oral–genital route and is caused by HSV-1 most commonly in the female who is seronegative to both HSV-1 and HSV-2.

Approximately 25% of the female population in the United States is infected with HSV-2, as determined using sensitive HSV type-specific antibody studies. HSV of the genital tract is one of the most prevalent viral sexually transmitted diseases (STDs) with an estimated 45 million men and women infected with genital herpes.

Pediatric, Adolescent, & Young Adult Gynecology. Edited by
A. Altchek and L. Deligdisch. © 2009 Blackwell Publishing,
ISBN: 978-1-4051-5347-8.

Approximately 1.6 million new cases of genital herpes occur annually. Most cases of HSV infection are asymptomatic. The genital tract of the female or male patient can be infected with HSV type 1 or type 2 virus. In the United States, the majority of genital infection is from HSV-2 virus. Up to 30% of first-episode cases of genital herpes are caused by HSV-1. The vast majority of primary genital infections are caused by HSV-2. Up to 40% of primary infection of the genital tract can be asymptomatic and produce no clinical disease.

Primary infection with clinical symptoms occurs 2–14 days after exposure and presents as a flu-like illness with a low-grade fever. It progresses to severe local disease with pain, multiple herpes lesions and inguinal adenopathy. After clinically apparent primary genital herpes infection with HSV-2, almost all patients will experience recurrences; however, recurrences with HSV-1 tend to be much less frequent. Type 2 antibodies usually appear first about the time of puberty and exhibit a significant increase during the prime reproductive years. The greatest incidence of type 2 infection occurs in women in their late teens and early twenties.

Infection

Primary infection

Primary genital infection due to HSV-2 may be asymptomatic or may be associated with severe symptoms. Genital lesions occur on the vulva, vagina, cervix, are multiple and larger than those observed in recurrent disease. Patients usually experience vaginal discharge, discomfort, and pain. Regional lymphadenopathy is the consequence of virus replication in the sites of lymphatic drainage. Systemic symptoms (malaise, myalgia, and fever) are virtually restricted to primary herpetic infection. These symptoms reflect the viremia during primary infection.

Recurrent infection

Limitation of lesions to one area of the vulva, vagina or cervix is more common in recurrent forms of the disease. The lesions tend to be limited in size and number. Cervical involvement may occur as a diffuse cervicitis or as a single large ulcer. Local symptoms predominate over systemic symptoms, with increased vaginal discharge or pain being the usual presenting complaint. In certain women, it can be demonstrated that once it is involved, the genital tract is the site of intermittent virus replication. Virus shedding without a lesion (asymptomatic shedding) can occur from the vulva and cervix intermittently in subsequent years after primary infection. Asymptomatic shedding of virus lasts an average of 1.5 days; however, a susceptible partner can acquire this virus during times of asymptomatic shedding. Shedding of virus without any symptoms or signs of clinical lesions (asymptomatic shedding) makes this viral STD difficult to control and prevent.

Patients will experience recurrent disease after clinical or asymptomatic primary HSV genital infection. Recurrences of genital HSV infection can be symptomatic or asymptomatic and there is significant variation from patient to patient in the frequency, severity, and duration of symptoms and viral shedding. Young adult women tend to acquire the first episode of genital herpes between the ages of 20 and 24 years.

Diagnosis

Isolation of virus by cell culture remains the standard and most sensitive test for the detection of infectious herpes virus from clinical specimens. Numerous factors in sampling and transport of the specimen determine the sensitivity of this technique. False-negative cultures are not uncommon in patients with recurrent infection or healing lesions. Newer techniques such as polymerase chain reaction (PCR) are three to four times more sensitive than culture techniques. As in cultures, false-negative results may occur. Because of cost and availability, PCR testing has not yet completely replaced virus isolation techniques. Early first-episode ulcers yield virus in 80% of patients,

whereas ulcers from recurrent infections are less likely to be culture positive and only 25% of crusted lesions contain recoverable virus.

In culturing for HSV, overt lesions that are not in the ulcerated state should be unroofed and the fluid sampled. Virus isolation can be readily achieved in many primary or continuous human tissue culture cell lines. The newly available serologic type-specific glycoprotein G (gG)-based assays can distinguish infection between HSV type 1 and 2 antibodies. These new immunoglobulin G (IgG) tests have excellent sensitivity (80–98%) and specificity (up to 96%) in comparison with Western blot assay; however, early in the course of infection, false-negative tests may occur. The older nonspecific antibody tests are of limited value owing to the frequency of cross-reacting antibodies to heterologous virus. IgM antibody test for HSV-1 and HSV-2 should not be used to diagnose acute infection. HSV-2 is considered to reside primarily in the genital tract. A demonstration of HSV-2 type-specific antibodies by a gG-based assay is deemed evidence of genital tract infection.

The newer gG-based test requires three weeks to turn positive and should not be repeated for at least 8–12 weeks to test for serologic conversion. One-third of the patients with recurrent herpes mount an IgM response. IgM testing for HSV cannot differentiate new from recurrent infection.

Therapy

Varied options are available to the healthcare provider to treat patients with genital herpes. Nucleoside analogs selectively inhibit viral replication and produce few or minimal effects on the cell. The first drug developed in this classification was aciclovir. This drug possesses a high safety profile and is selective against herpes virus-infected cells. Further advances with antiviral therapy have focused on the pharmacokinetics of the medications leading to better absorption and higher plasma levels of compound with fewer daily doses of medication.

Aciclovir

The drug stops HSV viral DNA replication and acts selectively against a viral-coded protein, thymidine kinase. The drug has been shown to be very safe, with few side effects. However, it has poor oral absorption; only approximately 20% of an oral dose is absorbed. The Food and Drug Administration (FDA) has approved aciclovir for the treatment of primary genital herpes and episodes of recurrent disease. Approximately 3% of isolates obtained from healthy patients demonstrate *in vitro* resistance to aciclovir. The frequency of *in vitro* resistance has not changed from that prior to its introduction. Foscarnet, a phosphonate viral DNA inhibitor, and cidofovir, an acyclic nucleoside phosphonate, have been used in infected AIDS patients with aciclovir-resistant isolates of herpes virus.

Valaciclovir

This agent is only for oral administration and, because there is an enzyme in the gut that cleaves the valine, the bioavailability is three to five times greater than oral aciclovir. The safety profile is that of aciclovir with a less frequent dosing schedule. The FDA has approved valaciclovir for the treatment of primary genital herpes, treatment of episodes of recurrent disease, daily treatment for suppression of outbreaks of recurrent genital herpes, and reduction of transmission of genital herpes to a susceptible sexual partner.

Famciclovir

Bioavailability is good, but its clinical long-term use is less than that of aciclovir. Famciclovir requires less frequent dosing than aciclovir, but more frequent dosing than valaciclovir.

All cases of primary genital herpes should be treated with antiviral medication. The bioavailability of the newer agents, valaciclovir and famciclovir, is greater so they may require a less frequent dosing schedule to achieve good therapy for primary infection to reduce the increased symptomatic and asymptomatic shedding.

A long-term safety and efficacy study was carried out in which more than 1140 immunocompetent patients with frequent recurrences of genital herpes (more than 12 episodes per year) were treated with aciclovir for the first ten years of the study and then valaciclovir in the 11th year. Goldberg et al summarize the first five-year data from that study [1]. There was a statistically significant reduction in recurrent disease when aciclovir was used at 400 mg twice a day. There was a 75–90% reduction in recurrent disease in each three-month quarter over the five-year period. This long-term study provides major

insights and information concerning suppressive therapy. Adverse reactions to the medication were minimal and, after the first year, less than 2% of patients reported any side effect. Nausea, diarrhea, headache, and rash were seen during the study.

Fife et al showed that six years of continuous daily aciclovir suppressive therapy did not produce the emergence of aciclovir-resistant isolates in immunocompetent patients [2]. Approximately 3% of patients required a higher dose to control symptoms than the standard dose of 400 mg aciclovir twice a day.

Suppressive therapy

Suppressive therapy can reduce the frequency of genital recurrences by 70–80% among individuals with frequent recurrences (six or more per year). Daily oral aciclovir therapy not only significantly reduces symptomatic recurrences but also suppresses asymptomatic viral shedding. Valaciclovir 500–1000 mg orally once a day or famciclovir 250 mg orally twice a day is effective in suppressing recurrent genital herpes. Patients on long-term suppressive therapy with oral aciclovir 400 mg twice a day can be changed to valaciclovir 500 mg once a day and maintain the safety and effectiveness of this therapy. Valaciclovir 500 mg once a day may be less effective than its higher dose or aciclovir dosing regimens in women who experience ten or more outbreaks in a year.

Daily valaciclovir (500 mg) has been shown to suppress overt acquisition of HSV-2 in susceptible sexual partners. Overall acquisition, symptomatic and asymptomatic, was reduced by 48% in the valaciclovir group compared with the placebo group [3].

Herpes in pregnancy

Distinguishing primary and recurrent genital herpes

The distinction between primary and secondary herpetic infections appears to be more difficult than previously assumed in pregnancy. Hensleigh et al evaluated 23 women with severe first clinical outbreak of genital herpes in the second and third trimesters of pregnancy [4]. Only one of the 23 women with clinical illnesses consistent with primary genital HSV infections had serologically verified primary infection. This primary infection was caused by HSV type 1. Three women had nonprimary type 2 infections, and 19 women had recurrent infections. This report demonstrates the need for careful serologic evaluation of all cases of presumed first episode of genital herpes in pregnant women.

Disseminated maternal herpetic infection and pregnancy

Disseminated disease in adults is thought to represent primary infection in a partially immunocompromised host. There are several patient populations in whom disseminated disease may occur: neonates, immunocompromised adults, particularly individuals with thymic dysplasias, and pregnant women. Disseminated herpetic infection in pregnancy is an extremely rare event. The manifestations of systemic dissemination in pregnancies tend to be viscerotropic rather than neurotropic. Its principal presentation is that of a fulminating hepatitis. Herpetic hepatitis is extremely rare, with a maternal mortality rate of 43%.

Classically, disease occurs in the third trimester. Often there is viral-like prodromal illness in association with vulvar or oropharyngeal vesicular or vesiculopustular lesions. Despite elevated liver enzymes, most of the cases are anicteric. In some cases, no clinically overt site of primary herpetic infection can be identified. Herpetic hepatitis should be included in the differential diagnosis of hepatic dysfunction in the third trimester. Any pregnant patient with primary infection in the third trimester should be closely watched for any evidence of disseminated disease. Once the diagnosis is made, aciclovir should be initiated to reduce maternal mortality. Both type 1 and 2 HSV viruses have been isolated from gravidas with disseminated disease in pregnancy.

Transmission to the newborn

Breast milk

Breastfeeding in the immediate postpartum period has been complicated by the demonstration of neonatal HSV-1 infection. Serologic studies demonstrated postnatal acquisition of infection for which breast milk was the vehicle of dissemination. The mother was found to have HSV-1 in her breast milk. She had no history of genital lesions and viral cultures of cervix, vagina, and throat were negative for HSV-1. Careful attention to hygiene measures must be implemented to adequately protect the infant. The nipple should be examined to exclude the presence

of herpetic lesions. In view of the occult transmission of HSVs in breast milk, it may be wise to individualize each case.

Other routes

The two most important variables that determine the probability of neonatal infection are the amount of virus present and the duration of labor. Both variables must function to achieve neonatal involvement. In the presence of one or more lesions, it is our recommendation that cesarean section be performed. The main point of therapy is that delivery must not occur through the birth canal harboring virus. Cesarean section prior to rupture of membranes is effective in reducing neonatal infection. Once the fetal membranes have been ruptured, both HSV-1 and HSV-2 have the ability to ascend and infect the fetus *in utero*.

With the advent of antiviral therapy of the newborn, the duration of rupture of membranes is not the important clinical factor, but rather the estimated time of delivery once the mother presents in labor. Scott et al reported a small, randomized, double-blind clinical trial in which women with clinically first-episode genital herpes during pregnancy received daily aciclovir treatment initiated in week 36 of gestation [5]. They were able to demonstrate a reduced need for cesarean section. Sheffield et al evaluated the efficacy of valaciclovir suppression late in pregnancy [6]. In this study, 170 women were treated with valaciclovir and 168 with placebo. At delivery, 13% of gravidas in the placebo group required cesarean section delivery as opposed to 4% in the valaciclovir group. Despite an over-representation of women with recurrent genital herpes, with only 6% of study participants having primary genital herpes, the investigators suggested the data show that valaciclovir suppression significantly reduced HSV shedding that required cesarean delivery.

The CDC and Glaxo-Wellcome have maintained a voluntary registry of women who have received aciclovir or valaciclovir during pregnancy (1-800-722-9292). Women who received aciclovir in the first trimester and whose birth outcomes were known had a 2.3% prevalence of birth defects as compared to a background rate of 3%.

Influence of primary genital herpes during pregnancy

Brown et al prospectively followed 29 patients who had acquired genital herpes during pregnancy [7]. While

15 patients had a primary episode of genital HSV-2, 14 had a nonprimary first episode. Six of the 15 gravida with primary genital herpes, but none of the 14 with nonprimary first episode infection, had infants with serious perinatal morbidity. Four of the five infants whose mothers acquired primary HSV in the third trimester had perinatal morbidity, which included prematurity, intrauterine growth retardation, and neonatal infection with HSV-2. Perinatal complications occurred in one of the five infants whose mothers acquired primary HSV-2 during the first trimester as well as one of the five infants who had primary HSV-2 during the second trimester. Around 50–70% of neonates with HSV infection are born to mothers who do not have a history of genital herpes infection. Unless a portal of infection is incidentally established, i.e. scalp electrode site, and in the absence of lesions in the periparturition period, the probability of ensuing neonatal disease appears to be exceedingly low. Prior disease that antedates this gestation is not a sensitive predictor of ensuing fetal disease. HIV-positive women have an increased tendency for genital shedding of virus; herpetic lesions persist longer and may become chronic ulcerations.

Therapy in pregnancy

In the United States 1500–2000 newborns contact neonatal herpes each year. Infections occur in the perinatal period from contact with infected maternal secretions in the majority of cases. Pregnant women who do not know they are infected with genital herpes and shed the virus without lesions or symptoms give rise to most infected newborns. New management of these women to prevent the transmission of this virus is being studied. Antiviral therapy of the mother to prevent maternal symptomatic and asymptomatic viral shedding during the intrapartum period is now recommended by the ACOG. Aciclovir, valaciclovir, and famciclovir are class B medications as categorized by the FDA. When aciclovir or valaciclovir is given by the oral or intravenous route to the mother, the drug crosses the placenta, is concentrated in amniotic fluid and breast milk, and reaches therapeutic levels in the fetus.

Starting in 1984, an aciclovir pregnancy registry has been compiled. The CDC published data in 1993 showing there was no increase in fetal problems in women who received aciclovir in the first trimester of their pregnancy. Studies on newer recommendations to reduce the number of newborns infected with HSV will combine serologic testing of all pregnant women for antibodies to

HSV-1 and HSV-2 using a type-specific glycoprotein gG-based test and the use of antiviral therapy starting at 36 weeks in selected cases. Intervention is aimed primarily at preventing primary infection in those women at risk for HSV.

Prevention of sexual transmission of herpes simplex virus

Suppressive antiviral therapy with valaciclovir reduces transmission of infection to sexual partners in discordant couples. In theory, using a condom may afford another layer of protection. Serologic type-specific testing of the partner is advised. Information and its sharing are the keys to prevention. An HSV-infected woman needs to know about the risk that HSV can be sexually and orally transmitted, how to detect the earliest symptoms of disease, the availability of suppressive therapy, the ability to obtain type-specific testing of sexual partners, and the potential dangers to the newborn when disease is present at parturition. Pregnant women who are not infected with HSV-2 should be advised to avoid intercourse during the second half of pregnancy. Pregnant women who are not infected with HSV-1 should be counseled to avoid oral sex with any partner with prior oral herpes and genital intercourse with a partner with genital HSV-1 infection.

References

1. Goldberg LK, Kaufinan R, Kurtz TO et al. Long-term suppression of recurrent genital herpes with aciclovir. *Arch Dermatol* 1993;**129**:582.
2. Fife KH, Crumpacker CS, Mertz GJ et al and the Aciclovir Study Group. Recurrence and resistance patterns of herpes simplex virus following cessation of >6 years of chronic suppression with aciclovir. *J Infect Dis* 1994;**169**:1338.
3. Corey L, Wald A, Patel R et al. Once daily valacyclovir to reduce the risk of transmission of genital herpes. *N Engl J Med* 2004;**350**:11–20.
4. Hensleigh PA, Andrews WW, Brown Z et al. Genital herpes during pregnancy: inability to distinguish primary and recurrent infections clinically. *Obstet Gynecol* 1997;**89**:891.
5. Scott LL, Sanchez PI, Jackson GJ et al. Aciclovir suppression to prevent cesarean delivery after first-episode genital herpes. *Obstet Gynecol* 1996;**87**:69.

6. Sheffield JS, Hill JB, Hollier LM et al. Valaciclovir prophylaxis to prevent recurrent herpes at delivery. *Obstet Gynecol* 2006;**108**:141.

7. Brown ZA, Gardella C, Wald A et al. Genital herpes complicating pregnancy. *Obstet Gynecol* 1986;**106**:845.

Further reading

Herpes and pregnancy

American College of Obstetricians and Gynecologists. *Practice Bulletin. Management of Herpes in Pregnancy. No.82.* Washington, DC: American College of Obstetricians and Gynecologists, 2007.

Ashley RL. Sorting out the new HSV type specific antibody tests. *Sex Trans Infect* 2001;**77**:232.

Arvin AM, Hensleigh PA, Prober CG et al. Failure of antepartum maternal cultures to predict the infant's risk of exposure to herpes simplex virus at delivery. *N Engl J Med* 1986;**315**:796.

Baker D, Brown Z, Hollier LM et al. Cost-effectiveness of herpes simplex virus type 2 serologic testing and antiviral therapy in pregnancy. *Am J Obstet Gynecol* 2005;**192**:483.

Benedetti J, Corey L, Ashley R. Recurrence rate in genital herpes after symptomatic first-episode infection. *Ann Intern Med* 1994;**121**:847.

Brown ZA, Gardella C, Wald A et al. Genital herpes complicating pregnancy. *Obstet Gynecol* 1986;**106**:845.

Bryson Y, Dillon K, Bernstein DI et al. Risk of acquisition of genital herpes simplex virus type 2 in sex partners of persons with genital herpes: a prospective couple study. *J Infect Dis* 1993;**167**:942–967.

Hensleigh PA, Andrews WW, Brown Z et al. Genital herpes during pregnancy: inability to distinguish primary and recurrent infections clinically. *Obstet Gynecol* 1997;**89**:891.

Koelle DM, Benedetti J, Langenberg A, Corey L. Asymptomatic reactivation of herpes simplex virus in women after the first episode of genital herpes. *Ann Intern Med* 1992;**116**:433.

Kulhanjian JA, Soroush V, Au DS et al. Identification of women at unsuspected risk of primary infection with herpes simplex type 2 during pregnancy. *N Engl J Med* 1992;**326**:916.

Scott LL, Sanchez PI, Jackson GJ et al. Aciclovir suppression to prevent cesarean delivery after first-episode genital herpes. *Obstet Gynecol* 1996;**87**:69.

Wald A, Zeh J, Selke S, Ashley RL, Corey L. Virologic characteristics of subclinical and symptomatic genital herpes infections. *N Engl J Med* 1995;**333**:771.

Whitley R, Arvin A, Prober C et al. Predictors of morbidity and mortality in neonates with herpes simplex infection. *N Engl J Med* 1991;**324**:450.

Whitley R, Corey L, Arvin A et al. Changing presentation of herpes simplex virus infection in neonates. *J Infect Dis* 1988;**158**:109.

Nosocomial herpes

Adams G, Purohit DM, Bada HS, Andrews BR. Neonatal infection by herpes virus hominis type 2: a complication of intrapartum fetal monitoring. *Pediatr Res* 1975;**9**:337.

Augenbraun M, Feldman J, Chirgwin K et al. Increased genital shedding of herpes simplex type 2 in HIV-seropostive women. *Ann Intern Med* 1995;**123**:845.

Chatelain S, Neumann DE, Alexander SM. Fatal herpetic hepatitis in pregnancy. *Obstet Gynecol* 1994;**1**:246.

Douglas JM, Schmidt O, Corey L. Acquisition of neonatal HSV-1 infection from a paternal source contact. *J Pediatr* 1983;**103**:908.

Dunkle LM, Schmidt RR, O'Connor DM. Neonatal herpes simplex infection possibly acquired via maternal breast milk. *Pediatrics* 1979;**63**:250.

Francis DP, Hermann KL, MacMahon JR et al. Nosocomial and maternally acquired herpesvirus hominis infections: a report of four cases of neonates. *Am J Dis Child* 1975;**129**:889.

Golden SM, Merenstein GB, Todd WA, Hill JM. Disseminated herpes simplex neonatorum: a complication of fetal monitoring. *Am J Obstet Gynecol* 1977;**129**:917.

Goldkrand JW. Intrapartum inoculation of herpes simplex virus by fetal scalp electrode. *Obstet Gynecol* 1982;**59**:163.

Hammerberg O, Watts J, Chernesky M et al. An outbreak of herpes simplex virus type 1 in an intensive care nursery. *Pediatr Infect Dis* 1983;**2**:290.

Kilbrick S. Herpes simplex virus in breast milk. *Pediatrics* 1979;**64**:290.

Light IJ. Postnatal acquisition of herpes simplex virus by the newborn infant: a review of the literature. *Pediatrics* 1979;**63**:480.

Pannuti CS, Finck MCDS, Grimbaum RS et al. Asymptomatic perinatal shedding of herpes simplex virus type 2 in patients with acquired immunodeficiency syndrome. *Arch Dermatol* 1977;**133**:180.

Therapy

Baker DA. Valaciclovir in the treatment of genital herpes and herpes zoster. *Exp Opin Pharmacother* 2002;**3**:51.

Baker DA, Blythe JG, Miller JM. Once daily valaciclovir for suppression of recurrent genital herpes. *Obstet Gynecol* 1999;**94**:103.

Centers for Disease Control. Pregnancy outcomes following systemic aciclovir exposure. June 1, 1984–June 30, 1993. *Morb Mortal Wkly Rep* 1993;**42**:806.

Dracker JL, Miller JM, and The International Valaciclovir Study Group. Once-daily valaciclovir sustains the suppressive efficacy and safety record of aciclovir in recurrent genital herpes. Proceedings of the First European Congress of Chemotherapy, Glasgow, UK, 1996.

Fife KH, Crumpacker CS, Mertz GJ et al and the Aciclovir Study Group. Recurrence and resistance patterns of herpes simplex virus following cessation of >6 years of chronic suppression with aciclovir. *J Infect Dis* 1994;**169**:1338.

Goldberg LK, Kaufinan R, Kurtz TO et al. Long-term suppression of recurrent genital herpes with aciclovir. *Arch Dermatol* 1993;**129**:582.

Lavoie SL, Kaplowitz LG. Management of genital herpes infections. *Semin Dermatol* 1994;**13**:248–255.

Patel R, Crooks JR, Bell AR and the International Valaciclovir Study Group. Once-daily valaciclovir for the suppression of recurrent genital herpes – the first placebo controlled clinical trial. Presented at the First European Congress of Chemotherapy, Glasow, UK, 1996.

Sarag P, Chastong C, Bertin L et al. Efficacy and safety equivalence of 1000 mg once-daily and 500 mg twice daily valaciclovir in recurrent genital herpes. Proceedings of the 36th ICAAC, New Orleans, 1996.

Scott LL, Sanchez PJ, Jackson GL et al. Aciclovir suppression to prevent cesarean delivery after first episode genital herpes. *Obstet Gynecol* 1996;**87**:69.

Sheffield JS, Fish DN, Hollier LM et al. Acyclovir concentration in human breast milk after valaciclovir administration. *Am J Obstet Gynecol* 2002;**186**:100.

Sheffield JS, Hill JB, Hollier LM et al. Valaciclovir prophylaxis to prevent recurrent herpes at delivery. *Obstet Gynecol* 2006;**108**:141.

Tyring SK, Baker D, Snowden W. Valaciclovir for herpes virus infection: long term safety and sustained efficacy after 20 years' experience with aciclovir. *J Infect Dis* 2002;**186** (suppl 1): 40s.

Wald A. New therapies and prevention strategies for genital herpes. *Clin Infect Dis* 1999;**28** (suppl 1):4.

Wald A, Zeh J, Barnum G et al. Suppression of subclinical shedding of herpes simplex virus type 2 with aciclovir. *Ann Intern Med* 1996;**124**(1, pt 1):8–15.

CHAPTER 40

Sexually Transmitted Infections

Rhoda Sperling

Mount Sinai School of Medicine, New York, NY, USA

What is a sexually transmitted infection?

What is the definition of a sexually transmitted infection (STI)? A simple enough question, but the answer is somewhat arbitrary. More than 20 different infectious agents can be acquired and/or spread by various types of sexual contact (e.g. vaginal intercourse, anal intercourse, hand–genital contact, oral–genital contact or oral–anal contact). These agents include bacteria, viruses, and protozoa (Box 40.1). For many of these agents, sexual contact is one of several possible modes of spread of infection.

What is the global burden of sexually transmitted infection?

STIs are among the most common infections worldwide. They are hyperendemic in many developing countries. In 1995, the World Health Organization estimated that the global burden of four curable STIs (syphilis, gonorrhea, chlamydia, and trichomoniasis) had reached more than 340 million new cases per year; this estimate includes 151 million cases in South/Southeast Asia, 38 million in Latin America, and 69 million in Africa. In many developing countries, the increasing numbers of cases have been fueled by the economic and societal disruption of the human immunodeficiency virus (HIV) pandemic. Although prevalence rates for many of these infectious agents vary widely by geographic region, changes in migration,

immigration, and travel patterns during the past 50 years have ensured that almost any STI can be acquired anywhere in the world.

What is the the burden of sexually transmitted infections in the United States?

STIs remain a major public health challenge in the United States. While substantial progress has been made in preventing, diagnosing, and treating certain STIs in recent years, the Centers for Disease Control and Prevention (CDC) estimates that 19 million new infections occur each year in the United States with almost half of these among young people aged 15–24. In addition to the physical and psychologic consequences of STIs, these diseases also exact a tremendous economic toll. Direct medical costs associated with STIs in the United States are estimated at $13 billion annually.

In the United States, the legal requirements for disease reporting provide the foundation for STI surveillance. Healthcare providers, healthcare facilities, laboratories, veterinarians, food services establishments, child daycare facilities, and schools are all mandated to notify local health jurisdictions or local health departments of suspected or confirmed conditions within a specified period of time. In turn, these local health officials must report their data to the CDC. However, only some STIs are notifiable diseases. National trends in notifiable STIs – chlamydia, gonorrhea, and syphilis – are tracked by the CDC and are available online at www.CDC.gov/STD/stat. These data, which are useful for examining overall trends as well as trends among populations at risk, represent only a small proportion of the true national burden of

Pediatric, Adolescent, & Young Adult Gynecology. Edited by A. Altchek and L. Deligdisch. © 2009 Blackwell Publishing, ISBN: 978-1-4051-5347-8.

Box 40.1 Infectious agents that can be spread through sexual contact

Viral diseases	Hepatitis A virus (HAV)
	Hepatitis B virus (HBV)
	Hepatitis C virus (HCV)
	Herpes viruses
	Herpes simplex virus types 1 & 2 (HSV-1, HSV-2)
	Cytomegalovirus (CMV)
	Epstein–Barr virus (EBV)
	Human lymphotropic virus (HTLV-1)
	Human immunodeficiency virus (HIV-1, HIV-2)
	Human papillomavirus (HPV)
	Molluscum contagiosum
Bacterial diseases	Bacterial vaginosis
	Klebsiella granulomatis (granuloma inguinale, donovanosis)
	Chlamydia trachomatis
	Serovars A–K (urethritis, cervicitis, PID)
	Serovars L1, L2 or L3 (lymphogranuloma venereum (LGV))
	Haemophilus ducreyi (chancroid)
	Neisseria gonorrhoeae (GC)
	Treponema pallidum (syphilis)
Fungal infections	Candida species (vulvovaginal candidiasis)
	Histoplasma capsulatum (histoplasmosis)
Parasitic diseases	*Entamoeba histolytica*
	Trichomonas vaginalis (trichomoniasis)
	Phythirus pubis (pediculosis pubis, pubic lice)
	Sarcoptes scabiei (scabies)

Table 40.1 Health consequences of common sexually transmitted bacterial infections

Pathogen	Health consequences
Chlamydia	If untreated, 30–40% of women will develop pelvic inflammatory disease (PID)
	If PID develops, ~20% risk of infertility and ~20% with chronic pelvic pain
	If untreated and exposed to HIV, 5 times more likely to become HIV infected
	If pregnant, increased risk of ectopic pregnancy
	If untreated and pregnant, high risk for delayed postpartum endometritis
	If untreated and pregnant, newborn at risk for conjunctivitis and pneumonia
Gonorrhea (GC)	If untreated, majority of women will develop PID
	If PID develops, ~20% risk of infertility and ~20% with chronic pelvic pain
	If untreated and exposed to HIV, 3–5 times more likely to become infected
	If pregnant, increased risk of ectopic pregnancy
	If untreated and pregnant, increased risk for disseminated GC (an acute dermatitis/tenosynovitis syndrome, which can be complicated by arthritis, meningitis or endocarditis)
	If untreated and pregnant, risk of premature delivery
	If pregnant and untreated, newborn at risk for severe sight-threatening conjunctivitis and rarely, sepsis with associated meningitis, endocarditis or arthritis
Syphilis	If early syphilis is untreated, risk of latent syphilis
	If untreated and pregnant, risk of intrauterine fetal demise
	If untreated and pregnant, risk of premature delivery
	If untreated and pregnant, newborn at risk for congenital syphilis

STIs. Many cases of notifiable STIs go undiagnosed, and some highly prevalent viral infections, such as human papillomavirus and genital herpes, are not reportable conditions.

Why worry about sexually transmitted infections?

Untreated STIs have acute morbidity as well as long-term health consequences (Table 40.1). For women of reproductive age, an important additional consideration is the risk of mother-to-child transmission. Also, many STI pathogens (including those listed in Table 40.1) may facilitate the acquisition and transmission of HIV.

Can you recognize and treat the common sexually transmitted syndromes?

Recognition of common STI syndromes is important and allows for more efficient diagnosis and treatment. Treatment guidelines generally advocate the use of regimens that are simple to use (once daily), have few side effects (high patient acceptability), have low costs (global availability), and minimize the development of antimicrobial resistance. Table 40.2 summarizes both disease manifestations and recommended regimens for common STIs.

Table 40.2 Recognition and treatment of common STIs

STI syndrome	Possible causative pathogens	Appropriate investigation	Appropriate treatment regimen by pathogen
Vaginal discharge	Candida sp.[1]	Vaginal pH and microscopy	Intravaginal azoles ((butoconazole, clotrimazole, miconazole, tioconazole, or terconazole), or intravaginal nystatin, or fluconazole 150 mg oral tablet, one tablet in single dose
	Bacterial vaginosis[2]	Vaginal pH, microscopy and whiff test, or Gram stain	Metronidazole 500 mg orally twice a day for 7 days, or metronidazole gel, 0.75%, one full applicator (5 g) intravaginally, once a day for 5 days, or clindamycin cream, 2%, one full applicator (5 g) intravaginally at bedtime for 7 days
	Trichomonas vaginalis	Vaginal pH and microscopy; sensitivity of microscopy is low (~60%) so consider vaginal culture or antigen-based detection test if disease is suspected	Metronidazole or tinidazole, both 2 g orally in a single dose
Cervicitis	Chlamydia trachomatis	Endocervical swab or urine samples – nucleic acid amplification tests (NAAT)[3]	Azithromycin 1 g orally in a single dose or doxycycline 100 mg orally twice daily for 7 days[4]
	Neisseria gonorrhoeae	Endocervical swab for culture, or endocervical swab or urine samples – nucleic acid amplification tests (NAAT)[3]	Ceftriaxone 125 mg IM in a single dose or cefixime 400 mg orally in a single dose[5] Treat for chlamydia co-infection if chlamydial infection has not been ruled out
Genital ulceration	Herpes simplex virus (HSV) 1 & 2	Ulcer exudate – test for HSV by viral culture, antigen detection kits or nucleic acid amplification by PCR Serology – type-specific tests for specific glycoproteins (G1 for HSV-1 and G2 for HSV-2)[6]	Valaciclovir, aciclovir, and famciclovir all approved for the treatment of initial and recurrent episodes or as suppressive therapy[3] First clinical episode – valaciclovir 1 g orally twice a day for 7–10 days[7] Recurrent genital herpes – valaciclovir 1 g orally once a day for 5 days[7]
	Haemophilus ducreyi	Ulcer exudate – isolation of H. ducreyi using special culture media	Azithromycin 1 g or ceftriaxone 250 mg IM or ciprofloxacin 500 mg orally twice a day for 3 days
	Treponema pallidum	Ulcer exudate – evidence of T. pallidum by dark-field examination Serology – serologic test for syphilis performed at least 7 days after onset of ulcers; a nontreponemal screening test (such as the VDRL or RPR) must be confirmed by a specific treponemal test (such as a FTA-ABS or TP-PA)	Primary, secondary, and early syphilis – benzathine penicillin G 2.4 million units IM in a single dose Latent syphilis or syphilis of unknown duration – benzathine penicillin G 2.4 million units IM q weekly for 3 doses[8]

[1] Candidaisis is not considered a sexually transmitted infection.

[2] It has been debated whether BV is a sexually transmitted infection. Treatment of male partners is beneficial in preventing recurrence.

[3] For nongenital sites, culture should be used.

[4] Alternative regimens for chlamydia cervicitis include erythromycin and quinolone antibiotics. For drug, dosage, and duration of treatment consult the 2006 CDC STD treatment guidelines.

[5] Cefixime is no longer available as a tablet, only a suspension. After the publication of the 2006 CDC STD treatment guidelines, fluoroquinolones were dropped as recommended first-line agents.

[6] Median detection of antibodies in bloodstream (seroconversion) has been 25 days for HSV-1 and 23 days for HSV-2.

[7] For first clinical episode of genital herpes, other recommended regimens include aciclovir 400 mg orally three times a day for 7–10 days, or aciclovir 200 mg orally five times a day for 7–10 days, or famciclovir 250 mg orally three times a day for 7–10 days. For recurrent episodes of genital herpes, other recommended regimens include aciclovir 400 mg orally three times a day for 5 days, aciclovir 800 mg orally twice a day for 5 days, aciclovir 800 mg three times a day for 2 days or famciclovir 125 mg orally twice daily for 5 days or famciclovir 100 mg orally twice daily for 1 day.

[8] For penicillin-allergic patients, patients with neurosyphilis, newborns, older children, HIV-infected individuals, consult the 2006 CDC STD treatment guidelines.

Diseases characterized by vaginal discharge

Vaginitis is usually characterized by a vaginal discharge and/or vulvar itching and irritation. A vaginal odor may or may not be present. The three diseases most frequently associated with vaginal discharge are bacterial vaginosis (BV), trichomoniasis, and candidiasis. Various diagnostic methods are available to identify the etiology of an abnormal vaginal discharge. Laboratory testing fails to identify the cause of vaginitis in a minority of women. The type of vaginitis a patient has can usually be determined by pH and microscopic examination of fresh samples of discharge.

BV is the most prevalent cause of vaginal discharge. BV results from the replacement of the normal H_2O_2-producing *Lactobacilli* species of the vagina with high concentrations of anaerobic micro-organisms – *Mycoplasma hominis* and *Gardnerella vaginalis*. BV can be diagnosed by the use of clinical criteria or by Gram stain. Clinical criteria require three of the following four symptoms or signs: (1) homogeneous, thin, white discharge that smoothly coats the vaginal walls; (2) presence of clue cells on microscopic examination; (3) pH of vaginal fluid >4.5; and (4) a fishy odor of vaginal discharge before or after addition of 10% KOH (i.e. the whiff test). When a Gram stain is used, determining the relative concentration of lactobacilli (long Gram-positive rods), Gram-negative and Gram-variable rods and cocci (i.e. *G. vaginalis*, *Prevotella*, *Porphyromonas*, and peptostreptococci), as well as curved Gram-negative rods (*Mobiluncus*) characteristic of BV is considered the gold standard laboratory method for diagnosing BV. Culture of *G. vaginalis* is not recommended as a diagnostic tool because it is not specific.

BV is associated with multiple adverse outcomes. Pregnancy-related complications include premature rupture of the membranes, preterm labor, preterm birth, intra-amniotic infection, and postpartum endometritis. Treatment of pregnant women with BV who are at high risk for preterm delivery might reduce the risk for prematurity. BV is also causally linked to endometritis, pelvic inflammatory disease, and vaginal cuff cellulitis following invasive procedures (endometrial biopsy, hysterectomy, hysterosalpingography, and placement of an intrauterine device (IUD)). Treatment of BV with metronidazole substantially reduces the risk of postabortion endometritis. Some specialists suggest that before performing surgical abortion or hysterectomy, providers should screen for and treat women with BV even if routine antimicrobial prophylaxis is given.

Recommended BV treatment regimens for nonpregnant adults include: metronidazole 500 mg orally twice a day for seven days; metronidazole gel, 0.75%, one full applicator (5 g) intravaginally, once a day for five days; clindamycin cream, 2%, one full applicator (5 g) intravaginally at bedtime for seven days. Patients should be advised to avoid consuming alcohol during treatment with metronidazole and for 24 hours afterwards. Clindamycin cream is oil based and theoretically could weaken latex condoms and diaphragms. Topical clindamycin preparations should not be used in the second half of pregnancy. Recommended regimens for pregnant women include: metronidazole 500 mg orally twice a day for seven days; metronidazole 250 mg orally three times a day for seven days; or clindamycin 300 mg orally twice a day for seven days.

Trichomoniasis is very common, causing over 170 million infections in women worldwide. Trichomoniasis is not a reportable STI condition in the United States. Epidemiology studies suggest that this infection is actually more common in older women than in adolescents and young adults.

Trichomoniasis is caused by the protozoan *T. vaginalis*. Infected women typically have symptoms characterized by a diffuse, malodorous, yellow-green vaginal discharge with vulvar irritation. However, some women have minimal or no symptoms. Diagnosis of vaginal trichomoniasis is usually performed by microscopy of vaginal secretions, but this method has a sensitivity of only approximately 60–70% and requires immediate evaluation of wet preparation slides for optimal results. FDA-approved point-of-care tests also are available. Although these tests tend to be more sensitive than vaginal wet preparations, false-positive test results might occur, especially in low-prevalence populations. Culture remains the most sensitive and specific commercially available method of diagnosis. In women in whom trichomoniasis is suspected but not confirmed by microscopy, vaginal secretions should be cultured for *T. vaginalis*.

The recommended treatment regimen for trichomoniasis is either metronidazole 2.0 g orally in a single dose or tinidazole 2.0 g orally in a single dose. An alternative metronidazole regimen is 500 mg orally twice a day for seven days. Patients should be advised to avoid consuming alcohol during treatment with metronidazole or tinidazole. Abstinence from alcohol should continue for 24 hours after completion of metronidazole or 72 hours after completion of tinidazole.

Candidiasis is usually not transmitted sexually; however, it is frequently diagnosed in women being evaluated for STIs and management of candidiasis continues to be included in the CDC treatment guidelines. Treatment of partners may be considered in adolescents who have recurrent infection.

Diseases characterized by cervicitis and pelvic inflammatory disease

At the time of a vaginal speculum examination, the two major diagnostic signs of cervicitis can be identified: (1) purulent or mucopurulent cervical discharge and (2) endocervical bleeding induced by gentle probing of the endocervical canal. Either or both signs may be present. Cervicitis may be asymptomatic but women often will complain of abnormal vaginal discharge or intermenstrual bleeding. The most frequently isolated organisms associated with cervicitis are *Chamydia trachomatis* (*C. trachomatis*, chlamydia) or *Neisseria gonorrhoeae* (*N. gonorrhoeae*, GC). However, in the majority of cases of cervicitis no organism is ever isolated.

Chlamydia cervicitis is caused by *C. trachomatis*, one of three *Chlamydia* species (*C. trachomatis*, *C. psittaci*, and *C. pneumoniae*) that are recognized to be human pathogens. The causative agent is a nonmotile, Gram-negative bacteria with a obligate intracellular life cycle. The anatomic sites that can be infected by *C. trachomatis* include the mucosal surfaces of the cervix, urethra, rectum, throat, and conjunctiva.

In the United States, chlamydia genital infections are the most frequently reported infectious disease, with the highest prevalence rates reported in women <26 years of age (Fig. 40.1). In 2005, the overall rate of reported chlamydia infection among women in the United States (496.5 cases per 100,000 females) was over three times higher than the rate among men (161.1 cases per 100,000 males), likely reflecting a greater number of women screened for this infection. Females aged 15–19 had the highest rates followed by females aged 20–24. African-American and other minority group women are also disproportionately affected by chlamydia. Data from chlamydia screening programs run by family planning clinics across the United States indicate that roughly 6% of 15–24-year-old females in these settings are infected.

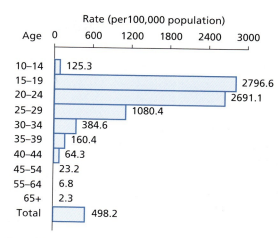

Figure 40.1 Chlamydia in females. Age- and sex-specific rates, United States, 2005.

Neisseria gonorrhoeae is a nonmotile, nonspore-forming, Gram-negative coccus that characteristically grows in pairs (diplococci) with adjacent sides flattened. It is a member of the genus *Neisseria* which contains a number of different species, most of which are nonpathogenic commensal flora in humans. Whenever it is isolated, *N. gonorrhoeae* is considered a pathogen. Similar to *C. trachomatis*, uncomplicated *N. gonorrhoeae* infections are usually confined to the mucosa of the cervix, urethra, rectum, and throat. In females, *N. gonorrhoeae* infections are often asymptomatic.

Neisseria gonorrhoeae is the second most commonly reported communicable infection in the United States. The age distribution of *N. gonorrhoeae* infections is similar to that for *C. trachomatis* infections (Fig. 40.2). In 2005, gonorrhea rates continued to be highest among adolescents and young adults. The overall gonorrhea rate was highest for 20–24 year olds (506.8 per 100,000 population), which is over four times higher than the national gonorrhea rate. Among females in 2005, 15–19 and 20–24 year olds had the highest rates of gonorrhea (624.7 per 100,000 and 581.2 per 100,000 population, respectively).

In adolescent females, *C. trachomatis* and *N. gonorrhoeae* urogenital infections are most reliably diagnosed by testing either urine or an endocervical swab specimen using the most sensitive and specific test available (a nucleic acid amplification test (NAAT)). Adolescents with cervicitis also should be evaluated for BV and trichomoniasis. Because of the high rates of chlamydia

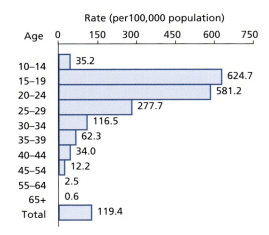

Figure 40.2 Gonorrhea in females. Age- and sex-specific rates, United States, 2005.

infection in women <26 years of age, routine screening of asymptomatic women in this age group is recommended as standard of care. The treatment of choice for chlamydia cervicitis is either a single dose of oral azithromycin or a seven-day course of oral doxycycline. Except for pregnant women, the CDC does not recommend performing routine test of cures (repeat testing 3–4 weeks after completing therapy). Current antimicrobial resistance patterns support the use of cephalosporins as first-line treatment for uncomplicated GC. The treatments of choice are ceftriaxone 125 mg intramuscularly or cefixime given as a single 400 mg oral dose. However, currently, 400 mg tablets of cefixime are not available in the United States and cefixime is only available in a suspension formulation. Some evidence suggests that a single oral dose of cefpodoxime 400 mg or cefuroxime axetil 1 g are adequate alternatives for the treatment of urogenital and anorectal gonorrhea. Single-dose fluoroquinolone regimens (ofloxacin and levofloxacin) are no longer recommended because of increasing and widespread prevalence of quinolone resistance.

Adolescent patients presenting with clinical cervicitis should be treated presumptively for both chlamydia and GC pending the results of NAAT. Since upper genital tract infections (pelvic inflammatory disease, PID) occur in ~10% of patients with chlamydia cervicitis, adolescents who are treated for cervicitis should be carefully assessed for signs of PID.

If untreated, both chlamydia cervicitis and GC cervicitis can lead to PID. The microbiologic etiology of PID also includes the micro-organisms associated with BV. PID occurs when lower genital tract infections ascend to the upper reproductive tract causing endometritis and/or salpingitis and/or peritonitis. The ascension of infection to the endometrium and fallopian tubes may cause lower abdominal pain and menstrual abnormalities. Chlamydia, alone or in combination with other micro-organisms, has been isolated from 5–50% of women seeking care for symptoms of PID. Both the diagnosis and the treatment of PID are unsatisfactory: ~20% of women treated for PID will become infertile, an equal proportion will experience chronic pelvic pain as a result of infection and 10% who do conceive will have an ectopic pregnancy.

Risk factors for PID have been identified. A prior episode of PID increases the risk of another episode. Women who douche may have a higher risk of developing PID compared with women who do not. Research has shown that douching changes the vaginal flora and can force bacteria into the upper reproductive organs from the vagina. Women who have an IUD inserted may have an increased risk of PID near the time of insertion; this risk is greatly reduced if a woman is tested and, if necessary, treated for STIs before an IUD is inserted.

Diseases characterized by genital ulceration

In the United States, the majority of young, sexually active patients with genital ulcer disease (GUD) have genital herpes, syphilis or chancroid. The frequency of each condition differs by geographic area and among different patient populations. In the United States, genital herpes is the most prevalent of these diseases. Although each condition has a classic appearance, diseases can be confused and co-infections can exist. Adolescents presenting with genital ulcers should be tested for both herpes and syphilis. In high-prevalence areas, testing for chancroid should also occur. Donovanosis and lymphogranuloma venereum, which are causes of GUD in other parts of the world, are very uncommon in the United States.

Herpes

Genital herpes, which is caused by infection with either herpes simplex virus type 1 (HSV-1) or type 2 (HSV-2), has reached epidemic proportions in the United States and other countries. Diagnosis and management are reviewed in detail in Chapter 39. The classic signs of disease include red macules that progress to a vesicular eruption. Lesion formation is often preceded by prodromal symptoms including local parasthesisas as well as localized burning and/or itching. Many patients do not experience these classic signs or symptoms but instead present with less severe lesions such as minor perigenital or perianal chafing or fissuring. In addition, many individuals are HSV seropositive (have serologic evidence of past infection) but lack any clinical history suggestive of genital herpes. Because genital herpes is an incurable, remitting-recurring disease, the focus of therapy is on symptom reduction, prevention of recurrences, and suppression of transmission.

Asymptomatic seropositive individuals can intermittently shed virus and when this asymptomatic shedding occurs, transmission to others is possible. Almost one in five individuals aged 12 or older in the US is seropositive for HSV-2 and the proportion of individuals with genital herpes caused by HSV-1 continues to rise. Without intervention, some public health experts estimate that HSV-2 seroprevalence will increase to 39% among men and 49% among women by 2025.

Syphilis

Syphilis is a systemic disease caused by the spirochete bacteria *Treponema pallidum*. Primary infection is characterized by an ulcer (chancer) at the site of infection. Secondary infection is characterized by constitutional symptoms, lymphadenopathy, mucocutaneous lesions, and a skin rash. Tertiary syphilis is characterized by cardiac, ophthalmic, auditory or gummatous lesions. CNS involvement can occur during any stage of syphilis. A patient who has clinical evidence of neurologic involvement with syphilis (for example, cognitive dysfunction, motor or sensory deficits, ophthalmic or auditory symptoms, cranial nerve palsies, and symptoms or signs of meningitis) should have a spinal tap for a CSF examination prior to treatment. Often the clinical manifestations of syphilis are missed and the disease is only diagnosed by serology. Syphilis that is diagnosed serologically within the previous year is referred to as early syphilis; syphilis of greater than one year's duration is referred to as latent syphilis.

Syphilis rates in women are highest in the 20–24 year age group – 3.0 cases per 100,000 population in 2005 (Fig. 40.3). The rate of primary and secondary (P&S) syphilis – the most infectious stages of the disease –

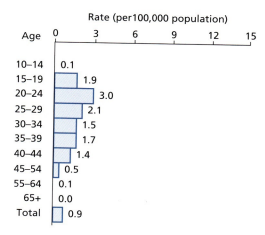

Figure 40.3 Primary and secondary syphilis in females. Age- and sex-specific rates, United States, 2005.

decreased throughout the 1990s, and in 2000 reached an all-time low (Fig. 40.4). However, over the past four years the syphilis rates in the United States have leveled out in women and have been increasing in men. The treatment of choice remains intramuscular, long-acting penicillin.

Chancroid

Chancroid is the least common of the three genital ulcer conditions seen in the United States. The disease is caused by infection with the bacteria *Haemophilus ducreyi* and is characterized by painful genital ulceration and tender, inflammatory inguinal adenopathy. The presence of suppurative inguinal adenopathy is almost pathognomonic. The treatment of choice is either oral azithromycin or intramuscular ceftriaxone. Patients should be re-examined 3–7 days after initiation of therapy to assess improvement of symptoms.

Human papillomavirus infection

Human papillomavirus (HPV) is the most prevalent viral STI. More than 100 different HPV viral types have been identified; ~30 viral types infect the anogenital area. HPV types are classified as low risk or high risk based on their oncogenic potential. Low-risk HPV types are associated with anogenital condyloma and low-grade cervical dysplasia (low-grade squamous intraepithelial lesions or CIN 1). High-risk HPV types are associated with high-grade dysplasia (high-grade intraepithelial lesions or CIN 2/3) and with invasive cervical cancer.

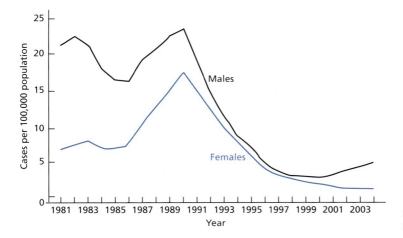

Figure 40.4 Primary and secondary syphilis. Rates by sex, 1981–2004.

Most HPV infections (with both high-risk and low-risk types) will clear spontaneously. HPV infection with high-risk types is necessary but not sufficient for the development of cervical cancer. There are multiple suspected cofactors including: long-term use of oral contraceptives; high number of full-term pregnancies; tobacco smoking; and past infection with HSV-2 and *Chlamydia trachomatis.*

Five HPVs – types 16, 18, 31, 33, and 45 – are responsible for most cervical cancers worldwide. In addition to cervical cancer, these oncogenic HPV types are associated with neoplasms of the vulva, penis, larynx, nasopharynx, and perhaps other sites as well.

Information and recommendations for the use of preventive HPV vaccines are included in the Prevention of STIs section later in the chapter.

Hepatitis B virus infection

Hepatitis B (HBV) is a small DNA virus which primarily infects hepatocytes. HBV makes its entry into hepatocytes through a liver cell-specific receptor, consistent with the strict hepatotropism exhibited by this and other members of the hepadnaviridae. The outcome of infection and spectrum of illness vary widely. During the acute phase, infections range from asymptomatic hepatitis to icteric hepatitis, including fulminant hepatitis. When chronic infection is established, the spectrum of illness ranges from the healthy carrier state to all the sequelae of chronic hepatitis, including cirrhosis and hepatocellular carcinoma.

More adults are killed by HBV every year than by any other vaccine-preventable disease.

HBV is highly contagious. It is found in blood as well as in other body fluids such as tears, saliva, semen, and vaginal secretions. The hepatitis B virus is 100 times more infectious than HIV, the virus which causes AIDS. The presence of virus in saliva makes even simple contact with a hand towel or toothbrush a possible means of transmission. The silent nature of the disease makes it difficult to know who is infected, and therefore, from whom you could catch the virus.

Sexual intercourse is the most common route of transmission of hepatitis B in developed countries. HBV primarily infects teenagers and young adults, high risk or not. The estimated annual incidence is 200,000 new cases in the US and 1,000,000 new cases in Europe. In endemic areas in the rest of the world, perinatal and childhood infections are still the most important route of transmission.

Information and recommendations for the use of HBV vaccines are included in the Prevention of STIs section later in the chapter.

Human immunodeficiency virus (HIV)

Infection with HIV produces a spectrum of disease that progresses from a latent, asymptomatic state to AIDS, a late manifestation. Of acute HIV infections 40–90% are associated with a mononucleosis-like illness characterized by fever, lymphadenopathy, sweats, myalgias, arthralgias, rash, malaise, lethargy, sore throat, anorexia, nausea/vomiting, diarrhea, headache, photophobia, and mucocutaneous ulcers. The acute infection is followed by a period of latency. The natural history of HIV progression can vary considerably from person to person. If untreated, the time between infection with HIV and the development of AIDS ranges from a few months to as long as 17 years (median 10 years). AIDS is defined by the development of serious opportunistic infections, neoplasms or other life-threatening manifestations resulting from progressive HIV-induced immuno-suppression. Multidrug antiretroviral regimens are used to control HIV viral replication and have led to a significant decrease in HIV-related morbidity and mortality. If HIV infected, pregnant and untreated, the risk of mother-to-child HIV transmission is >25%. In the United States, antiretroviral treatment that is provided antepartum, intrapartum, and in the newborn period has significantly reduced the risk of mother-to-child HIV transmission (<1%).

Heterosexually acquired HIV infections represent 35% of all new HIV cases; 64% of heterosexually acquired HIV infections now occur in females. Recent CDC surveillance data have found the proportion of HIV-infected females was highest among sexually active girls aged 13–19 years, consistent with a previous finding. Survey data suggest that females in this age group engage in behaviors that place them at increased risk for acquiring HIV infections; the high proportion of infected females might be associated with sexual contact with older males, who are more likely to be infected.

There are important biologic interactions between HIV and other STIs. STIs, especially those that cause genital ulceration, increase the risk of acquiring HIV if exposed. Also, in those who are already HIV infected, treatment of STIs reduces the shedding of HIV in genital secretions and plasma, and therefore decreases the risk of transmitting HIV to others.

Special considerations in diagnosing and treating common sexually transmitted infections

Treating exposure
When patients report that STI exposures have occurred, treatment should be given. Do not wait for positive screening tests to treat.

Child abuse
Management of children who have STIs requires co-operation between clinicians, laboratories, and child protection agencies. Some diseases (GC, chlamydia, and syphilis), if acquired after the neonatal period, are considered indicative of sexual contact. Other diseases, for example HPV and vaginitis, may or may not be indicative of sexual contact.

Studies suggest that almost one-third of sexually experienced adolescent girls and one-tenth of sexually experienced adolescent boys have been sexually abused. Adolescents with a history of sexual abuse report greater sexual risk taking than those without such a history.

Drug resistance
In addition to the higher prevalence rates of STIs in the developing world, a steadily increasing proportion of infections acquired abroad are resistant to standard antibiotics. Disease surveillance for antimicrobial resistance is conducted on an ongoing basis by local health departments and the CDC.

Prevention of sexually transmitted infections

Prevention of STIs is an important aspect of clinical care for adolescents and young adults. Prevention is preferable to treatment. Public health strategies employed to reduce the spread of STIs include abstinence counseling, health education to reduce at risk behaviors, provision of condoms, periodic screening of at-risk teens, treatment of partners, and preventive vaccinations.

In all 50 states and the District of Columbia, medical care for STIs can be provided to adolescents without parental consent or knowledge. In addition, in the majority of states, adolescents can consent to HIV counseling and testing. Current laws for vaccination of adolescents vary from state to state.

General screening recommendations
The highest prevalence of bacterial STIs occurs in females aged 15–24. Twenty five percent of sexually experienced teens will in fact develop an STI prior to graduating from high school; among adolescents, a past history of a STI remains the single best predictor of having a subsequent STI. Public health efforts should be directed to promoting

---

Box 40.2 General approach to STI evaluations in adolescents and young adults

- Prevention is always preferable to treatment
- Partner notification/treatment may be legally required and is essential to prevent reinfection and disease spread
- Condoms reduce the risk of most, but not all, STIs
- Evaluation of STIs should include appropriate use of cultures and serology
- Cultures and serology should not be used to guide treatments following exposures
- When available, cultures and serology should guide choice of treatment
- Prompt diagnosis and therapy can reduce both complications and spread of STIs
- The presence of one STI should signal the need to screen for other STIs
- Global resistance patterns should be considered when choosing therapy

---

preventive behavior among adolescents newly diagnosed with an STI.

Since many infected individuals may be asymptomatic, the CDC recommends screening sexually active adolescents for STIs every six months. Adherence to bi-yearly examinations may be problematic and recent studies have demonstrated both the utility and the acceptability of self-collected vaginal specimens among teenagers as an alternative strategy. The CDC continues to recommend that all persons who seek evaluation and treatment for STIs be screened for HIV infection.

Chlamydia screening recommendations

Chlamydia screening has been shown to be highly effective. Data from a study in a managed care setting suggest that chlamydia screening and treatment can reduce incidence of PID by over 50%. Unfortunately, many sexually active young women are not being tested for chlamydia, in part reflecting a lack of awareness among some providers and limited resources for screening. Recent research has shown that a simple change in clinical procedures – coupling chlamydia tests with routine Pap testing – can sharply increase the proportion of sexually active young women screened. Stepping up screening efforts is critical to preventing the serious health consequences of

this infection, particularly infertility. Chlamydia screening and reporting are likely to continue to expand further in response to the Health Plan Employer Data and Information Set (HEDIS) measure for chlamydia screening of sexually active women 15 through 25 years of age who receive medical care through managed care organizations or Medicaid.

HIV testing recommendations

The CDC now recommends routine HIV testing in multiple healthcare settings. The objectives of these recommendations are to increase HIV screening of patients, including pregnant women, in healthcare settings; foster earlier detection of HIV infection; identify and counsel persons with unrecognized HIV infection and link them to clinical and prevention services; and further reduce perinatal transmission of HIV in the United States. Under the new CDC guidelines:

- HIV screening is recommended for patients in all healthcare settings after the patient is notified that testing will be performed unless the patient declines (opt-out screening)
- persons at high risk for HIV infection should be screened for HIV at least annually
- separate written consent for HIV testing should not be required; general consent for medical care should be considered sufficient to encompass consent for HIV testing
- prevention counseling should not be required with HIV diagnostic testing or as part of HIV screening programs in healthcare settings.

For pregnant women:

- HIV screening should be included in the routine panel of prenatal screening tests for all pregnant women
- HIV screening is recommended after the patient is notified that testing will be performed unless the patient declines (opt-out screening)
- separate written consent for HIV testing should not be required; general consent for medical care should be considered sufficient to encompass consent for HIV testing
- repeat screening in the third trimester is recommended in certain jurisdictions with elevated rates of HIV infection among pregnant women.

Condoms

Male condoms are widely promoted as an essential component of STI control programs. Consistent, correct use without breakage or slippage should protect an uninfected person from acquiring a primary infection or transmitting a secondary infection to a partner. Male latex condoms are expected to provide different levels of protection for various STIs, depending upon how diseases are transmitted. Because condoms block the discharge of semen or protect the male urethra against exposure to vaginal secretions, a greater level of protection is provided for the discharge diseases. A lesser degree of protection is provided for GUD or HPV because these infections are transmitted by exposure to areas that are not necessarily covered by condoms.

Vaccination recommendations

Hepatitis B

The first vaccine that protected against an STI was the hepatitis B virus (HBV) vaccine. This is a recombinant, subunit vaccine given in a series of three intramuscular injections over the course of six months.

In the United States, infants have been routinely inoculated with the HBV vaccine since 1991 and HBV vaccine has been integrated successfully into the childhood vaccination schedule. Infant vaccination coverage levels for HBV now are equivalent to those of other vaccines in the childhood schedule. Vaccination coverage among adolescents also has increased substantially; preliminary data from 2003 indicated that approximately 50–60% of adolescents aged 13–15 years have records indicating vaccination (with three doses) against hepatitis B. From 1990 to 2005, the incidence of acute hepatitis B in the United States declined 78%. The greatest decline (96%) occurred among children and adolescents, coincident with an increase in hepatitis B vaccination coverage.

Hepatitis B vaccine should be offered to all unvaccinated adolescents. Because HBV infection is frequently sexually transmitted, hepatitis B vaccination should be part of the routine treatment plan for all unvaccinated, uninfected adolescents being evaluated for a STI.

Human papillomavirus

It is helpful to review the genomic organization of HPV in order to understand the efficacy of the new HPV vaccines. HPV is a nonenveloped DNA virus. The genomic organization of all HPV types is generally similar and consists of:

- an early (E) region that codes for proteins that control DNA replication (oncoproteins E6 and E7 and replication proteins E1 and E2)
- a late (L) region that codes for the major capsid protein (L1) and a minor capsid protein (L2)
- a noncoding upstream regulatory region.

In cell expression systems, the L1 protein can self-assemble into virus-like particles (VLPs). Vaccination with L1 VLPs produces very potent type-specific antibody responses. A quadrivalent HPV vaccine (Gardasil®, Merck, New Jersey, USA) was approved in 2006. This is a L1 VLP vaccine against HPV types 6, 11, 16 and 18. HPV-6 and -11 are associated with 90% of genital warts and HPV-16 and -18 are associated with 70% of cases of high-grade cervical dysplasia and cervical cancer. In previously unexposed women, this vaccine offers a high level of type-specific protection against HPV. GlaxoSmithKline (Middlesex, UK) has filed for FDA approval of Cervarix®, a bivalent HPV-16/18 VLP vaccine; Cervarix has been approved for use in women and children in 67 countries around the world. The latter may have some cross-protection against other oncogenic HPV types. Because the most aggressive cervical cancers are associated with HPV-16 and HPV-18, it has been estimated that with a highly effective HPV-16/18 vaccine, the level of protection from death due to cervical cancer could exceed 95%. If vaccination targeted only young women before they became sexually active, a reduction in the incidence of cervical cancer would not be expected to become apparent for at least a decade.

Studies of the quadrivalent HPV vaccine have demonstrated that the vaccine is highly effective for the prevention of HPV-6, -11, -16, and -18 related persistent infection, vaccine type-related cervical intraeptihelial neoplasia (CIN), high-grade dysplasia (CIN 2/3), as well as external genital lesions (genital warts, vulvar intraepithelial neoplasia (VIN) and vaginal intraepithelial neoplasia (VaIN). The vaccine was not effective in those with baseline evidence of infection to the vaccine types. Efficacy in men is being studied but has not yet been determined.

The quadrivalent HPV vaccine is administered in a three-dose schedule. The second and third doses should be administered two and six months after the first dose. The dose of quadrivalent HPV vaccine is 0.5 mL, administered intramuscularly (IM), preferably in the deltoid muscle.

The Advisory Committee on Immunization Practices (ACIP) recommends routine vaccination of females aged 11–12 years with three doses of quadrivalent HPV vaccine.

The vaccination series can be started as young as age nine years. Vaccination also is recommended for females aged 13–26 years who have not been previously vaccinated or who have not completed the full series. Ideally, vaccine should be administered before potential exposure to HPV through sexual contact; however, females who might have already been exposed to HPV should be vaccinated. Sexually active females who have not been infected with any of the HPV vaccine types would receive full benefit from vaccination. Vaccination would provide less benefit to females if they have already been infected with one or more of the four vaccine HPV types. However, it is not possible for a clinician to assess the extent to which sexually active persons would benefit from vaccination, and the risk for HPV infection might continue as long as persons are sexually active. Pap testing and screening for HPV DNA or HPV antibody are not needed before vaccination at any age.

Genital herpes vaccines

Vaccines against HSV remain under development and to date have only shown partial protection in women who are serologically naive to both HSV-1 and HSV-2 (double seronegative individuals) prior to vaccination.

Microbicides for the prevention of STIs

Microbicides are products that can be applied to either the vaginal or rectal mucosa in order to prevent (or significantly reduce) the risk of acquiring STIs, including HIV. Multiple candidate microbicides are under development and there are large-scale efficacy trials being conducted internationally. It is feasible that there may be one or more licensed microbicides available by the end of the decade.

Further reading

CDC. A comprehensive immunization strategy to eliminate transmission of hepatitis B virus infection in the United States. Recommendations of the Advisory Committee on Immunization Practices (ACIP) Part II: Immunization of Adults. *Morbid Mortal Wkly Rep* 2006;**55**(RR16):1–25.

CDC. *Fact Sheet for Public Health Personnel: Male Latex Condoms and Sexually Transmitted Diseases.* Available at: www.cdc.gov/nchstp/od/condoms.pdf.

CDC. Quadrivalent human papillomavirus vaccine. Recommendations of the Advisory Committee on Immunization Practices (ACIP). *Morbid Mortal Wkly Rep* 2007;**56**:1–24.

CDC. Revised recommendations for HIV testing of adults, adolescents, and pregnant women in health-care settings. *Morbid Mortal Wkly Rep* 2006;**55**(RR14):1–17.

CDC. Sexually transmitted diseases treatment guidelines 2006. *Morbid Mortal Wkly Rep* 2006;**55**(No.RR-11):1–94.

CDC. *STD Surveillance 2005 National Report.* December 2006. Available at: www.cdc.gov/std/stats/toc2005.htm.

CDC. Update to CDC's *Sexually Transmitted Diseases Treatment Guidelines, 2006*: fluoroquinolones no longer recommended for treatment of gonococcal infections. *Morbid Mortal Wkly Rep* 2007;**56**(14):332–336.

Crosby R, Leichliter J, Brackbill R. Longitudinal prediction of sexually transmitted diseases among adolescents. Results from a national survey. *Am J Prev Med* 2000;**18**(4):312–317.

Gerbase AC, Rowley JT, Mertens TE. Global epidemiology of sexually transmitted diseases. *Lancet* 1998;**381**(suppl III):2–4.

Low, N, Broutet N, Adu-Sarkodie Y, Barton P, Hassain M, Hawkes S. Sexual and reproductive health 5. Global control of sexually transmitted infections. *Lancet* 2006;**368**:2001–2016.

McGowan I. Microbicides: a new frontier in HIV prevention. *Biologicals* 2006;**34**:241–255.

Ward BJ, Plourde P. Travel and sexually transmitted infections. *J Travel Med* 2006;**13**(5):300–318.

Weinstock H, Berman S, Cates W Jr. Sexually transmitted diseases among American youth: incidence and prevalence estimates, 2000. *Perspect Sex Reprod Health* 2004;**36**(1):6–10.

CHAPTER 41

Imaging

Sabah Servaes[1] *& Monica Epelman*[2]

[1] The Children's Hospital of Philadelphia, Philadelphia, PA, USA
[2] University of Pennsylvania, Philadelphia, PA, USA

Introduction

Ultrasound has played a central role in the gynecologic evaluation of patients. Although transabdominal and endovaginal approaches are often available, an endovaginal exam is not always feasible, particularly in young patients. Excellent visualization of the pelvis can be obtained with the bladder serving as an acoustic window for transabdominal exams. Many institutions utilize radiography of the abdomen and pelvis and then ultrasound prior to the use of computed tomography (CT) in young females with acute abdominal or pelvic pain. The rationale for this approach is that ultrasound is an excellent study to aid in the diagnosis of many of the likely etiologies for acute abdominal pain in a young female without exposing the patient to radiation.

In the nonacute setting, magnetic resonance imaging (MRI) is emerging as a more frequently utilized modality in the evaluation of gynecologic issues. Tissue characterization is unparalleled. As with ultrasound, no ionizing radiation is utilized. One area in which MRI has become instrumental is in the evaluation of Müllerian duct developmental abnormalities. Fluoroscopic examination is often a useful adjunct.

Radiography is a simple first study that proves invaluable in the acute setting and in the identification of pelvic calcifications which are often present with teratomas. Mass effect upon bowel loops or the stomach is easily demonstrated with an abdominal radiograph.

Oncologic evaluations most often require the use of CT. Also utilized with the acute abdomen, CT provides excellent spatial resolution and characterizes tissues. With faster CT scanning equipment and higher resolution imaging acquisition, coronal and sagittal planes may be reformatted with anatomic results helpful for surgical planning.

Normal variants

The normal endometrium varies in appearance during the phases of menses and is well seen with ultrasound or MRI. The proliferative phase is characterized by a thin, echogenic endometrium early with ultrasound with progressive thickening of the endometrium to nearly 1 cm in thickness. The echogenic endometrium is surrounded by a relatively hypoechoic functional layer. During the secretory phase, the functional layer becomes echogenic and the endometrium thickens to >1.5 cm thickness (Fig. 41.1).

The normal ovaries are lateral to the uterus and typically posterior. There are peripheral follicles in the otherwise homogeneous echotexture of the ovary. The follicle which will ovulate may increase to over 2 cm in diameter and later involute (Fig. 41.2).

Congenital abnormalities

Müllerian duct

The normal development of the uterus, cervix, and vagina arises from fusion of the Müllerian (paramesonephric) ducts. Congenital abnormalities result from failure of resorption of the median septum (septate uterus), failure of fusion (didelphys or bicornuate uterus) or failure to form (absence of the uterus or unicornuate uterus). These abnormalities are associated with renal abnormalities.

Pediatric, Adolescent, & Young Adult Gynecology. Edited by A. Altchek and L. Deligdisch. © 2009 Blackwell Publishing, ISBN: 978-1-4051-5347-8.

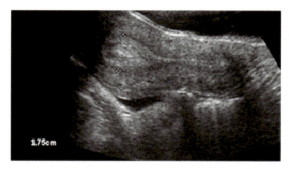

Figure 41.1 Ultrasound image of normal thickened secretory endometrium, marked by calipers and measuring 1.75 cm.

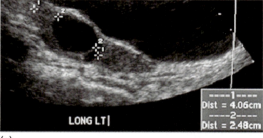

(a)

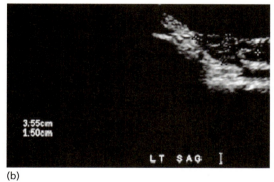

(b)

Figure 41.2 (a) Ultrasound image of dominant follicle measuring over 2 cm within the ovary (the ovary is delineated by calipers marked 1). The dominant follicle is hypoechoic, consistent with simple fluid and delineated by the calipers marked 2. (b) Three weeks later the dominant follicle is no longer seen (calipers delineate the margins of the ovary).

Uterine abnormalities give rise to obstetric issues. MRI outperforms ultrasound in these evaluations, although three-dimensional ultrasound is narrowing the gap (Figs 41.3–41.6). Mayer–Rokitansky–Küster–Hauser syndrome consists of the absence of a vagina, a Müllerian duct abnormality secondary to failure of formation, renal abnor-

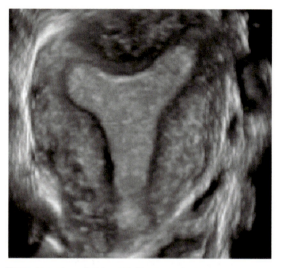

Figure 41.3 Three-dimensional ultrasound of an arcuate uterus, considered a normal variant, and results from incomplete resorption of the uterovaginal septum.

mality, and skeletal abnormality (usually vertebral). This syndrome can be imaged utilizing ultrasound or MRI. There are intersex issues that arise secondary to complex abnormalities involving the development of male and female genitalia. Fluoroscopic imaging in combination with ultrasound and MRI is helpful to unravel the anatomy (Fig. 41.7).

Hydrocolpos is vaginal dilation secondary to a congenital obstruction. Hydrometrocolpos is the term used if there is concomitant dilation of the uterus. In a patient who has started menstruating, there are also blood products causing dilation and hematometrocolpos is the term used. A common and benign cause is imperforate hymen. Atresia of the vagina or a vaginal septum are alternative etiologies which are likely to be associated with other anomalies. Radiography is a simple method to demonstrate a midline pelvic mass displacing bowel loops (Fig. 41.8a). Ultrasound is the next test of choice to characterize a pelvic mass identified in a child or in the evaluation of suspected hydrometrocolpos (Fig. 41.8b). CT and MRI can also demonstrate these findings (Fig. 41.8c–e).

Metanephric blastema and ureteral bud

Uterine abnormalities can be associated with renal abnormalities such as ectopic kidney. Ectopic kidney

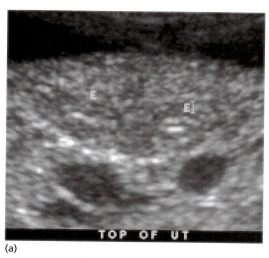

(a)

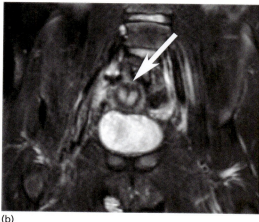

(b)

Figure 41.4 (a) Transverse ultrasound of septate uterus demonstrating two echogenic endometrial canals, marked by E, with intervening uterine tissue. (b) Coronal T2 fat-saturated MRI of partial septate uterus with arrow pointing towards uterine fundus given a heart shape by low-signal septum seen within the high-signal endometrium. Note that the septum does not extend to the cervix.

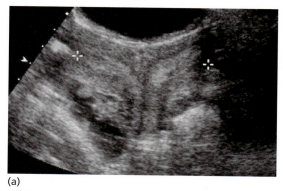

(a)

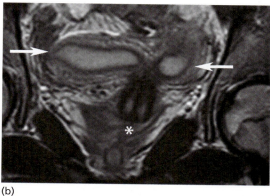

(b)

Figure 41.5 (a) Ultrasound of uterus didelphys with widely divergent uterine horns delineated by calipers. Note the two separate echogenic endometrial canals. (b) Coronal T2-weighted MRI of uterus didelphys with arrows pointing to the divergent uterine horns and * at the cervices, which demonstrate a mild degree of fusion medially. Note the zonal anatomy of the uterus which is demonstrated on T2-weighted images with the high-signal endometrium, low-signal junctional zone and intermediate-signal myometrium, which blends with the serosa.

results from failed migration of the metanephric blastema and ureteral bud to the renal fossa. When uterine abnormalities are identified, the kidneys should be imaged to assess for any associated abnormality. Ultrasound can easily be performed to evaluate the kidneys. Often, prenatal imaging detects a renal abnormality which may be identified prior to the uterine abnormalities (Fig. 41.9). If the metanephrogenic blastema fuse prior to ascent, a horseshoe kidney results. There is an association with other anomalies including rectovaginal fistula and Müllerian abnormalities (Fig. 41.10).

Wolffian duct

The remains of the Wolffian (mesonephric) ducts are Gartner duct cysts found around the vagina. They may be associated with urinary tract or genital tract abnormalities. These cysts are anechoic on ultrasound. The cysts contain proteinaceous material which impacts their appearance on MRI (high in signal on both T1- and T2-weighted imaging) (Fig. 41.11).

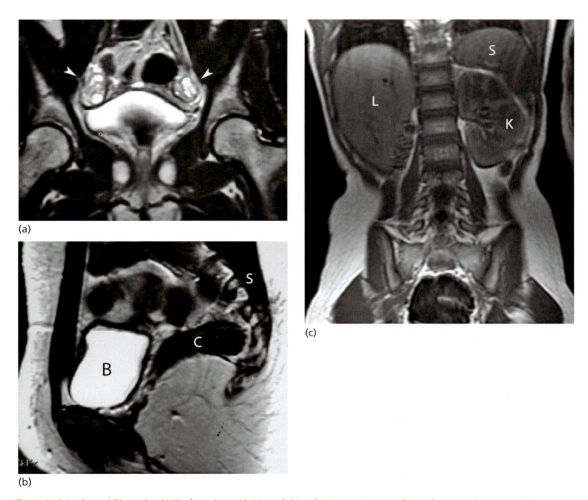

(a)

(b)

(c)

Figure 41.6 (a) Coronal T2-weighted MRI of a patient with Mayer–Rokitansky–Kuster–Hauser syndrome demonstrating two ovaries (*arrowheads*) with absence of the uterus. (b) Lateral T2-weighted MRI demonstrating bladder (B) with colon (C) posterior and no uterus. The sacrum is marked by an S. (c) This same patient also has congenital absence of the right kidney as demonstrated in this coronal MRI. L, liver; K, left kidney; S, spleen.

Location distinguishes Gartner duct cysts from Nabothian cysts, which are mucus-filled cysts on the cervix (Fig. 41.12). Nabothian cysts arise secondary to squamous metaplasia from obstructed endocervical glands.

Cloaca and allantois

The cloaca and allantois give rise to the urachus which normally closes in the last half of gestation. There are four types of abnormalities which result from a urachal rem-

nant: patent urachus, sinus between the umbilicus and urachus, vesicourachal diverticulum, and urachal cyst. Infection is the main issue which brings this abnormality to clinical attention, although there is drainage from the umbilicus in the case of a patent urachus (Fig. 41.13).

Processus vaginalis

The parietal peritoneal membrane extends into the internal inguinal ring during development, forming the processus vaginalis. An indirect inguinal hernia may result if

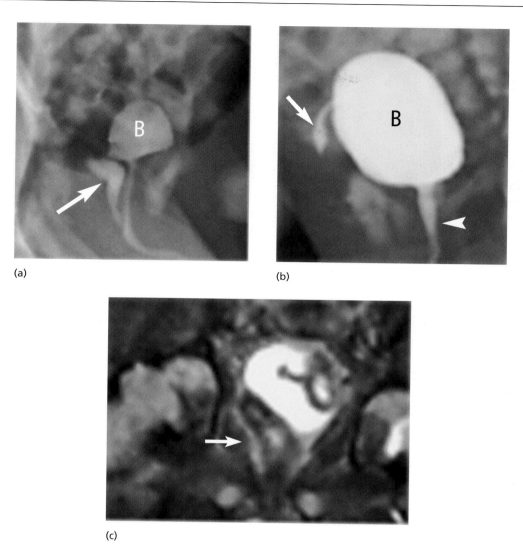

(a)

(b)

(c)

Figure 41.7 (a) Fluoroscopic lateral spot image of a patient with ambiguous genitalia and contrast administered via the solitary orifice anterior to the rectum. Contrast opacifies the bladder labeled with B and arrow points to the opacified vagina which connects to the anatomically male urethra. (b) Fluoroscopic frontal spot image of the same patient demonstrates the opacified bladder (B), right unicornuate uterine horn (*arrow*), and urethra (*arrowhead*). (c) Coronal T2 fat-saturated MRI of right unicornuate uterus, with arrow pointing to uterus.

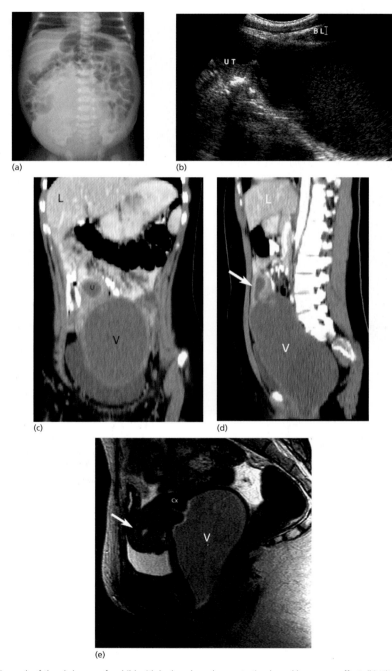

Figure 41.8 (a) Radiograph of the abdomen of a child with hydrocolpos demonstrating bowel loop mass effect. (b) Ultrasound demonstrates the fluid-distended vagina which may contain echoes secondary to cellular debris, mucus, and blood. UT, uterus; BL, bladder. (c) Coronal and (d) sagittal reformats from CT examination of a patient with hydrometrocolpos (uterus, U in (c) and arrow in (d); V, vagina; L, liver). (e) Sagittal T2 MRI of hydrometrocolpos (uterus delineated by arrow; V, vagina; Cx, cervix).

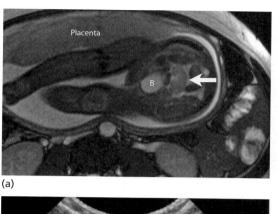

(a)

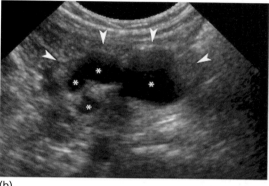

(b)

Figure 41.9 (a) Fetal MRI demonstrates a pelvic kidney (*arrow*) located posterior to the bladder (B). (b) A different patient with a multicystic dysplastic kidney identified in the pelvis (arrowheads outline the kidney and * denote the multiple cysts within the kidney).

the processus vaginalis remains patent. Bowel, an ovary or a fallopian tube may herniate (Fig. 41.14).

Etiologies of pelvic pain

There are a multitude of causes of pelvic pain. En-dometriosis is one cause of chronic pelvic pain. There are several purported theories regarding the etiology of the presence of functional endometrial tissue outside the uterus, with two of the favored including retrograde men-struation via the fallopian tubes and dissemination via lymphatics. Diagnosis is best made with laparoscopy, but there is some success with ultrasound and MRI (Fig. 41.15).

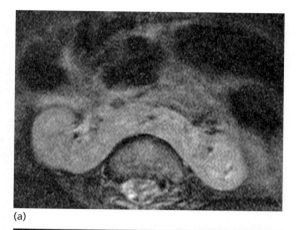

(a)

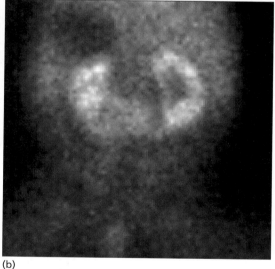

(b)

Figure 41.10 Horseshoe kidney. (a) Axial T2 MRI. (b) Nuclear renal scan.

Acute pelvic pain is a frequent cause for emergency room visits. Despite myriad etiologies, the presentations may be similar but, fortunately, imaging can help to re-solve the true cause. A girl with right lower quadrant pain should have a pelvic ultrasound, especially if she is peripubertal. Often the basis for the pain is ovarian and the appendix may also be evaluated, particularly in slim patients. CT is less sensitive in assessing the adnexa and exposes the patient to ionizing radiation. Ovarian torsion most frequently is demonstrated by an asymmetrically enlarged ovary. Doppler interrogation is unreliable in

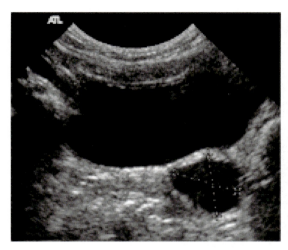

Figure 41.11 Transverse ultrasound of bladder and vagina with adjacent anechoic Gartner duct cyst delineated by calipers.

assisting with this diagnosis (Fig. 41.16). The enlarged ovary may also have an associated cyst or mass such as a teratoma, which is the likely cause of the torsion (Fig. 41.17). Massive ovarian edema is an entity thought to be secondary to intermittent torsion and another etiology for pelvic pain. The ovary is enlarged but, unlike torsion, extensive edema is demonstrable with MRI (Fig. 41.18).

Other ovarian etiologies for pain include a hemorrhagic cyst that may rupture (Fig. 41.19). Hydrosalpinx and tubo-ovarian abscess are well demonstrated with ultrasound. A tortuous anechoic tubular structure represents the fluid-filled, dilated fallopian tube. A fluid–fluid

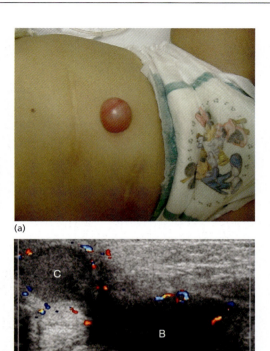

(a)

(b)

Figure 41.13 Infected urachal cyst. (a) Clinical presentation of child with bulging red mass at umbilicus. (b) Ultrasound demonstrating complex cyst (C) at the dome of the bladder (B). Doppler demonstrates the absence of flow within the cyst and relative hyperemia at the periphery.

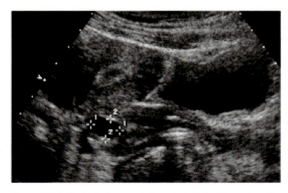

Figure 41.12 Sagittal ultrasound of anechoic Nabothian cyst on the cervix with calipers delineating the cyst.

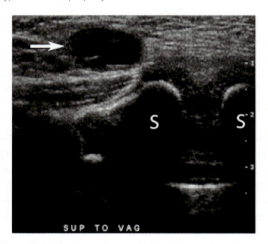

Figure 41.14 Transverse ultrasound of ectopic ovary (*arrow*) adjacent to pubic symphysis (S).

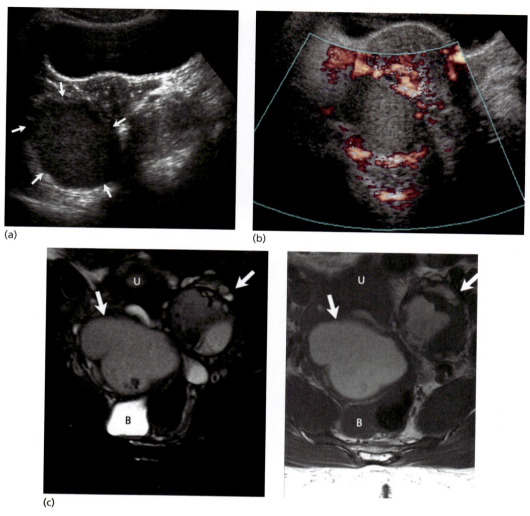

Figure 41.15 Adnexal endometriosis. (a) Ultrasound of adnexal endometrioma (*arrows*). (b) No flow is demonstrated within the lesion using power Doppler. This appearance is similar to a hemorrhagic cyst, but is unlikely to change considerably over time with an endometrioma in contradistinction to the hemorrhagic cyst. (c) MRI of adnexal lesions (*arrows*) which are high in signal on both T1- (right image) and T2- (left image) weighted imaging, consistent with blood products within the cysts. U, uterus; B, bladder.

level may be seen in the presence of organizing pus. The abscess typically has internal complexity with peripheral hyperemia, but no internal flow with Doppler. Gas may be present causing shadowing. The appearance may be similar to an adnexal neoplasm, but the clinical history helps to resolve this difference (Fig. 41.20).

An abnormal appendix can often be identified in the right lower quadrant as a dilated (>6), blind-ending tubular, aperistaltic, hyperemic structure which does not com-

press. An echogenic appendicolith may be seen casting a posterior acoustic shadow. If the appendix has already ruptured, there may be free fluid, phlegmonous changes or abscess (Fig. 41.21). A ruptured appendix can cause abscess within the pelvis and symptoms which the gynecologist may encounter (Fig. 41.22). Radiography is helpful to diagnose intraperitoneal pathology, but CT provides the extent of disease. Acute renal pathology such as obstructing calculi or infection can cause pelvic pain.

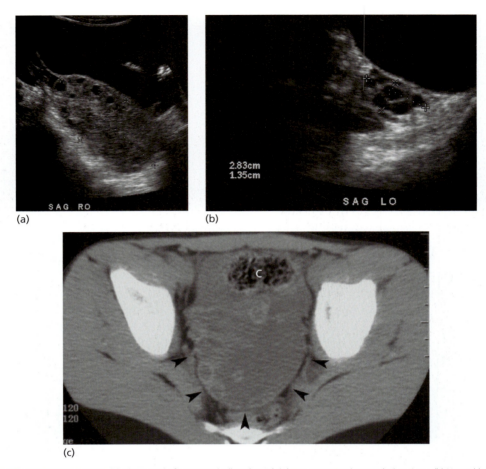

(a)

(b)

(c)

Figure 41.16 Right ovarian torsion. (a) Ultrasound of asymmetrically enlarged right ovary measuring nearly 8 × 4 cm. (b) Normal left ovary ultrasound. (c) The patient had undergone a CT at another institution prior to the ultrasound demonstrating the torsed right ovary.

Ultrasound is excellent at detecting an obstructed renal collecting system and can identify calcified calculi. Visualization of the ureters is more easily accomplished with CT. Acute pyelonephritis is often radiologically occult, but may be manifest as renal enlargement with poor corticomedullary differentiation. A renal abscess can be assessed with ultrasound which may be utilized for an interventional procedure. CT is often the modality utilized for patients in whom the site suspected of pathology is not known (Fig. 41.23). A cervical hematoma may resemble a malignancy, but the clinical scenario or follow-up examination can distinguish between these entities (Fig. 41.24).

Pelvic neoplasms

Ovarian neoplasms

Germ cell neoplasms

The most common malignant ovarian neoplasms in children and young women are of germ cell origin. All three germ cell layers, ectoderm, mesoderm, and endoderm, are present in these tumors. However, they are often called dermoid cysts because there is a preponderance of ectodermal components. The subtypes are: mature teratoma, immature teratoma, dysgerminoma, endodermal sinus tumor, embryonal carcinoma, and choriocarcinoma.

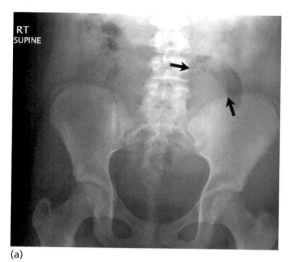

(a)

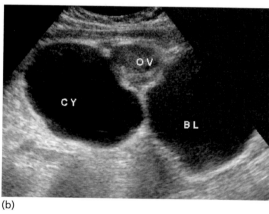

(b)

Figure 41.17 Paraovarian cyst with torsion. (a) Thirteen-year-old girl presented with acute abdominal pain and this radiograph of the abdomen demonstrating mass effect on the bowel (*arrows*). (b) Ultrasound of this same patient demonstrates a paraovarian cyst with torsion. CY, paraovarian cyst; OV, ovary; BL, bladder.

The mature teratoma is the only benign tumor in this group, but also the most common. Mature cystic teratomas are generally unilocular with hair, muscle, teeth, bone, and skin lining the wall and predominating at the Rokitansky nodule on pathologic examination. Mature teratomas vary in appearance at imaging, ranging from cystic to echogenic mass or heterogeneous mass. Some of the characteristic signs include the "tip of the iceberg" in which an echogenic mass is identified with shadowing that obscures visualization of the entire lesion. Fat–fluid

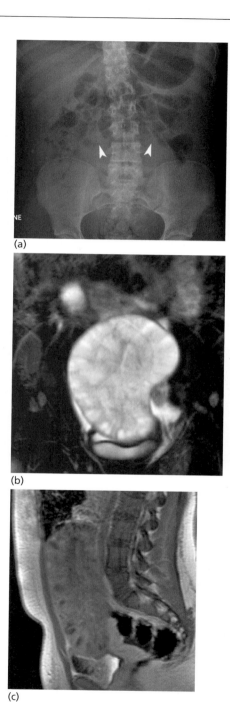

(a)

(b)

(c)

Figure 41.18 Massive ovarian edema. (a) Radiograph of abdomen demonstrating mass effect (*arrowheads*) from enlarged ovary. (b) Coronal and (c) sagittal MRI of enlarged ovary secondary to massive edema.

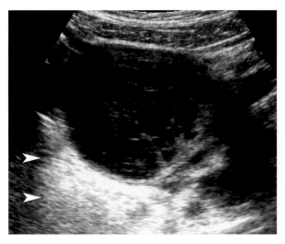

Figure 41.19 Ultrasound of hemorrhagic cyst illustrates meshwork of clot within the cyst and increased through transmission posteriorly (*arrowheads*).

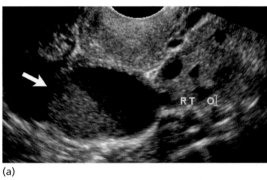

(a)

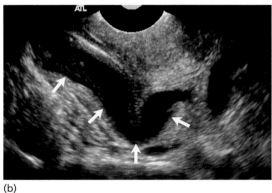

(b)

Figure 41.20 (a) Ultrasound of tubo-ovarian abscess (*arrow*) with fluid–fluid level and ovary = RT OV. (b) Ultrasound of hydrosalpinx (*arrows*).

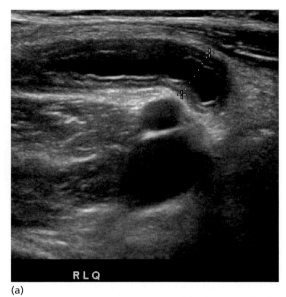

(a)

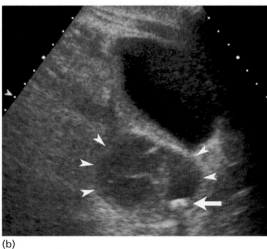

(b)

Figure 41.21 (a) Ultrasound of inflamed appendix with calipers measuring the diameter as 9 mm. (b) Ultrasound of a fallen appendicolith (*arrow*) with surrounding phlegmon (*arrowheads*).

or hair–fluid levels may be seen. Hair fibers floating in the cyst produce the "dermoid mesh" which is typical for a mature teratoma (Fig. 41.25).

Rarely, gliomatosis peritonei results from immature teratomas despite the absence of malignancy. Peritoneal implants may be seen with ovarian carcinoma, which is rare in patients less than 20 years of age.

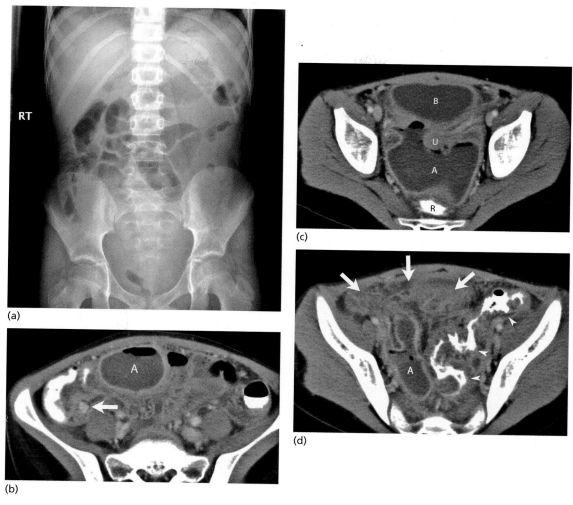

Figure 41.22 Ruptured appendicitis with abscess. (a) Radiograph of the abdomen demonstrating prominent bowel loops and a paucity of bowel gas in the pelvis. (b) Axial CT demonstrates a rim-enhancing abscess (A) and appendicolith (*arrow*). (c) Axial CT of bladder (B), uterus (U), abscess (A), and rectum (R). (d) Axial CT of abscess (A), adjacent phlegmon (*arrows*), and inflamed bowel (*arrowheads*).

CT or MRI is the modality of choice for imaging spread of tumor. Small peritoneal implants may be difficult to see, but become more apparent in the presence of ascites. Implants have a 30% chance of being calcified with serous cystadenocarcinoma (Fig. 41.26). Dysgerminomas represent the most common pelvic malignancy in girls following rhabdomyosarcoma. Malignant germ cell tumors are typically large with a significant solid component. Laboratory values such as elevated levels of serum α-fetoprotein and human

chorionic gonadotropin (hCG) are supportive of the diagnosis.

Epithelial neoplasms

Although rare in the prepubescent population, epithelial tumors are the most common ovarian neoplasm in women. The subtypes of epithelial ovarian neoplasms are: serous, mucinous, endometrioid, clear cell, and Brenner, with serous and mucinous tumors the most common. Mucinous tumors are usually multilocular cystic masses

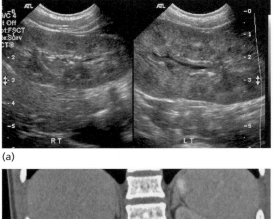

(a)

(b)

Figure 41.23 (a) Split-screen ultrasound sagittal imaging of the kidneys demonstrates asymmetric enlargement with poor corticomedullary differentiation in this patient with left pyelonephritis. (b) Coronal CT reformat of right renal abscess (*arrow*).

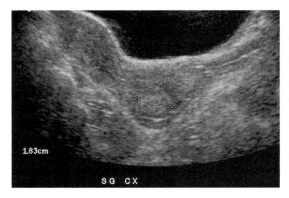

Figure 41.24 Sagittal ultrasound demonstrates a cervical hematoma (*calipers*) following rape.

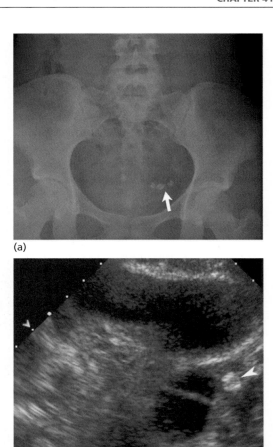

(a)

(b)

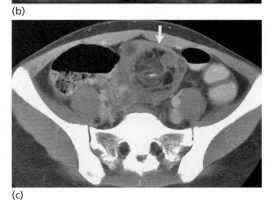

(c)

Figure 41.25 Teratoma. (a) Radiograph of the pelvis demonstrating irregular-shaped calcifications on the left (*arrow*). (b) Ultrasound exam demonstrates a predominantly cystic structure with an echogenic focus (*arrowhead*) casting a posterior acoustic shadow consistent with calcification. (c) Axial CT is characteristic for a teratoma with a mass containing fat, fluid, and calcification (*arrow*).

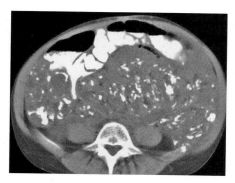

Figure 41.26 Axial CT of calcifications throughout the peritoneum in gliomatosis peritonei.

with thin septa and heterogeneity of the cystic components. Serous cystadenomas may be unilocular or multilocular cystic masses with thin septa and homogeneity of the cystic components (Figs 41.27, 41.28).

Sex cord stromal neoplasms

This group of tumors arises from the embryonic gonad sex cord and/or ovarian stroma and includes the following subtypes: granulosa cell, Sertoli–Leydig cell, thecoma, and fibroma. The juvenile granulosa cell tumor secretes estrogen and causes precocious puberty in premenarchal girls. No features typical of this lesion have yet been reported (Fig. 41.29).

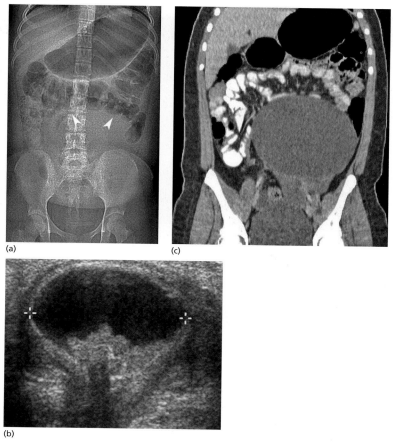

(a)

(b)

(c)

Figure 41.27 (a) A scout view of the abdomen demonstrates mass effect upon the bowel (*arrowheads*) consistent with a mass arising from the pelvis. (b) Transverse ultrasound of a unilocular cystic mass arising from the ovary. (c) Coronal CT reformat demonstrates a homogeneous, unilocular cystic mass consistent with the diagnosis of serous cystadenoma.

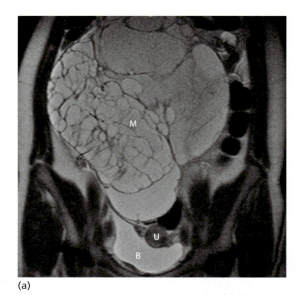

(a)

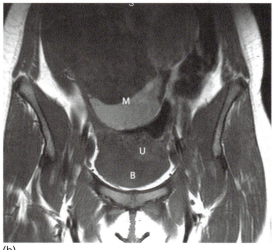

(b)

Figure 41.28 Coronal MR images demonstrate a multilocular heterogenous cystic mass arising from the pelvis consistent with a mucinous cystadenoma. B, bladder; U, uterus; M, mass. (a) HASTE; (b) T1.

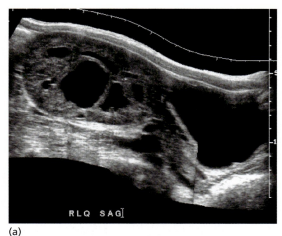

(a)

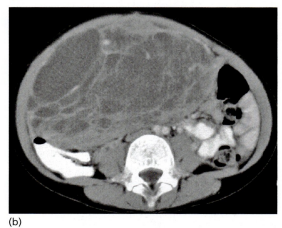

(b)

Figure 41.29 (a) Ultrasound of complex adnexal mass. (b) Axial CT of complex solid and cystic septated mass found to be a granulosa cell tumor.

Rhabdomyosarcoma

Rhabdomyosarcoma is the most common soft tissue sarcoma in the pediatric population. This tumor can arise nearly everywhere but most commonly arises in the pelvis in children. Common sites include the genitourinary tract (urinary bladder is most common), vagina, uterus, pelvic floor or perineum. Ultrasound is useful to identify the lesion. CT and MRI demonstrate the extent of the tumor (Fig. 41.30).

Adrenocortical neoplasms

Adrenocortical neoplasms are a potential cause of virilization in girls. Clinical features in young girls are typically abnormal size and strength secondary to increased muscle mass, clitoromegaly, advanced bone age, and pubic hair. Ultrasound is an excellent modality to evaluate for a suprarenal mass. The mass is well circumscribed. CT is the other modality commonly utilized to image this tumor

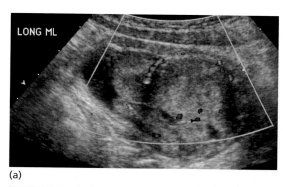

(a)

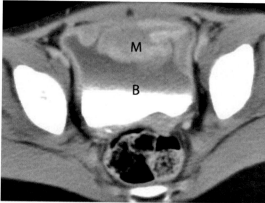

(b)

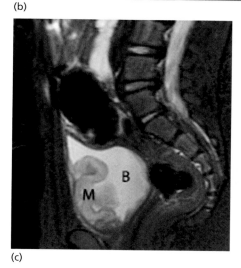

(c)

Figure 41.30 (a) Ultrasound of a solid mass with flow arising from the bladder. (b) Delayed axial CT of bladder (B) demonstrating rhabdomyosarcoma (M). (c) Sagittal T2 MRI also illustrates the bladder rhabdomyosarcoma.

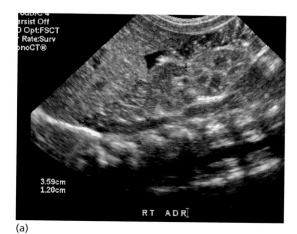

(a)

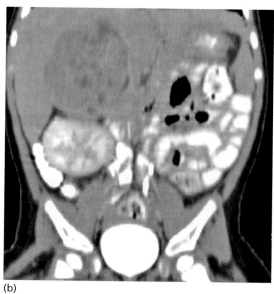

(b)

Figure 41.31 (a) Sagittal ultrasound demonstrates suprarenal mass (*calipers*). (b) Coronal CT reformat demonstrates the large right suprarenal mass.

(Fig. 41.31). Other lesions affecting the adrenals of children include neuroblastoma, adrenal hemorrhage, and pheochromocytoma, but the clinical history or follow-up examination can help refine the diagnosis.

Further reading

Agrons GA, Wagner BJ, Lonergan GJ, Dickey GE, Kaufman MS. From the archives of the AFIP. Genitourinary rhabdomyosarcoma in children: radiologic-pathologic correlation. *Radiographics* 1997; **17**(4):919–937.

Agrons GA, Lonergan GJ, Dickey GE, Perez-Monte JE. Adrenocortical neoplasms in children: radiologic-pathologic correlation. *Radiographics* 1999; **19**(4):989–1008.

Benacerraf BR, Eichhorn JH. Case records of the Massachusetts General Hospital. A one-month-old girl with an intraabdominal mass found on prenatal ultrasonographic examination. *N Engl J Med* 1995; **332**(8):522–527.

Bennett GL, Slywotzky CM, Giovanniello G. Gynecologic causes of acute pelvic pain: spectrum of CT findings. *Radiographics* 2002; **22**(4):785–801.

Blask AR, Sanders RC, Rock JA. Obstructed uterovaginal anomalies: demonstration with sonography. part II. teenagers. *Radiology* 1991; **179**(1):84–88.

Brody JM, Koelliker SL, Frishman GN. Unicornuate uterus: imaging appearance, associated anomalies, and clinical implications. *Am J Roentgenol* 1998; **171**(5):1341–1347.

Donaldson SS, Anderson J. Factors that influence treatment decisions in childhood rhabdomyosarcoma. Intergroup Rhabdomyosarcoma Study Group of the Children's Cancer Group, the Pediatric Oncology Group, and the Intergroup Rhabdomyosarcoma Study Group Statistical Center. *Radiology* 1997; **203**(1):17–22.

Imaoka I, Wada A, Kaji Y et al. Developing an MR imaging strategy for diagnosis of ovarian masses. *Radiographics* 2006; **26**(5):1431–1448.

Jaramillo D, Lebowitz RL, Hendren WH. The cloacal malformation: radiologic findings and imaging recommendations. *Radiology* 1990; **177**(2):441–448.

Jeong YY, Outwater EK, Kang HK. Imaging evaluation of ovarian masses. *Radiographics* 2000; **20**(5):1445–1470.

Jung SE, Lee JM, Rha SE, Byun JY, Jung JI, Hahn ST. CT and MR imaging of ovarian tumors with emphasis on differential diagnosis. *Radiographics* 2002; **22**(6):1305–1325.

Kawamoto S, Urban BA, Fishman EK. CT of epithelial ovarian tumors. *Radiographics* 1999; **19**:S263–264.

Kim SK, Rozanski R. Massive edema of the ovary. *Radiology* 1976; **118**(3):689–690.

Kinkel K, Hricak H, Lu Y, Tsuda K, Filly RA. US characterization of ovarian masses: a meta-analysis. *Radiology* 2000; **217**(3):803–811.

Kuligowska E, Deeds L 3rd, Lu K 3rd. Pelvic pain: overlooked and underdiagnosed gynecologic conditions. *Radiographics* 2005; **25**(1):3–20.

Lang IM, Babyn P, Oliver GD. MR imaging of paediatric uterovaginal anomalies. *Pediatr Radiol* 1999; **29**(3):163–170.

Lee AR, Kim KH, Lee BH, Chin SY. Massive edema of the ovary: imaging findings. *Am J Roentgenol* 1993; **161**(2):343–344.

Levsky JM, Mondshine RT. Hematometrocolpos due to imperforate hymen in a patient with bicornuate uterus. *Am J Roentgenol* 2006; **186**(5):1469–1470.

Mintz MC, Thickman DI, Gussman D, Kressel HY. MR evaluation of uterine anomalies. *Am J Roentgenol* 1987; **148**(2):287–290.

Nishimura K, Togashi K, Itoh K et al. Endometrial cysts of the ovary: MR imaging. *Radiology* 1987; **162**(2):315–318.

Ombelet W, Verswijvel G, de Jonge E. Ectopic ovary and unicornuate uterus. *N Engl J Med* 2003; **348**(7):667–668.

Outwater EK, Siegelman ES, Hunt JL. Ovarian teratomas: tumor types and imaging characteristics. *Radiographics* 2001; **21**(2):475–490.

Raga F, Bauset C, Remohi J, Bonilla-Musoles F, Simon C, Pellicer A. Reproductive impact of congenital mullerian anomalies. *Hum Reprod* 1997; **12**(10):2277–2281.

Reed MH, Griscom NT. Hydrometrocolpos in infancy. *Am J Roentgenol Radium Ther Nucl Med* 1973; **118**(1):1–13.

Rosenberg HK, Sherman NH, Tarry WF, Duckett JW, Snyder HM. Mayer-Rokitansky-Kuster-Hauser syndrome: US aid to diagnosis. *Radiology* 1986; **161**(3):815–819.

Siegel MJ. Pediatric gynecologic sonography. *Radiology* 1991; **179**(3):593–600.

Siegelman ES, Outwater EK. Tissue characterization in the female pelvis by means of MR imaging. *Radiology* 1999; **212**(1):5–18.

Strubbe EH, Willemsen WN, Lemmens JA, Thijn CJ, Rolland R. Mayer-Rokitansky-Kuster-Hauser syndrome: distinction between two forms based on excretory urographic, sonographic, and laparoscopic findings. *Am J Roentgenol* 1993; **160**(2):331–334.

Tanaka YO, Tsunoda H, Kitagawa Y, Ueno T, Yoshikawa H, Saida Y. Functioning ovarian tumors: direct and indirect findings at MR imaging. *Radiographics* 2004; **24**(suppl 1):S147–166.

Troiano RN, McCarthy SM. Mullerian duct anomalies: imaging and clinical issues. *Radiology* 2004; **233**(1):19–34.

Woodward PJ, Sohaey R, Mezzetti TP Jr. Endometriosis: radiologic-pathologic correlation. *Radiographics* 2001;**21**(1):193–216; questionnaire 288–294.

Wootton-Gorges SL, Thomas KB, Harned RK, Wu SR, Stein-Wexler R, Strain JD. Giant cystic abdominal masses in children. *Pediatr Radiol* 2005; **35**(12):1277–1288.

Yu JS, Kim KW, Lee HJ, Lee YJ, Yoon CS, Kim MJ. Urachal remnant diseases: spectrum of CT and US findings. *Radiographics* 2001; **21**(2):451–461.

CHAPTER 42

Preservation of Fertility

Michelle Tham & Alan B. Copperman
Mount Sinai Medical Center, New York, NY, USA

Introduction

The diagnosis of malignancy in a young patient is devastating. In 2005, approximately 1.3 million people were diagnosed with cancer, of whom 4% were under the age of 35. Due to advances in chemotherapy and radiation, five-year survival for those with childhood cancer has recently approached 80% [1]. With this success, however, a new challenge, achieving an acceptable quality of life in adulthood, has risen. In the United States, one in 900 people between the ages of 20 and 45 are cancer survivors [1]. For the women in this cohort, a consequence is often compromised fertility as a result of undergoing life-saving therapy.

Childhood cancer

After 20 weeks gestation, when the female fetus has approximately 6–7 million oocytes, progressive atresia of germ cells continues until menopause. This natural progression can be accelerated by cancer treatments. A 90% reduction in germ cells prior to age 14 leads to ovarian failure by age 27 [2]. The therapeutic regimen for many childhood malignancies, of which acute lymphoblastic leukemia is the most common, can irreversibly damage a young girl's fertility. The majority of cancers prior to age 40 include cervical and breast cancer, melanoma, non-Hodgkin lymphoma and leukemia. Cures for these malignancies have varying effects on ovarian function [3].

A bimodal age distribution of infertility is noted in these patients. Acute ovarian failure (AOF) occurs at the time of treatment or within five years, while progressive loss of function prior to age 40 is termed premature ovarian failure (POF). AOF shows a correlation with age, diagnosis of Hodgkin lymphoma, and exposure to alkylating agents or pelvic irradiation [4]. Chemotherapeutic agents are classified as high, intermediate or low risk based on gonadotoxicity. Alkylating agents such as cyclophosphamide, busulfan, and chlorambucil are high risk and increase the chances of POF ninefold; methotrexate, bleomycin and vincristine are low-risk agents [5]. The cause of failure is believed to be either depletion of primordial follicles or induction of apoptosis in granulosa cells, which causes a significant decline in endocrine and reproductive function. After therapy, adolescents have a fourfold increase in the risk of POF, while patients treated between 21 and 25 years of age have a 27-fold increase in risk [6].

Patients receiving high-dose chemotherapy combined with total body irradiation have the highest risk for POF, with rates approaching 92%. A 50% reduction in ovarian follicle count will occur after 4 Gy of radiation exposure. A 20 Gy dose will cause complete cessation of ovarian function in women younger than 40 years, but only 6 Gy is needed to deplete ovarian reserve in older women. In addition to depletion of function, pelvic radiation can also significantly diminish uterine volume [7].

Gynecologic malignancy

Twenty one percent of gynecologic malignancies occur in women of child-bearing age. Recent advances in surgical technique and surveillance options have afforded young women more conservative options for cure and preservation of fertility [8].

Pediatric, Adolescent, & Young Adult Gynecology. Edited by A. Altchek and L. Deligdisch. © 2009 Blackwell Publishing, ISBN: 978-1-4051-5347-8.

Cervical cancer may be managed in its early stages (1A1) with cold knife conization which can enable subsequent child bearing if desired. Since the presence of lymph vascular space involvement or stage IA2 disease carries a higher risk of lymph node spread (5–9%), stage IA2 and IB disease are usually treated with radical hysterectomy and node dissection. However, alternative management with radical trachelectomy with laparoscopic lymphadenectomy may spare reproductive function. Vaginal trachelectomy includes vaginotomy and paracervical dissection, ligation of the descending branches of the uterine artery and amputation of the distal cervix. The body of the uterus is left intact and a cerclage is placed in the portion of remaining cervix. Interval child bearing may be at high risk for prematurity, preterm labor and cervical incompetence and should be managed by a high-risk obstetrician [8].

Endometrial cancer is frequently viewed as a disease of the postmenopausal woman, yet 2–14% of patients with this diagnosis are <45 years old. Cure rates exceed 95% in those with early-stage, well-differentiated adenocarcinoma. Standard treatment for parous women includes hysterectomy and bilateral salpingo-oophorectomy with lymph node dissection/biopsy at the discretion of the gynecologic oncologist. Conservative treatment with high-dose medroxyprogesterone, gonadotropin-releasing hormone (GnRH) agonists and progestin-containing intrauterine devices (IUDs) may be options for those who want to postpone hysterectomy for child bearing. An extensive discussion of risk of recurrence and possibility of concurrent ovarian malignancy must be held with the patient, and close surveillance must be a part of this treatment plan. To date, over 100 cases of conservative management have been reported. These patients must be carefully selected and adequately counseled about all implications of this alternative therapy [8].

Epithelial ovarian cancer is predominantly a postmenopausal entity. Treatment usually involves debulking with staging laparotomy, total abdominal hysterectomy, bilateral salpingo-oophorectomy, lymphadenectomy, omentectomy, peritoneal biopsy and pelvic washings followed by chemotherapy as warranted. McHale et al have described conservative management via unilateral salpingo-oophorectomy, omentectomy, washings and lymph node biopsy in those patients with well-differentiated serous, mucinous, endometrioid or mesonephric carcinoma that is presumed to be confined to the ovary [9]. Based on

stage, subsequent treatment with chemotherapy may or may not be warranted. Recurrence risk is associated with histologic grade and is equivalent between those staged conservatively or by a radical procedure.

Borderline tumors (ovarian tumors with low malignant potential) are characterized by lack of stromal invasion, younger age of onset, and earlier stage at presentation. Overall five-year survival is 90%. Conservative staging may be implemented in these patients as well, with most studies reporting excellent fertility outcomes [8].

Fertility options

The desire for future fertility should not impede or significantly delay treatment. For very young patients there are few successful or well-studied options for fertility preservation, though reproductive-age women with partners may have more opportunities for child bearing. When discussing preservation options, an integrated approach with the patient, oncologist, parent, pediatrician and reproductive endocrinologist is warranted. There are five broad categories of fertility preservation in addition to the conservative staging methods for gynecologic malignancy.

Embryo cryopreservation

Embryo cryopreservation is the most widely studied and utilized of fertility options. Ovulation induction protocols are the same as for those without malignancy in nonestrogen-related cancers and usually include gonadotropin therapy, serial sonography and ultrasound-guided aspiration of follicles. *In vitro* fertilization and cryopreservation of embryos allows transfer to be delayed until cancer remission. When estrogen-responsive tumors occur, ovarian stimulation agents such as tamoxifen or letrozole may be utilized to decrease risk of inadvertent co-stimulation of cancer cells. A progestin-releasing IUD is placed at the time of ovarian stimulation to prevent activation of the endometrium in patients with endometrial malignancies. Pregnancy rates after transfer of cryopreserved embryos is 20–30% when 2–3 embryos are transferred. However, this therapy is only applicable to reproductive-age women with partners or to patients who are willing to use donor sperm for fertilization of their gametes. A delay of up to six weeks for chemotherapy may be acceptable in some instances. This delay, however, may not be an option for the pediatric patient [10].

Oocyte cryopreservation

The first reported pregnancy following oocyte preservation was in 1986. Oocyte cryopreservation represents another option for women of reproductive age. Stimulation protocols are the same as for embryo cryopreservation but may be more acceptable to a woman without a male partner or to those who are disinclined to use donor sperm.

Unfertilized oocytes, however, are more susceptible to temperature damage than embryos. Disruption of the meiotic spindle during freeze/thaw cycles may increase the risk of aneuploidy. The zona pellucida may also become hardened during this process, making traditional fertilization more challenging; however, the use of intracytoplasmic sperm injection (ICSI) has since overcome this obstacle. As of 2005, 120 deliveries had been reported with a 2% live birth rate per thawed oocyte [3]. Various methods of freezing have been demonstrated in the animal model. Vitrification, or conversion of fluid surrounding the tissue to a glass-like state during cooling via elevation of viscosity, may avoid ice cystallization and may help to preserve fragile oocytes [5].

Some institutions now collect immature oocytes. Unlike metaphase II oocytes, germinal vesicles do not have a spindle apparatus and so may be less susceptible to cooling damage. This technique is highly experimental and, until methods of *in vitro* maturation become more reliable, is only offered in a research setting [10].

More recently, advances in laboratory techniques have yielded better results with the slow-freeze protocol. In our center, a study was performed with four oocyte donors, to eliminate oocyte quality as a confounding variable. Seventy-nine metaphase II oocytes were frozen, stored frozen overnight in liquid nitrogen and then thawed. The post-thaw survival rate was 86.1%. Normal fertilization following ICSI occurred in 89% of the surviving oocytes. Cleavage was observed in 98% of normally fertilized oocytes. A total of 23 embryos were transferred to four recipient patients. A clinical pregnancy rate of 75% and an implantation rate of 26% were achieved [10].

Ovarian cryopreservation and transplantation

Although animal studies in ovarian cryopreservation were first described in the 1950s, the human model was not reported on until 1996. This may represent the only fertility option for the prepubertal female. Hundreds of immature oocytes may be cryopreserved in whole tissue. Ovarian stimulation is not performed, and therfore no delay in treatment of the malignancy is required. A single ovary or portion thereof is surgically removed via laparoscopy, and the cortex and stroma are separated prior to freezing.

Harvested tissue may be orthotopically (returned to original site) or heterotopically (extraovarian) replaced. After replacement, a finite time period of endocrinologic function occurs, with reports varying from nine months to three years [11]. Data on pregnancy and ovulation rates with this technology are limited.

A significant concern for patients who may choose to preserve ovarian tissue is the risk of cancer cell transmission. This treatment option should only be offered to patients with low risk of metastatic cancer to the ovary, as reintroduction of the primary malignancy after treatment could be disastrous. Cancers with low risk of ovarian involvement include Wilms' tumor, early-stage breast cancer, osteogenic sarcoma, Ewing sarcoma and non-Hodgkin and Hodgkin lymphoma, cervical cancer and nongenital rhabdomyosarcoma. Highest risk cancers include leukemia, neuroblastoma, Burkitt lymphoma and genital rhabdomyosarcoma. A comprehensive histologic assessment of all cryopreserved tissue should be made prior to autotransplantation [11].

Oophoropexy

Patients undergoing radiotherapy for Hodgkin disease may be exposed to as much as 2000 cGy. Transposition of ovarian tissue farther from the field of radiation is known as oophoropexy and may be used to preserve ovarian function. Oophoropexy may be performed at the time of laparotomy for cancer staging or as an interval laparoscopic, outpatient procedure. Typically, the ovary is transposed laterally after transection of the utero-ovarian ligament. Due to risk of possible migration of the ovaries, the surgery should be performed as close in timing to radiation therapy as possible. Overall success rates are somewhere around 50% with failure attributed to scatter radiation and diminished ovarian blood supply. The ovaries do not always need to be returned to their original location, as spontaneous pregnancies have been reported. If these patients do require oocyte retrieval, however, repositioning may be warranted to allow transvaginal versus percutaneous collection. Physicians caring for these patients must also remember that the ovaries may not be palpable on bimanual exam, masking ovarian pathology on clinical findings [3].

GnRH suppression

Although controversial, suppression of ovarian function at the time of chemotherapy has been described. Pretreatment with GnRH is presumed to place ovaries in a quiescent state and decrease the effects of alkylating agents by decreasing the quantity of rapidly dividing cells. A second possible explanation for a decrease in chemotherapy-associated gonadotoxicity is that the hypoestrogenic state diminishes utero-ovarian perfusion and allows less exposure of the ovaries to chemotherapeutic injury. Most studies have used menstrual function as a primary outcome measure of gonadal protection, but with conflicting results. No clear guidelines have been outlined for their use [3].

Conclusion

Many of the techniques utilized in fertility preservation stem from a need to assist women of advanced reproductive age who have delayed child bearing. In the context of malignancy in young patients, this issue is a more complex entity, where decisions are made regarding future desires. Decisions to undergo laparoscopy or oocyte retrieval in the pediatric population, essentially elective surgical procedures, are the responsibility of the patient's guardians. The decision to withhold these options made by second parties may have unexpected psychosocial ramifications. The technology is advancing towards the possibility of offering fertility disassociated from chronologic age. The complex ethical scenarios that come with that ability and the application of this technology to those without malignancy will be controversial. Through clinical trials and innovative research we will soon be able to offer patients comprehensive fertility-preserving options to match clinical desires.

References

1. Burns KC, Boudreau C, Panepinto JA. Attitudes regarding fertility preservation in female adolescent cancer patients. *J Pediatr Hematol Oncol* 2006;**28**(6):350–354.
2. Kim SS. Fertility preservation in female cancer patients: current developments and future directions. *Fertil Steril* 2006;**85**(1):1–11.
3. Lee SJ, Schover LR, Partridge AH et al. American Society of Clinical Oncology recommendations on fertility preservation in cancer patients. *J Clin Oncol* 2006;**24**(18):2917–2931.
4. Chemaitilly W, Mertens AC, Mitby P et al. Acute ovarian failure in the Childhood Cancer Survivor Study. *J Endocrinol Metab* 2006;**91**(5):1723–1728.
5. Donnez J, Martinez-Madrid B, Jadoul P et al. Ovarian tissue cryopreservation and transplantation: a review. *Hum Reprod Update* 2006;**12**:519–535.
6. Blumenfeld Z, Eckman A. Preservation of fertility and ovarian function and minimizing chemotherapy-induced gonadotoxicity in young women. *J Soc Gyneol Invest* 1999;**6**(5):229–239.
7. Lobo TA, Rogerio A. Potential options for preservation of fertility in women. *N Engl J Med* 2005;**353**(1):64–73.
8. Liou WS, Yap OW, Chan JK, Westphal LM. Innovations in fertility preservation for patients with gynecologic cancers. *Fertil Steril* 2005;**84**(6):1561–1573.
9. McHale MT, DiSaia PJ. Fertility-sparing treatment of patients with ovarian cancer. *Comp Ther* 1999;**25**:144–150.
10. Baritt J, Luna M, Duke M et al. Donor oocyte cryopreservation resulting in high pregnancy and implantation rates. *Fertil Steril* 2006.
11. Shamonki M, Oktay K. Oocyte and ovarian tissue cryopreservation: indications, techniques, and applications. *Semin Reprod Med* 2005;**23**(3):266–276.

CHAPTER 43

Where Law and Medicine Meet

Rhea G. Friedman

New York State Family Court Judge (retired), New York, NY, USA

This chapter tracks a call from a mandated source (e.g. a physician or hospital social worker) of suspected child neglect or abuse which results in a case filed in the family court. Emphasis is placed on legal issues which recur frequently in medical practice: mandated reporting; physician–patient privilege and confidentiality; subpoenas; releases; and record-keeping. Chapter 44 addresses legal aspects of reproductive healthcare for minors and rights to privacy. Topics included are: minors' rights to consent to contraception; abortion; treatment for STDs; and treatment for HIV and AIDS. Confidentiality of information, and parental notice and parental access to information are addressed. References to HIPAA (the Health Insurance Portability and Accountability Act) (Public l. 104–191, 110 Stat 1936 [1996]) (codified as amended throughout sections 18, 26, 29, and 42 US Code) through its Privacy Rule (45 CFR parts 160, 164) are contained in both chapters.

This chapter and the next grew out of a series of presentations that I delivered at the Mount Sinai Hospital School of Medicine in New York City as part of the Annual Conference on Adolescent and Pediatric Gynecology chaired by Dr Albert Altchek. These talks reflected my experience as a New York City Family Court Judge, because it is in the family court that the worlds of the law and this type of medicine so often meet. That happens most importantly in child abuse and neglect cases.

It is vital that doctors understand the unique powers and rules of the family court in which they may often be called to testify, and which may often demand their records. Emphasis is placed on legal issues which recur frequently in medical practice.

Pediatric, Adolescent, & Young Adult Gynecology. Edited by A. Altchek and L. Deligdisch. © 2009 Blackwell Publishing, ISBN: 978-1-4051-5347-8.

This chapter describes New York State law and practice. Other jurisdictions will differ. However, New York is typical enough to be a very useful paradigm for other states and even for other countries.

What doctors report and what they say in court often decide the outcome of a case which profoundly affects children and families. A court can decide whether a child remains with the parent or guardian or is removed to foster care. The court can also decide that unless the child is removed, she is in danger. Numerous well-known cases show how vital it may be to remove a child. It is less publicized that removal itself can harm a child, so a court must be careful to weigh evidence for removal. In each case a diagnosis or misdiagnosis of child abuse or neglect is a key factor in a court's decision.

Child abuse and neglect cases are also called child protective or child dependency cases. They are adjudicated in a family court or a juvenile division. This placement of jurisdiction has implications. The standard of proof these courts use is the civil standard rather than the criminal standard familiar from movies and press accounts. In a criminal case, the standard is proof "beyond a reasonable doubt." In a civil case, it is the preponderance of the credible evidence, which can mean no more than a minimum of 51% in layman's terms. Because they are also adjudicated in civil courts, much of what this chapter addresses applies to other types of cases, such as child custody and medical malpractice, but remember that this chapter is about child protective cases (neglect and abuse).

The impact of a doctor's testimony in a family court is greater than in other courts because there is no jury. The judge is the sole decider of fact. Unlike the members of a jury, a judge has often seen hundreds or thousands of cases, and thus may be more familiar with the nature of medical testimony. The unusual character of the family court is not well known even in the legal world.

That should be kept in mind by any doctor choosing a lawyer with whom to consult about a family court case.

The family court's power in child protective cases is awesome. It can remove a child from his or her home on a finding of "imminent danger," even before any allegations have been proven. Given a finding of neglect or abuse, the court can keep the child and any siblings in placement for an initial period of up to six months, subject to annual extensions until the child is 18. Alternatively, the child can be released to a relative, such as the spouse or ex-spouse, with an order of protection against the abusive parent, which may severely restrict or prohibit contact with that child, until the child is 18.

If the foster care agency proves, in a separate proceeding, that the parent has failed to plan for the child, has abandoned the child or is too mentally ill to care for the child, the family court can terminate parental rights. The child can be freed for adoption – taken away from the parent on a permanent basis. Such orders are reserved for the most serious of child abuse cases. Ultimately these cases turn on medical evidence. Diagnosis or misdiagnosis must often determine the outcome of such cases – with enormous impact on children and their families.

The specialized rules governing child protective cases magnify the importance of what a doctor reports to child protective authorities. Medical evidence is the most critical information available to the court. Moreover, the court usually has to act quickly. If a child is being abused, he or she should be removed at once to a place of safety. Court proceedings may later review or reverse that decision, but early evidence is very important. Recent changes in procedure place greater weight on the court's decision to remove a child. Almost always orders removing children are issued on the same day that charges are filed against parents or guardians. In New York State, the preliminary hearing is within 72 hours of the removal.

The statutes favor proof other than a child's testimony. Generally the only witnesses to abuse are the abuser and the victim. Often the victim is too young to speak or too impaired to be able to testify. The statute, moreover, envisages quick removal of the victim followed by therapy. It would be cruel to force a child to relive painful events after therapy had begun to repair the damage they suffered. Such recall might well reverse the effects of the therapy. Cross-examination in court, which is an essential feature of sworn testimony, would likely make matters even worse. New York State does envisage testimony from unsworn witnesses (children, in accord with a special rule of evidence, may give unsworn testimony), but that must be corroborated. Medical evidence can supply such corroboration for a child's admissible out-of-court statements. Credibility is vital in cases of such significance to the future of child and parents.

The courts therefore seek alternative sources of information. They have adopted specialized rules of evidence:
• out-of-court statements by children about alleged occurrences are admissible
• the usual physician–patient privilege is abrogated, along with other statutory privilege blocks against admitting information
• the *res ipsa* presumption is accepted. That is, if abuse is recognized, and any of several people may have committed it, all of them are required to go forward with their own evidence to rebut the presumption which would otherwise obtain.

These rules are radically different from those in criminal courts.

Difficulties in obtaining testimony from those involved make doctors' testimony much more important. The court obtains doctors' information primarily in four ways:
• subpoenas requesting testimony and/or medical files
• releases, requesting records
• pretrial depositions
• testimony.

Doctors have particular impact in a case of child abuse, because so often theirs is the decisive evidence. Typically only the child and the abuser are involved, and the law often recognizes that a child's testimony generally cannot be sufficient. Often it cannot even be given great weight if admitted into evidence. Thus a court finds itself relying on medical testimony. It is vital that doctors realize how important their evidence can be, and also how difficult it is for the lay court to appreciate possible ambiguities in what they have seen – ambiguities which other doctors may instantly understand.

Let us turn to the specialized rules of evidence which impact not only on court cases, but also on the practice of medicine. Keep in mind that these rules in general are biased towards making it easier to prove abuse charges, given the tender years of most victims and the secrecy of most acts of abuse.

There is no physician–patient privilege in family court abuse and neglect cases. Your patient's statements to you are not confidential. Your records are an open book.

Physicians and other medical personnel are mandated reporters of suspected child abuse or neglect in all jurisdictions. State law requires that you, as a medical provider, call in a report of suspected abuse to the state central registry. Failure to do so in New York State is a misdemeanor. Good-faith callers are given both civil and criminal immunity by law. And the statute presumes good faith.

The physician–patient privilege is abrogated by statute in most jurisdictions in child neglect and abuse cases in the family court. Keep in mind that privilege exists in all other family court cases, including custody and visitation cases. Because child abuse is so repugnant, allegations of abuse, sometimes originating as suggestions to young children, have become weapons in child custody warfare. Again, the presence or absence of medical evidence can be vital to a judge who has to confirm or deny the child's version. Physicians, therefore, must zealously safeguard confidential information about their patients or risk liability.

Confidentiality pitfalls exist for the unwary. Privacy protections under statutes such as HIPAA are the subject of numerous journal articles, treatises and case law and are beyond the scope of this chapter. Information pertaining to HIV/AIDS is strictly controlled by statute in terms of confidentiality. It is vital to consult with attorneys trained in this area before such information is released. A HIPAA-compliant release form signed by or on behalf of a patient is a great asset to a doctor who must protect his or her patient's confidential communications.

A 2007 decision issued by New York's highest court, the Court of Appeals, is a good illustration of potential pitfalls in patient confidentiality. In the case of *Arons v. Jutkowitz*, the court answered the question of whether the defense attorney may be permitted to interview, ex parte and without a record, the plaintiff's or decedent's treating physician in personal injury, wrongful death, and medical malpractice cases. The court held that, even after formal discovery proceedings were over, the defendant has the right to ask the physician for the interview. It also addressed any role HIPAA would play in this scenario. Such HIPAA-compliant authorizations would be court-ordered if not freely given by the plaintiff. While the initial reaction might be that plaintiff directs her treating physician not to comply with the interview, it may be that this leads instead to time-consuming court-ordered depositions. Again, a doctor in this position needs to seek legal advice.

This caveat about the need to protect confidential information applies to the various methods by which courts and lawyers obtain information from doctors. Subpoenas can be "so ordered" by the court or issued by attorneys. The sanctions for noncompliance and the procedures for enforcement of the different types of subpoenas vary but again, be wary of confidentiality pitfalls in the information you provide. For instance, a New York subpoena issued in child protective cases most frequently states that the information is to be redacted for protected information pursuant to Public Health Law 2780-81 (AIDS & HIV information). Many subpoenas are not for your personal appearance but, rather, for your medical records (subpoena "duces tecum"). Records, accompanied by a proper certification (and delegation of certification authority, if necessary) that the records were kept in the ordinary business of the institution or office, that it was in the ordinary course of the business to keep such records, and that the entries in the records were made at or about the time of the occurrence (i.e. the "business records rule" in New York State), usually obviate the need for a doctor's personal appearance.

These considerations also pertain to other types of pretrial discovery. These include examinations before trial, pretrial depositions and interrogatories. It is foolish to attend a pretrial examination or to answer pretrial interrogatories without consulting an attorney. The scope of the questions may range far beyond the immediate case at hand. Particularly because child protective cases often move beyond the trial stage much more quickly than related civil cases (such as medical malpractice or insurance investigations into, e.g., use or misuse of diagnostic codes for billing purposes), discovery efforts may actually be geared towards future litigation.

The other specialized evidentiary rule which is worthwhile to highlight is the *res ipsa* presumption, again common to most jurisdictions. This means, literally, that the act speaks for itself. Would that it were so easy! Say an injury happens to a child which would not occur naturally or accidentally, such as a spiral fracture in a very young child. The mere fact that the injury happened shifts the burden of explaining what did happen to the parents or other caretakers charged with abuse or with neglect. If they do not know what happened, and if this is the only thing they can say, they lose.

Say a parent comes home from work or picks up a baby from day care, and later finds that the child's head is swollen or that the arm is painful and swollen, and that parent rushes the child to a doctor or to an emergency room and a fracture is diagnosed. If, when asked what happened, the parent says "I don't know" or says "well, two weeks ago, the baby fell off the bed or changing table," a report of suspected abuse will be sent to the state central registry. The parent will likely be charged with abuse; the child, and quite possibly all of the child's siblings under 18 living at home, will likely be removed from home and placed in foster care. Eventually, if nothing else happens, the parent will be found to have abused or neglected the child. This process will take many months, in all likelihood (hopefully services, such as parenting skills and anger management if appropriate, geared to reuniting the family, will have begun). This process leaves anyone who knows anything about it wondering whether there is a better way to find out which parents are a danger to their children.

The *res ipsa* presumption is so powerful because it calls on one to imagine that in certain cases the evidence of abuse or neglect is so "objective" that there can be no questions. Yet, case law belies that assumption. There are many reported cases where recognized experts have disagreed on whether a condition or injury is the result of neglect or abuse; for example, whether a child is being starved or whether there are metabolic or other medical issues precluding proper absorption of food; whether a child has been physically abused or whether he suffers from some variant of a brittle bone disease; or whether anal warts in a very young child can be explained only by sexual contact with an infected person. Or take the case of a baby born at 26 weeks suffering from, *inter alia*, congenital abnormalities such as severe bilateral congenital glaucoma (followed by two eye surgeries) who was also hydrocephalic and macrocephalic and had various chromosomal abnormalities. The case was reported to the registry by his pediatrician and by a pediatric ophthalmologist because of suspected shaken baby syndrome, with specific symptoms of retinal hemorrhages and subdural hematomas. It took additional testimony by two pediatric neurologists to conclude that this was not a case of shaken baby syndrome. Both specialists, for instance, detailed a lack of shearing; the unusual location of the hematoma when compared with hematomas in known shaken baby syndrome cases; the greatly increased risk that a child with such congenital problems would suffer hematomas with normal handling; and also concluded that the retinal hemorrhages and the hematomas did not occur simultaneously.

In a case of suspected sexual abuse based solely upon the (mis)infomation reported to the registry, that the baby's anal warts could have resulted only from sexual contact with an infected person, the child was initially removed from the parent and placed in foster care until the court obtained corrected information.

To reiterate, doctors have a particular impact in a case of child abuse, because theirs is so often the decisive evidence. Particularly because of specialized rules of evidence in child protective cases, doctors must be vigilant about the information they report to the registry as suspected abuse or neglect, as the initial report is often the most critical factor in the court's determination as to whether to remove the child and any siblings from the home. It is extremely helpful to a court to include, if possible, assessment as to whether the parent or caretaker's explanation(s) of the condition or injury is consistent with the type of injury. An assessment of the child's relationship with the parent(s) and of the child's desire to go home is also helpful to the court's determination.

Time spent in obtaining a correct diagnosis is time very well spent. There is no penalty for taking the necessary time to run tests and to consult with specialists. There is never a penalty for using your best medical judgment. The alternatives are unacceptable – either children removed unnecessarily from their families or children left in dangerous situations.

It is vital that doctors realize how important their evidence can be, and also how difficult it is for the lay court to appreciate possible ambiguities in what they have seen – ambiguities which other doctors may instantly understand.

An invaluable, albeit somewhat dated, resource is *A Guide to the Law on Minors' Rights in New York State*, by the Reproductive Rights Project of the New York Civil Liberties Union. Their web address is: www.nyclu.org.

CHAPTER 44

Minors' Rights to Reproductive Healthcare and Privacy

Rhea G. Friedman

New York State Family Court Judge (retired), New York, NY, USA

Minors' rights to reproductive healthcare vary from jurisdiction to jurisdiction; the area is often subject to intense controversy and the law is in constant flux. These rights derive from federal, state, local public health, and educational laws; from local health regulations; and from constantly changing court decisions, up to and including decisions by the US Supreme Court. In countries covered by the European Convention on Human Rights, the rights and obligations set forth by Article 8, for example, may also obtain. The topic is closely linked with privacy law. It would be impossible to describe the current state of the law in a volume several times the size of this one, and moreover such a volume would have to be updated on a monthly, perhaps a weekly, basis. Instead, this chapter constructs a framework within which the changing law can be understood.

A major reason why adolescents, more than any other age group, do not access needed healthcare is their fear that the medical providers will tell their parents or guardians. Recognizing how vital medical care is, the law does allow minors the right to obtain certain medical treatment, including reproductive healthcare, without their parents' involvement or even their parents' knowledge. In the overwhelming majority of cases (incest being an obvious exception), healthcare professionals should encourage youngsters to communicate with their parents or, if impossible, with other responsible adults such as family members or social workers, rather than confront these problems on their own. If this proves impossible,

the priority is for the minor to obtain healthcare even without adult involvement rather than no healthcare at all. Thus, the law has carved out exceptions to the general rule that the consent of a parent or guardian or custodian is necessary for minors to receive medical treatment.

This chapter addresses minors' rights to consent to certain types of healthcare based upon two factors:
- legal status – including adolescents who are married, pregnant or who are themselves parents
- type of procedure: sexually transmitted diseases (STD) testing or treatment; HIV/AIDS testing or treatment; contraception; and abortion.

The reader should keep in mind that every jurisdiction has a set of complex laws and regulations addressing the areas of minors' rights and healthcare providers' obligations in the areas of sexual offense victims, substance abuse, and mental health treatment. These areas are beyond the scope of this chapter, but there may be overlapping issues. Other topics beyond the scope of this chapter include additional problems faced by minors in foster care when they seek confidential treatment, as well as the interplay of health insurance, public and private, with minors' rights to privacy.

Consent

The place to begin any inquiry in this area is with the issue of consent by minors (in New York State, for purposes of medical treatment, a minor is a person under 18). Consent means *informed* and *willing* consent. Consent means a knowing and a voluntary agreement to a proposed medical treatment. At a minimum, in order to establish that

Pediatric, Adolescent, & Young Adult Gynecology. Edited by A. Altchek and L. Deligdisch. © 2009 Blackwell Publishing, ISBN: 978-1-4051-5347-8.

the provider did not adequately inform the patient, the patient must demonstrate that (1) the provider failed to disclose alternatives to treatment and failed reasonably to alert the patient to foreseeable risks and benefits involved that the similarly situated reasonable provider would have disclosed in terms permitting the patient to make a knowledgeable assessment; (2) a "reasonably prudent person" in the patient's position would not have undergone the treatment or procedure if fully informed; and (3) the lack of informed consent was a proximate cause of the injury or condition for which the patient seeks recovery (PHL 2805-d).

If you, as healthcare provider, think that your patient, the minor, is not capable of consenting, it is irrelevant that she falls within the appropriate status (e.g. married) or that the appropriate medical service (e.g. treatment related to her pregnancy) is at issue. If, in your opinion, she is incapable of giving consent, do not perform the procedure, do not offer the treatment. You may be wary because she appears limited or under the influence of drugs or alcohol, or coerced. Whether that minor is giving you a knowing, willing and informed consent is your judgment call.

The first basis for the rights of minors to consent to medical services and treatments derives from their status. This analytic framework is based on New York State law. New York law is in the majority rule for most jurisdictions; practitioners must check the law in their jurisdiction. States may not accord their citizens fewer rights than those provided by the United States Supreme Court.

The following categories of minors can always consent to healthcare (*caveat*: remember that the consent must be informed and willing). Married minors and minors who are parents can always consent to healthcare; minors who are parents can also consent to healthcare for their children; pregnant minors can always consent to healthcare for services related to pregnancy, a "right" with its own set of issues.

There are recurring references in the literature to "emancipated" and "mature" minors as also being able to consent to reproductive healthcare (e.g. American Academy of Pediatrics. Policy statement: informed consent, parental permission, and assent in pediatric practice (RE9510). *Pediatrics* 1995;**314**:95, advising physicians to seek informed consent directly from patients "in cases involving emancipated or mature minors with adequate decision-making capacity, or when otherwise permitted

by law. . . ."). There is a paucity of case law in all jurisdictions addressing the terms "emancipated" and "mature" minors. These cases deal primarily with emancipation in terms of parental child support obligations (where the law defines minors as under 21). There are almost no written court orders which issue declaring such a status. Moreover, very few cases have relied on this status as one allowing minors to consent to healthcare and this case law has not developed in any meaningful way since the Academy's 1995 policy statement. A note of caution is therefore in order to the physician or provider relying solely on the minor's consent based on her status as mature or emancipated.

The second basis for the right of minors to consent to medical treatments and services derives from the type of medical procedure.

Sexually transmitted diseases

Parental consent is unnecessary in New York State in order for a minor to obtain testing or treatment for STDs (PHL 2504). Confidentiality is mandated unless the minor consents to release of testing and results. There are reporting requirements (PHL 2101(1)) to the district office where the STD occurred. There are additional notification requirements by the patient or by the Department of Health to partners of exposure to STDs. Reporting requirements for STDs in the communicable disease category (syphilis, chlamydia, and gonorrhea) offer greater anonymity for patients than do reporting requirements for other communicable diseases, as the regulation allows reporting of the patient's initials only unless the full name and address is specifically requested by the authorized public health officer. Additional reporting requirements for county health clinics require them to send information about all patients diagnosed with and/or treated for STDs to the New York State Department of Health. However, this information, apparently, may be in aggregate form with no specific patient-identifying information. Reporting requirements must be checked jurisdiction by jurisdiction.

HIV/AIDS

Regarding HIV/AIDS testing or treatment (PHL 2780-81), confidentiality is the keyword. There are extensive and strict statutory protections from disclosure. Minors may consent, or refuse to consent, to HIV testing *except* for mandatory testing of all newborns and, by extension, mothers. In New York, minors appear to have the right to consent to treatment, although the statute should be clearer.

Confidential HIV/AIDS-related information is permitted only in very limited circumstances (PHL 2782). These circumstances include certain third-party reimbursers, persons complying with court orders, and correctional facilities and their employees under some circumstances. In general, once certain authorized facilities and individuals have received such information, they are not permitted to redisclose it. The prohibition against disclosure applies to physicians, other health professionals, health facilities and social workers, not to those who obtain this information in nonprofessional capacities, although this is a potential case law area for civil breach of privacy suits.

Contraception

Minors' right to consent to contraception applies to both contraceptive services and prescriptions, including emergency contraception. According to the New York State Department of Health protocol, a minor who is a victim of a sexual assault should be offered emergency contraception where medically appropriate. Federal programs offering contraception services are governed by rules guaranteeing minors' rights. Local Department of Education regulations also must be referenced. Minors in foster care enjoy the same rights as minors living at home.

In the United States, the Federal Family Educational Rights and Privacy Act (FERPA)(20 USCA 1232g)(2001) is an important law in this area. Among other provisions, FERPA denies funds to schools that refuse to allow parents of students under 18 access to student records which contain information about a student and are kept by or on behalf of the school. Thus, "education records" may be subject to parental disclosure. If a school provides services such as contraceptives to a student, commentators have pointed out that records of such confidential health information (this may also include counseling records) should be kept separate from educational records available to a parent. This would arguably go a long way towards obviating the conflict between FERPA's requirement of parental disclosure and state confidentiality laws.

Nothing in the law requires a minor seeking confidential reproductive healthcare or pregnancy or STD services to reveal the identity of their partners. Of course, if the minor does reveal that the sex partner is a family member, that will trigger mandated reporting requirements.

Abortion

Abortion has been legal in New York State since 1970, three years before the lead US Supreme Court case of *Roe v. Wade*. States may give their citizens greater rights than does the Supreme Court. Again, the laws for the particular jurisdiction one is in need to be consulted. In New York, a minor can obtain an abortion without parental or spousal consent or notification. In a long line of cases beginning with *Belloti v. Baird* (1979), the United States Supreme Court has ruled that parental consent requirements for abortion are not constitutional unless they provide a judicial bypass procedure or an opportunity for a court order. This procedure must be both confidential and expeditious. There is no provision for such a bypass procedure in New York or in the majority of states. While there is no New York law which explicitly permits abortions for minors, they may get them without parental consent. The literature tells us that the majority of minors do involve at least one parent in this decision, and this, unless inappropriate, they should be encouraged to do by healthcare professionals. There is no waiting period requirement in New York State. Hospitals need not allow abortions to be performed, but must provide referral information to a patient as to where an abortion can be obtained (10 NYCRR 905.10(a)). Since most minors have incomes below the poverty level, they would be eligible for payment under a variety of government insurance programs for any abortion.

Release of records to parents or others of abortions performed on minors is prohibited, without the consent of the minor.

Protecting minors' health information privacy

A healthcare provider who discloses confidential information without patient authorization or court order or statutory authority may be subject to professional as well as legal sanctions. Such a disclosure is deemed professional misconduct (NYCRR 29.1(8); see also NY Educ. L. 6509(9)). This duty to preserve confidentiality exists if there is a provider–patient relationship; if the information was obtained in the course of treatment; and if this information was necessary for treatment.

Bear in mind that when seeking to protect minors' health information, it is the *minor* who exercises rights of the individual over the health information if: (1) the minor consented and no other consent is necessary, (2) a court or another authorized person consented or (3) the parent assented to confidentiality.

Regarding parental access to minors' health information, if the *minor* exercises the rights of the individual over the health information: (1) parents are not allowed access unless state or other law explicitly requires or permits parental notification or access; (2) if state law is silent, the provider has discretion to grant parental access, if the parent so requests; and (3) the provider always has discretion to deny parental access if the minor's safety is at stake.

Confidentiality issues are impacted by the Health Insurance Portability and Accountability Act (HIPAA). HIPAA is a complex statute and already has an extensive litigation history and commentaries. A doctor must be able to recognize a potential HIPAA issue and know when to consult with counsel.

Conclusion

In relation to legal aspects of reproductive healthcare for minors, parental (and spousal) consent is not needed for testing and treatment of minors for STDs; for HIV/AIDS; for contraception services and prescriptions; or for abortions. There is no waiting period required in New York State for abortions. Confidentiality must be strictly preserved. Some minors can *always* consent to healthcare based on their legal status. Use your best informed medical judgment about whether the consent proffered is informed, knowing and voluntary.

CHAPTER 45

Human Papillomavirus Infection and Cervical Neoplasm Pathology in Adolescents

Liane Deligdisch

Mount Sinai Medical Center, New York, NY, USA

Introduction

Human papillomavirus (HPV) infection elicits cytopathic effects in the uterine cervical epithelium ranging from koilocytosis (degenerating squamous epithelial cells with nuclei studded with HPV as an episomal infection, mostly due to low-risk HPV) to dysplasia or cervical intraepithelial neoplasia (CIN) (potential cancer precursors, with HPV strands integrated in the nuclear chromatin, due to high-risk HPV). Cervical biopsies from HPV-infected adolescents often display marked nuclear atypia representing an overload of a primary viral infection rather than preneoplastic change. This infection is considered to be transitory and should not be overtreated. Vaccination and cytologic screening are preventive means for sexually active adolescents.

Uterine cervical cancer is the most frequent malignant neoplasm of the female pelvis in the world, and still a common and lethal malignant tumor in the United States, despite its spectacular decline during the past decades. It is now well documented that this cancer is causally associated with a viral infection that contains strains of HPV. Even before the identification of HPV in the histogenesis of cervical cancer and precancer, statistical evidence pointed toward an infectious origin of this neoplasm, in particular, a sexually transmitted infection with a prolonged subclinical asymptomatic phase [1]. The neoplas-

Pediatric, Adolescent, & Young Adult Gynecology. Edited by A. Altchek and L. Deligdisch. © 2009 Blackwell Publishing, ISBN: 978-1-4051-5347-8.

tic tissue is diagnosed many years or even decades after the infection took place, and is represented most commonly by invasive squamous cell carcinoma originating in the exocervix. Precancerous changes of the uterine cervical tissue are diagnosed some time between the primary infection and the development of overt cancer.

Statistics demonstrate that the two most common epidemiologic risk factors in the development of cervical cancer are the young age of the patients at the time of the first sexual intercourse and multiple sexual partners [2]. It therefore seems appropriate to investigate the issue of adolescent sexually transmitted infections in order to understand the mechanism of carcinogenic transformation of the infectious process, and the means to prevent it.

Precursors of cervical cancer

Precursors of cervical cancer have been described for over 100 years. Carcinoma *in situ* of the cervix is probably the first noninvasive malignancy that pathologists and gynecologists encountered because the uterine cervix is easily accessible to both clinical and laboratory examination. Preinvasive changes in the uterine cervix have been described as dysplasias, classified into mild, moderate and severe, according to the percentage of epithelial layers involved (lower, middle and upper third respectively) and carcinoma *in situ* in which the entire thickness of the squamous epithelium is transformed into a neoplastic epithelium that is confined by the presence of an intact basement membrane. The colposcopically

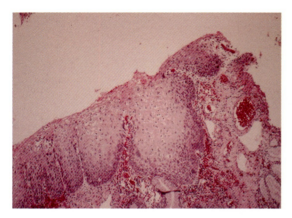

Figure 45.1 Cervical biopsy of HPV lesion in 15-year-old patient. Koilocytes are present in all layers of the squamous epithelium. H&E × 40.

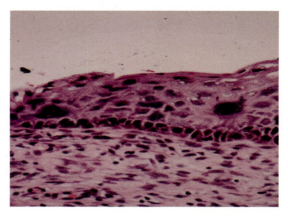

Figure 45.2 Cervical biopsy of the same patient. Koilocytes with large bizzare-shaped nuclei in the lower half of the squamous epithelium. H&E × 400.

directed histologic examination is diagnostic. It is based on microscopic changes that include architectural modifications such as arrest or loss of maturation, disarray of the epithelial layers, and cytologic changes such as an increased nuclear/cytoplasmic ratio, hyperchromatic nuclei with coarse chromatin pattern, thickened nuclear membrane, prominent and multiple nucleoli, and abnormal proliferative pattern consisting of the presence of mitotic cell divisions throughout the thickness of the squamous epithelium (Fig. 45.1). These changes were considered to represent progressive stages of dysplasia, evolving from mild to severe and potentially invasive, over a period of months or years.

Whether the progression toward malignancy was leading to invasive cancer in individual patients was not clear. It seemed imperative, however, to use some means of early detection by screening the susceptible female population with a relatively simple and unexpensive method which was elaborated in the 1950s – the Papanicolaou cytologic screening or Pap test. The result of systematic implementation of Pap tests was a spectacular decline of invasive cervical cancer, in terms of both morbidity and mortality, mostly in the North American continent and in Europe.

Human papilloma virus (HPV)

Despite this major success in preventing development of a malignant tumor by diagnosing and eliminating its precursors, the natural history of cervical cancer was only

clarified after the identification of HPV infection in the late 1970s [3,4]. Although often encountered in vulvar and vaginal lesions diagnosed as genital warts, HPV infection of the uterine cervix has been confirmed mostly in flat, nonwarty lesions, by the presence of cytopathic changes in the squamous epithelium often associated with dysplastic changes. The cytopathic effect of the HPV infection consists chiefly of the presence of koilocytes, squamous epithelial cells infected by HPV. These cells have irregular, enlarged nuclei surrounded by clear zones (perinuclear halos) and occasional individual cell keratinization (Fig. 45.2). Ultrastructurally, the nuclear content is studded with viruses displaying a honeycomb appearance, composed of hexagonal double-stranded DNA material. The koilocytes are degenerating squamous epithelial cells containing HPV, fully assembled virions, and represent an episomal nuclear infection.

Molecular biologic research identified by cross-hybridization the "footprints" of HPV infection in dysplastic and cancer cells, integrated in the host nuclear DNA. The presence of HPV in the cell nuclei is detected by a number of methods ranging from Southern blot hybridization and *in situ* hybridization to the polymerase chain reaction which amplifies the DNA sequences, making it the most sensitive technique. Over 80 subtypes of HPV have been detected, the most common being HPV-16, -18, -33, -31, -45, -52, and -58, associated with precursors and cancerous cervical lesions, considered as high-risk viral infections. HPV-6 and -11 are associated with genital warts and considered nononcogenic or low risk.

Classification

The tissue response to these infections, however, does not necessarily correspond to the type of HPV infection in individual cases. In other words, not every person infected with high-risk HPV develops high-grade dysplastic changes. The classification used at present by most cytology laboratories into high-grade squamous intraepithelial lesions (HSIL) and low-grade intraepithelial lesions (LSIL) is generally not applied for the histopathologic diagnosis which is based on a three-tier classification into mild, moderate and severe dysplasia or CIN grade 1, 2 and 3. CIN 3 includes both severe dysplasia and carcinoma *in situ* because the presence of neoplastic features in the upper third of the squamous epithelium should be considered equivalent to the involvement of the entire thickness of the squamous epithelium and managed accordingly.

Carcinogenesis

As in other preinvasive, precancerous lesions, it is not possible to predict progression to overt cancer. The oncogenic potential of the HPV is related to the early transcriptional units (open reading frames E1, E2, E4, E6 and E7) that play a role in the epithelial cell replication and possible oncogenic mutations [5]. Host factors such as cigarette smoking, herpes virus infections, and immunologic competence may be involved to various degrees in the oncogenic transformation of the HPV-infected cervical epithelium. Less common than squamous cell carcinoma of the cervix is adenocarcinoma originating in the endocervical glands. This cancer is less commonly detected in early stages because of its location in a less accessible area, the endocervical canal, which is not visualized in its entirety on examination by speculum and on colposcopy. Cytologic screening may also be eluded by endocervical malignant cells. The etiopathogenesis of endocervical neoplasms is also closely related to HPV infection, especially HPV-18. Hormonal factors such as pregnancy and contraceptive therapy may stimulate the proliferation of endocervical glands and may be involved in the carcinogenesis of this less common type of cervical neoplasm. Histologically, endocervical cancers are most often composed of mucin-secreting glands or endometrioid type glands. Less common are clear cell and small cell endocervical carcinomas. The precursors of these neoplasms are more difficult to diagnose than those of squamous cell carcinoma. Cytologically, suspicious cells of endocer-

vical origin are included in the rather vague term AGUS (atypical glandular cells of unknown significance), more recently divided into low and high grade.

Histologically, adenocarcinoma *in situ* (AIS) is a challenging entity consisting of atypical glandular cells with mitotic activity, high nuclear cytoplasmic ratio, loss of mucin secretion, lining endocervical glands without stromal invasion. The transition area between exo- and endocervical epithelium (T-zone) is an area of heightened metabolic activity due to the common shifting and replacement of squamous epithelium (squamous metaplasia) from the exocervix and glandular epithelium (eversion) from the endocervix, during the reproductive period of life. HPV infection is most commonly found in the T-zone, probably due to the increased DNA replication in this area. The HPV infection prevents cell differentiation and promotes p53 degradation, playing a role in the progression of the HPV infection to a malignant cell transformation, usually starting in the T-zone [6]. Excisional biopsies and conization are performed to remove this area in order to prevent a potential progression to overt neoplasm.

HPV infection in adolescents

In adolescents the HPV infection is characterized by condylomatous changes which are often histologically different from those seen in adult patients, probably reflecting a primary infection acquired at a young age. The koilocytes seen in the condylomatous lesion, often associated with intraepithelial neoplastic lesions of low or high grade, display unusually large, bizarre nuclei and are often multinucleated (Fig. 45.3). The increase in size and alteration in shape of the nuclei are evident in koilocytes found throughout the thickness of the squamous epithelium, often in the basal and parabasal layers (Fig. 45.4). This is in contrast with condylomatous lesions diagnosed in more mature women. Biopsies taken from cervical HPV-related lesions in the latter group show koilocytes mostly in the superficial, more mature layers of keratinocytes mature enough to permit a full assembly of viral particles, with antigenic expression of their capsid, characteristic of the episomic viral infection. In adolescents the bizarre nuclei of koilocytes often do not express capsid antigens. The much enlarged and bizarre nuclei studded with HPV represent a productive primary hyperinfection, different

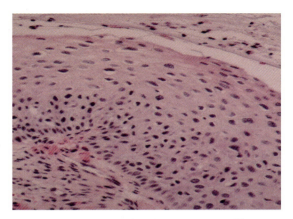

Figure 45.3 Cervical biopsy of HPV lesion in a 37-year-old patient. Koilocytes are present in the superficial layers.

from the HPV infection seen in patients of an older age group.

A morphometric study compared condylomatous, HPV-related cervical lesions from biopsies taken from adolescent patients age 14–20 with lesions found in cervical biopsies from women age 35–64, in order to quantify the findings and assess their significance [7]. The nuclei in the lesions from adolescents were found to be on average twice as large as those seen in older women, and they often were located in the lower half of the squamous epithelium. The nuclei were further analyzed for their texture by computerized image analysis using the autocorrelation

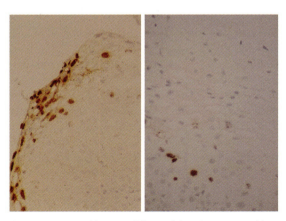

Figure 45.4 Cervical biopsies of flat condyloma in a 37-year-old patient (*left*) and a 16-year-old patient (*right*). Immunohistochemical positive stain for HPV-16/18 involved superficial layers (*left*) and basal layers (*right*). × 100.

factor [8]. The nuclear structure of the largest nuclei in the biopsies from adolescent patients was markedly different from that of the largest nuclei seen in biopsies from older women. Their tridimensional image revealed a smooth surface, consistent with a homogenous structure due to the presence of a large load of HPV while the large nuclei (although half as large on average) from koilocytes seen in the biopsies from older women had a tridimensional spiked surface, reflecting the irregular chromatin pattern, consistent with dysplastic, precursor changes [7].

It was concluded that the major atypical changes in condylomatous lesions diagnosed in adolescent females reflect the presence of an overload of HPV and have no or little precancerous significance since there is no basic alteration in the host's nuclear chromatin. Therefore, these lesions should not be overtreated. This is in accordance with the 2002 guidelines of the American Cancer Society [9] asserting the transient, reversible nature of the HPV infection in adolescents despite cytologic and histologic atypical changes. It seems that at a young age the infection is highly productive but does not elicit a short-term oncogenic effect. Adolescents with HPV infection, however, are at higher risk of developing cervical neoplasms in later decades, perhaps due to reinfections or reflaring of previous HPV infections related to poorly understood host factors.

The increased HPV load in cervical condylomatous lesions in adolescents is significant for their primary infection and suggests a higher infectious potential. It is now considered that HPV infection in adolescents is often transient and reversible. However, this group of young patients is highly vulnerable, capable of spreading the

---

Quick Take 45.1

HPV infection in adolescents

- Cervical cancer in women less than 19 years is rare.
- Patients aged 10–19 years have 18% HSIL.
- Most HPV infections are transient: 90% low risk, 70% high risk regress.
- LSIL regress more often in adolescents: 90% vs 50–80% in adults over 30 years.
- More benign nature of HPV infection in adolescents. Avoid overtreatment.
- Risk of progression of HSIL still unknown (54–60 months?).
- Screening to begin at three years from potential exposure to HPV (age cap 21).

Quick Take 45.2

Cytopathic effect of HPV in adolescents

- Large, bizarre-shaped, often multinucleated cells present throughout the thickness of the squamous cervical epithelium.

- Nuclear texture significantly more homogeneous than that of dysplastic cells.

- Findings suggestive of increased viral load (highly productive HPV infection) rather than dysplastic change.

- Oncogenic potential? HPV-infected adolescents at high risk for cervical carcinoma.

infection, and at risk for later carcinogenesis. Therefore, prevention has been emphasized recently by using the approach of forming type-specific neutralizing antigens, directed mostly against the high-risk types of HPV. Cell-mediated immunity develops in adolescents and young women and declines further with age.

Vaccination

Now approved by FDA and ready for use is a vaccine directed against HPV infections, proposed to be used in preadolescent females and males in order to avoid lesions that are highly infectious during the adolescent period in life and potentially carcinogenic in later life. This new approach to preventing HPV-related lesions should by no means deter the implementation of screening programs by cytologic and colposcopically directed biopsies in use, which accomplished a dramatic decrease in cervical cancer

morbidity and mortality in recent decades. It should be emphasized that most invasive cervical cancer cases are diagnosed in women who had not been screened for five years or more.

References

1. Munoz N, Bosch FX, de Sanjose S et al. Epidemiologic classification of human papilloma virus types associated with cervical cancer. *N Engl J Med* 2003;**348**:518–527.

2. Ho GYF, Bierman R, Beardsley L, Chang C, Burk RD. Natural history of cervico-vaginal papilloma virus infection in young women. *N Engl J Med* 1998;**338**:423–428.

3. Ferenczy A, Braun L, Shah K. Human papilloma virus (HPV) in condylomatous lesions of the cervix. *Am J Surg Pathol* 1981;**5**:661–670.

4. Schiffman M, Castle PE. Human papilloma virus: epidemiology and public health. *Arch Pathol Lab Med* 2003;**127**:930–934.

5. Moscicki A-B. Human papilloma virus infection in adolescents. *Pediatr Clin North Am* 1999;**46**:783–807.

6. Zur Hausen H. Papilloma virus and cancer: from basic studies to clinical application. *Nature Rev* 2002;**2**:342–350.

7. Deligdisch L, Miranda C, Wu H, Gil J. Human papilloma virus-related cervical lesions in adolescents: a histologic and morphometric study. *Gynecol Oncol* 2003;**89**:52–59.

8. Deligdisch L, Gil J, Kerner H, Wu H, Beck D, Gershoni-Baruch R. Ovarian dysplasia in prophylactic oophorectomy specimens. *Cancer* 1999;**86**:1544–1550.

9. Saslov D, Runowitz CD, Solomon D et al. American Cancer Society guideline for early detection of cervical neoplasia and cancer. *CA Cancer J Clin* 2002;**52**:342–362.

CHAPTER 46

Endometrial Pathology in Young Patients

Liane Deligdisch
Mount Sinai Medical Center, New York, NY, USA

Introduction

Endometrial tissue is a sensitive target for steroid hormones, able to modify its structural characteristics with promptness and versatility.

Before puberty the endometrial tissue is inactive. It is composed of short tubular glands, a dense fibroblastic stroma and thin blood vessels. The advent of cyclic pituitary and ovarian hormonal activity at puberty results in endometrial cyclic morphologic changes involving the three compartments: glands, stroma, and blood vessels. The presence of sex steroid receptors in the cells of the endometrium is responsible for the prompt translation of hormonal impulses into structural changes. During the estrogenic stimulation taking place in normal cycles, the endometrial glands grow and become tortuous due to the active proliferation of epithelial cells. Numerous mitoses are present in both glands and stroma, the nuclei increase in size, and the nucleoli become prominent. The individual cell mass increases, as does the nuclear/cytoplasmic ratio.

After ovulation the secretion of progesterone inhibits the proliferative activity in the endometrium and induces a complex secretory activity starting with the polarization of glycogen at a subnuclear location followed by its transport via microfilaments to the apical region of the cell. Secretory granules are eventually expelled into the glandular lumen. Secretory changes take place only in an estrogen-primed endometrium. The morphologic changes of the

Pediatric, Adolescent, & Young Adult Gynecology. Edited by
A. Altchek and L. Deligdisch. © 2009 Blackwell Publishing,
ISBN: 978-1-4051-5347-8.

postovulatory endometrium consist of glandular secretion, thickening and convoluting of the arteries which become spiral arterioles, and decidual transformation of the stromal cells. The secretory phase normally lasts 14 days and each day the histologic pattern of the endometrium is different. These structural changes prepare the endometrium for possible implantation of a fertilized egg. In the absence of implantation the withdrawal of estrogen and progesterone results in the menstrual shedding of the endometrium.

Absence of ovulation (anovulatory cycles)

The first postmenarchal cycles are often anovulatory, manifested clinically by irregular vaginal bleeding and/or amenorrhea, and histologically by the absence of secretory changes in the endometrium. Prolonged anovulation in young patients occurs in polycystic ovarian disease (PCOD). It may also occur with obesity, diabetes or other metabolic/genetic disorders leading to extragonadal endogenous estrogen production by aromatization. The prolonged and uninterrupted (by progesterone) estrogenic stimulation of the endometrium may cause glandular hyperplasia and occasionally endometrial neoplasia. Endometrial hyperplasia resulting from unopposed estrogenic stimulation is classified into three degrees of increasing severity:
• simple glandular hyperplasia that consists of an exaggeration of the proliferative changes with glandular crowding, piling up of epithelial layers, active mitotic activity

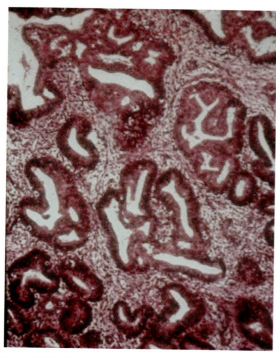

Figure 46.1 Endometrial complex glandular hyperplasia in a 19-year-old patient with polycystic ovarian disease. H&E ×100.

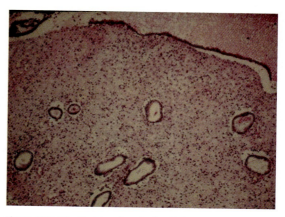

Figure 46.2 OC effect: inactive glands and stromal decidualization. H&E ×100.

• complex glandular hyperplasia displaying glandular crowding (back-to-back arrangement) due to a markedly reduced stromal tissue and glandular "complex" lumina with protruding and outpouching epithelial folds (Fig. 46.1)

• atypical glandular hyperplasia with loss of polarity of the epithelial cells, the glands being lined by irregular and atypical cells with hyperchromatic nuclei exhibiting coarse chromatin and prominent nucleoli. Mitotic activity is not necessarily correlated with the degree of severity of the hyperplasia.

Iatrogenic hormonal effects on the endometrium

Endometrial changes in women receiving hormone therapy may encompass a wide variety of histologic changes that vary with the dosage, duration and individual hormone receptor activity and do not fit the classically described cyclic patterns. Iatrogenic endometrial changes in young women are most often related to contraceptive therapy, and less commonly to ovulation stimulation, to replacement and to antineoplastic hormone therapy [1].

Oral contraceptives (OC)

Over 10 million women in the USA use OC as an effective and accessible method of contraception. Most contraceptives contain small dosages of estrogens and testosterone-derived progesterone, whereas some contain only progestins. Historically, OC were used initially in a sequential manner, with estrogen alone in the first half of the cycle, which was associated with a number of endometrial malignancies diagnosed in young women [2]. This method was discontinued in the USA in 1976.

The mechanism of preventing pregnancy is based on the notion that the presence of one pregnancy prevents the onset of another pregnancy. Therefore the administration of hormones secreted during pregnancy (estrogens and progesterone) should suppress ovulation and implantation.

The progesterone effect predominates on the endometrium which does not resemble histologically any "natural" phase or spontaneous pathologic endometrial changes. The unique pattern of OC-induced endometrial changes consists of inactive or atrophic glands, sometimes containing an "abortive" secretion in the lumen, and an abundant stroma with decidual transformation of the fibroblasts which become plump decidual cells (Fig. 46.2). The blood vessels may be thin, tortuous or

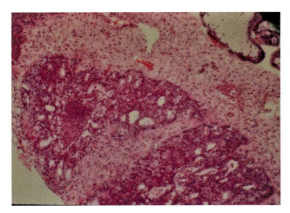

Figure 46.3 Ovulation stimulation for PCOD: patient became pregnant with triplets, aborted and endometrial curettings showed chorionic villi (*upper right corner*), decidua (*middle*) and endometrial adenocarcinoma (*lower half*). H&E ×100.

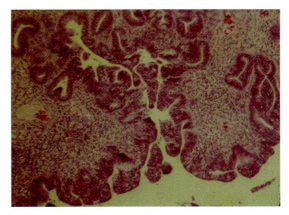

Figure 46.4 Endometrial atypical glandular hyperplasia in patient with Turner disease, treated with estrogens. H&E ×40.

hyperplastic, with thickened walls due to smooth muscle hyperplasia. Occasional telangiectatic vessels with thrombosis are associated with bleeding during prolonged use of OC.

Ovulation stimulation therapy

Infertility due to irregular or infrequent ovulation in young women is treated by augmentation of endogenous gonadotropins aimed at creating endometrial cycling changes resembling spontaneous natural cycles. However, this therapy may result in a disparity between the more advanced stromal development and the glandular secretion which lags behind. The endometrial accelerated maturation is often associated with hosting multiple gestations due to the recruitment of oocytes from multiple ovulating follicles. In rare cases of treated anovulatory cycles, especially those related to PCOD, persistent endometrial hyperplasia is seen along with secretory changes induced by the ovulatory cycles. In a 27-year-old patient diagnosed previously with PCOD and atypical glandular hyperplasia who became pregnant with triplets after ovulation stimulation therapy and aborted at six weeks gestation, histologic examination of the products of conception revealed chorionic villi, decidua and endometrial complex atypical glandular hyperplasia with areas of well-differentiated endometrioid adenocarcinoma (Fig. 46.3).

Hormonal substitution therapy

Young patients are rarely treated with estrogens alone, which represents a therapeutic modality for postmenopausal symptoms due to ovarian failure. However, adolescents diagnosed with Turner syndrome and associated disorders related to genetic abnormalities (XO monosomy), characterized by gonadal failure to develop into normal ovaries, need hormone replacement therapy at the time of puberty. Estrogen therapy promotes the development of secondary sexual characteristics and stimulates the growth of an otherwise infantile uterus. The effect on the endometrium is positively related to the duration of therapy, causing proliferation, hyperplasia, and even neoplasia. These young patients may present with alternating periods of amenorrhea and vaginal bleeding. One such patient developed, at age 17, an atypical endometrial hyperplasia with well-differentiated adenocarcinoma that was treated surgically by hysterectomy (Fig. 46.4). The patient was subsequently treated with replacement estrogen therapy for the rest of her life.

Premature ovarian failure is an ovarian disorder characterized by amenorrhea, elevated serum gonadotropins and hypoestrogenemia in women by the age of 30. The causes are diverse (genetic, iatrogenic, metabolic, antoimmune). Associated conditions include thyroid disorders and diabetes mellitus. These patients are treated with hormone replacement therapy, i.e. estrogens and cyclic progestins that will elicit proliferative and secretory endometrial changes. If ovarian function resumes

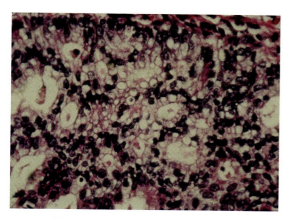

Figure 46.5 Endometrial carcinoma in a 26-year-old patient, treated with progesterone: secretory changes and quiescent epithelial cells in a well-differentiated adenocarcinoma.

spontaneously, the endometrium can host the implantation of a fertilized ovum in these patients.

Hormonal antitumoral therapy

Endometrial carcinoma is unusual in young and premenopausal women [3]. It may occur in patients suffering from PCOD because of failing ovulation, in morbidly obese patients because of the excessive extragonadal estrogen production, and rarely in patients with strong family histories of cancer and/or multiple primary neoplasms. Progesterone therapy is considered as an adjuvant therapy for endometrial carcinoma but in some cases, in young patients desirous of future fertility, a conservative, nonsurgical approach with high-potency progestational agents is attempted, especially for cases of well-differentiated endometrial carcinomas [4]. The endometrial histologic pattern may be profoundly changed under the influence of high-potency progesterone therapy, the glands becoming quiescent, with no mitotic activity, a regular epithelial lining and stromal decidual reaction imitating gestational endometrium. However, glandular crowding, cribriforming and irregularities persist as architectural changes characteristic of carcinoma (Fig. 46.5). Endometrial hyperplasia of varying degrees of severity in young women, associated with anovulation, is usually treated successfully with progesterone, reverting the hyperplastic endometrium to a quiescent, secretory endometrium. It is controversial whether endometrial carcinoma, even when well differentiated, can be reverted with progesterone

therapy. However, when diagnosed early, endometrial carcinoma in young women has a rather favorable prognosis.

An antitumoral hormonal therapy not frequently used in young women is that with Lupron (GnRH agonist) for uterine leiomyomas (fibroids) that elicits a shrinking of the myometrium and fibroids, and a temporary atrophy of the endometrium with temporary cessation of the cyclic changes. This therapy induces a precocious menopause in young women and is not indicated for more than a few months [5].

Hormone therapy widely prescribed for breast neoplasms, with tamoxifen, a nonsteroidal, synthetic triethylene estrogen derivative, is relatively rarely used in younger women as an adjuvant therapy, along with radiation and other chemotherapeutic agents. It has an antiestrogenic effect on the breast tissue but may also have an estrogen-agonist effect on the uterus. The endometrial changes depend on the duration of therapy. In most cases the endometrium becomes inactive or remains functional in younger women. About 24% of patients develop endometrial polyps manifested by vaginal bleeding. About 4.71% of patients treated with tamoxifen for over five years develop endometrial carcinoma, mostly in the polyps, with histologic features of high-risk, nonendometrioid carcinoma in about two-thirds of the cases. It was generally concluded that the benefits of tamoxifen therapy for breast cancer outweigh the risk of endometrial pathologic conditions [6,7].

Conclusion

Endometrial pathology in children is unusual; with the advent of ovarian hormonal influences during puberty, the endometrial histology may reflect abnormalities of gonadal development and hormonal stimulation. Anovulation is the most common abnormality causing functional vaginal bleeding in adolescents and young women due to endometrial hyperplasia resulting from prolonged and unopposed estrogen effects. Iatrogenic influences on the endometrium in young females include most frequently the effect of oral contraceptives, less commonly that of replacement hormone therapy with estrogens and progesterone, and antitumoral hormone therapy with progesterone, Lupron or tamoxifen. Fortunately endometrial malignancies are unusual in this age group and, when diagnosed early, are amenable to cure.

References

1. Deligdisch L. Hormonal pathology of the endometrium. *Mod Pathol* 2000;**13**:285–294.

2. Silverberg SG, Makowski EL. Endometrial carcinoma in young women taking oral contraceptive agents. *Obstet Gynecol* 1975;**46**:503–506.

3. Farhi DC, Nosanchuk J, Silverberg SG. Endometrial carcinoma in women under 25 years of age. *Obstet Gynecol* 1986;**67**:741–745.

4. Randall TC, Kurman RJ. Progestin treatment of atypical hyperplasia and well differentiated carcinoma of the endometrium in women under age 40. *Obstet Gynecol* 1997;**90**:434–440.

5. Deligdisch L, Hirschman S, Altchek A. Pathologic changes in gonadotropin releasing hormone agonist analogue treated uterine leiomyomata. *Fertil Steril* 1997;**67**:831–841.

6. Sclesinger C, Kamoi S, Ascher S, Kendell M, Lage JM, Silverberg SG. Endometrial polyps: a comparison study of patients receiving tamoxifen with two control groups. *Int J Gynecol Pathol* 1998;**17**:302–311.

7. Deligdisch L, Kalir T, Cohen CJ et al. Endometrial histopathology in 700 patients treated with tamoxifen for breast cancer. *Gynecol Oncol* 2000;**78**:181–186.

CHAPTER 47

Ovarian Tumor Pathology in Children, Adolescents, and Young Women

Liane Deligdisch

Mount Sinai Medical Center, New York, NY, USA

Introduction

Ovarian tumors may be benign, malignant or of low malignant potential (borderline). They are classified according to their origin into epithelial, sex cord and germ cell tumors. There is a radical difference in the distribution of the various types of ovarian tumors according to the age of the patient, with the younger age group being afflicted more often by malignancies that are rather uncommon overall. Conversely, the most common ovarian malignant tumors overall are almost nonexistent in children and adolescents and rare in young adult females.

Ovarian tumors of epithelial origin arise on the surface epithelium which is an extension of the peritoneal mesothelium and often invaginates into the ovarian stroma, forming inclusion cysts from which the vast majority of both benign and malignant tumors arise, forming neoplasms with partly cystic and partly solid components.

Histologically, the lining of these cysts is most often a ciliated epithelium, similar to the lining of the fallopian tubes, in serous cysts, followed in frequency by mucin-secreting epithelium similar to the lining of the endocervix and/or colon, and by endometrial-like glandular epithelium. Benign ovarian cystic neoplasms are rarely seen in children; young adult females, however, are not uncommonly diagnosed with ovarian serous and mucinous cystadenomas, often manifested clinically as twisted (torsioned) cysts. Endometriotic cysts, although generally not considered as neoplasms, may occasionally be associated with neoplastic glandular proliferation and affect young women.

Pediatric, Adolescent, & Young Adult Gynecology. Edited by A. Altchek and L. Deligdisch. © 2009 Blackwell Publishing, ISBN: 978-1-4051-5347-8.

> **Box 47.1 Ovarian tumors of children, adolescents and young adults**
>
> • Different distribution from overall (all ages) patients
> • Most common: germ cell tumors
> • Least common: carcinomas (epithelial)
> • Some associated with abnormal sexual development and/or abnormal hormonal activity
> • Most malignant tumors responsive to chemotherapy

> **Box 47.2 Ovarian tumors, classification**
>
> • Epithelial origin: serous, mucinous, endometrioid, clear cell tumors
> • Germ cell origin: dermoid, dysgerminoma, teratoma, yolk sac tumor, embryonal tumors
> • Sex cord origin: granulosa cell, thecoma, Sertoli and Sertoli–Leydig cell, steroid cell tumors

---

Epithelial ovarian tumors

Malignant tumors of epithelial origin are the most common malignant ovarian tumors, representing about 90% of all ovarian malignancies. Most are serous followed by endometrioid and mucinous adenocarcinomas. Fortunately, children are generally not involved by this group of neoplasms which is the fourth in frequency but the first in lethality of all cancers of the female pelvis.

A subgroup of epithelial tumors are the group of borderline ovarian tumors (BOT) or tumors of low malignant potential including mainly serous and mucinous tumors, both of which are not uncommon in young female adults, raising challenging questions regarding their management in terms of preserving future fertility.

The diagnosis of serous borderline ovarian tumor is based on the findings of piled-up serous-type epithelium with papillary excrescences and detached clusters of epithelial cells displaying moderate nuclear atypia (Fig. 47.1). The hallmark of this tumor is a lack of stromal invasion, despite a florid cell proliferation into the cystic cavity or on the ovarian surface. These ovarian tumors are associated in 15–20% of cases with papillary implants of the peritoneum. The implants are most often noninvasive and do not alter the rather favorable prognosis of BOT. Invasive implants have a more ominous significance and are considered to be more often associated with

BOT in which the predominant pattern is micropapillary. The histopathologic diagnosis of a BOT with micropapillary features associated with invasive implants in the peritoneum in a young woman usually represents an indication for radical surgery, chemotherapy and possible loss of future fertility.

Germ cell ovarian tumors

The group of ovarian tumors most often encountered in children, adolescents, and young women are the germ cell tumors. Sixty percent of all ovarian neoplasms of children and adolescents are germ cell tumors, encountered in both the female and male gonads. They represent approximately 20% of all ovarian tumors in Europe and North America. Their incidence is much higher in Africa and Asia where epithelial ovarian tumors are uncommon. Fortunately again, the great majority of germ cell tumors are benign, with mature cystic teratomas (dermoids) being the most common (90%) of the group. About 80% of these teratomas occur in patients aged less than 35 years.

Gonadal germ cell tumors derive from primitive germ cells and represent a histologically diverse group of tumors. The most common germ cell tumors, the mature teratomas or dermoid tumors, frequently but not always involving young patients, are composed of a mixture of endo-, meso- and ectodermal-derived tissues, the latter predominating with elements of mature skin and skin adnexa, and neural tissue. The tumors are usually unilateral (15% are bilateral), cystic in most cases with a uniloculated cavity containing sebum and hair (Figs 47.2, 47.3).

Histologic sections reveal a mixture of heterogeneous tissue with no axial arrangement but displaying a certain

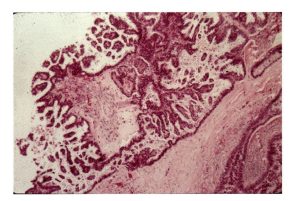

Figure 47.1 Ovarian serous papillary tumor of borderline malignancy composed of papillary excrescences and detached clusters of epithelial cells. H&E ×40.

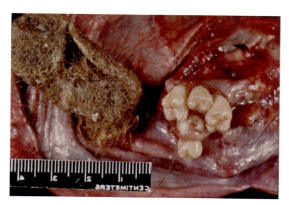

Figure 47.2 Ovarian benign cystic teratoma (dermoid). The cystic cavity contains hair and teeth.

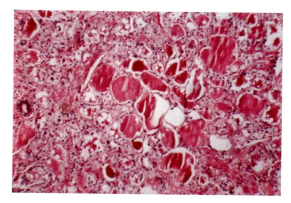

Figure 47.4 Struma ovarii (monodermal teratoma) composed of mature thyroid tissue. H&E ×40.

"induction" of adjacent structures, such as for example thyroid tissue next to cartilage, choroid plexus next to neural tissue, sebaceous glands with hair follicles, etc. All tissues are mature, therefore benign.

Solid mature teratomas are rare. They are seen in younger patients and have to be extensively sampled histologically to rule out immature elements. Monodermal teratomas consist of tumors composed of only one type of tissue, the most common being thyroid (struma ovarii) (Fig. 47.4) and carcinoid.

Immature ovarian teratomas

Immature ovarian teratomas are uncommon, compared to the mature ones. The presence of immature tissues in teratoma implies a malignant nature of the tumor, the degree of malignancy being related to the extent and sever-

ity of the immature components of the tumor (Fig. 47.5). Since the most constant component of these teratomas is neural tissue, the degree of malignancy is established according to the proportion and degree of immaturity of the neuroectodermal tissue (Fig. 47.6). Immature ovarian teratomas are classified into three grades that represent significant criteria for the patient's management. Mature elements are usually intermingled with the immature, the tumors are generally larger than the mature benign teratomas and are solid or partly cystic. Immature teratomas are sometimes admixed with other germ cell tumor elements such as dysgerminoma, embryonal, yolk sac or trophoblastic tumors.

Dysgerminoma

Dysgerminoma is the most common malignant germ cell tumor, pure or combined with other germ cell tumor

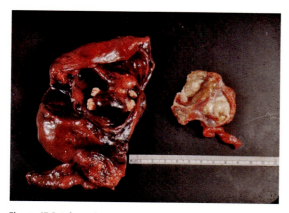

Figure 47.3 Infarcted, tortioned dermoid with teeth. The tumor is hemorrhagic and necrotic.

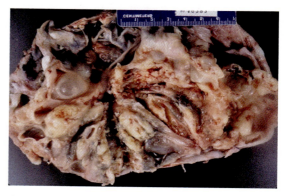

Figure 47.5 Immature ovarian teratoma. Solid and partly cystic tumor composed of a mixture of mature and immature tissue.

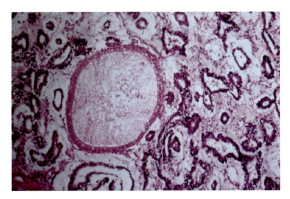

Figure 47.6 Immature teratoma: cyst surrounded by immature neuroectodermal tubules. H&E ×100.

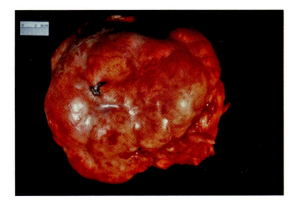

Figure 47.8 Dysgerminoma (left gonad) of same true hermaphrodite patient.

elements. This tumor is diagnosed most often in individuals younger than 30 years; it is encountered in the gonads of both sexes and named seminoma in the male testes. Ovarian dysgerminomas affect mostly adolescent and young female adults, with a peak incidence in the second and third decade.

About 5–10% of patients with dysgerminoma have an associated gonadal maldevelopment (Figs 47.7, 47.8), some with chromosomal abnormalities, manifested clinically by amenorrhea or other hormonal abnormalities. Rarely dysgerminomas are associated histologically with gonadoblastoma. Dysgerminoma, because of the age of the patients, is the most common malignant ovarian tumor associated with pregnancy. The patients may come

to medical attention because of torsion of the tumor, with acute abdomen, as do other ovarian tumors.

Ovarian dysgerminomas are usually unilateral (only 10% are bilateral); they are solid gray-tan soft tumors with a shiny external capsule and grow rapidly to large sizes. Microscopically, they are composed of mostly uniform large tumor cells of germ cell origin, with large nuclei containing a double DNA amount (Fig. 47.9).

The tumor cells are arranged in sheets and nests, separated by fibrovascular septa infiltrated by plasma cells and lymphocytes, often with granulomatous reaction and multinucleated giant cells. Tumor cells from dysgerminoma and testicular seminoma stain with placental specific alkaline phosphatase (PLAP). Occasional coexisting syncytiotrophoblastic cells may produce human chorionic gonadotropin (hCG); in the case of dysgerminoma

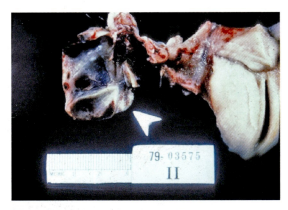

Figure 47.7 Ovotestis (right gonad) of a 27-year-old true hermaphrodite patient with contralateral dysgerminoma (see Fig. 47.8).

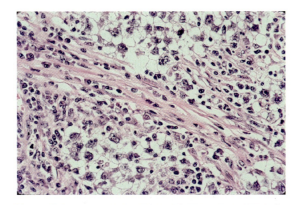

Figure 47.9 Dysgerminoma composed of large primitive germ cells separated by fibrovascular septa. H&E ×100.

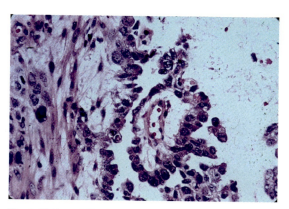

Figure 47.10 Ovarian endodermal sinus tumor (yolk sac tumor) of 20-year-old patient. Sinuses lined by malignant cells surround blood vessel (Schiller–Duvall bodies). H&E ×400.

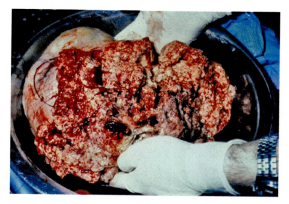

Figure 47.11 Embryonal carcinoma of 11-year-old patient who received chemotherapy and is alive and free of tumor 10 years later.

combined with nongestational choriocarcinoma, the level of hCG is very high. Other germ cell tumors such as yolk sac (endodermal sinus) tumors or embryonal carcinoma may also be admixed with dysgerminoma.

The biologic behavior is that of an aggressive tumor with destructive infiltration of the ovary and surrounding tissues which is also highly radio- and chemosensitive.

Yolk sac tumor (endodermal sinus tumor)

Yolk sac tumor (endodermal sinus tumor) is most frequently diagnosed in patients in their second and third decade and rarely in older women. This is a rapidly growing tumor with a lobulated appearance, often necrotic and hemorrhagic, usually unilateral, sometimes associated with teratoma. Histologically, this tumor may display a wide variety of microscopic patterns including polyvesicular, hepatoid, primitive intestinal as well as papillary, solid and especially endodermal sinus patterns, the latter with perivascular tumor cells (Schiller–Duvall bodies) (Fig. 47.10). Glandular structures and a myxoid stroma can also be present, as are eosinophilic hyaline globules staining positive for α-fetoglobulin (AFP) by immunohistochemistry. The presence of AFP in the serum is a reliable tumor marker of this neoplasm which is highly malignant, invasive and metastatic.

Embryonal carcinoma

Embryonal carcinoma is an uncommon tumor of the ovary, less so of the testis, which is often mixed with other germ cell tumors, especially the yolk sac tumor and choriocarcinoma. These tumors are unilateral, rapidly growing and metastasizing; they are seen in the first 2–3 decades of life (half of the patients are prepubertal) and are responsive to chemotherapy (Fig. 47.11). In about half of the cases the patients present with endocrine abnormalities such as isosexual pseudoprecocity. Histologically, the tumors are composed of primitive cells with glandular and papillary structures, high mitotic activity, and immunoreactivity to PLAP, hCG, AFP and cytokeratin.

Ovarian sex cord tumors

This group of tumors are uncommon at any age. Of all ovarian tumors, they most often are associated with abnormal endocrine manifestations due to estrogen and/or androgen secretion. Their origin is in the gonadal sex cord bipotential elements.

In the ovary the most common neoplasms in this group are the feminizing granulosa cell tumors and

---

Box 47.5 Ovarian sex cord tumors

- Rare overall. Some associated with hormone effects
- Juvenile granulosa cell tumor: 80% present with isosexual pseudoprecocity, rare virilization
- Sertoli and Sertoli–Leydig cell tumor: 75% in first 3 decades, 1/3 virilization, malignancy varies with stage
- Steroid cell tumors: rare, benign

thecomas, followed by the masculinizing Sertoli cell tumor and Sertoli–Leydig cell tumor. The tumors are generally composed of sex cord-derived cells and ovarian stromal cells. In rare cases there is a mixture of testicular and ovarian elements in the same tumor which is named gynandroblastoma.

Ovarian granulosa cell tumors

Ovarian granulosa cell tumors are unusual in children and young women, with the exception of juvenile granulosa cell tumors (JGCT) which are rare and occur in the first three decades of life. About 80% of these patients present with isosexual pseudoprecocity, while patients in the reproductive years develop menstrual irregularities or amenorrhea and postmenopausal women present with vaginal bleeding. Rare cases present with virilization. Inhibin is the tumor marker that monitors these neoplasms.

Grossly, granulosa cell tumors are predominantly unilateral and may reach large sizes. They are solid and cystic, soft, often yellowish and hemorrhagic, with necrosis (Fig. 47.12). Most JGCT are diagnosed in stage I. Histologically, they are composed of solid sheets and nodules of cells with scattered follicles. The tumor cells resemble luteinized granulosa cells with more abundant cytoplasm than those from adult granulosa cell tumors, and dark nuclei, less often grooved than in the latter (Fig. 47.13). Also, compared to the adult granulosa cell tumor, the juvenile tumor displays more irregular follicles, surrounded by a mantle of cells with nuclear atypia and mitotic activity, without this implying necessarily a worse prognosis. Stage is probably the single most significant prognostic factor

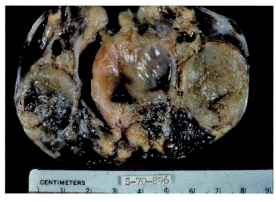

Figure 47.12 Granulosa cell tumor, solid and cystic, with areas of necrosis and hemorrhage.

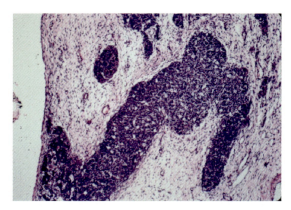

Figure 47.13 Juvenile granulosa cell tumor from 14-year-old patient with precocious pseudopuberty. Infiltrating sheets of tumor cells with dark nuclei. H&E ×40.

for this unusual group of tumors in adolescents and young adults.

Fibromas

Fibromas are rarely seen in patients younger than 30 years. They are benign tumors, usually not hormonally active and occasionally associated with Meig syndrome and basal cell nevus syndrome.

Sclerosing stromal tumors

Sclerosing stromal tumors are rare tumors but they occur most commonly in the first three decades of life. They may be asymptomatic or present clinically as menstrual irregularities or abdominal pain. They are usually unilateral, solid, sometimes edematous, with cystic spaces and hemorrhage. Microscopically, they are composed of cellular zones separated by fibrous tissue with a rich vascular network. The tumor cells are oval to spindle-shaped with indistinct cell borders, vesicular nuclei and rare mitoses. All reported cases have been benign.

Sertoli cell tumors

Sertoli cell tumors occur more often in young female adults than in older women, with an average onset at 30 years. They may be estrogenic and elicit isosexual pseudoprecocity, and are rarely androgenic. These tumors are unilateral, solid yellow-brown and composed of tubules lined by Sertoli cells with cytoplasmic vacuoles and often lipid rich (Fig. 47.14). Most are benign; there are few reported malignancies.

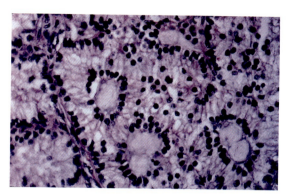

Figure 47.14 Sertoli cell tumor composed of seminiferous tubules lined by Sertoli cells. H&E ×400.

Sertoli–Leydig tumors

Sertoli–Leydig tumors are also relatively rare tumors which occur predominantly in young individuals, 75% in the first three decades of life, on average at age 25. Virilization is associated with about one-third of these tumors, most being nonfunctional and rarely estrogenic. Presenting symptoms include amenorrhea, atrophy of breasts, acne, hirsutism, clitoromegaly, deepening of voice, temporal balding, and rarely menorrhagia.

The majority of these tumors are diagnosed in stage I, are solid and cystic, yellowish-tan with necrotic areas. Histologically, they are well, intermediately and poorly differentiated, and retiform. They are composed of solid or hollow tubules surrounded by Leydig cells, in various degrees of differentiation, nuclear atypia and mitotic activity. Heterologous elements (cartilage, epithelium) may be present in the poorly or intermediately differentiated tumors.

Most of these tumors are unilateral. Those tumors diagnosed in higher than stage I are malignant and may recur early, with metastases.

A rare tumor has been described as a subtype of Sertoli tumors, as sex cord tumor with annular tubules (SC-TAT), associated or not with Peutz–Jeghers syndrome. These tumors are also seen in younger patients (on average 27 years). They are usually benign but in 20% of cases with Peutz–Jeghers syndrome there is a malignant course.

These tumors are usually small, up to 3 cm, and composed of annular tubules forming rings around eosinophilic globules of basement membrane material. In tumors without Peutz–Jeghers syndrome, granulosa cells and Sertoli–Leydig cells may be associated histologic elements.

Gynandroblastomas are exceedingly rare, composed of a mixture of granulosa and Sertoli cells, and are benign.

Steroid (lipid) cell tumors, stromal luteoma and Leydig cell tumors rarely involve younger females. The only tumor in this group occasionally seen in children and adolescents is the steroid cell tumor, NOS, which may present clinically with virilization and rarely Cushing syndrome or hyperestrogenism. The tumors are solid, yellow and are composed of lipid-containing cells with central vesicular nuclei. The presence of high mitotic activity is seen in clinically malignant tumors more often affecting younger patients (16 or older).

Further reading

Deligdisch L. Epithelial ovarian neoplasms. In: Altchek A, Deligdisch L, Kase N (eds) *Diagnosis and Management of Ovarian Disorders*, 2nd edn. New York: Academic Press, 2003, 83–93.

Silverberg S, Bell D, Kurman RJ et al. Borderline ovarian tumors: key points and workshop summary. *Hum Pathol* 2004;**35**:910–948.

Talerman A. Germ cell tumors of the ovary. In: Kurman RJ (ed) *Blaustein's Pathology of the Female Genital Tract*, 5th edn. New York: Springer-Verlag, 2002, 967–1033.

Arroyo JG, Harris W, Laden SA. Recurrent mixed germ cell–sex cord stromal tumor of the ovary associated with isosexual precocious puberty. *Cancer* 1988;**61**;2122–2133.

Scully RE. Sex cord-stromal tumours. In: *Histological Typing of Ovarian Tumours*, 2nd edn. Berlin: World Health Organization/Springer-Verlag, 1999, 19–28.

Malmstrom H, Hogberg T, Bjorn R, Simonsen E. Granulosa cell tumors of the ovary: prognostic factors and outcome. *Gynecol Oncol* 1994;**52**:50–55.

Lappohn RE, Burger HG, Bouma J et al. Inhibin as a marker for granulosa-cell tumor. *N Engl J Med* 1989;**321**:790–793.

CHAPTER 48

Gestational Trophoblastic Diseases Pathology in Adolescents and Young Adults

Liane Deligdisch
Mount Sinai Medical Center, New York, NY, USA

Introduction

The biology and physiopathology of the trophoblast represent a unique and fascinating aspect of reproductive and tumor pathobiology.

The trophoblast originates in the outer layer of the blastocyst. Its function during the early stages of embryonal development is to contact, penetrate and invade the maternal organism. The trophoblast is alien to the maternal tissues both genetically and antigenically. Its survival, tumultuous growth and nonrejection during normal pregnancy still represent an unsolved mystery. There are three types of trophoblast cells:
• cytotrophoblast composed of large cuboidal cells with high proliferative activity
• syncytiotrophoblast composed of multinucleated cells capable of performing multiple functions during gestation, such as secreting hormones (hCG, estrogen, progesterone, thyroid-stimulating hormone, etc.) by replacing the endocrine functions of the maternal pituitary and ovary
• intermediate trophoblast that invades maternal blood vessels by replacing their endothelial lining, and maintains the structural integrity of the anchoring villi.
The growth pattern of the trophoblast during the process of implantation is a unique biologic phenomenon because it represents the growth of one biologic individual entity

into another. The fact that there is no rejection by the maternal host and that the invasion of the maternal tissues by the trophoblast is self-limited makes gestation the perfect successful allograft. Indeed, once implantation is achieved, the trophoblast stops its aggressive penetration of the uterus and maternal blood vessels and becomes a highly differentiated tissue capable of replacing lungs, kidneys, endocrine glands, etc. in the complex maternal–fetal exchanges during the development of normal gestation.

Chromosomal defects of the trophoblast are the cause of major anomalies of gestation ranging from spontaneous abortions, which are relatively common, to trophoblastic neoplasms such as hydatidiform mole and choriocarcinoma which are fortunately rare.

Classification, epidemiology and pathogenesis of trophoblastic diseases

Complete hydatidiform mole is a disorder of pregnancy recognized since ancient history and described as a pregnancy without a fetus. Its geographic distribution in the world is variable, ranging from one case per 80 pregnancies in some countries in the Far East (Taiwan, Philippines, China) to one per 1000–2000 pregnancies in the United States, Australia and Western Europe.

Hydatidiform moles are more common at the two age extremes of the reproductive years: in pregnant adolescents under 20 years and in women over 40. Hydatidiform moles are complete or partial.

Pediatric, Adolescent, & Young Adult Gynecology. Edited by A. Altchek and L. Deligdisch. © 2009 Blackwell Publishing, ISBN: 978-1-4051-5347-8.

It has been demonstrated that the 46XX karyotype identified in the majority of complete hydatidiform moles, far from being a normal female karyotype, actually represents an aberration due to the fact that both X chromosomes are of paternal origin and that the maternal karyotype is nonexistent because of the complete and early inactivation of the oocyte [1].

The oocytes are more vulnerable in older and in very young pregnant women and therefore are more easily inactivated by diploid sperm, which is encountered more frequently in Asian males. The absence of a maternal component in the molar tissue is incompatible with the development of a fetus, so in complete hydatidiform moles fetal tissues are almost always absent. Therefore, the complete hydatidiform moles in their vast majority are androgenic, with two paternal sets of chromosomes and no maternally imprinted genetic contribution. The empty egg is fertilized by diploid or two spermatozoids.

Partial hydatidiform moles have been recognized more recently [2] and are usually associated with a severely malformed fetus. The estimated prevalence is 1:700 pregnancies but may be higher since most of these gestations are aborted and not properly evaluated. The origin of this abnormality lies in the fertilization of a normal oocyte by diploid or two spermatozoids resulting in a monogynic, diandric triploidy. Partial hydatidiform mole may be seen in pregnant women of all ages since it is not related to an inactivation of vulnerable oocytes, as is the case in the very young and in older pregnant women. Most partial moles are triploid (69XXY most often, 69XXX or XYY less commonly).

Invasive moles may follow complete and, less often, partial hydatidiform moles. They represent a more advanced form of gestational trophoblastic disease, probably representing a breakdown of the local barriers that prevent trophoblastic invasion of the myometrium. Molar villi may be present occasionally in extrauterine locations (lungs, pelvis).

Choriocarcinoma is the most malignant of the trophoblastic neoplasms, relatively uncommon in the USA and Western Europe (about 1 per 20,000–40,000 pregnancies but about ten times as common in Southern Asia, and in some African and Latin American countries). Cytogenetic studies revealed frequent aneuploidy, not unlike other poorly differentiated neoplasms. The histogenesis of this tumor of the trophoblastic cells in which villous structures are usually absent is possibly related to the growth of villous intermediate trophoblast, along with cyto- and syncytiotrophoblast.

Placental site trophoblastic tumor is a relatively rarely diagnosed condition in which intermediate trophoblastic cells are implanted in the myometrium, following usually a normal pregnancy.

Clinical and pathologic aspects of gestational trophoblastic diseases

Partial, complete and invasive mole, choriocarcinoma and placental site trophoblastic tumor are different forms of trophoblastic diseases, representing increasing degrees of severity.

Complete hydatidiform mole

Complete moles may progress to invasive moles; choriocarcinoma and placental site trophoblastic tumors may occur at a variable time (up to 20 years!) after a molar or a normal pregnancy or, rarely, after an extrauterine pregnancy. By no means, however, do these entities represent necessarily progressive stages of disease in individual patients.

Complete hydatidiform moles consist of a grossly abnormal development of the placenta which is composed of innumerable cystic, grape-like vesicles filling the uterine cavity, some attached to the uterus wall, some free-floating in the cavity, usually associated with blood and, as mentioned before, without a fetus (Fig. 48.1). The diagnosis

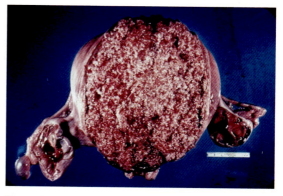

Figure 48.1 Complete hydatidiform mole. The uterine cavity is filled with vesicular, grape-like structures (hydropic chorionic villi). No fetus is present. Both ovaries are enlarged, with luteal cysts.

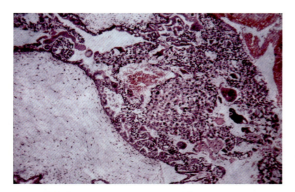

Figure 48.2 Complete hydatidiform mole. Chorionic villus with hydropic degeneration, absent fetal vessels and marked proliferation of syncytio- and cytotrophoblastic cells.

can be made as early as 8–12 weeks of pregnancy by ultrasound showing a "snowstorm" pattern, and by high levels of human chorionic gonadotropins (hCG), especially the β-subunit of hCG in both the serum and urine. The fetal chorionic villi are filled with fluid and microscopically display edema and hydropic degeneration of the villous stroma, with central "cisterns," absence of a fetal vasculature (since there is no fetus and no fetal placental circulation) and, most importantly, a marked proliferation of the trophoblast with a circumferential pattern, as opposed to the normal proliferation of the early trophoblast which is polarized and directed toward the site of implantation (Fig. 48.2). There is an active proliferation of both cyto- and syncytiotrophoblast, reminiscent of the early stages of normal implantation, even though the molar tissue originates from a second-trimester pregnancy, as is the case with spontaneous molar abortions in patients who were not diagnosed clinically in early stages.

Despite the technology (sonography, MRI, bio-immunologic tests) that offers the possibility of early diagnosis, some very young pregnant patients, adolescents in many cases, who do not have prenatal care may present during the second trimester of pregnancy with spontaneous abortions of molar tissue. The uterus containing a complete hydatidiform mole is larger than the corresponding age of gestation and the patient experiences symptoms of hypergestosis with increased morning sickness, as well as hypertension, pre-eclampsia and/or hyperthyroidism. The ovaries are enlarged due to the presence of luteal cysts stimulated by high luteinizing hormone (LH). The symptoms are related to the secretion by the trophoblast of excessive amounts of hormones (hCG,

TSH, FSH, LH, steroids). It should be mentioned that hCG secretion has a lymphopenic effect, notable also in normal pregnancies but increased in molar pregnancies: this explains the nonrejection of the molar placenta, with spontaneous abortion occurring relatively late, during the second trimester. The high levels of hCG may persist after the evacuation of the mole, up to 60 days.

Interestingly, in molar pregnancies the pathway of degenerative changes induced by genetic and developmental defects may join the pathway of neoplasia. About 82% of complete hydatidiform moles have a benign outcome. The neoplastic, often histologically quite atypical growth pattern is self-limited. The patient is cured in most cases, requiring chemotherapy only in the presence of metastatic lesions and/or very high persistent hCG titers, with no deleterious influence on her obstetric future.

In the remaining 18% of cases, however, a complete hydatidiform mole can be followed by invasive mole, choriocarcinoma or placental site trophoblastic tumor.

Partial hydatidiform moles

The placental tissue may appear grossly unremarkable, although a careful examination, with a magnifying glass, may reveal cystic structures and vesicles. There is a gestational sac and/or embryo or fetus, most often severely malformed. Histologically, there are two populations of chorionic villi: large hydropic, irregular and small immature, often with fetal blood vessels containing nucleated red blood cells (Fig. 48.3). The chorionic villi are irregular, with scalloped borders and stromal trophoblastic inclusions. The trophoblastic hyperplasia is usually mild. The

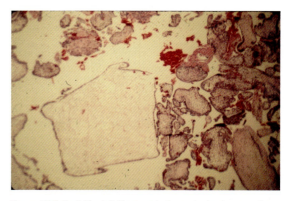

Figure 48.3 Partial hydatidiform mole. Large, hydropic, avascular villus and normal-sized chorionic villi with minimal trophoblastic hyperplasia.

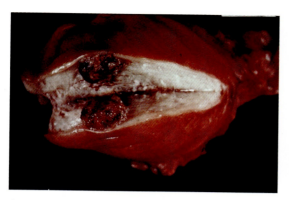

Figure 48.4 Invasive mole penetrating the uterine wall as a hemorrhagic mass with hydropic villous structures.

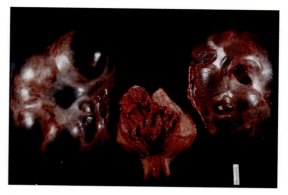

Figure 48.5 Choriocarcinoma presenting as a pelvic hemorrhagic mass, with no visible uterine lesion. The ovaries are enormously enlarged due to multiple luteal cysts resulting from elevated LH production by the trophoblast.

main differential diagnosis is hydropic abortion in which the abnormal villous morphology may be associated with other genetic abnormalities, such as trisomy. This distinction is important because of the higher risk of persistent gestational trophoblastic disease in molar pregnancy. The risk is lower in partial versus complete hydatidiform mole (0.5–4% versus 15–20%). Choriocarcinoma is rare after partial moles.

Following all cases with serum hCG levels in serum is mandatory in both partial and complete hydatidiform moles.

Invasive mole

Invasive mole is diagnosed by the presence of molar chorionic villi surrounded by a highly aggressive growth of the trophoblast, invading the myometrial wall (Fig. 48.4) and occasionally resulting in perforation with hematoperitoneum. Distant metastases are rare, however. This condition is diagnosed by sonography and persistent, high titers of hCG and hemorrhage after the evacuation of a molar pregnancy.

Choriocarcinoma

Choriocarcinoma is the most malignant of all gestational trophoblastic diseases and used to be a highly lethal disease before the advent of chemotherapy in the mid 1950s. It is a fascinating and unique disease because it represents the malignant growth of tissue from one individual into another one. It also represents the first solid malignant tumor completely cured by chemotherapy. Another

unique feature of choriocarcinoma is the occurrence of spontaneous remission in about 5% of cases.

This neoplasm is first clinically diagnosed in half of the cases by its metastases which are manifested by bleeding (Fig. 48.5). Actually, only in about half of the cases there is a lesion in the uterus that presents as a hemorrhagic mass. Microscopically, there is a diffuse invasion of the maternal tissues by biphasic (cyto- and syncytiotrophoblastic tissue) without chorionic villi, surrounded by hemorrhagic and necrotic tissues, with no lymphocytic reaction reflecting a loss of host defenses (Fig. 48.6). Patients with choriocarcinoma seem to be immunologically deprived. They have an impaired rejection reaction against their

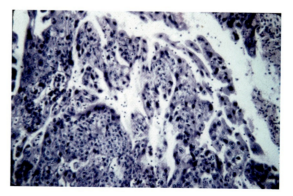

Figure 48.6 Choriocarcinoma composed of highly malignant biphasic cyto- and syncytiotrophoblastic tissue, with no chorionic villi.

husband's skin grafts. These patients are very sick, with symptoms related to the various metastases characterized by profuse bleeding. The most frequent sites of metastases are the pelvis, lungs, brain, liver, gastrointestinal tract; other areas that may harbor metastatic choriocarcinoma are bones, muscle, mediastinum, and gingiva.

In children and adolescents nongestational choriocarcinoma may be diagnosed as a component of germ cell tumors, especially of embryonal type, in which trophoblastic cells, immunoreactive to hCG, may be found along with endodermal sinus tumor elements, immunoreactive to α-fetoproteins. To diagnose a lesion as choriocarcinoma, the trophoblastic components should predominate and serum hCG titers should be elevated. Nongestational choriocarcinoma is not as responsive to chemotherapy as gestational choriocarcinoma. The epithelioid choriocarcinoma, histologically similar to poorly differentiated carcinomas, is occasionally diagnosed in very young patients after abortions and full-term deliveries.

Placental site trophoblastic tumors

Placental site trophoblastic tumors are diagnosed uncommonly and their clinical and biologic characteristics are still not well defined. Patients may present with bleeding and elevated hCG titers after an abortion or full-term pregnancy. Histologically, there is a monomorphic trophoblastic cell infiltration of the myometrium that splits muscle bundles and may invade vascular walls. The trophoblastic cells are variable in size, shape and mitotic activity. The immunoreactivity of these cells is positive for hCG, as are the other trophoblastic tumors, and for human placental lactogen (HpL).

Management

The working classification of the gestational trophoblastic diseases, for purposes of management, is different from the didactic histopathologic classification (see Tables 48.1 and 48.2).

The single most significant factor in the prognosis of gestational trophoblastic diseases is the inception of chemotherapy, with methotrexate and actinomycin. The earlier the diagnosis, the more effective the chemotherapy, with most cases treated early achieving complete cure, without surgical removal of the uterus, thus not affecting the reproductive future of the patient.

Table 48.1 Gestational trophoblastic diseases histopathologic classification

- Partial hydatidiform mole
- Complete hydatidiform mole
- Invasive hydatidiform mole
- Choriocarcinoma
- Placental site trophoblastic tumor
- Recently proposed entities:
  - Epithelioid trophoblastic tumor
  - Placental site nodule

Table 48.2 Gestational trophoblastic diseases clinical classification

- Non-metastatic trophoblastic disease
- Metastatic trophoblastic disease

Good prognosis
- Early inception of therapy (<4 months)
- HCG < 40.000
- Lung and pelvic metastases
- No antecedent term pregnancy

Poor prognosis
- Late inception of therapy (>4 months)
- HCG > 40.000
- Liver and brain metastases
- Antecedent term pregnancy

It should be emphasized that the youngest patients with gestational trophoblastic diseases are those who may not be diagnosed early because of lack of prenatal care, lack of awareness that their symptoms may be related to pregnancy in some adolescents in whom, because of their young age, the ova were inactivated by a fertilization with diploid or double sperms, resulting in molar pregnancy.

Conclusion

Gestational trophoblastic diseases are a unique group of disorders with an etiopathogenesis that includes genetic and developmental defects and that may evolve to oncogenic processes.

The spectrum of trophoblastic diseases including spontaneous abortions, partial, complete and invasive hydatidiform mole, choriocarcinoma and placental site trophoblastic tumors represents a succession of abnormalities with distinct clinical manifestations. However, they share elements of a developmental aberration leading, at one extreme, to destruction and elimination by natural selection of a malformed conceptus and at the other extreme, to invasion and, if not treated, to destruction of the host. Study of these diseases suggests that gestation and tumors share some biologic and morphologic characteristics, being the only situations in which the host tolerates the growth of an allogenic tissue. In both pregnancy and malignancy, this growth is made possible by the escape of both the conceptus and tumor tissue from the host's rejection mechanism, by eluding a destructive immune reaction through the masking of their respective antigens.

The mechanism of the paradoxic function of specific antibodies protecting rather than destroying the growth of these tissues is still not completely clear. The self-limited growth of the trophoblast in normal pregnancies is profoundly different from the loss of control in the growth of malignant tumors. The study of the abnormal trophoblastic growth and its regression to a primitive extraembryonal tissue in a way analogous to the regression of tumor tissues may provide an insight into some basic biologic characteristics shared by early reproductive and carcinogenic mechanisms.

References

1. Kajii T, Ohama K. Androgenetic origin of hydatidiform mole. *Nature* 1977;**268**:714–716.
2. Szulman AE, Surti U. The clinicopathologic profile of the partial hydatidiform mole. *Obstet Gynecol* 1982;**59**(5):597–602.

Further reading

Deligdisch L. Trophoblastic disease. A bridge between pregnancy and malignancy. In: Gleicher N (ed) *Reproductive Immunology*. New York: Alan R Liss, 1981, 323–337.

Gillespie AM, Liyim D, Goepel JR et al. Placental site trophoblastic tumor: a rare but potentially curable cancer. *Br J Cancer* 2000;**82**:1186.

Kajii T, Ferrier A, Niikawan N et al. Anatomic and chromosomal anomalies in 639 spontaneous abortuses. *Hum Genet* 1980;**55**:87–98.

Shih IM, Kurman RJ. The pathology of intermediate trophoblastic tumors and tumor-like lesions. *Int J Gynecol Pathol* 2001;**20**:31–47.

CHAPTER 49

Rhabdomyosarcoma of the Vagina and Cervix

Frédérique Penault-Llorca,[1] *Hinde El Fatemi,*[2] *&*
Florence Mishellany[1]

[1] Centre Jean Perrin, Clermont-Ferrand, France
[2] Hassan II Teaching Hospital, Fez, Morocco

Incidence

Rhabdomyosarcoma (RMS) is the most common soft tissue sarcoma in children and young adults (40–60% of all sarcomas) and accounts for 4–6% of all malignancies in this age group. Two peak ages are encountered: before five years and 15–18 years. The pelvis and lower genital tract are the most common sites of RMS (39%), then head and neck (31%). Vaginal primary RMS are five times more frequent than cervical primaries, and the mean age at diagnosis is two years. Almost all occur in children under the age of five. The peak incidence for cervical RMS is the second decade of adolescence.

Clinical presentation

The most common symptom is vaginal bleeding. Presentation is a swelling which may be around the vagina (with or without hemorrhagic discharge), uterus, and occasionally in the limbs. In infants it is detected because of intermittent bloody stains on the diaper. The occurrence of repetitive vaginosis or compression symptoms for deep tumors has been reported. If the tumor is large, it may distend the lumen of the vagina and protrude through the introitus as a soft polypoid grape-like mass (see Chapter 8, Figs 8.1, 8.2).

Pediatric, Adolescent, & Young Adult Gynecology. Edited by
A. Altchek and L. Deligdisch. © 2009 Blackwell Publishing,
ISBN: 978-1-4051-5347-8.

On cut sections, the grape-like mass is edematous and watery. Its colour is gray to tan.

Histopathology

This highly malignant tumor originates from striated muscle. As skeletal muscle is not normally present in the genital tract, RMS are heterologous tumors. RMS have been classified into three major histopathologic subtypes by the Intergroup Rhabdomyosarcoma Study Group (IRS) and the International Society of Pediatric Oncology:
• embryonal type: the most common; often arises in the head or neck region, or in genitalia in childhood. The bótryoid type occurs in the female genitourinary tract and is a variant of the embryonal type, usually demonstrating a submucosal lesion with a typical grape-like appearance
• alveolar type: often arises in the limbs
• undifferentiated.
The tumor cells are rhabdomyoblasts, elongated spindle cells with prominent cytoplasmic cross-striations. Classically, a dense zone of rhabdomyoblasts is found beneath the surface epithelium called the cambium layer (characteristic) (see Chapter 8, Fig. 8.3). The tumor is edematous and involves the lamina propria of the vagina diffusely. The stroma is loose and myxoid. Some tumors lack a cambium layer so a superficial surface biopsy may show only normal vaginal mucosa. Diagnosis should be performed by multiple deep vaginal biopsies to avoid false-negative biopsies.

Box 49.1 IRS clinical grouping classification

Group I (75% of patients)	A. Confined to organ or muscle of origin
Localized disease, completely resected	B. Infiltration of the external organ or muscle of origin; regional nodes not involved
Group II	A. Grossly resected tumors with microscopic residual tumor
Compromised or regional resections of three types including	B. Regional disease, completely resected, in which nodes may be involved and/or extension of tumor into an adjacent organ present
	C. Regional disease with involved nodes, grossly resected, but with evidence of microscopic residual tumor
Group III	Incomplete resection or biopsy widely gross residual disease
Group IV	Distant metastases, present at onset

Quick Take 49.1

Rhabdomyosarcoma

RMS is the most frequent sarcoma in childhood

Most of them occur before the age of two years

Vagina > cervix

Polypoid grape-like appearance

Multiple deep biopsies for diagnosis

Histologically, cambium layer is characteristic but may be lacking

Myogenin positivity on immnohistologic stain

Multimodality combined approaches with conservative surgery

Nonmetastatic botryoid RMS have an excellent prognosis

RMS are positive for desmin in 95% of cases, but myogenin positivity is required for the positive diagnosis of RMS. Molecular biology can be used to exclude an aggressive form of RMS such as the alveolar RMS with a translocation t(1;13)(p36;q14). This RMS requires specific chemotherapeutic regimens.

Evolution

RMS is a rapidly growing tumor, with local invasion. The recurrences occur mainly in the site of the primary tumors. Metastases occur mainly in the lungs and bones. Group I and II tumors have an overall survival of 90%. Favorable prognosis parameters in group I RMS are single polyp, embryonal histologic subtype and localized disease without deep myometrial invasion. The worst prognosis is associated with alveolar RMS.

The prognosis has improved greatly since the introduction of the combined modality approach of multiagent chemotherapy, radiotherapy and conservative surgery, especially if the tumor is group I. Extensive surgery does not improve survival in patients with stage I disease. Vaginal lesions have a better prognosis than cervical lesions with survival rates of 80–96% and 60% respectively.

Further reading

Gruessner SE, Omwandho CO, Dreyer T et al. Management of stage I cervical sarcoma botryoides in childhood and adolescence. *Eur J Pediatr* 2004;**163**(8):452–456.

Leuschner I, Harms D, Mattke A et al. Rhabdomyosarcoma of the urinary bladder and vagina: a clinicopathologic study with emphasis on recurrent disease: a report from the Kiel Pediatric Tumor Registry and the German CWS Study. *Am J Surg Pathol* 2001;**25**(7):856–864.

Martelli H, Oberlin O, Rey A et al. Conservative treatment for girls with nonmetastatic rhabdomyosarcoma of the genital tract: a report from the Study Committee of the International Society of Pediatric Oncology. *J Clin Oncol* 1999;**17**(7):2117–2122.

Zeisler H, Mayerhofer K, Joura E et al. Embryonal rhabdomyosarcoma of the uterine cervix: case report and review of the literature. *Gynecol Oncol* 1998;**69**:78–83.

CHAPTER 50

Benign Ovarian Disorders

Frédérique Penault-Llorca, Erika Rivera-Serrano, &
Wassim Essamet

Centre Jean Perrin, Clermont-Ferrand, France

Introduction

Benign cysts are usually functional cysts and should re-solve without treatment. Multiple cysts of follicular ori-gin are common in the neonate and in the immediate postmenarchal years. They are usually asymptomatic and regress spontaneously. Multiple follicular cysts may be part of a syndrome such as the Donahue syndrome. Symp-tomatic cysts are less frequent. The diagnosis of ovarian neoplastic tumors must be considered in children, espe-cially in those with solid or complex masses or large masses that do not regress (teratoma, germ cell tumors). Usually neoplastic tumors are associated with clinical signs, rather than with incidental ultrasound findings.

Follicular cysts

Clinical features

The prevalence of follicular cysts is difficult to appreciate because they are usually asymptomatic. A study evalu-ating their prevalence in a population of 139 girls aged 10–19, treated in hospital for another reason, found the prevalence of ovarian cysts by routine ultrasound exam-ination was 12%, with a mean diameter of 47 mm, and 98% were asymptomatic. Rarely, the follicular cysts may independently and spontaneously secrete estrogen, result-ing in precocious puberty. Sometimes it is part of the McCune–Albright syndrome of polyostotic fibrous dys-plasia of bones, café-au-lait patches and isosexual pre-

Pediatric, Adolescent, & Young Adult Gynecology. Edited by
A. Altchek and L. Deligdisch. © 2009 Blackwell Publishing,
ISBN: 978-1-4051-5347-8.

cocious puberty. Persistent, complex cysts or solid neo-plasms may cause pain, vomiting, diarrhea and constipa-tion, from ovarian torsion.

Diagnosis

Diagnosis relies upon ultrasound examination. Normal ovaries in teenagers are usually large, asymmetric and multifollicular (until the cycles are established). Follicu-lar cysts are single or, rarely, multiple, thin walled, with smooth surfaces and larger than 3 cm.

Histopathologic features

Usually the four normal layers of granulosa cells above the basal lamina have disappeared. In Figure 50.1 the corpus luteum cyst is involuting with a smooth internal contour and inapparent lining of cells of follicular origin. Shed granulosa cells in the lumen are useful guides to diagnosis.

Corpus luteum cysts

These may be found in postmenarchal girls, but also rarely in neonates. On ultrasound they are frequently misinter-preted as a tumor. The wall is thick and irregular, and sometimes a neovascularization is found. The blood clots give an image of either a solid tumor or pseudovege-tations. The evolution of the lesions (regression within three months) confirms their benignity.

Corpus luteum cysts are often seen on routine ul-trasound in early pregnancy. They are sometimes pal-pable and tender and may be confused with ectopic pregnancy.

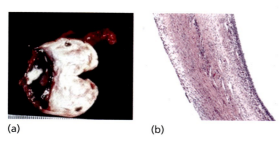

(a)   (b)

Figure 50.1 (a) Corpus luteum cyst. (b) Corpus luteum cyst wall.

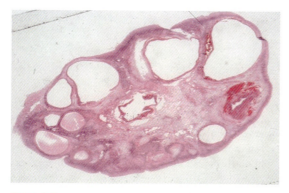

Figure 50.2 Polycystic ovary syndrome.

Ultrasound descriptions of corpus luteum cysts are often "complex ovarian cysts." This may cause concern because in the postmenopausal woman such a description is suspicious of malignancy.

Quick Take 50.1

Benign ovarian disorders

- An ovarian cyst in a child or an adolescent should be considered "functional" until proved otherwise.
- Consider repeating the ultrasound after six weeks.
- Alert patient to symptoms of torsion.
- Management is based on close observation and conservative treatment.

Polycystic ovary syndrome

This is a familial syndrome of chronic hyperandrogenic anovulation affecting at least 10% of reproductive women in the family and manifests a unique form of insulin resistance. It is suspected clinically in a context of hirsutism, amenorrhea, and excessive weight gain. Ultrasound examination shows enlarged ovaries with multiple cortical cysts (more than ten peripheral small follicles and associated increased stroma) (Fig. 50.2; see also Chapter 22).

Further reading

Brandt ML, Helmrath MA. Ovarian cysts in infants and children. *Semin Pediatr Surg* 2005;**14**:78–95.

Strickland JL. Ovarian cysts in neonates, children and adolescents. *Curr Opin Obstet Gynecol* 2002;**14**:459–465.

CHAPTER 51

The History of Pediatric and Adolescent Gynecology in the United States

Alvin F. Goldfarb

Jefferson Medical College of Thomas Jefferson University, Philadelphia, PA, USA

Pediatric and adolescent gynecology has been a special interest area for gynecologists and adolescent medicine people for the past half century. Before that, there was very little interest in this subject as we did not have the tools to measure the onset of puberty: the genetic studies to allow us to divide sexing and congenital anomalies and endocrine testing for the various sex hormones, pituitary hormones or hypothalamic hormones. In addition, it was not until the advent of small instruments for laparoscopic surgery that we were able to develop techniques for pediatric and adolescent surgery. The individuals who took an interest in this special area were adolescent medicine folk and gynecologists, mainly those involved in reproductive endocrinology.

Prior to the middle of the last century, there were very few gynecologists interested in pediatric and adolescent gynecology. Those who were included John Huffman of Chicago, Vincent Capraro of Buffalo, New York, and C. Schauffler from Portland, Oregon. In addition, much work in endocrinology was done by Lawson Wilkins at Johns Hopkins, Mel Grumbach at the Columbia University School of Medicine in New York, Roy Greep at the Harvard Dental School and Robert Greenblatt at the Medical College of Georgia. In addition, Howard Jones and Georgianna Jones at Johns Hopkins did much work on the problems of the androgenized female.

With the defining of hormone studies for the various sex hormones, we were able to study the awakening of ovarian and adrenal function. Ovarian function as seen in urinary estrogen studies and vaginal cytology could slowly predict the appearance of the secondary sexual characteristics in the female population as they went from pediatric age into adolescence. It was Tanner in England who defined the various stages in the appearance of breast tissue and pubic hair as young girls approached puberty and menarche, which became known as the Tanner classification, with 5 being a fully matured woman and 1 being prepubertal. With this common language, using the Tanner classification, we could follow the progress of pubertal changes in the female. A similar classification was made for the development of the male.

In the 19th century the average age of menarche in Western Europe and America was approximately 15–16 years of age. In the course of one century, this decreased to 12.5–13. Other factors influenced menarche and it became apparent that weight and height as described by Frisch at Harvard also affected pubertal development and the age of onset of menarche. In addition, chronic diseases such as tuberculosis will influence the onset of menarche.

In the mid 1950s Barr of Canada introduced cytologic tests that could give us information as to the genetics of the individual. All girls of less than normal stature for age and with absence of secondary sexual development should be evaluated for the possibility of gonadal dysgenesis. The simplest and least expensive test is the buccal

Pediatric, Adolescent, & Young Adult Gynecology. Edited by A. Altchek and L. Deligdisch. © 2009 Blackwell Publishing, ISBN: 978-1-4051-5347-8.

smear. While the technique is not difficult, it does require correct preparation and interpretation on the part of the laboratory. The presence of sex chromatin near the nuclear membrane (Barr body) must be seen in 30% or more of the cells returned to indicate a female. Although or undetermined count should occasion a determination of the karyotype. Properly conducted, this will better reveal XO gonadal dysgenesis and various forms of mosaicism. The studies when dealing with individuals who had primary amenorrhea and were suspect of some anomalies that developed in the gonads.

The early 1960s saw the advent of the oral contraceptives. One of the questions that had to be evaluated was whether or not the postpubertal female with a normal menstrual cycle could use oral contraceptives. As time has proved, there was no reason why an adolescent could not use oral contraceptives to modify her menstrual cycle and treat some of the problems associated with menstrual irregularities.

As we moved into the 1970s and 1980s, society was changing and adolescents were increasing their alcohol consumption and drug use. In addition, the number of unintended pregnancies rose, as did the number of sexually transmitted diseases. The HIV/AIDS epidemic also affected the adolescent population.

Family life was changing. There were more single parents than previously and in the 1980s the development of computers and the Internet gave the adolescent a tool for privacy. These societal changes influenced adolescents and their health.

We know that smoking is more prevalent in adolescent girls than in adolescent boys. We also know that alcohol is being increasingly used by young women, and problems with drugs and nutritional problems are more prevalent. While obtaining a history, the physician should ask about these problems. The nutritional problems of obesity, bulimia, and anorexia are associated with menstrual irregularities, which may lead many patients to visit the gynecologist. Thus gynecologists need to be able to recognize eating disorders and know how to treat them or at least know who to refer them to.

Harold Lief at the University of Pennsylvania discussed the problems in sexuality that existed among adolescents. We saw an increased number of unintended pregnancies, as adolescents were poor contraceptive users. However, it is interesting to report that in the last few years of the 20th century, unintended pregnancies and voluntary

interruption of pregnancies in the adolescent population declined.

I have written on several occasions that sexual dysfunction in our society is strictly related to the fact that we do not educate our adolescent population concerning human sexuality. We rather moralize about it. Today, the adolescent obtains most of her information about health on the Internet, not in school and not from families or in places of worship.

North American Society of Pediatric and Adolescent Gynecology

In 1983, Sir John Dewhurst wrote me about developing an international meeting on pediatric and adolescent gynecology in the United States. In 1984, I presented this problem to a friend, Ervin Nichols, Associate Director of the American College of Obstetricians and Gynecologists. After deliberation with the ACOG and their leadership, they allowed us to use the College as a secretariat for this meeting. Ingred Ablatt was assigned to be the secretary for the organization. Thus the 8th International Congress on Pediatric and Adolescent Gynecology was held in Washington, DC in April 1986.

Those involved in organizing the meeting included Jean Emans, Susan Coupey, David Muram, and Albert Altchek. In addition, Susan Pokorney and Donald Goldstein were active on the Committee. The meeting was a success and allowed those of us who are interested in pediatric and adolescent gynecology to finally meet face to face and exchange ideas.

Six months after the meeting concluded, the North American Society of Pediatric and Adolescent Gynecology was incorporated. Members of the Board included some of those who were on the committee who organized the International Meeting in Washington plus Ezra Davidson of Los Angeles and John Spence of Canada. The first Board elected me as President while Paul McDonough became the editor of its peer-reviewed journal entitled *The Journal of Pediatric and Adolescent Gynecology*.

The organization has grown over the course of the last two decades and includes gynecologists, adolescent medicine specialists, nurse practitioners and PhDs who are interested in the health of our adolescent population. The society holds an annual clinical meeting, and an annual postgraduate course has been created. It allows gynecologists and pediatricians to meet together for the common purpose of improving the healthcare of the pediatric and adolescent female population, exchanging ideas regarding the health of this population and making every effort to set high standards for the health of these individuals.

We now understand more about psychosexual development and its evaluation, the examination of the young adolescent female, and how to use the initial examination as an educational tool during the course of the first visit. Much of this work has been done by Yordan and Yordan in Hartford, CT, and Susan Pokorney at Baylor College in Houston, Texas.

Conclusion

We must spend more time in educating the adolescent and have them participate in their own healthcare to avoid the use of tobacco and the risk factors of many diseases. The use of alcohol and other drugs to excess is a problem that must be addressed by every practitioner. We as physicians have this responsibility and should introduce a discussion of these points in the management of all our adolescent gynecologic patients.

Further reading

Dynamics and abnormalities of puberty. Ed. by Alvin F. Goldfarb, M.D. Published by Hoeber Med Division of Harper Row in Clinical Obstetrics and Gynecology. September: 755–878:1968.

Pediatric and Adolescent Gynecology: In Clinical Obstetrics and Gynecology pub. Med. Dept. Harper and Row. September: Vol. 20: 531–667:1977.

Bitleyman R. Tobacco, alcohol and other drugs. In: Coupey SM (ed) *Primary Care of Adolescent Girls*. Philadelphia: Hanley and Belfus, 2000: 187–202.

Brown R. Adolescent sexuality. In: Goldfarb AF (ed) *Clinical Problems in Pediatric and Adolescent Gynecology*. Chapman and Hall, 1996: 71–76.

Frisch RE, McArthur JW. Menstrual cycles: fatness as determinant of minimum weight for height necessary for their maintenance or onset. *Science* 1974;**185**:149–151.

Lee P. Normal pubertal development. In: Goldfarb AF (ed) *Clinical Problems in Pediatric and Adolescent Gynecology*. Chapman and Hall, 1996: 49–60.

Lief H. Sexual behavior in adolescence. In: Bongiovanni AM (ed) *Adolescent Gynecology*. Plenum Medical, 1983: 55–87.

Marshall WA, Tanner JM. Variations in pattern of prepubertal changes in girls. *Arch Dis Child* 1969;**44**:291.

Yordan EE, Yordan RA. The early historical roots of pediatric and adolescent gynecology. *J Pediatr Adolesc Gynecol* 1997;**4**:183–191.

CHAPTER 52

A History of the International Federation of Infantile and Juvenile Gynecology (FIGIJ)

Irmi Rey-Stocker
University of Lausanne, Switzerland

Laszlo von Dobszay (d.1983), a Hungarian pediatrician and the director of the state asylum for children at Gyula, was the pioneer of pediatric gynecology. Prior to his contribution, knowledge of diseases of the genital organs of children was limited to atresia of the vagina and other malformations, precocious puberty, ovarian tumors and severe genital infections such as gonorrhea. Dobszay examined hundreds of children and found that the genital organs of young girls do not remain, as was generally believed, in a state of rest from birth to puberty but are modified by the presence or absence of estrogens. He observed that these hormonal variations cause typical modifications of the hymen, the vaginal epithelium and the uterus long before any other clinical sign appears. He further noticed that vaginal discharge may be a physiologic event. However, because genital infections also cause discharge, a correct diagnosis necessitates a gynecologic examination of the child. In order to visualize the vagina, to observe a possible inflammation or to extract a foreign body without pain and without hurting the hymen, Dobszay developed a special vaginoscope.

In 1939, he wrote the first monograph on pediatric gynecology, published in German and entitled *Beiträge zur Physiologie und Klinik der weiblichen Genitalorgane im Kindesalter* (*Contribution to the physiology and clinic of the female genital organs during childhood*), Acta Literarum

ac Scientiarum Regiae Universitatis Hungaricae Francisco Josephinae, Fasc. 3, Vol. VIII, Published by Barth, Leipzig.

Thanks to Dobszay the medical world became aware of the existence of a specific gynecologic pathology during childhood and adolescence and some physicians immediately started to explore this new medical field.

In Prague, at the Czech Hospital for Children, the gynecologist, Rudolf Peter, introduced gynecologic consultations for young and adolescent girls. In 1940, he inaugurated the first independent Clinic for Pediatric and Adolescent Gynecology in Europe, composed of eight beds for premenarchal and eight beds for postmenarchal girls. In 1953, the Charles University of Prague appointed Peter to the new position of Chair of Obstetrics and Adult and Pediatric Gynecology, the first in the world in this new discipline. From then on, all students of medicine in Prague were trained in pediatric and adolescent gynecology. Peter's reputation spread and attracted numerous students, mainly from Eastern Europe, and Prague became the center of teaching in this new medical field.

In 1956, Denys Sersiron at the Hôpital Bretonneau in Paris started the first consultations in pediatric and adolescent gynecology in France. In 1965, in Czechoslovakia, 12 regional consultant posts in the field were established by law. In 1966, Rudolf Peter and Karel Vesely wrote *Kindergynäkologie (Pediatric Gynecology)* Thieme, Leipzig.

In Eastern Europe, pediatric and adolescent gynecology was not limited to a particular person or hospital. It rapidly became an integral part of the state's health service and was provided in every major town. By 1962, Brno

Pediatric, Adolescent, & Young Adult Gynecology. Edited by A. Altchek and L. Deligdisch. © 2009 Blackwell Publishing, ISBN: 978-1-4051-5347-8.

(Czechoslovakia) had developed a hospital unit with 12 beds for young gynecologic patients.

Nearly at the same time as Dobszay and Peter, other physicians started to practice pediatric and adolescent gynecology in their own clinics and began to publish their experiences. In 1942, in the USA, C. Schauffler edited *Pediatric Gynecology* (YearBook, Chicago). This was followed by two books in 1963: Dewhurst's *Gynecological Disorders of Infants and Children* (Cassell, London) and Mitolo and Bellone's *Ginecologia Paediatrica* (Minerva Medica, Torino).

In 1966 (at the same time as Peter and Vesely) Jones, Heller and Heald wrote books in the same field: Jones and Heller *Pediatric and Adolescent Gynecology* (Williams and Wilkins, Baltimore) and Heald *Adolescent Gynecology* (Williams and Wilkins, Baltimore).

These were followed in 1967 by Lang et al *Pediatric and Adolescent Gynecology* (Academy of Sciences, New York) and in 1968 Huffman *The Gynecology of Childhood and Adolescence* (W. B. Saunders, Philadelphia). This became a famous textbook world-wide.

In contrast with Eastern Europe, in the Anglo-Saxon countries pediatric and adolescent gynecology was practiced by individual physicians who had acquired knowledge in this medical field and successfully achieved institutional support for their work.

By the middle of the 20th century three main centers had been established for the study, practice and teaching of gynecology in childhood and adolescence: one in Eastern Europe based in Prague, one based in Chicago (J.W. Huffman, North Western University) and another in New York (A. Altchek, Mount Sinai Hospital). They developed more or less independently. The two streams were brought together in Switzerland.

In 1969, Irmi Rey-Stocker, who was trained by Karel Vesely and by John Huffman in Chicago, started regular consultations in this specialist field at the University Clinic, CHUV, in Lausanne.

At the International Federation of Gynecology and Obstetrics (FIGO) World Congress in New York in 1970, she met Professor Robert Contamin from Grenoble (France) and Professor John Huffman from Chicago. Contamin was interested in the uterus' growth during childhood and puberty because its hypotrophy was one of the reasons for sterility and abortion in adulthood. Huffmann had just published his textbook on pediatric and adolescent gynecology. The three agreed that many gynecologic troubles of the adult are related to their apparently benign manifestations during childhood. In order to promote the study of the female genital organs from birth to the end of adolescence, they decided to found an association to bring together pediatricians, gynecologists and other physicians interested in this medical field.

The First International Symposium on Pediatric and Adolescent Gynecology took place in Lausanne on 5 February 1971. It brought together around 300 pediatricians and gynecologists from all over the world. The International Federation of Infantile and Juvenile Gynecology (FIGIJ) was founded. Professor R Contamin was elected President, Professor John Huffman Vice President and Irmi Rey-Stocker Secretary General.

A few months later, at the World Congress of the FIGO in Dublin, the FIGIJ became one of the joint committees of the FIGO for the study of gynecologic problems in childhood and adolescence. The new subspecialty of gynecology spread rapidly. National groups for infant and juvenile gynecology arose in many parts of the world. They constituted the FIGIJ and they determined its statutes. Composed of national organizations and individual members, the aim of the FIGIJ is to promote research and to educate physicians by national and international meetings on themes associated with pediatric and adolescent gynecology and by the organization of a world congress every three years. Members of the FIGIJ are invited to create specialized centers for the gynecologic examination and treatment of children and youngsters within a friendly environment.

Among the numerous national groups of the FIGIJ are the following.

1 European groups
Eastern Europe
- Czech Republic, Slovak Republic, Poland, Hungary, Lativa, Lithuania, Russia

Other parts of Europe
- Italy: Società Italiana di Ginecologia dell'Infanzia e dell'Adolescenza (SIGIA) since 1971
- Switzerland: Schweizerische Arbeitsgemeinschaft für Kinder- und Jugendgynäkologie (GYNEA) since 1972
- France: Groupement Français de Gynécologie de l'Enfant et de l'Adolescente since 1972
- Belgium: Groupement Belge de Gynécologie de l'Enfant et de l'Adolescente since 1972

- Germany: Arbeitsgemeinschaft für Kinder- und Jugendgynäkologie since 1972 German Democratic Republic; since 1978 Federal Republic of Germany; since 1990 together
- Greece: Hellenic Society of Pediatric and Adolescent Gynecology since 1977
- Austria: Oesterreichische Arbeitsgemeinschaft für Kinder – und Jugendgynäkologie since 1978
- Finland: Finnish Society of Pediatric and Adolescent Gynecology (SLANGY) since 1983
- Great Britain: The British Society for Paediatric and Adolescent Gynecology (Brit SPAG) since 1999
- EURAPAG: 2008, during the XI European Congress of Pediatric and Adolescent Gynecology in St Petersburg, the European Association of Pediatric and Adolescent Gynecology was founded. It covers European national groups of FIGIJ and individual physicians interested in this special field.

2 American groups

North America (USA and Canada)

- The North American Society of Pediatric and Adolescent Gynecology (NASPAG) was founded in 1986. Its more than 400 members reside in the United States and in some countries abroad. The Society has a most prestigous journal, the *Journal of Pediatric and Adolescent Gynecology*, which was first published in 1987 by Elsevier.

South America

- Asoción Latinoamericana de Obstetricia y Ginecologia Infantil y de la Adolesecente (ALOGIA). Argentina's Society of Infantile and Juvenile Gynecology, and the Bolivian Society were founded in 1972. In 1993, ALOGIA was created with the participation of Brazil, Colombia, Cuba, Costa Rica, Chile, Ecuador, Salvador, Guatemala, Mexico, Panama, Dominican Republic, Peru, Paraguay, Uruguy, and Venezuela. It has currently 19 country members and approximately 4000 individual members.

3 Asian and Pacific groups

- Japan: Society of Pediatric and Adolescent Gynecology since 1976
- India: Academy of Juvenile and Adolescent Gynecology since 1984
- Singapore: Society of Pediatric and Adolescent Gynecology since 1985
- Philippines: Society of Pediatric and Adolescent Gynecology of the Philippines (PAGSPHIL) since 2004

with a training center in Manila and Quezon city, and IFEPAG exams in 2006
- Australia: with a training center in Victoria

4 Middle East Groups
- Israel: Israel Society of Pediatric and Adolescent Gynecology since 1995.

Since its beginning, the FIGIJ has had its own journal. The first was *Gynécologie Pratique* (Vigot Frères, Paris), later replaced by *Gynécologie* (Masson, Paris). In 2007 the prestigous official journal of the North American Society of Pediatric and Adolescent Gynecology (NASPA) also became the official journal of the FIGIJ.

The FIGIJ offers a training program and an International Examination of Pediatric and Adolescent Gynecology (IFEPAG). It created an International Fellowship (IFA) for those who have successfully passed the examination. In 2008, IFA has 163 active members. This postgraduate exam is accepted as an academic qualification for the practice of pediatric and adolescent gynecology by some universities:

- Charles University Prague: Department of Obstetrics and Adult and Pediatric Gynecology
- University of Debrecen (Hungary), School of Medicine
- National University of Venezuela, School of Medicine
- University of Chile, Faculty of Medicine
- University of Buenos Aires, Faculty of Medicine.
- University of Athens, Greece
- University of Florence, Italy
- University of Toronto, Canada

There are other important training centers in North America, Europe and Asia where pediatric and adolescent gynecology is taught but without being formally recognized as a specialty.

Since its foundation in Lausanne in 1971, the FIGIJ has held the following World Congresses:

- 1972 Bordeaux
- 1976 Lausanne
- 1978 Florence
- 1979 Tokyo
- 1981 Punta del Este (Uruguay)
- 1982 Athens
- 1985 Budapest
- 1986 Washington, DC
- 1989 Bombay
- 1992 Paris

- 1995 Singapore
- 1998 Helsinki
- 2001 Buenos Aires
- 2004 Athens
- 2007 Sao Paolo (Brazil)
- 2010 Montpellier (France)

Eleven European congresses have been held on this specialty:

- 1981   Munich
- 1985   Budapest
- 1987   Florence
- 1988   Rhodes
- 1990   Dresden
- 1993   Budapest
- 1997   Vienna
- 2000   Prague
- 2002   Florence
- 2006   Budapest
- 2008   St Petersburg

Since the founding of the FIGIJ numerous publications have appeared on the subject of pediatric and adolescent gynecology. The following are some of the more significant in this field.

- 1974

  Sersiron, D. *Gynécologie de l'Enfance et de l'Adolescence* (Delachaux et Niestlé, Neuchâtel), followed by a second edition in 1983
- 1977

  Emans S, Goldstein DP. *Pediatric and Adolescent Gynecology* (Little Brown, Boston)

  Huber A, Hiersche H. *Praxis der Gynäkologie im Kindes- und Jugendalter* (Thieme, Stuttgart)

  McDonough PG. *Pediatric and Adolescent Gynecology* (YearBook, Chicago)

  De Zeiguer B. *Ginecologia Infanto Juvenil* (Panamerican, Buenos Aires)

  Tourinho C. *Ginecologia de Infancia e Adolescencia* (BYK-Procienx, Rio de Janeiro)
- 1978

  Kessler K et al. *Adolescent Obstetrics and Gynecology* (YearBook, Chicago)
- 1980

  Dewhurst JC. *Practical Pediatric and Adolescent Gynecology* (Marcel Dekker, New York)

  Domini R. *Progressi in Ginecologia Pediatrica* (Minerva Medica, Torino)

- 1981

  Brookman R. *Pediatric and Adolescent Gynecology Case Studies* (Medical Examination Publishing Co., New York)
- 1982

  Barwin N, Belisk S. *Pediatric and Adolescent Gynecology* (Masson, New York)

  Bruni V. *Pediatric and Adolescent Gynecology* (Academic Press, New York)

  Hoyme S, Heinz M. *Gynäkologie des Kindes-und Jugendalters* (Enke, Stuttgart)
- 1985

  Heinz M. *Gynäkologie im Kindes- und Jugendalter* (Thieme, Leipzig)

  Lavery J, Sanfilippo J. *Pediatric and Adolescent Obstetrics and Gynecology* (Springer, New York)
- 1987

  Stolecke H, Terruhn V. *Pädiatrische Gynäkologie* (Springer, Berlin)
- 1990

  Bellone F, Bruni V. *Ginecologia dell'Infancia e dell'Adolescenza* (Soc. Editr. Univ., Rome)

  Horejsi J. *Detska Gynekologie* (Avicenum, Prague)
- 1990

  Koehler Carpenter SE, Rock J. *Pediatric and Adolescent Gynecology* (Raven Press, New York)

  Salomon Y, Thibaud E, Rappaport R. *Gynécologie Médico-Chirurgicale de l'Enfant et de l'Adolescente* (Doin, Paris)
- 1993

  Enfoque actual de la Adolescente por el ginecólogo. José Maria Mendez Ribas y cols. Editorial ASCUNE, Hnos. Buenos Aires Argentina, 2° Edición. 2005

  Manual de Ginecologia Infanto Juvenil. Sociedad Argentina de Ginecologia Infanto Juvenil. 2° Edición. Editorial ASCUNE, Buenos Aires Argentina, 2003
- 1994

  Rey-Stocker I. *Kinder- und Adoleszentengynäkologie* (Bäbler, Bern)

  Sociedad Argentina de Ginecologia Infanto Juvenil. *Manual de Ginecologia Infanto Juvenil* (Escune HNOS, Buenos Aires)
- 1995

  Sanfilippo G. *Pediatric and Adolescent Gynecology* (Saunders, Philadelphia)
- 1996

  Goldfarb A. *Clinical Progress in Pediatric and Adolescent Gynecology* (Hodder Arnold, London)

Wolf A, Esser Mittag J. *Kindergynäkologie und Jugendgynäkologie in Sprechstunde und Klinik* (Deutscher Ärzteverlag, Köln)

- 1999
  Sultan C. *Gynécologie de l'Enfant et de l'Adolescente* (Flammarion, Paris)

- 2000
  Bruni V, Dei M. *Ginecologia dal Periodo Neonatale all'eta Evolutiva* (SEE, Firenze)
  Sánchez la Crus B. *Ginecologia Infanto Juvenil* vol I and II (Atrepoca, Caracas)

- 2003
  Amy J. *Pediatric and Adolescent Gynecology* (Elsevier, Munich)

- 2004
  Creighton S et al. *Pediatric and Adolescent Gynecology* (Cambridge University Press, Cambridge, UK)

- 2007
  Compendio De Ginecologia Infanto Juvenil. Diagnostico e Tratamento: Maria de Lourdes Caltabiano de Magalhaes, Joao Tadeu Leite dos Reis. (EDBOOK, Editoria Cientifica, Ltda., Rio de Janeiro, Brasil)

Pediatric and adolescent gynecology continues to develop, especially in Latin America, and knowledge in this field is increasing rapidly. It promises better care of young and adolescent girls world-wide with respect to their gynecologic health in adulthood. By 2008, the FIGIJ consisted of more than 6000 members in total.

Index